RECENT ADVANCES IN ENDOCRINOLOGY

RECENT ADVANCES IN ENDOCRINOLOGY

RECENT ADVANCES IN ENDOCRINOLOGY

PROCEEDINGS OF THE
SEVENTH PAN-AMERICAN CONGRESS
OF ENDOCRINOLOGY
SÃO PAULO, BRAZIL, 16-21 AUGUST, 1970

Editors:

EMILIO MATTAR
GABY DE BRONG MATTAR
VIVIAN H. T. JAMES

1971
EXCERPTA MEDICA
AMSTERDAM

INTERNATIONAL CONGRESS SERIES NO. 238

ISBN 90 219 0181 1

EXCERPTA MEDICA OFFICES

Amsterdam	Herengracht 362-364
London	Chandos House, 2 Queen Anne Street
Princeton	Nassau Building, 228 Alexander Street

Printed in The Netherlands by Trio, The Hague

CONGRESS OFFICERS

Honorary Presidents

BERNARDO HOUSSAY

THALES MARTINS

ALEJANDRO LIPSCHUTZ

President of the Local Committee

A. B. DE ULHÕA CINTRA

Congress General Secretary

EMILIO MATTAR

Program Committee

CARLOS GUAL, President (Mexico)

ELIAS ZISMAN (Venezuela)

FEDERICO MONCLOA (Peru)

HECTOR CROXATTO (Chile)

ERNST KNOBIL (U.S.A.)

ROBERTO CALDEYRO BARCIA (Uruguay)

ROBERTO SOTO (Argentina)

ROMULO RIBEIRO PIERONE (Brasil)

OFFICERS OF THE PAN-AMERICAN FEDERATION OF ENDOCRINE SOCIETIES

President

JORGE LITVAK (Chile)

Vice-President

CARLOS GUAL (Mexico)

Secretary

ROBERTO SOTO (Argentina)

Members

SHELDON SEGAL (U.S.A.)

ROGER GUERRA GARCIA (Peru)

EDUARDO GAITAN (Colombia)

ACKNOWLEDGMENT

The Organizing Committee are very grateful to the Fundação de Amparo à Pesquisa do Estado de São Paulo, the State of São Paulo Research Assistance Foundation, for the grant which has made the publication of this book possible.

CONTENTS

INTRODUCTION

Endocrinology has attained such a broad scope that it cannot be fully covered by any single meeting. A Congress of Endocrinology is a coming together of people working in completely different areas of research. It was unavoidable, as it has happened in all previous endocrine congresses and as it will happen more and more in the future ones, that this gathering should bring together scientists from many fields of biology and medicine. Anatomists, histologists, zoologists, embryologists, mingled with biochemists, physiologists, pharmacologists, with clinicians, neurosurgeons, gynecologists and even with that ill-defined specimen, the endocrinologist.

The Program Committee of any meeting on endocrinology have to select the subjects to fit a certain schedule and time. The VII Pan-American Congress of Endocrinology met during 5 full days to hear 163 free communications and 58 lectures by invited speakers. Judging from all the comments heard and received, the Congress was highly successful. Only one note of sadness pervaded the meeting due to the untimely death of one guest speaker, Shawn Schapiro, in a plane crash on his way to the Congress. A short summary of his lecture is included in these proceedings.

These Proceedings contain most of the lectures presented by invited speakers at the different symposia. Some of the papers have implications in more than one field of endocrinology, such as those dealing with the fundamentals of radioimmunoassays, the function of plasma membranes, the significance of bradykinins, the secretion of catecholamines, and the contraceptives, and they have been brought together under the heading of general endocrinology. Some of the newer and more fundamental developments were masterfully presented in the lectures which comprised the Symposia on Thyroid, Steroids, Gonadotrophins, Androgens, Thyrocalcitonin, Hypothalamic Hormones, Growth Hormone, Insulin Secretion, Lipid Metabolism and Diabetes Mellitus.

The reader of these proceedings will find a considerable amount of new and interesting material, critical and timely reviews of fascinating work in the field presented by authors who have contributed with original thoughts and research. Furthermore, for those who attended the Congress we hope that these Proceedings will recall the happy and fruitful days they spent in São Paulo.

EMILIO MATTAR
GABY DE BRONG MATTAR

GENERAL ENDOCRINOLOGY

CONTENTS

THE THYROID PLASMA MEMBRANE AND ITS PROTEIN COMPONENTS*

J. B. STANBURY and J. V. WICKEN

Unit of Experimental Medicine,
Department of Nutrition,
Massachusetts Institute of Technology, Cambridge, Mass., U.S.A.

Electron micrographs of the thyroid parenchymal cell have shown that it is bounded by the usual double-layered plasma membrane (Heiman, 1966). At the base of the cell the membrane is in apposition to the basement membrane of the follicle. Laterally, adjacent membranes are closely approximated and occasionally appear to fuse to form the desmosomes. The follicular surface is thrown into projections which are the microvilli, important in the process of endocytosis wherein the colloid is entrapped to be formed into vesicles for digestion of the contained thyroglobulin.

While it is clear that much of the business of the cell is transacted in and through the plasma membrane, studies of these membranes have been hampered by methodological problems and the difficulty of ascertaining the source of particulate fractions obtained by fractionation of broken cells. The thyroid presents unique problems because of the fact that its parenchymal cells are embedded in a tough, fibrous supporting structure which makes disruption difficult. The particles which are obtained when a cell is broken vary in size depending upon their nature, the amount of sheer exerted during the homogenizing process, and the ionic strength and composition of the medium (Wallach *et al.*, 1966). These factors in turn govern the sedimenting properties. Clearly the content of a centrifugal pellet will depend upon the resultant of these factors and the adherent and entrapped protein, as well as on the density of the supporting medium, the centrifugal field force-time factor, and the temperature.

METHODS AND RESULTS

In preparing thyroid membranes we have adapted the method of Kamat and Wallach for Ehrlich ascites cells (Kamat *et al.*, 1965; Stanbury *et al.*, 1969). Bovine thyroids are perfused through an afferent artery to rid them as completely as possible of blood elements, cut into 3 to 5 mm pieces, and pressurized for 20 minutes in 0.26 M sucrose under 800 PSI of nitrogen. Sudden release of pressure disrupts the tissue, leaving most of the nuclei intact, but no remaining unbroken cells. The 10^5g-min sediment is discarded. A pellet is prepared from the supernatant by centrifuging at $10^5 \times g$ for 45 minutes, and is then repeatedly washed in low ionic-strength buffer and EDTA. It is then resuspended and layered over ficoll density 1.096 and centrifuged overnight in the Spinco SW 25.3 rotor at 24,000 r.p.m. This separates the membranous structures into two fractions, one just at and below the barrier and the other at

* Supported by NIH grant AM 10992 from the National Institutes of Health.

the bottom of the tube. These are recovered, repeatedly dialyzed and washed, and stored in the frozen state. Wallach *et al.* (1966) have presented evidence that membrane vesicles derived from the endoplasmic reticulum shrink and aggregate more in low ionic-strength buffer and in the presence of divalent cations than do the plasma membrane vesicles, and accordingly are more dense than those derived from the plasma membrane. This is borne out by the finding that with the Ehrlich ascites cells the membranes at the ficoll barrier have a higher Na^+–K^+ ATPase specific activity (per mg protein) and a lower NADH-diaphorase activity than the pelleted membranes. These are the enzymatic properties thought to be associated with the plasma membranes and those of the endoplasmic reticulum, respectively.

The thyroid membranes behave similarly. The results of assays for Na^+–K^+ ATPase, NADH-diaphorase, neuraminic acid, 5′-nucleotidase, and other enzymes appear in Table I.

TABLE I

Enzyme activities in calf thyroid membranes

Enzyme	Activity (μmoles/mg protein/hr) at barrier	in pellet
Na^+-K^+-activated ATPase	3.95	0.19
Mg^{++}-dependent ATPase	9.46	3.09
NADH-diaphorase[a]	0.12	0.41
Phosphodiesterase (bis-(p-nitrophenyl)-phosphate)	2.22	0.89
Phosphodiesterase (cyclic AMP)	0.085	0.021
Alkaline phosphatase	2.04	0.66
UDPase	2.89	2.02
5′-Nucleotidase	1.37	0.16

It may be seen that the specific activities of the 5′-nucleotidase, the salt-activated ATPase and the neuraminic acid are several fold higher in the membranes from the ficoll barrier than in those from the pellet. We take these findings as indicating that there is selective enrichment of the fraction at the barrier by membranous elements derived from the plasma membrane.

Electron micrographs of pelleted membranes from the ficoll barrier and pellet disclosed vesicular structures free of mitochondria and without entrapped debris. These varied in diameter from 1,000 to 2,000 Å. The larger vesicles in the preparation were derived from the gradient barrier. Scanning electron micrographs disclosed comparable vesicular structures (Fig. 1). These were prepared by spreading a thin film of the suspended membranes on a glass platform, coating with gold, and scanning in the scanning electron microscope.

These membranes have been solubilized in 5% sodium dodecyl sulfate (SDS), dialyzed against 0.1% SDS, and separated into protein components by electrophoresis on 3.5 to 7.5% gradients of polyacrylamide. The advantage of the gradient is that the SDS components of the membranes vary widely in mobility (and presumably molecular weight). If uniform gels are used the number of components obtained is considerably less than with the gradient gels. These gels can be calibrated with proteins of known molecular weight (Fig. 2). The disaggregated proteins from the plasma membrane fraction vary in molecular weight from approximately 20,000 to 150,000.

Much effort has been expended in endeavoring to reduce the background staining by the Coomassie brilliant blue dye used in these experiments. This presumably results from minute amounts of protein in various states of disaggregation, or to random aggregation. While some advantage was achieved by use of mercaptoethanol or dithiothreitol or by performing the electrophoresis in the cold, or by warming the membranes to 70° before electrophoresis,

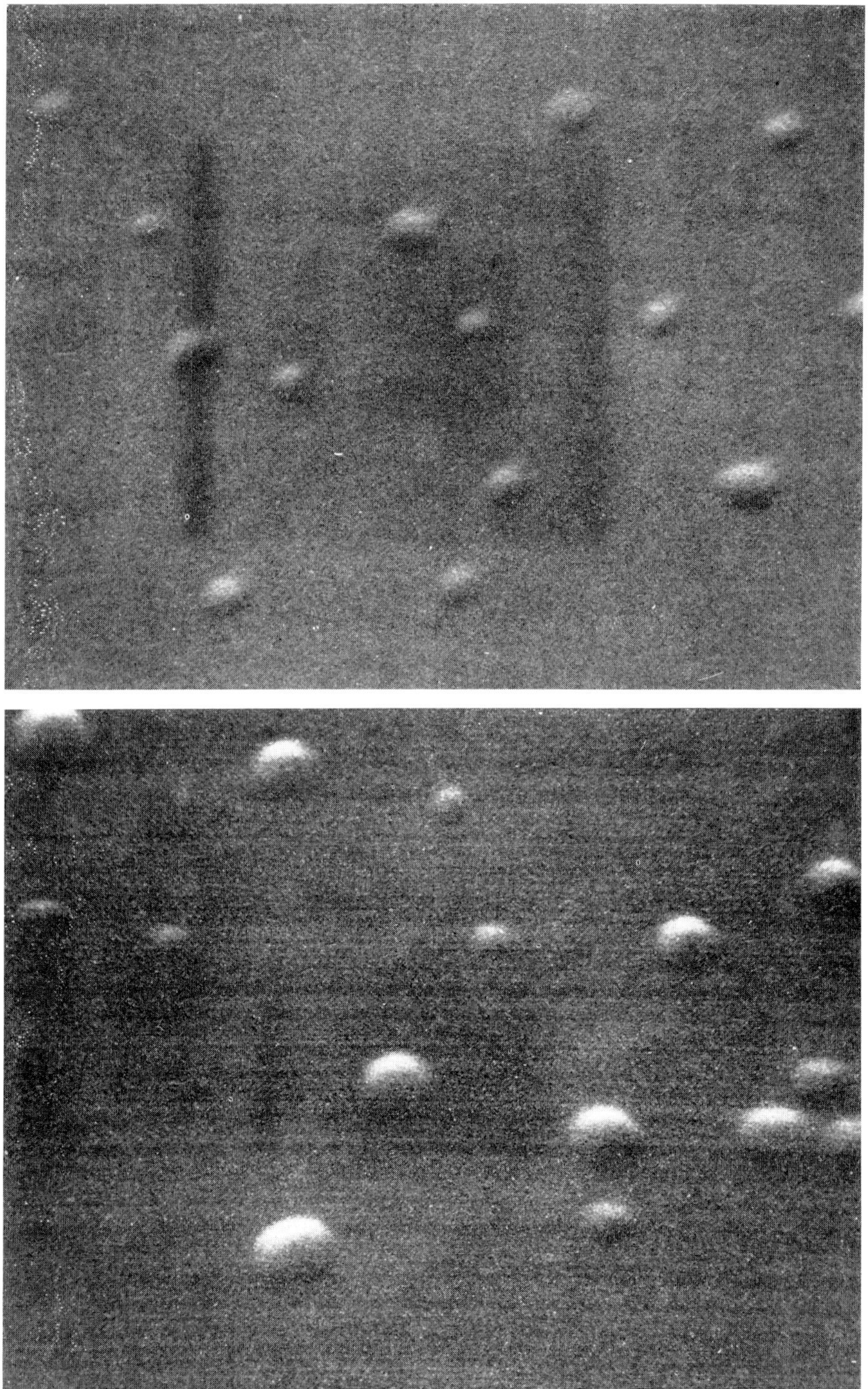

Figs. 1a + b. Scanning electron micrographs showing vesicular structures from thyroid homogenates. Fig. 1a: from the endoplasmic reticulum fraction; Fig. 1b: from the plasma membrane fraction. Magnification: approx. 22,000×; reduced for reproduction 50%.

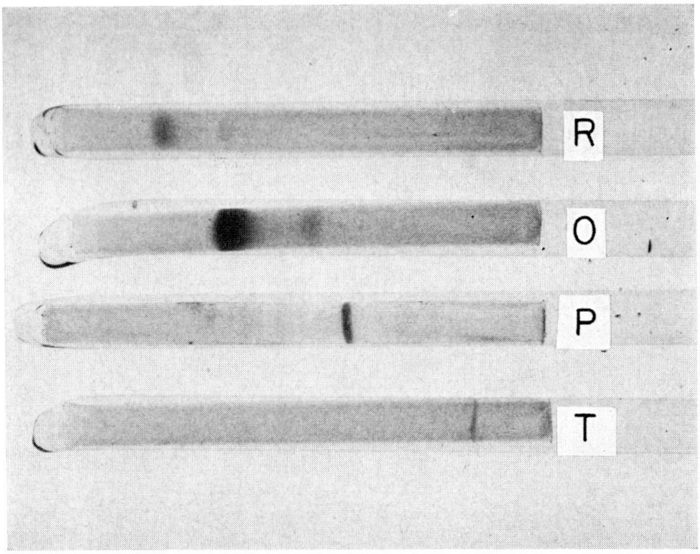

Fig. 2. Polyacrylamide gels of thyroglobulin, phosphorylase, ovalbumin, and RNAase. The gels were in gradient mode from 3.5% at the top to .5% at the bottom.

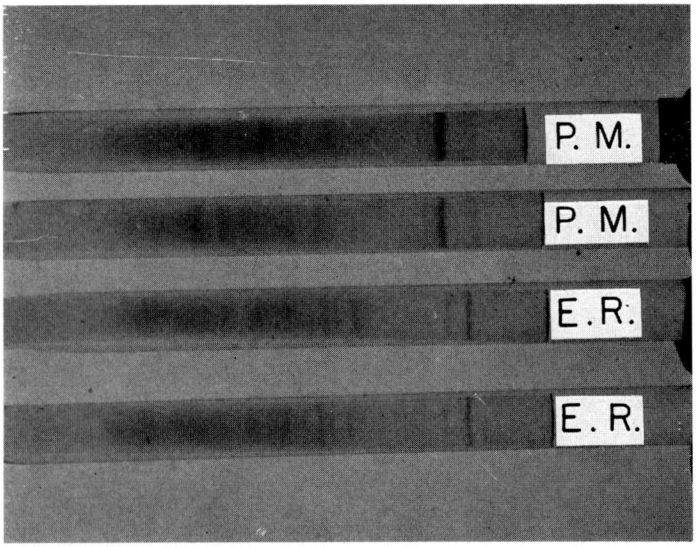

Fig. 3. Polyacrylamide gels in SDS of cell membranes corresponding to the plasma membrane fraction (upper two) and the endoplasmic reticulum (lower two). The dilute end of the gel is to the right.

or by varying the salt content of the buffers, none of these was found to be particularly helpful.

The patterns of protein distribution of membranes derived from the ficoll barrier and the pellet appear in Figures 3 and 4. Regularly there were approximately 15 well-delineated bands from the barrier membranes, and a few more from the pellet membranes. The banding and the relative density of similar bands were distinctly different between the two classes.

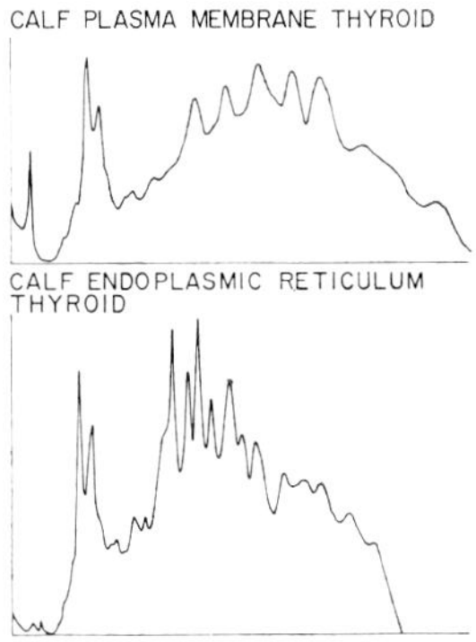

Fig. 4. Scans of polyacrylamide gradient gels of thyroid membranes. Ordinate = optical density at 5,500 mm. The dilute end of the gel is to the left.

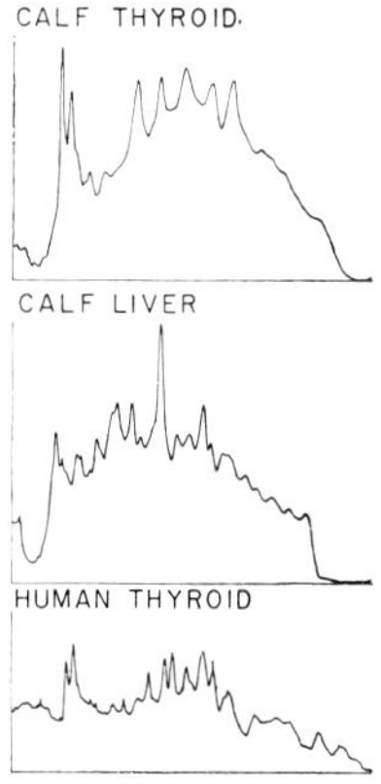

Fig. 5. Scans of polyacrylamide gradient gels of plasma membrane fraction. Top, calf thyroid; center, calf liver; and bottom, human thyroid.

These scans were obtained with the Gilford linear drive spectrophotometer recording at 5,500 mm. The patterns from the barrier membranes were less complex than those from the pellet. These patterns are quite reproducible from one preparation to the next.

The protein patterns of membranes prepared from bovine thyroid were considerably less complex and the number of bands fewer than those prepared from bovine liver or adrenal (Fig. 5). The patterns differed also from that obtained from a human thyroid. Differences in gel patterns of protein in SDS from different organs has also been noted by Kiehn and Holland (1970).

DISCUSSION

Most of the adenyl cyclase activity of cells resides in the plasma membrane (Robison *et al.*, 1968). Also, there is strong support for the concept that most if not all the effects of TSH on the thyroid are mediated through enhancement of cyclase activity and synthesis of cyclic AMP (Zor *et al.*, 1969; Liberti and Stanbury, 1971). Logically, one might conclude that the effect of TSH is exerted at the plasma membrane where it activates adenyl cyclase. This appears to be well substantiated.

Pastan *et al.* (1966) first demonstrated that thyroid cells exposed to TSH and then washed showed a persistent increase in 1-^{14}C-glucose metabolism, but if these cells were exposed after washing to anti-TSH antibody or to trypsin the effect was much reduced or obliterated. The antibody used in these experiments had a molecular weight of approximately 150,000, and accordingly must have been effective on the TSH entrapped on the cell surface. The effect of the antibody or trypsin was not due to cell damage because neither altered glucose metabolism of untreated cells or their ability to respond to TSH after they were removed by washing. Pastan and his colleagues concluded that the initial interaction of the thyroid cell with TSH is rapid, firm binding with an estimated equilibrium constant of 3×10^8, and that the binding is on the cell surface. They calculated that approximately 3% of the binding sites of the resting thyroid are occupied, and that stimulation of glucose metabolism is detectable at an occupancy of 38%. Similar findings have been reported with adrenal and fat cells in relation to ACTH (Schimmer *et al.*, 1968; Taunton *et al.*, 1967; Rodbell, 1967). Corroborating evidence has been that ACTH, firmly bound covalently to a large insoluble cellulose resin which could not conceivably pass the plasma membrane, was effective in stimulating the adrenal cell (Schimmer *et al.*, 1968). Microscopically visible rounding up of adrenal cells when stimulated is further evidence of conformational change in the plasma membrane in response to tropic hormone. Vasopressin binding to kidney membranes through disulfide linkage is a necessary prelude to the action of the hormone (Fong *et al.*, 1967). Glucagon interacts with plasma membrane fractions from hepatic cells to stimulate adenyl cyclase activity (Pohl *et al.*, 1969).

Exposure of the thyroid cell to lecithinase C abolishes the response to TSH stimulation of both 1-^{14}C glucose metabolism and phosphate incorporation into phospholipid, without affecting basal metabolic activity (Burke, 1969; Macchia *et al.*, 1970). This reduced the lecithin content by about 50%. When thyroid slices were similarly treated with purified sphingomyelinase there was no blocking. Neither enzyme blocked stimulation by dibutyryl cyclic AMP (Macchia *et al.*, 1970). The effect of lecithinase is exerted both on TSH and LATS stimulation (Burke, 1969). There is competitive interaction between LATS and TSH for binding sites at the thyroid cell surface (Burke, 1968). Furthermore, the thyroids of patients with high plasma LATS levels fail to respond to TSH (Adams *et al.*, 1969).

The electrical properties of thyroid membranes have been studied by Williams (1970). Endogenous production of TSH was stimulated by administration of propylthiouracil or by cold stress. Both measures induced a fall in transmembrane potential. Rabbits pretreated with propylthiouracil had a higher capacitance and lower resistance than controls, possibly related to a larger membrane area. Addition of TSH to the perfusion fluid of thyroids *in vitro* also caused a rapid fall in resistance and an increase in capacitance.

The effects of stimulating hormones on 'ghosts' of responsive cells have been studied. These are prepared by exposure of cells to hypotonic solution. Rodbell (1967) has studied the properties of ghosts prepared from isolated fat cells. Some of the formed elements contained nuclei, and most of them contained undefined particles and vesicles. The preparation responded to ACTH with an increase in adenyl cyclase activity. The specific activity of the adenyl cyclase of the ghosts was 2½ times that of the intact cells. This suggested enrichment in plasma membranes. The ghosts contained 62% of the total adenyl cyclase activity, the rest being in a 'mitochondrial' fraction, which may well have contained fragments of plasma membrane. Thyroid cell 'ghosts' prepared by Maayan *et al.* (1970) retained a remarkably large repertoire of responses to TSH in metabolizing iodine but had lost ability to increase glucose metabolism. A 10-fold increase in the specific activity of 5'-nucleotidase activity suggested preferential retention of plasma membrane components. These results do not imply that iodine metabolism is a property of the plasma membrane.

The transport of iodide into the thyroid cell is against an electrochemical gradient and requires an expenditure of work. The process is closely related to the Na^+–K^+-dependent ATPase activity of the cell, since it is inhibited by absence of either ion and is blocked by concentrations of ouabain which also block the salt-dependent ATPase (Wolf, 1960). Similarly, many of the responses of the thyroid to TSH are inhibited by the absence of Na^+ and by ouabain. These findings suggest that at least part of the TSH effect is exerted on the plasma membrane, since there is abundant evidence that the Na^+–K^+ ATPase activity resides largely in the surface membrane of the cell.

Whole homogenates of thyroid glands (Pastan and Katzen, 1967; Zor *et al.*, 1969) and particulate preparations (Yamashita and Field, 1970) respond to TSH with an increase in adenyl cyclase activity. This appears within one minute. The effect is on the adenyl cyclase system, not the phosphodiesterase which degrades cyclic AMP to 5′-AMP. The antibiotic nystatin inhibits the TSH stimulation of adenyl cyclase activity in particulate preparations (Butcher and Serif, 1969). Yamashita and Field (1970) prepared membranes on sucrose gradients which had Na^+–K^+ ATPase and adenyl cyclase specific activities which were 10 times that of the crude homogenate. Cyclase activity was stimulated fivefold by TSH. By electron microscopy the fraction contained minimal contaminating elements. An active membrane fraction has also been obtained by Wolff by density gradient centrifugation. Adenyl cyclase was purified 60- to 140-fold and was stimulated by TSH but not by other peptide hormones (Wolff, 1970).

From the foregoing it may be seen that strong evidence supports the locus of action of ACTH, vasopressin, glucagon and TSH on the plasma membranes of the adrenal cortical, renal tubular, hepatic and thyroid follicular cells, respectively. Studies with enzymes and antibiotics which are apparently acting on the cell surfaces suggest that specific conformations in the micro-architecture of the plasma membrane determine tropic hormone binding. The interaction somehow activates adenyl cyclase which is either part of the plasma membrane or closely related to it; cyclic AMP is produced, and a train of intracellular events begins which is characteristic of the special cell.

Much more information is needed about the components of the plasma membrane. Methods are not yet available for obtaining pure isolated plasma membranes, but steps toward significant enrichment of fractions have been taken. The methods which we and others have employed have yielded fractions which are enriched in Na^+–K^+ ATPase and 5′-nucleotidase activity, functions which are thought to reside exclusively or largely in the plasma membrane.

The plasma membrane fraction which we have obtained from bovine thyroids can be separated into approximately 15 clearly visible and separate protein components by gradient polyacrylamide gel electrophoresis. Presumably, these are the monomers of a number of proteins. The distribution patterns differ from those of membranes similarly prepared from liver and adrenal of the same species, from the thyroid of man, and from the membrane fraction corresponding to the endoplasmic reticulum from the same gland. It will be of interest to study the binding properties of these fractions for TSH and the correspondence of the individual polyacrylamide bands to enzyme activity.

SUMMARY

Thyrotropin, as well as certain other polypeptide hormones exert their action by initially binding to receptor sites on the plasma membranes of the target cells, wherein they activate adenyl cyclase to increase synthesis of cyclic AMP. There is scanty evidence of any other role of these hormones.

A number of methods have been employed for preparing plasma membranes of thyroid cells. Indicators of preferential enrichment include Na^+–K^+ ATPase and 5′-nucleotidase activity, and absence of enzymes associated with the cell sap and intracellular organelles.

A plasma membrane fraction of calf thyroid has yielded approximately 15 protein bands on electrophoresis in sodium dodecyl sulfate on gradient polyacrylamide gels. The banding pattern differs from that obtained from plasma membrane fractions of liver and adrenal, as well as from the thyroid of man.

REFERENCES

ADAMS, D. D., COUCHMAN, K. and KILPATRICK, J. A. (1969): Lack of response to TSH injections in euthyroid patients with high LATS levels. *J. clin. Endocr.*, *29*, 1502.

BURKE, G. (1968): On the competitive interaction of long-acting thyroid stimulator and thyrotropin *in vivo*. *J. clin. Endocr.*, *28*, 286.

BURKE, G. (1969): The cell membrane: A common site of action of thyrotropin (TSH) and long-acting thyroid stimulator (LATS). *Metabolism*, *18*, 720.

BUTCHER, F. R. and SERIF, G. S. (1969): The influence of polyenes on cyclic 3′, 5′-AMP formation and glucose utilization in thyroid. *Biochim. biophys. Acta (Amst.)*, *192*, 409.

FONG, C. T. O., SILVER, L., CHRISTMAN, D. R. and SCHWARTZ, I. L. (1960): *Proc. nat. Acad. Sci. (Wash.)*, *46*, 1273.

HEIMAN, P. (1966): Ultrastructure of human thyroid. *Acta endocr. (Kbh.)*, *53*, *Suppl.*, 110.

KAMAT, V. B. and WALLACH, D. F. H. (1965): Separation and partial purification of plasma-membrane fragments from Ehrlich ascites carcinoma microsomes. *Science*, *148*, 1343.

KIEHN, E. D. and HOLLAND, J. J. (1970): Membrane and nonmembrane proteins of mammalian cells. Organ, species, and tumor specificities. *Biochemistry (Wash.)*, *9*, 1729.

LIBERTI, P. and STANBURY, J. B. (1971): The pharmacology of substances affecting the thyroid. *Ann. Rev. Pharmacol.*, p. 113.

MAAYAN, M. L., SHAPIRO, R. J. and INGBAR, S. H. (1970): Metabolic functions of thyroid cell 'ghosts'. Paper presented at VIth International Thyroid Conference, Vienna, 1970.

MACCHIA, V., TAMBURRINI, O. and PASTAN, I. (1970): Role of lecithin in the mechanism of TSH action. *Endocrinology*, *86*, 787.

PASTAN, I. and KATZEN, R. (1967): Activation of adenyl cyclase in thyroid homogenates by thyroid-stimulating hormone. *Biochem. biophys. Res. Commun.*, *29*, 792.

PASTAN, I., ROTH, J. and MACCHIA, V. (1966): Binding of hormone to tissue: The first step in polypeptide hormone action. *Biochemistry (Wash.)*, *56*, 1802.

POHL, S. L., BIRNBAUMER, L. and RODBELL, M. (1969): Glucagon-sensitive adenyl cyclase in plasma membrane of hepatic parenchymal cells. *Science*, *164*, 566.

ROBISON, G. A., BUTCHER, W. R. and SUTHERLAND, E. W. (1968): Cyclic AMP[1]. *Ann. Rev. Biochem.*, *37*, 149.

RODBELL, M. (1967): Metabolism of isolated fat cells. *J. biol. Chem.*, *242*, 5744.

SCHIMMER, B. P., UEDA, K. and SATO, G. H. (1968): Site of action of adrenocorticotropic hormone (ACTH) in adrenal cell cultures. *Biochem. biophys. Res. Commun.*, *32*, 806.

STANBURY, J. B., WICKEN, J. V. and LAFFERTY, M. L. (1966): Preparation and properties of thyroid cell membranes. *J. Membrane Biol.*, *1*, 459.

TAUNTON, O. D., ROTH, J. and PASTAN, I. (1967): The first step in ACTH action: Binding to tissue. *J. clin. Invest.*, *46*, 1122.

WALLACH, D. F. H., KAMAT, V. B. and GAIL, M. H. (1966): Physicochemical differences between fragments of plasma membrane and endoplasmic reticulum. *J. Cell Biol.*, *30*, 601.

WILLIAMS, J. A. (1970): Effects of TSH on thyroid membrane properties. *Endocrinology*, *86*, 1154.

WOLF, J. (1960): Thyroidal iodide transport. I. Cardiac glycosides and the role of potassium. *Biochim. biophys. Acta (Amst.)*, *38*, 316.

WOLFF, J. (1970): Enzymatic properties of thyroid membranes. Paper presented at VIth International Thyroid Conference, Vienna, 1970.

YAMASHITA, K. and FIELD, J. B. (1970): Preparation of thyroid plasma membranes containing a TSH-responsive adenyl cyclase. *Biochem. biophys. Res. Commun.*, *40*, 171.

ZOR, U., BLOOM, G., LOWE, I. P. and FIELD, J. B. (1969): Effects of theophylline, prostaglandin E_1 and adrenergic blocking agents on TSH stimulation of thyroid intermediary metabolism. *Endocrinology*, *84*, 1082.

ZOR, U., KANEKO, T., LOWE, I. P., BLOOM, G. and FIELD, J. B. (1969): Effect of thyroid-stimulating hormone and prostaglandins on thyroid adenyl cyclase activation and cyclic adenosine 3′, 5′-monophosphate. *J. biol. Chem.*, *244*, 5189.

NEW ASPECTS OF THE PHYSIOLOGICAL IMPORTANCE OF BRADYKININ*

M. ROCHA E SILVA

Department of Pharmacology, Faculty of Medicine, U.S.P., Ribeirão Prêto, São Paulo, Brazil

In the short time allowed in this symposium, we can only consider a few aspects of such an extensive subject as the physio-pathological importance of kinins. For a wider source of information we would refer to our monograph *Kinin Hormones*, published recently (Rocha e Silva, 1970).

Since this is a congress on endocrinology, I have to stress the point that bradykinin has been classified as a tissue hormone, and in our recent monograph we tried to define a class of vasoactive polypeptides, including bradykinin and angiotensin, as Kinin Hormones. This name was chosen to distinguish such polypeptides from the other peptide hormones secreted by the neuro-hypophysis, namely oxytocin and the vasopressins. This circumstance, I suppose, was the main reason why the organizers of this congress chose the Kinins as one of the main topics to be dealt with in this section of General Endocrinology.

Let us start with some generalities on the physiological or pharmacological actions of the kinins of the bradykinin family, namely with some points about the relationship between structure and activity. There are now about a hundred derivatives and analogs of bradykinin, but we shall consider here those found in the mammalian body, that might properly be called Kinin Hormones, such as bradykinin (Bk), lysyl-bradykinin (Lys-Bk) (or kallidin), and methionyl-lysyl-bradykinin (Met-Lys-Bk), which were found to be released from bradykininogen in mammalian plasma. Figure 1 gives a picture of the bradykininogen molecule from the α_2-globulin fraction with the formulae of the peptides derived from bradykinin as well as the mechanism of release, by the action of trypsin and other hydrolytic enzymes found in the body and in the venom of *Bothrops jararaca*. Of the tissue hormones, bradykinin has been one of the best studied from the point of view of its mechanism of release, but again we have to refer to our monograph (Rocha e Silva, 1970*b*) to cover the large literature on the subject. Other references should also be consulted (Erdös, 1970; Sicuteri *et al.*, 1970).

I wish to refer here to very recent data on structure-activity relationships. It has been well established (Schröder and Lübke, 1966; Stewart and Woolley, 1967) that if we lengthen the chain of amino acids at the NH_2-terminal, the activity on smooth muscle falls to one half with Lys-Bk and to one third with Met-Lys-Bk. On the other hand, as far as the effect on blood pressure is concerned, the activity increases by about the same proportion and in the reverse direction, in such a way that we have the following sequences:

Rat uterus: Bk > Lys-Bk > Met-Lys-Bk

Guinea-pig ileum: Bk > Lys-Bk > Met-Lys-Bk

Rabbit blood pressure: Met-Lys-Bk > Lys-Bk > Bk

* Aided in part by a grant from FAPESP (Fundação de Amparo à Pesquisa do Estado de São Paulo).

We have recently analysed in a comparative manner (Reis *et al.*, 1970) the actions of a new kinin with 13-amino-acid residues:

Gly-Arg-Met-Lys-Bk (GAML-Bk)

and found that it conforms well to the above series, being less potent than Met-Lys-Bk upon the smooth muscle of the guinea-pig ileum and rat uterus and more potent upon the rat's blood pressure, when given i.v.

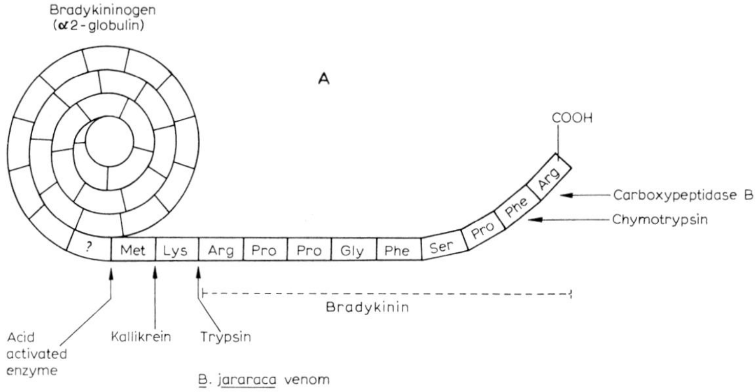

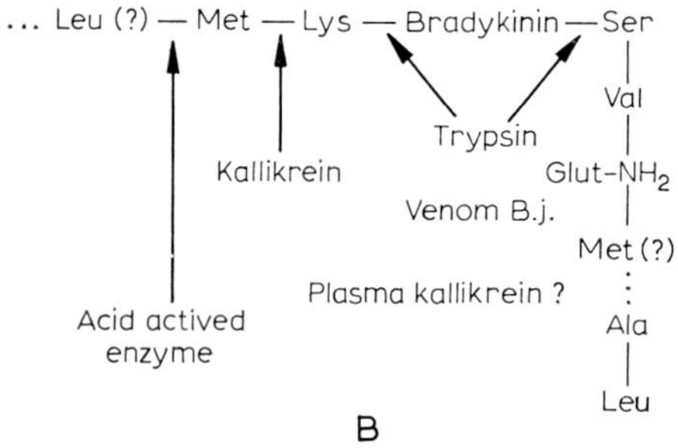

Fig. 1. Diagrammatic representation of the structure of bradykininogen showing the attachment of the bradykinin molecule. A. Bradykinin and derived peptides at the end of an α_2-globulin molecule. According to the specificity of the releasing enzyme, an increasing number of amino acid residues can remain attached to the N-terminal of bradykinin. B. The structure of bradykininogen according to Habermann (1966).

It is known that when Bk is given intravenously its effect upon the blood pressure is 7 to 8 times less than if given into the artery, in such a way that the ratio artery/vein is approximately 7 or 8 for Bk. This was explained by Ryan *et al.* (1968) as indicating that Bk is rapidly destroyed in a single passage through the lung and therefore by the action of kininases, *i.e.*, enzymes present in the lung lining which rapidly inactivate Bk. As shown in Figure 2 after

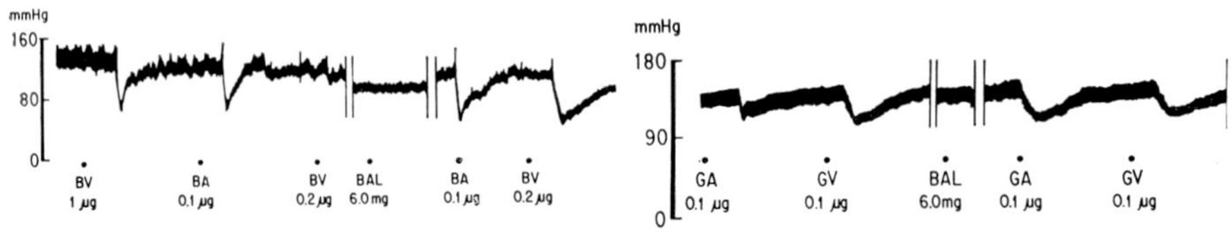

Fig. 2. Rat systemic blood pressure. BV and BA indicate bradykinin administered by venous or arterial route, respectively, before and after the injection of 6.0 mg of BAL. GA and GV indicate GAML-Bk administered by venous or arterial route, respectively, before and after the injection of 6.0 mg of BAL. Note that BAL affected strongly the ratio artery/vein for bradykinin but not for GAML-Bk.

previous treatment of the animal with BAL, a known protecting agent blocking kininases, the ratio becomes approximately 1.0.

If Met-Lys-Bk or Gly-Arg-Met-Lys-Bk are injected intravenously and intra-arterially, the ratio 'artery/vein' is approximately 0.9 to 1.0, indicating that these kinins are more resistant to destruction by kininases than Bk or Lys-Bk. Furthermore, if BAL is given to the animal before the injection of the larger kinins, no change in the ratio can be observed, as shown in Figure 2.

Let us now calculate the so-called index of discrimination BP/guinea-pig ileum, when the effects of the kinins injected intravenously on the blood pressure, or applied to the isolated ileum of the guinea pig, are compared. Taking the sensitivity of Bk as 1.0 in both preparations, the index BP/ileum will increase to 21 to 24 for Met-Lys-Bk or Gly-Arg-Met-Lys-Bk. It is obvious that if we are faced with a new principle extracted from body fluids, and find it much more active upon blood pressure than upon the ileum of the guinea pig we would be inclined to assume that the material is not a kinin, though it is clear now that the pharmacological effects of a kinin can shift to very low levels when tested on smooth muscle and still be very active, or more active, on the blood pressure, when given intravenously.

To show that the activity depends upon the sequence that is characteristic of bradykinin, it is sufficient to treat the peptide with trypsin, which will release bradykinin. In this case, an increase of 4 times was found for Met-Lys-Bk and 8 times for Gly-Arg-Met-Lys-Bk, as shown in Figure 3.

A still more interesting relationship refers to the comparative action of the larger kinins upon vascular (capillary) permeability, using the so-called blue test (Evans blue) in the rat's skin. Though Lys-Bk was not much more active than Bk itself, the other larger kinins Met-Lys-Bk and Gly-Arg-Met-Lys-Bk were about 10–20 times more potent than Bk. This will

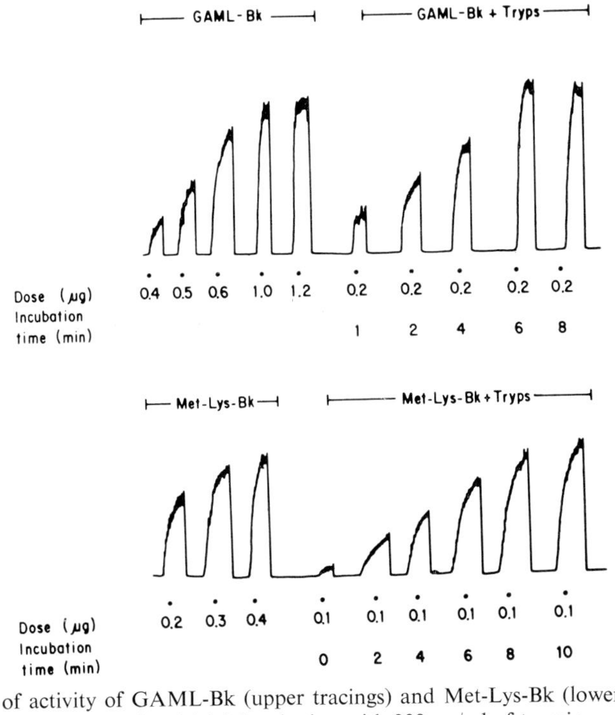

Fig. 3. Increase of activity of GAML-Bk (upper tracings) and Met-Lys-Bk (lower tracings) before (left) and after (right) incubation with 200 µg/ml of trypsin.

raise the discrimination index 'vascular permeability/guinea-pig ileum' to 150 to 300, since the larger kinins were 10 to 15 times less potent on the guinea-pig ileum than Bk.

Let us dwell a little longer on such a remarkable fact. If a large kinin, such as Met-Lys-Bk or GAML-Bk were tested on the smooth muscle of the guinea-pig ileum or the rat uterus, as is usually done in a first screening of activity, and then tested upon the skin of the rat, with the blue test, the ratio of 150 to 300 would probably disqualify the material as a kinin, and it would be labelled as a 'permeability factor', though we know that the active group in the molecule of GAML-Bk and Met-Lys-Bk is still bradykinin. Therefore we might suspect that some 'permeability factors' derived from globulins and that have been described in the literature as independent entities, might be just some of the larger kinins, giving such high discrimination indexes when tested by the vascular permeability test against the guinea-pig ileum or rat uterus.

Let us consider now the possibility of such a situation arising practically. We know that bradykininogen is a large globular protein belonging to the group of α_2-globulins, contained in the so-called pseudoglobulin fraction precipitated by half-saturation with ammonium sulfate. This is the precursor of kinins and of many permeability factors, such as the one described by Miles and Wilhelm (1960) and others.

We know that trypsin acting upon such a substrate releases free bradykinin. Also the proteases from the venom of *B. jararaca* and the so-called plasma kallikrein (kininogenin from plasma) release free bradykinin. However, we might think of other kininogenins, which might split other bonds and release Lys-Bk, as happens with the salivary and pancreas kallikreins, or Met-Lys-Bk, shown by Elliott and Lewis (1965) to be released by a plasma enzyme activated by acid treatment (pH = 2.0 at room temperature). To show that the release of different kinds of kinins by acid treatment might depend on whether the pseudoglobulin fraction is heated at pH = 2.0, or not heated at the same pH, followed by 3 days of dialysis at pH = 2.0, pH adjustment to 7.4 and incubation at 37°C for a few hours, we recently performed such an experiment with Dr. J. W. Ryan, in Miami (Ryan and Rocha e Silva, 1970). A bovine pseudoglobulin fraction was submitted to the acid treatment without heating (pH = 2.0) according to Elliott and Lewis (1965), obtaining Met-Lys-Bk, as compared to the method utilized by Rocha e Silva and Holzhacker (1959) and Hamberg (1962) of heating the globulin at pH = 2.0 for 5 minutes followed by the same treatment of 3 days dialysis and further incubation at pH = 7.4, 37°C. In this latter case *(after heating* at pH = 2.0) only bradykinin could be obtained after prolonged incubation, thus confirming the findings of Hamberg (1962). From the fraction kept at pH = 2.0 at room temperature for 3 days under dialysis and then adjusted to pH = 7.4 at 37°C for 5–6 hours, practically no free bradykinin could be obtained. Instead, a material, which was even more powerful in its effect on blood pressure than Met-Lys-Bk, but much less active upon the ileum of the guinea pig was found. Therefore, we had to conclude that different enzymes may be activated by acid treatment, depending on whether the material is heated or not at pH = 2.0. The splitting of different bonds in the bradykininogen sequence might of course explain the results of such experiments (Ryan and Rocha e Silva, 1970).

In conclusion I would like to stress the importance of such findings in explaining the participation of bradykinin in physio-pathological phenomena such as inflammation and shock, in which the main symptom is increased vascular permeability. We have found that Bk might play a role in acute inflammatory reactions produced by heat or by the injection of sulfated polysaccharides, such as cellulose sulfate, carragenin, dextran, etc. (Rocha e Silva *et al.*, 1969; Rocha e Silva, 1970*a*; Garcia Leme *et al.*, 1970). In particular the thermal edema produced in the rat's paw at 43–46°C, apparently is due mainly to a release of kinins. The importance of such phenomena to explain 'heat stroke' was studied in our laboratory by Dr. J. M. de Souza (Rocha e Silva *et al.*, 1969). However, what should be emphasized is the possibility of participation of kinins with larger molecular weights than bradykinin and having a predominant effect on vascular permeability and the systemic blood pressure.

Thus, a promising new field has been opened by such studies, which might lead to interesting results for the explanation of the important phenomenon of inflammation, in its broadest sense.

REFERENCES

ELLIOTT, D. P. and LEWIS, G. P. (1965): Methionyl-lysyl-bradykinin, a new kinin from ox blood. *Biochem. J.*, *95*, 437.

ERDÖS, E. G. (Ed.) (1970): Bradykinin, kallidin and kallikrein. In: *Handb. exp. Pharmakol.*, *25*. Springer Verlag, Berlin.

GARCIA LEME, J., HAMAMURA, L. and ROCHA E SILVA, M. (1971): Effect of anti-proteases and hexadimethrine bromide upon the release of a bradykinin-like substance during heating (46°C) of rat paws. *Brit. J. Pharmacol.*, *40*, 294.

HABERMANN, E. (1966): Enzymatic kinin release from kininogen and from low-molecular compounds. In: *Hypotensive Peptides*, p. 116. Editors: E. G. Erdös, N. Back and F. Sicuteri. Springer-Verlag, New York.

HAMBERG, U. (1962): Isolation of bradykinin from human plasma. *Ann. Acad. Sci. fenn. II*, *113*, 1.

MILES, A. A. and WILHELM, D. L. (1960): Globulins affecting capillary permeability. In: *Polypeptides which Affect Smooth Muscle and Blood Vessels*, p. 309. Editor: M. Schachter. Pergamon Press, Oxford.

REIS, M., OKINO, L. and ROCHA E SILVA, M. (1971): Comparative pharmacological actions of bradykinin and related kinins of larger molecular weights. *Biochem. Pharmacol.*, in press.

ROCHA E SILVA, M. (1970*a*): Direct evidences on the participation of bradykinin and related kinins in acute inflammatory reactions. In: *Advances in Experimental Medicine and Biology. Vol. VIII: Bradykinin and Related Kinins. Cardiovascular Biochemical and Neural Actions*, p. 507. Editors: F. Sicuteri, M. Rocha e Silva and N. Back. Plenum Press, New York.

ROCHA E SILVA, M. (1970*b*): *Kinin Hormones with Special Reference to Bradykinin and Related Kinins*. Charles C. Thomas, Springfield, Ill.

ROCHA E SILVA, M., GARCIA LEME, J. and DE SOUZA, J. M. (1969): The significance of the kinin system in inflammatory reactions. In: *Proceedings, International Symposium on Inflammation Biochemistry and Drug Interaction, Como 1968*, pp. 170–184. Editors: A. Bertelli and J. C. Houck. ICS 188. Excerpta Medica, Amsterdam.

ROCHA E SILVA, M. and HOLZHACKER, E. (1959): Liberation of bradykinin from plasma by treatment with peptone or by boiling with HCl. *Arch. int. Pharmacodyn.*, *122*, 168.

RYAN, J. W., ROBLERO, J. and STEWART, J. M. (1968): Inactivation of bradykinin in the pulmonary circulation. *Biochem. J.*, *110*, 795.

RYAN, J. W. and ROCHA E SILVA, M. (1971): Release of kinins by acidified bovine pseudoglobulin. *Biochem. Pharmacol.*, *20*, 459.

SCHRÖDER, E. and LÜBKE, K. (1966): *The Peptides*, *Vol. II*. Academic Press, New York.

SICUTERI, F., ROCHA E SILVA, M. and BACK, N. (Ed.) (1970): *Advances in Experimental Medicine and Biology. Vol. VIII: Bradykinin and Related Kinins. Cardiovascular Biochemical and Neural Actions*. Plenum Press, New York.

STEWART, J. M. and WOOLLEY, D. W. (1967): Bradykinin analogs. In: *Proceedings, International Symposium on Vaso-Active Polypeptides: Bradykinin and Related Kinins, Ribeirão Prêto, 1966*, p. 7. Editors: M. Rocha e Silva and H. A. Rothschild. Edart, São Paulo.

FUNDAMENTAL PRINCIPLES OF RADIOIMMUNOASSAY TECHNIQUES IN MEASUREMENT OF HORMONES

R. S. YALOW and S. A. BERSON

Radioisotope Service, Veterans Administration Hospital, Bronx, and
Department of Medicine, Mount Sinai School of Medicine, New York, N.Y., U.S.A.

The method of radioimmunoassay was originally developed for the measurement of insulin in plasma (Berson, 1957; Berson and Yalow, 1957, 1958, 1959; Yalow and Berson, 1959, 1960). Since this method is capable of yielding a sensitivity far beyond that generally obtainable by bioassay, it was soon applied to the measurement of other peptide hormones for which no bioassay was available – namely glucagon (Unger *et al.*, 1959), growth hormone (Utiger *et al.*, 1962; Greenwood *et al.*, 1963; Roth *et al.*, 1963; Glick *et al.*, 1963) and parathyroid hormone (Berson *et al.*, 1963) – and eventually to many others. In parallel with other advances in the fractionation and characterization of peptide hormones, radioimmunoassay has been used increasingly not only to measure hormone concentrations but also to detect the existence of multiple forms of hormones in blood and tissues; in several cases radioimmunoassay has been responsible for the discovery of new forms of the hormones.

Before discussing individual topics it would be well to review the principles on which radioimmunoassay is based and to outline briefly the present applications of the method.

The principles of radioimmunoassay are summarized in the set of competing reactions (Berson and Yalow, 1964):

LABELED ANTIGEN		SPECIFIC ANTIBODY		LABELED ANTIGEN-ANTIBODY COMPLEX
Ag* (F)	+	Ab	⇌	$\overline{\text{Ag* – Ab}}$ (B)
		+		
		Ag UNLABELED ANTIGEN in known standard solutions or unknown samples		
		⇅		
		$\overline{\text{Ag–Ab}}$ UNLABELED ANTIGEN-ANTIBODY COMPLEX		

Labeled hormone binds to its specific antibody to form a labeled antigen-antibody complex. Now let us suppose that the antiserum is diluted sufficiently so that there is just enough antibody present to bind about 50% of a small tracer quantity of added labeled hormone after incubation to equilibrium. If we should add to such a mixture a quantity of unlabeled hormone sufficient to occupy most of the combining sites on the antibody molecules present, the labeled hormone would be excluded by competition, and very little of it, much less than 50%, would attain the bound state. Thus, a reduction in the binding of labeled hormone provides evidence for the presence of unlabeled hormone, supposing, of course, that there are suitable controls to exclude non-specific inhibition of the immunochemical reaction. In radioimmunoassay we exploit the ability of unlabeled hormone in plasma or other solutions to compete with labeled hormone for antibody and thereby to inhibit the binding of labeled hormone. As a consequence of this competitive inhibition, the percent of bound labeled hormone, b, or the ratio (B/F) of antibody-bound hormone (B) to free labeled hormone (F) is progressively reduced as the concentration of unlabeled hormone is increased. For each assay, this relationship is established in a series of standard solutions containing known increasing concentrations of hormone, which permits the construction of a standard curve relating B/F ratio or b for labeled hormone to concentration of unlabeled hormone. Hormone concentration in an unknown sample is then determined by referring the observed B/F ratio or b in the unknown to the standard curve (Fig. 1). The standard hormone will usually be a highly purified preparation obtained from glandular extracts or may be a synthetic preparation. However, a crude preparation suffices for the determination of absolute concentrations if it has been assayed against a proper reference standard or in any other suitable manner independent of radioimmunoassay. For measurement of relative concentrations in different samples, no other reference is required and even a plasma specimen containing a high concentration of hormone can serve as a satisfactory standard.

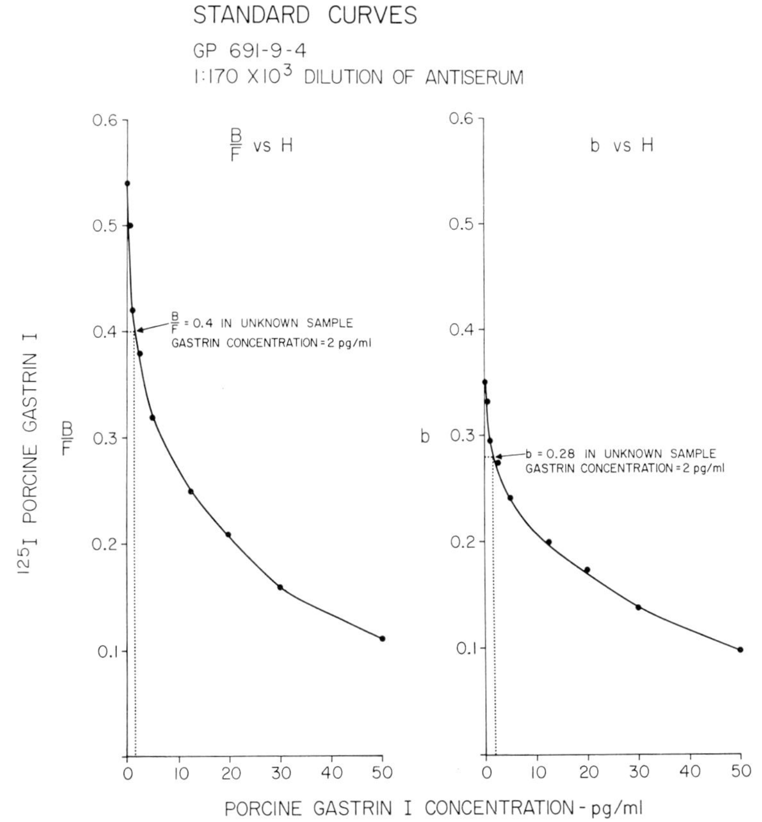

Fig. 1. Standard curves for gastrin. Hormone concentration in unknown sample is determined as shown. Synthetic human gastrin I had 80% of the potency of the porcine gastrin I used as standard.

An essential, although not sufficient, requirement for specificity of the reaction is that the unknown sample behaves on dilution like the standard hormone. Thus, when plasma containing a high hormone concentration is assayed at multiple dilutions and any one point is fixed to the standard curve, all other points must fall along the same curve (Fig. 2). If the

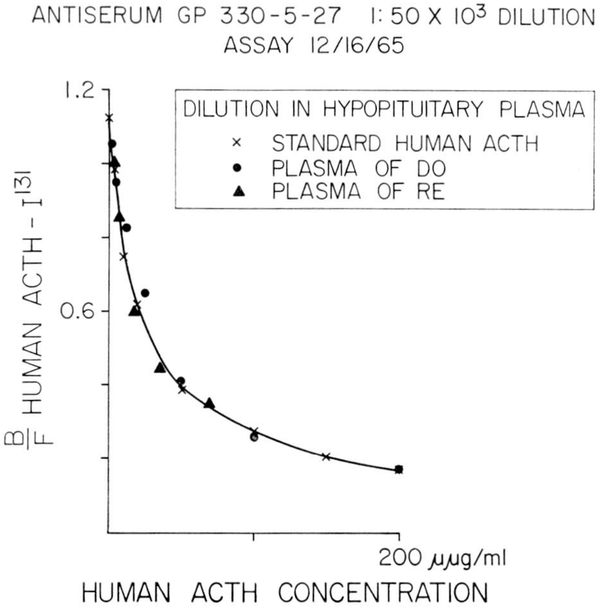

Fig. 2. Plasmas of two patients (Do. and Re.) with high concentrations of endogenous plasma ACTH were assayed at multiple dilutions by mixing with appropriate quantities of hypopituitary plasma. All tubes including standards contained plasma at 1 : 2.5 dilution in 0.02 M veronal buffer. The concentration in whole plasma was determined from the assay at 1 : 2.5 dilution. The concentrations at other dilutions were then calculated from the dilution factors and plotted against the observed B/F ratios. (From Berson and Yalow, 1968*b*).

points at either extremity diverge significantly in any direction from the curve, then clearly the competing plasma substance is not immunochemically identical with the standard hormone; plasma hormone and glandular hormone may, in fact, differ or the latter may have been altered from the native state. However, as we shall later discuss, even when identical curves are obtained there may be significant differences between plasma hormone and standard that are not reflected in obvious immunochemical dissimilarity.

Before proceeding further with peptide hormones, it is worth emphasizing that the principle of radioimmunoassay is not limited to peptides or proteins, to hormones, or indeed to immune systems. Extension of the principle of radioimmunoassay to non-immune and non-hormonal systems may be expressed by the general term, 'Competitive Radioassay' and in the more general set of equations:

$$\begin{array}{ccccc} S^* & + \text{ SPECIFIC REACTOR (R)} & \leftrightarrows & \overline{S^*\text{–}R} & \dashrightarrow \text{ PRODUCTS} \\ (F) & + & & (B) & (P) \\ & S & & & \\ & \uparrow\downarrow & & & \\ & \overline{S\text{–}R} & & & \\ & \downarrow & & & \\ & \text{PRODUCTS} & & & \end{array}$$

TABLE I

Competitive radioassay

Immune systems (antibody is the specific reactor)			
Peptide hormones		Non-hormonal substances	Non-peptide hormones
Insulin	LH	Intrinsic Factor	Testosterone
Growth H.	Vasopressin	Digoxin, Digitoxin	Estradiol
ACTH	Angiotensin	Morphine	Aldosterone
Parathyroid H.	Oxytocin	cAMP, cGMP, cIMP, cUMP	Estrone
Glucagon	Bradykinin	Australia Antigen	Dihydrotestosterone
TSH	Thyroglobulin	C_1 Esterase	
HCG	α MSH	Fructose 1, 6 Diphosphatase	
FSH	β MSH	Carcinoembryonic Antigen	
Placental lactogen	Gastrin	Rheumatoid Factor	
Proinsulin	Calcitonin	Human IgG	
Secretin	Proinsulin C-Peptide	Folic Acid	
	PZ-CCK	Neurophysin	
		TBG	

Non-immune systems			
Hormones	Specific reactor	Non-hormonal substances	Specific reactor
Thyroxine Cortisol Corticosterone Cortisone 11-Desoxycortisol Progesterone Testosterone	Specific binding proteins in plasma	Vitamin B_{12}	Intrinsic factor
		Folic Acid	F.A. reductase
		Cyclic AMP, GMP	Phosphodiesterases
		Messenger RNA	Complementary DNA (Competition-annealing)
ACTH	Adrenal receptor sites		

Here, S represents any substance to be measured, R a specific reactor for the substance and P the products that may result in the case when S and R are substrate and enzyme respectively. The term 'Competitive Radioassay' is not completely inclusive since the principle is applicable also to the use of 'markers' other than radioisotopic tracers though only the latter have been employed to the present time. Table I lists hormones and other substances which are presently being assayed according to the principles we have described. Herbert *et al.* (1960) devised an assay for Vitamin B_{12} in buffered solutions using intrinsic factor, and Rothenberg (1961) in our laboratory and Barakat and Ekins (1961) in London developed assays for Vitamin B_{12} in plasma using intrinsic factor and plasma protein binders, respectively, as specific reactors. Rothenberg (1965) later measured folic acid using folic acid reductase as specific reactor. Ekins (1960) and Murphy and Pattee (1964) have assayed thyroxine and Murphy *et al.* (1963) have assayed a variety of steroid hormones using the specific binding proteins in plasma as specific reactors. Because antigen-antibody reactions are frequently characterized by a very high affinity constant and are therefore potentially capable of great sensitivity and also because, with proper selection of antisera, a greater degree of specificity is frequently obtainable with antibody-binding than with other specific reactors, emphasis is eing placed on immunoassay even for steroid hormones and other substancese such as folic acid which were earlier measured by competitive radioassay in non-immune syst ms. A radioimmunoassay for folic acid has recently been reported by Rothenberg (DaCostaand Rothenberg, 1970) who earlier (Rothenberg, 1965) used enzyme as specific reactor. Radioimmunoassays have also been developed for the cyclic nucleotides (Steiner *et al.*, 1969, 1970) and for pharmaceutical agents such as the digitalis glycosides (Oliver *et al.*, 1968; Smith and Haber, 1969) and morphine (Spector and Parker, 1970). These small molecules, which are not in themselves antigenic, are first coupled to proteins to serve as haptenic antigens for immunization. A very sensitive and specific competitive radioassay for ACTH has recently been reported by Lefkowitz *et al.* (1970) in which adrenal cortical receptor sites serve as specific reactor. The first application of radioimmunoassay to a viral substance is that recently developed for Australia antigen in our laboratory (Walsh *et al.*, 1970).

Returning now to the peptide hormones, we wish to focus on the theme of the heterogeneity of plasma hormone, of which there has been an increasing awareness only over the past two or three years. The existence of several forms of MSH has been recognized for some time; Burgers (1961) had shown that two forms of β MSH, differing in a single amino acid substitution, may be extracted from single pituitary glands of individual animals from several species. Also, Gregory and Tracy (1964) have shown that two forms of gastrin, differing only in the presence (gastrin II) or absence (gastrin I) of an 0-sulfate substitution onto the tyrosyl residue in the 12th position, are extractable from the antral mucosa of the stomach in several species, although the presence of both forms in an individual antrum has not yet been demonstrated. When multiple forms of a hormone are produced in a single gland it might be anticipated that they will be represented in the plasma as well, although this has not yet been established for the examples cited. However, evidence for heterogeneity of another sort has been obtained in at least three cases – insulin, parathyroid hormone, and gastrin. In all cases the heterogeneity of the plasma hormone was discovered by radioimmunoassay; at least in the cases of insulin and gastrin, the second form of the hormone differs considerably in size and charge from the well-recognized form and has been identified in the tissues of origin as well as in the plasma.

Soon after Steiner's brilliant demonstration of proinsulin in the pancreas (Steiner and Oyer, 1967; Steiner *et al.*, 1967), Roth *et al.* (1968) identified an immunoreactive form of insulin emerging earlier than insulin on Sephadex column chromatography. These findings were shortly confirmed by Steiner's group (Rubenstein *et al.*, 1968) and ourselves (Goldsmith *et al.*, 1969) and it now appears very likely that the so-called 'big insulin' of Roth *et al.* (1968) is, in fact, proinsulin. Although usually present only as a minor component of plasma insulin, big insulin may predominate in some cases of insulinoma (Goldsmith *et al.*, 1969; Lazarus *et al.*, 1969). Other forms of insulin may also be present in plasma in trace quantities.

The evidence for heterogeneity of plasma parathyroid hormone is as yet restricted to that derived from immunochemical studies (Berson and Yalow, 1968*a*). We have already noted that an essential requirement for the validity of radioimmunoassay is that dose-response curves for standard hormone and for plasma hormone must be parallel. However, this condition is not critically *sufficient* for identity of plasma and standard hormone. As in all areas of science, complete identity can never be proven. We can only seek to show that two materials behave alike in a large number of systems and gain increasing assurance of their similarity according as the number of systems tested increases, but we must be prepared to find that any new system might detect differences in their behavior. In the case of parathyroid hormone, we found that dose-response curves for plasma and standard glandular hormone were indeed parallel in individual antisera. However, the values obtained for plasma concentration in terms of the standard in two antisera failed to agree with those obtained in another antiserum (Fig. 3). In essence, the antibodies in the different antisera to parathyroid hormone were reacting with different relative affinities towards the glandular and plasma hormones. These differences were most marked in cases of secondary hyperparathyroidism associated

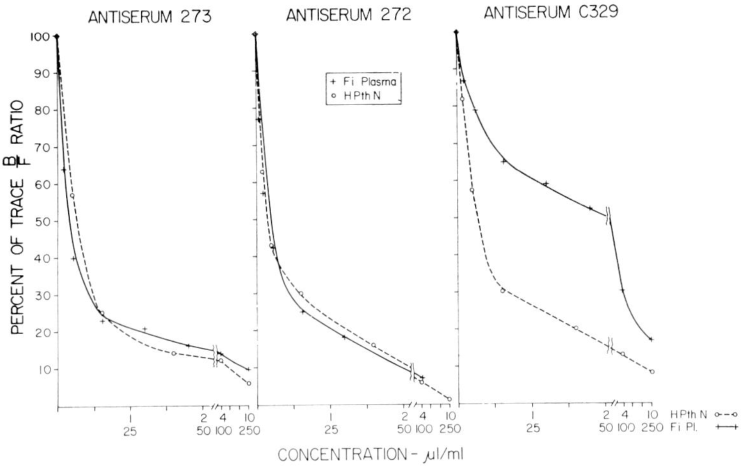

Fig. 3. Inhibition of binding of ^{125}I-Bpth in 3 antisera by pooled plasma from a patient with 2° hyperparathyroidism (+) and by extract of a normal parathyroid gland (o). (From Berson and Yalow, 1968*a*).

with long-standing renal insufficiency. One antiserum (# 273) reacted with high affinity to the plasma hormone and another antiserum (# C329) reacted with low affinity, although both antisera reacted very similarly with most preparations of hormone extracted from parathyroid adenomata or from normal human parathyroid glands. These characteristics are best illustrated by plotting the change in B/F ratio in one antiserum versus that in the second antiserum for a series of increasing concentrations of hormone. With seven different preparations, including two lots of highly purified bovine parathyroid hormone as well as extracts of human parathyroid hormone obtained from pooled adenomata or from individual normal glands, parathyroid adenoma or parathyroid carcinoma, the changes in B/F ratio were nearly the same in both antisera (Fig. 4a). In contrast, similar plots of data obtained from serial dilutions of plasmas from patients with secondary or tertiary hyperparathyroidism showed marked differences in behavior in the two antisera (Fig. 4b). Similar but much less marked differences were also observed with the plasma hormone from patients with primary hyperparathyroidism (Fig. 4c). It appears as if there are at least two forms of parathyroid hormone present in plasma, one behaving like the major fraction of the extracted glandular hormone and predominating in the plasmas of patients with primary hyperparathyroidism; the other fraction of the plasma hormone, which predominates in the plasma of patients with secondary or tertiary hyperparathyroidism, reacts weakly with antiserum C329 but strongly with 273. The concentration of hormone in normal plasma is too low to permit similar studies in normal subjects.

In a more extensive survey of guinea pig antisera to parathyroid hormone, we have since obtained two fairly large groups of antisera, one behaving like antiserum 273 and showing relatively good reactivity with the plasma hormone in secondary hyperparathyroidism compared to the glandular hormone, the other group behaving like C329 and showing relatively poor reactivity with the plasma hormone compared to the glandular hormone. Because of the strong adsorptive characteristics of parathyroid hormone it has been difficult to fractionate small quantities on chromatographic columns and other systems so that the further characterization of the various forms of the plasma and glandular hormone is progressing only very slowly. Gastrin does not suffer from this disadvantage and a more satisfying picture of the heterogeneity of plasma and tissue gastrin has emerged from recent studies, which will be discussed shortly.

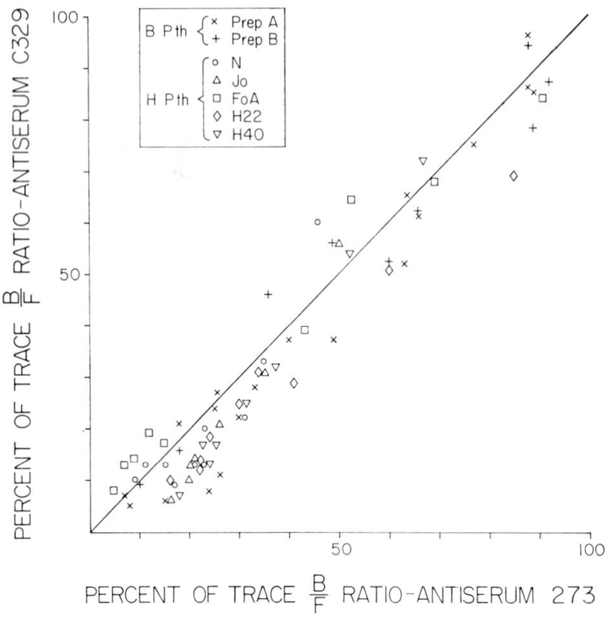

Fig. 4a. Inhibition of binding of ^{131}I- or ^{125}I-Bpth by various extracts of bovine (Bpth) and human (Hpth) parathyroid tissue. Extracts were assayed at multiple concentrations simultaneously in antisera C329 and 273. Trace B/F ratios were approximately 0.9–1.1 for both antisera in all assays. Results from 3 different assays are summarized. (From Berson and Yalow, 1968*a*).

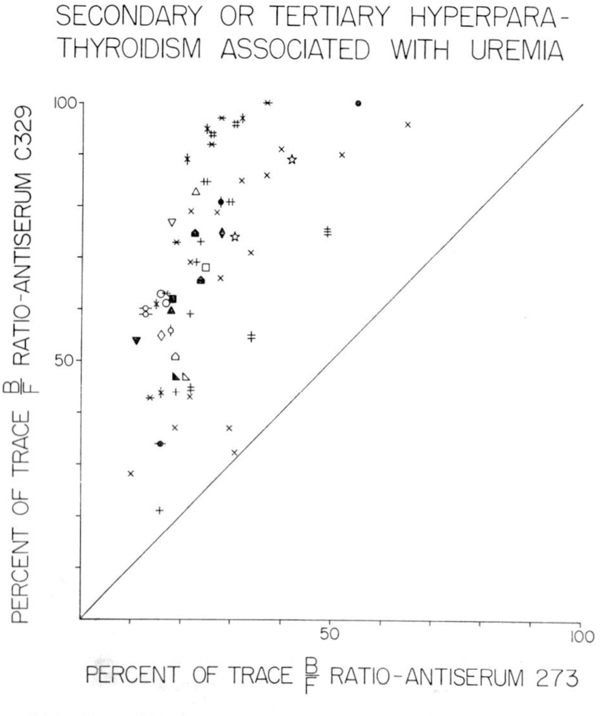

Fig. 4b. Inhibition of binding of ^{131}I- or ^{125}I-Bpth by plasmas from patients with 2° or 3° hyperparathyroidism. Different symbols represent different patients. Many plasmas were assayed at multiple dilutions. Results from several different assays are summarized. (From Berson and Yalow, 1968*a*).

The recent accomplishments of Gregory and Tracy (1964) in purifying gastrin and the subsequent elucidation of the structures and synthesis of gastrin I and II as highly acid heptadecapeptide amides, have permitted the development of radioimmunoassays for plasma

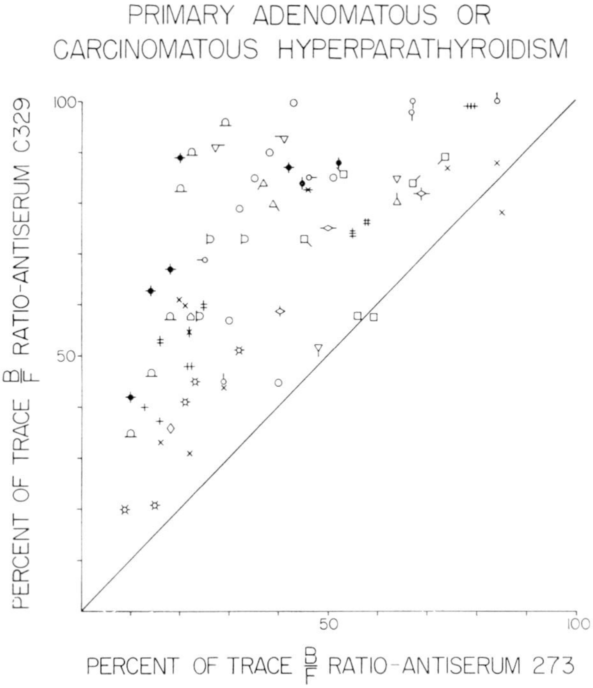

Fig. 4c. Same as Fig. 4b except that plasmas were from patients with 1° hyperparathyroidism. (From Berson and Yalow, 1968*a*).

gastrin (McGuigan, 1969; Charters *et al.*, 1969; Yalow and Berson, 1970*a*). Fortunately, crude gastrin is a good antigen, and antisera with 'titers' of 1 : 150,000 or greater and capable of measuring 1 pg gastrin or less per ml are now available (Yalow and Berson, 1970*b*). Aside from interest attached to the employment of radioimmunoassay for study of physiologic processes, the assay is of a distinct value in the diagnosis of Zollinger-Ellison syndrome (McGuigan and Trudeau, 1968; Yalow and Berson, 1970*a*; Berson *et al.*, 1971). In this disorder, gastrin, released in large quantities from non-beta islet cell tumors in the pancreas or in adjacent aberrant sites, stimulates an excessive secretion of gastric HCl which frequently results in the production of severe peptic ulcers in esophagus, stomach and small intestine. Often associated with other endocrine abnormalities, including pituitary tumors and hyperparathyroidism, the Zollinger-Ellison syndrome may exist as an isolated disorder and present a diagnostic problem. Characteristically, the plasma gastrin concentration is very high and readily distinguished from that observed in normal subjects or in patients with duodenal ulcer (Fig. 5a). The only other condition in which we have observed such high values is pernicious anemia (Yalow and Berson, 1970*a*). In the latter disease, the long-standing anacidity presumably leads to a chronic stimulation of gastrin-producing cells in antrum and duodenum. The high plasma gastrin concentrations in pernicious anemia reflect the physiologic compensatory hyperactivity in response to the absence of the normal feedback inhibitor, gastric HCl, whereas the coexistence of high plasma gastrin with marked hyperchlorhydria in Zollinger-Ellison syndrome is evidence of unregulated gastrin release from an autonomously secreting tumor. A parallel situation may be cited in the case of the parathyroid

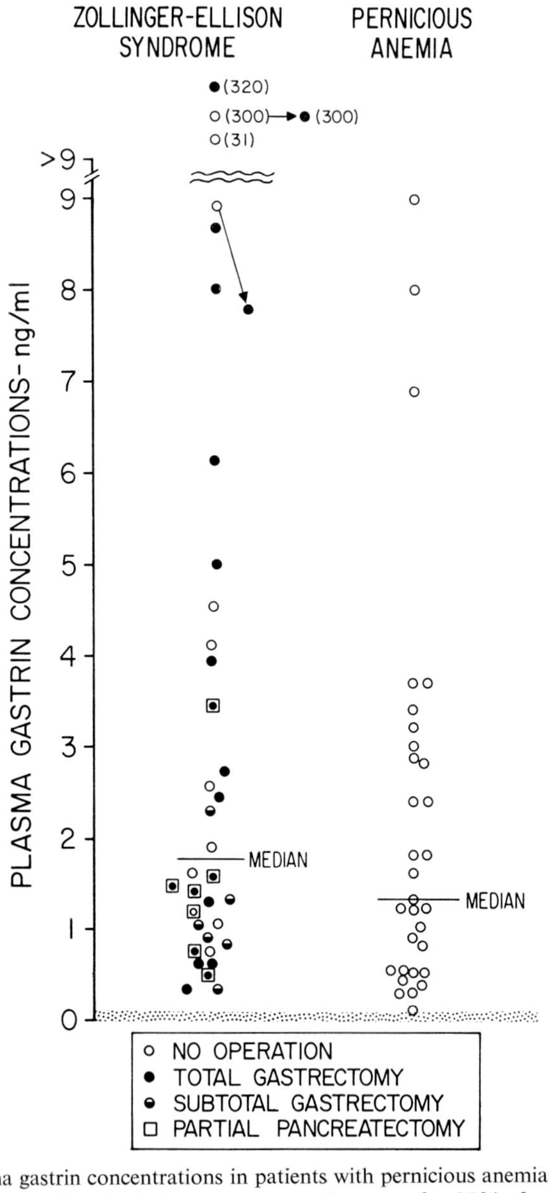

Fig. 5a. Basal plasma gastrin concentrations in patients with pernicious anemia (PA) and Zollinger-Ellison (Z-E) syndrome. The stippled area represents the range for 95% of normal and duodenal ulcer patients. (Data reproduced from Berson *et al.*, 1971).

glands. In the presence of longstanding hypocalcemia, as frequently obtains in chronic renal insufficiency, the parathyroids become markedly hyperplastic and plasma parathyroid hormone concentrations reach levels fully as high as or higher than those in primary hyperparathyroidism due to parathyroid adenoma or carcinoma (Fig. 5b) (Berson and Yalow, 1966). In the latter conditions, however, serum calcium levels are elevated, but are ineffective in inhibiting hormone output from the tumor. In secondary hyperparathyroidism, on the other hand, elevation of serum calcium either by calcium infusion (Fig. 6a) or by successful renal

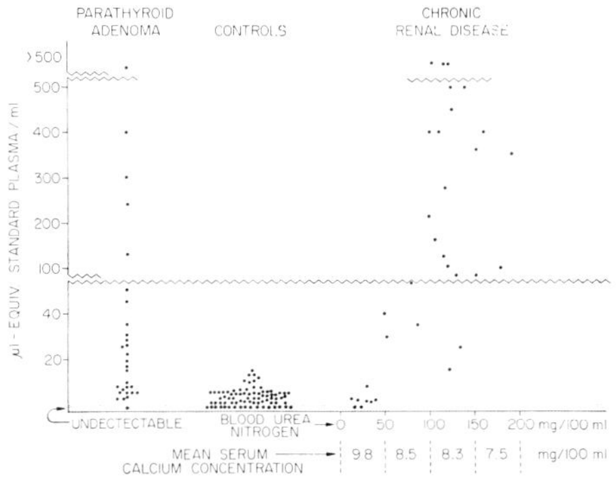

Fig. 5b. Plasma concentrations of parathyroid hormone in normal subjects and in patients with parathyroid adenoma or chronic renal disease. (Data reproduced from Berson and Yalow, 1966).

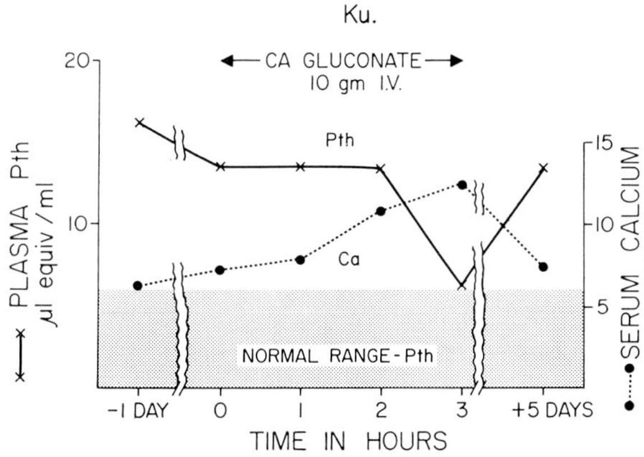

Fig. 6a. Effect of calcium infusion on plasma parathyroid hormone concentrations in a patient with uremia and secondary hyperparathyroidism.

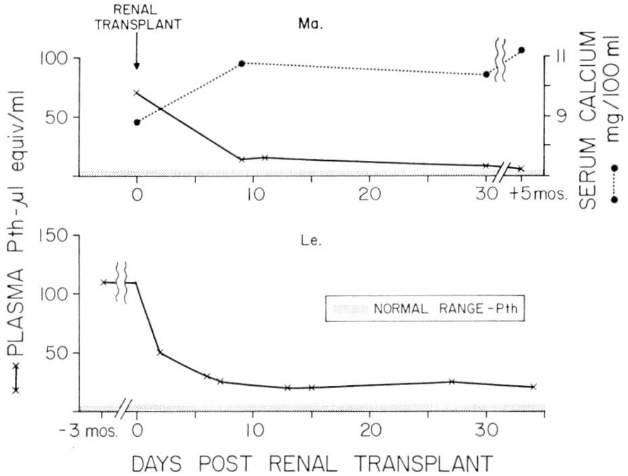

Fig. 6b. Effect of renal transplant on plasma parathyroid hormone concentrations in two patients with uremia and secondary hyperparathyroidism.

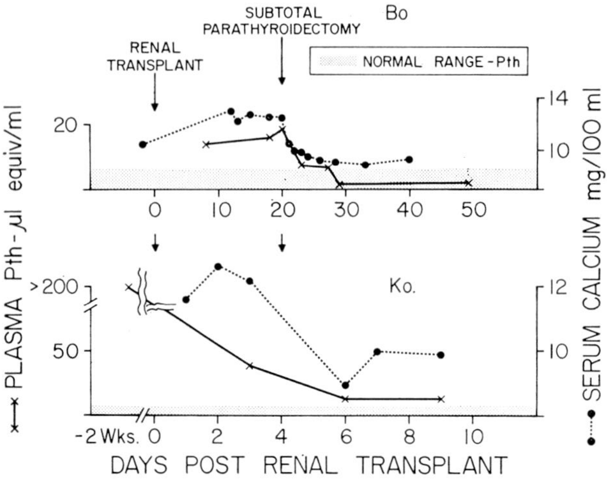

Fig. 6c. Effect of renal transplant and subtotal parathyroidectomy on plasma parathyroid hormone concentrations in two patients with uremia and secondary hyperparathyroidism.

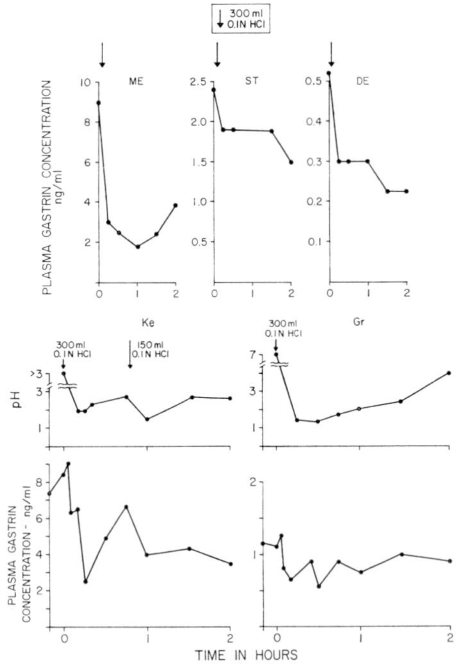

Figs. 7a, b. Effect of HCl administration on plasma gastrin concentrations of 5 patients with pernicious anemia. (a) Patients received 300 ml of 0.1 N HCl *per os*. (b) Patients received HCl by gastric instillation as indicated. pH of gastric contents was determined using a pH meter. (From Yalow and Berson, 1970*a*).

transplantation (Fig. 6b) frequently, but not always, brings about prompt suppression of hormonal secretion (Berson and Yalow, 1966). So too, in the secondary hypergastrinism of pernicious anemia, replacement of the missing physiologic inhibitor of secretion by oral administration of HCl results in a prompt fall in plasma gastrin levels (Yalow and Berson, 1970*a*) (Fig. 7). The failure to return completely to normal levels may reflect the inability of a large mass of cells to be totally suppressed. Again, there is a parallel in secondary hyperparathyroidism since plasma parathyroid hormone levels may not return completely to normal for some time following renal transplantation even when hypercalcemia ensues; in some cases subtotal parathyroidectomy has been performed to effect a more rapid return of calcium to normal levels and to protect the newly transplanted kidney (Fig. 6c).

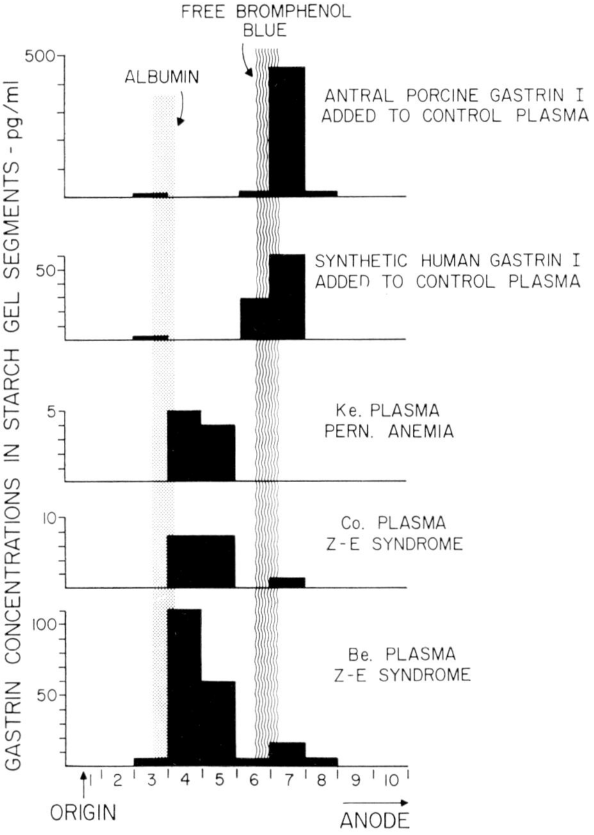

Fig. 8. Distribution of immunoreactive gastrin components, on starch gel electrophoresis, in plasmas from normal control subjects to which had been added heptadecapeptide porcine gastrin I or synthetic human gastrin I and in plasmas from patients with pernicious anemia and Zollinger-Ellison syndrome. Thirty-microliter samples of bromphenol blue-stained plasma and plasma-gastrin mixtures were placed in alternate slits of the starch gel and subjected to electrophoresis according to the method of Smithies (1959). After 8 hr at 2.5 v per cm, the serum albumin (stippled areas) had migrated approximately 3.5 cm and free bromphenol blue about 6.5 cm from the origin. The gel was placed on a transparent ruled paper grid and sliced in 1-cm sections along the path of migration as well as between the slits parallel to the path of migration. The gel segments were frozen for at least 3 hr; after thawing, gastrin was eluted by maceration in 1 ml of Veronal buffer (0.02 M, pH 8.4) containing 1 % human serum albumin. Gel particles were removed by centrifugation and the supernatant solutions were immunoassayed for gastrin. (From Yalow and Berson, 1970*b*).

We have earlier discussed the necessity for testing plasma at multiple dilutions to detect possible immunochemical differences between plasma hormone and standard hormone. Such differences could not be discerned in plasma gastrin since all antisera tested reacted with the same relative affinity towards the plasma hormone and heptadecapeptide gastrin when tested in this way (Yalow and Berson, 1970*a*). However, in previous studies with insulin and growth hormone, we had investigated the behavior of both plasma hormone and the purified standards in certain systems that distinguish proteins on the basis of size and charge in order to determine whether the plasma hormone existed in the free or the protein-bound state. In similar studies with plasma gastrin we were surprised to find that the plasma hormone behaved quite differently from the heptadecapeptide gastrins purified from antral extracts or made synthetically. Investigation revealed that this apparently anomalous behavior was not related to protein-binding of the plasma gastrin, but to the presence of a heretofore unsuspected gastrin component (Yalow and Berson, 1970*b*). On starch gel electrophoresis most of the plasma hormone migrates less rapidly than the heptadecapeptide gastrin (Fig. 8) and on Sephadex gel filtration the major fraction of plasma hormone emerges between proinsulin (M.W.8900) and insulin (M.W.5900) (Fig. 9) and therefore corresponds to a molecular weight of about 7000, whereas heptadecapeptide gastrin emerges much later, consistent with its molecular weight of 2100. A small fraction of the plasma gastrin exhibits characteristics of heptadecapeptide gastrin in both systems. A larger sampling of plasmas showed that the heptadecapeptide-like component, called H-LG, is present in significant abundance in some plasmas with a contribution that ranges from nearly zero to about 50% of the total immunoreactive plasma gastrin (Fig. 10) (Yalow and Berson, 1971). The size-charge relationships of the two components were unequivocally established by refractionating the components eluted from starch gel on Sephadex columns (Fig. 11). The less acidic component on electro-

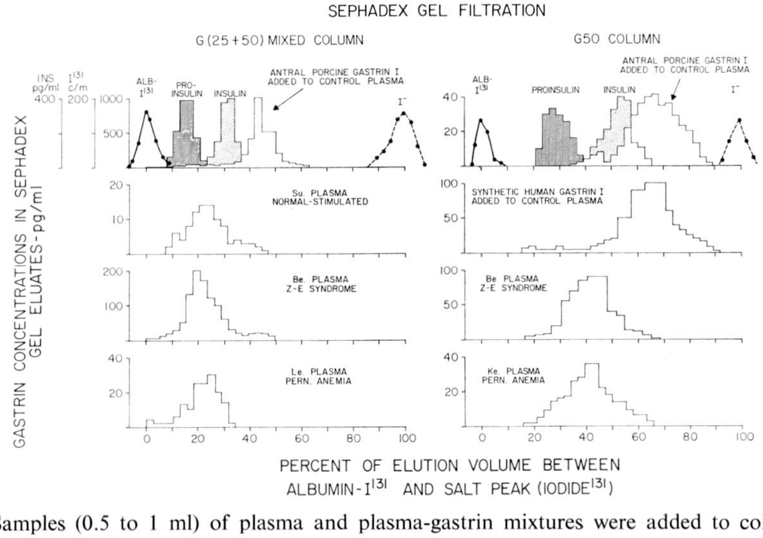

Fig. 9. Samples (0.5 to 1 ml) of plasma and plasma-gastrin mixtures were added to columns of Sephadex G-50 or mixtures of G-50 and G-25, prepared in 50 ml burettes approximately 50 cm in length, and were eluted with Veronal-albumin buffer. ^{131}I-labeled iodide and labeled human serum albumin were added to samples prior to application to columns. Crystalline porcine insulin (mol wt 5800) and porcine proinsulin (mol wt 9100) were added to some plasmas and plasma-gastrin mixtures before application to the columns and were measured in the eluates by radioimmunoassay. ^{125}I-labeled porcine gastrin I was added in negligible quantity and volume to some of the same samples undergoing fractionation. Labeled and unlabeled gastrin showed essentially the same elution volume. (From Yalow and Berson, 1970*b*).

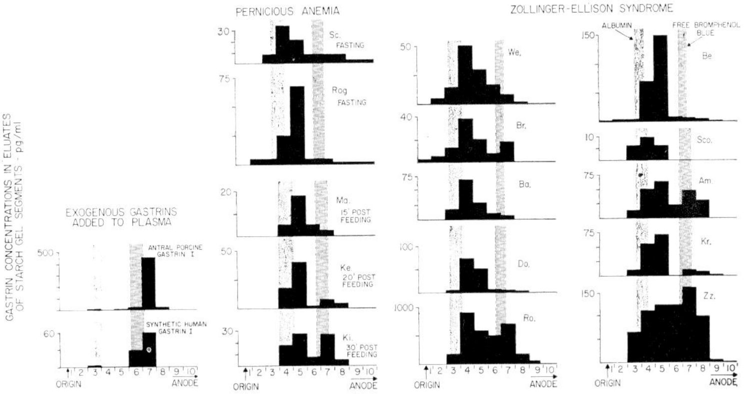

Fig. 10. Distribution of immunoreactive gastrin components, on starch gel electrophoresis, in plasmas from normal control subjects to which had been added heptadecapeptide porcine gastrin I or synthetic human gastrin I (left) and in plasmas from patients with pernicious anemia (middle) and Zollinger-Ellison syndrome (right). Experimental details are given in Fig. 8. (From Yalow and Berson, 1971).

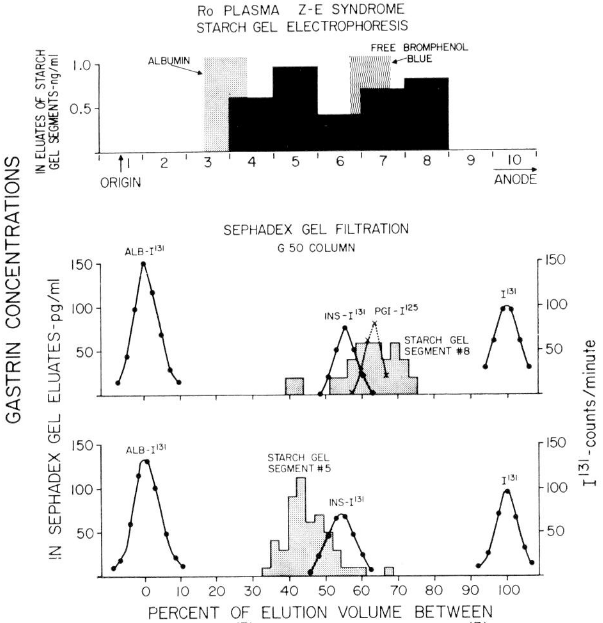

Fig. 11. Distribution of immunoreactive gastrin components in Ro plasma, on starch gel electrophoresis (top), and in eluates of starch gel segment #8 (middle) and segment #5 (bottom) on Sephadex gel filtration. Gastrin concentrations are shown in stippled bars. Distribution of labeled substances added to eluates prior to Sephadex filtration are also shown. (From Yalow and Berson 1971).

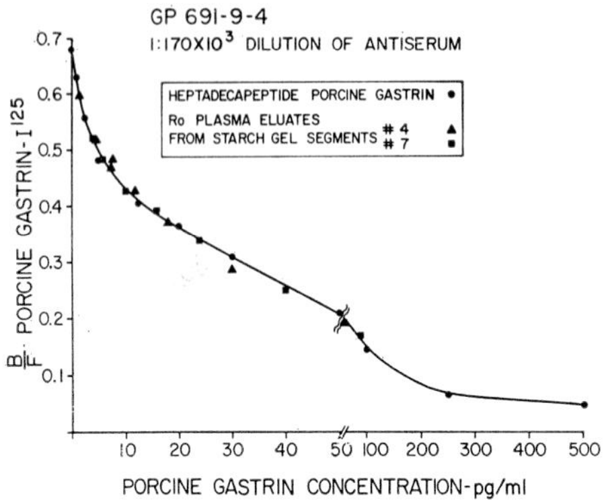

Fig. 12. Ratio of antibody-bound to free ^{125}I-porcine gastrin I as a function of the concentration of unlabeled porcine gastrin I (●—●). The gastrin concentrations in eluates from the starch gel electrophoresis were determined in the assay of the eluates at 1 : 600 dilution by reference to the standard curve of porcine gastrin; concentrations in all other dilutions were then calculated from the dilution factors employed. (From Yalow and Berson, 1971).

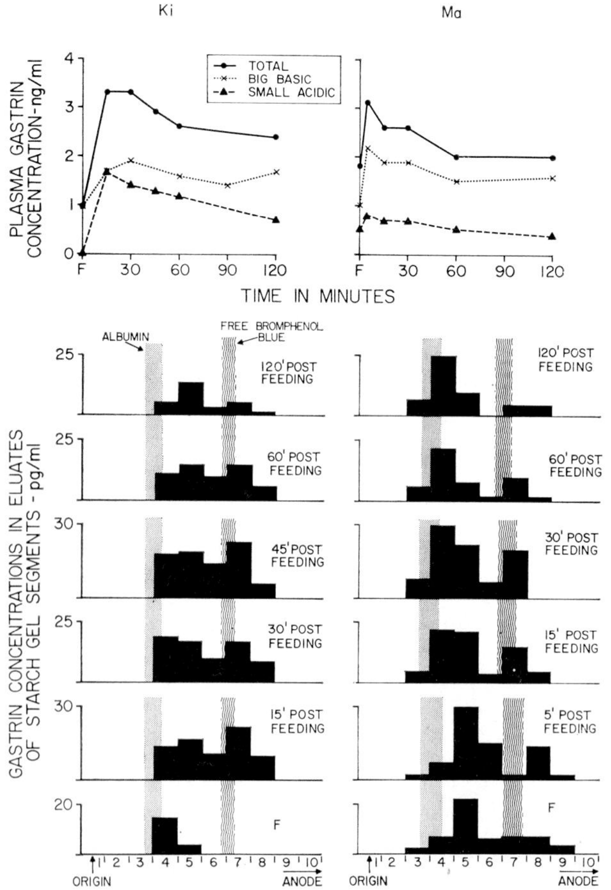

Fig. 13. Effects of feeding on concentrations of the two immunoreactive plasma gastrin components in 2 patients with pernicious anemia. (From Yalow and Berson, 1971).

phoresis corresponds to the big gastrin component, called BG, on gel filtration, and the acidic heptadecapeptide-like component on electrophoresis emerges in the region of authentic heptadecapeptide gastrin on gel filtration. When these components were individually tested in multiple dilutions in the radioimmunoassay, they proved to be immunochemically indistinguishable from each other and from native porcine heptadecapeptide gastrin (Fig. 12). Both components appear to be stimulated by feeding; BG may disappear from the plasma at a slower rate than H-LG (Fig. 13). We have found also that similar components are present

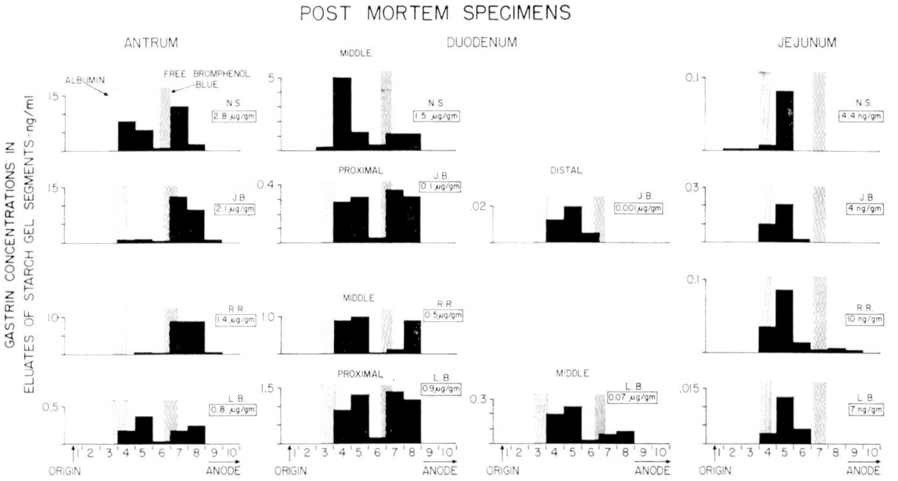

Fig. 14. Distribution of immunoreactive gastrin, on starch gel electrophoresis, in extracts of antrum, duodenum and proximal jejunum in postmortem material. The zones of migration of bromphenol blue-stained albumin and of free bromphenol blue were noted prior to sectioning of the gels. The total concentration of gastrin (boxed values) in the crude extract for each sample is expressed as micrograms or nanograms gastrin/g mucosa. Since gel eluates from different gels were assayed at different dilutions the absolute concentrations in the individual segments are to be ignored, only the relative abundance of the components in each gel being of importance. (From Berson and Yalow, 1971).

in extracts of antrum and proximal small bowel (Fig. 14) (Berson and Yalow, 1971). Some antral extracts contain little or no BG, but substantial amounts of this component are to be found in other antral extracts. In proceeding distally along the G.I. tract, BG becomes more and more prominent in relation to H-LG, and the first part of the jejunum contains only BG, although at relatively low concentration. The greater abundance of BG in peripheral plasma than in the antrum raises some interesting questions. Whether this picture is attributable to a preferential secretion of BG, to the more rapid removal of H-LG than of BG, or to a significant duodenal-jejunal contribution to plasma gastrin remains to be determined.

Again, a parallel with another hormone may be cited – in this case, proinsulin. In our experience with approximately 60 plasmas fractionated on Sephadex gel, the maximal contribution of big insulin did not exceed 20% of the total insulin except in several cases of insulin adenoma where as much as 75% of plasma insulin was big insulin. However, extracts of the islet cell tumors in these cases contained only a small fraction of big insulin (Fig. 15). Thus, here again, it appears as if there may have been preferential secretion of the big insulin component or a more rapid removal of the regular insulin from the circulation.

From the few examples presented it appears that further efforts must be directed towards the more complete characterization of plasma hormones as well as towards establishing the identity of all minor components of glandular hormone, in the anticipation that multiple forms of other hormones may likewise be brought to light.

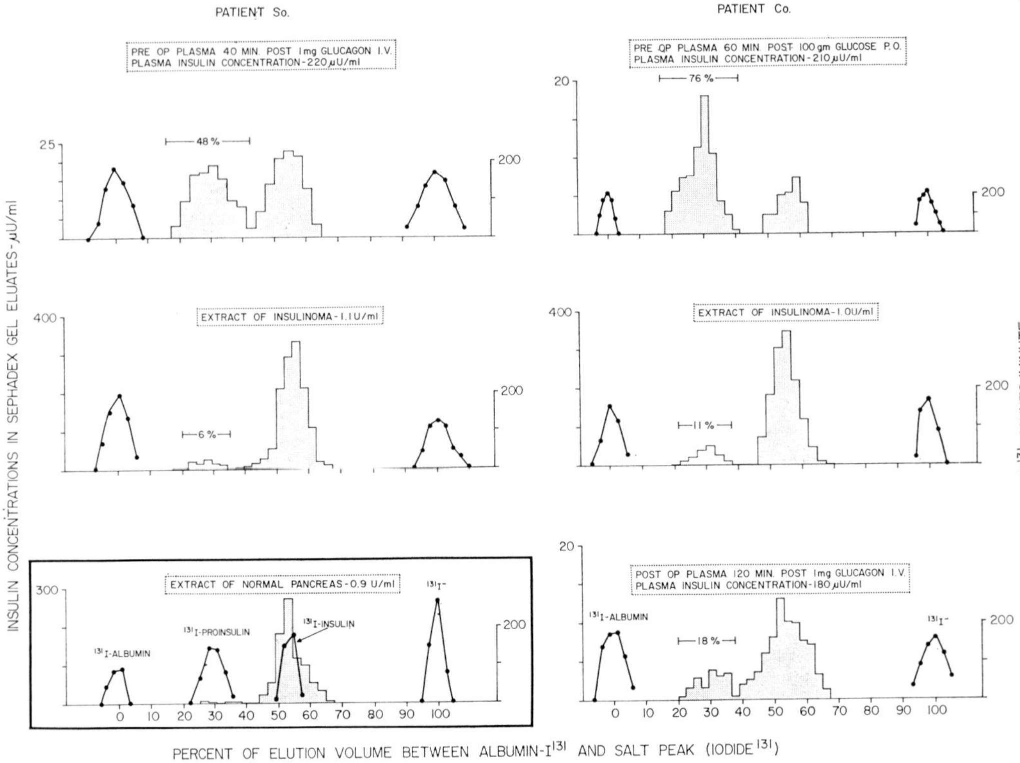

Fig. 15. Distribution of immunoreactive insulin in extracts of normal pancreas and insulinomas and in plasmas of patients with insulinoma. Stippled areas represent immunoreactive material.

REFERENCES

BARAKAT, R. M. and EKINS, R. P. (1961): Assay of vitamin B_{12} in blood, a simple method. *Lancet*, *2*, 25.

BERSON, S. A. (1957): In: *Resume of Conference on Insulin Activity in Blood and Tissue Fluids*, p. 7. National Institutes of Health, Bethesda, Md.

BERSON, S. A., WALSH, J. H. and YALOW, R. S. (1971): Radioimmunoassay of gastrin in human plasma and regulation of gastrin secretion. In: *Symposium on Frontiers in Gastrointestinal Hormone Research, 1970*. Special Nobel Symposia Series, Almqvist and Wiksell, Uppsala. To be published.

BERSON, S. A. and YALOW, R. S. (1957): Kinetics of reaction between insulin and insulin-binding antibody. *J. clin. Invest.*, *36*, 873.

BERSON, S. A. and YALOW, R. S. (1958): Isotopic tracers in the study of diabetes. *Advanc. biol. med. Phys.*, *6*, 349.

BERSON, S. A. and YALOW, R. S. (1959): Recent studies on insulin-binding antibodies. *Ann. N. Y. Acad. Sci.*, *82*, 338.

BERSON, S. A. and YALOW, R. S. (1964): In: *The Hormones*, *IV*, pp. 557–630. Editors: G. Pincus, K. V. Thimann and E. B. Astwood. Academic Press, New York, N.Y.

BERSON, S. A. and YALOW, R. S. (1966): Parathyroid hormone in plasma in adenomatous hyperparathyroidism, uremia, and bronchogenic carcinoma. *Science*, *154*, 907.

BERSON, S. A. and YALOW, R. S. (1968*a*): Immunochemical heterogeneity of parathyroid hormone in plasma. *J. clin. Endocr.*, *28*, 1037.

BERSON, S. A. and YALOW, R. S. (1968*b*): Radioimmunoassay of ACTH in plasma. *J. clin. Invest.*, *47*, 2725.

BERSON, S. A. and YALOW, R. S. (1971): Nature of immunoreactive gastrin extracted from tissues of gastrointestinal tract. *Gastroenterology, 60,* 215.

BERSON, S. A., YALOW, R. S., AURBACH, G. D. and POTTS JR, J. T. (1963): Immunoassay of bovine and human parathyroid hormone. *Proc. nat. Acad. Sci. (Wash.), 49,* 613.

BURGERS, A. C. J. (1961): Occurrence of three electrophoretic components with melanocyte-stimulating activity in extracts of single pituitary glands from ungulates. *Endocrinology, 68,* 698.

CHARTERS, A. C., ODELL, W. D., DAVIDSON, W. D. and THOMPSON, J. C. (1969): Gastrin: immunochemical properties and measurement by radioimmunoassay. *Surgery, 66,* 104.

DACOSTA, M. and ROTHENBERG, S. P. (1970): A radioimmunoassay for folic acid in serum and whole blood. *Clin. Res., 18,* 453.

EKINS, R. P. (1960): The estimation of thyroxine in human plasma by an electrophoretic technique. *Clin. chim. Acta, 5,* 453.

GLICK, S. M., ROTH, J., YALOW, R. S. and BERSON, S. A. (1963): Immunoassay of human growth hormone in plasma. *Nature (Lond.), 199,* 784.

GOLDSMITH, S. J., YALOW, R. S. and BERSON, S. A. (1969): Significance of human plasma insulin Sephadex fractions. *Diabetes, 18,* 834.

GREENWOOD, F. C., HUNTER, W. M. and GLOVER, J. S. (1963): The preparation of ^{131}I-labelled human growth hormone of high specific radioactivity. *Biochem. J., 89,* 114.

GREGORY, R. A. and TRACY, H. J. (1964): The constitution and properties of two gastrins extracted from hog antral mucosa. Part I. The isolation of two gastrins from hog antral mucosa. *Gut, 5,* 103.

HERBERT, V., CASTRO, Z. and WASSERMAN, L. R. (1960): Stoichiometric relations between liver-receptor, intrinsic factor and vitamin B_{12}. *Proc. Soc. exp. Biol. (N.Y.), 104,* 1960.

LAZARUS, N. R., TANESE, T. and RECANT, L. (1969): Proinsulin and insulin synthesis and release by human insulinoma. *Diabetes, 18,* 340.

LEFKOWITZ, R. J., ROTH, J., PRICER, W., PASTAN, I. (1970): ACTH receptors in the adrenal: Specific binding of ACTH ^{125}I and its relation to adenylcyclase. *Proc. nat. Acad. Sci. (Wash.), 65,* 745.

MCGUIGAN, J. E. (1969): Studies of the immunochemical specificity of some antibodies to human gastrin. *Gastroenterology, 56,* 429.

MCGUIGAN, J. E. and TRUDEAU, W. L. (1968): Immunochemical measurement of elevated levels of gastrin in the serum of patients with pancreatic tumors of the Zollinger-Ellison variety. *New Engl. J. Med., 278,* 1308.

MURPHY, B. E. P., ENGELBERG, W. and PATTEE, C. J. (1963): Simple method for the determination of plasma corticoids. *J. clin. Endocr., 23,* 293.

MURPHY, B. E. P. and PATTEE, C. J. (1964): Determination of thyroxine utilizing the property of protein-binding. *J. clin. Endocr., 24,* 187.

OLIVER JR, G. C., PARKER, B. M., BRASFIELD, D. L. and PARKER, C. W. (1968): The measurement of digitoxin in human serum by radioimmunoassay. *J. clin. Invest., 47,* 1035.

ROTH, J., GLICK, S. M., YALOW, R. S. and BERSON, S. A. (1963): Hypoglycemia: A potent stimulus to secretion of growth hormone. *Science, 140,* 987.

ROTH, J., GORDEN, P. and PASTAN, I. (1968): 'Big Insulin': A new component of plasma insulin detected by immunoassay. *Proc. nat. Acad. Sci. (Wash.), 61,* 138.

ROTHENBERG, S. P. (1961): Assay of serum vitamin B_{12} concentrations using Co^{57}-B_{12} and intrinsic factor. *Proc. Soc. exp. Biol. (N.Y.), 108,* 45.

ROTHENBERG, S. P. (1965): A radio-enzymatic assay for folic acid. *Nature (Lond.), 206,* 1154.

RUBENSTEIN, A. H., CHO, S. and STEINER, D. F. (1968): Evidence for pro insulin in human urine and serum. *Lancet, 1,* 1353.

SMITH, T. W. and HABER, E. (1969): Measurement of clinical blood levels of digoxin by radioimmunoassay. *J. clin. Invest., 6,* 78a.

SMITHIES, O. (1959): Zone electrophoresis in starch gels and its application to studies of serum proteins. *Advanc. Protein Chem., 114,* 65.

SPECTOR, S. and PARKER, C. W. (1970): Morphine: Radioimmunoassay. *Science, 168,* 1347.

STEINER, A. L., KIPNIS, D. M., UTIGER, R. and PARKER, C. (1969): Radioimmunoassay for the measurement of adenosine 3′, 5′-cyclic phosphate. *Proc. nat. Acad. Sci. (Wash.), 64,* 367.

STEINER, A. L., PARKER, C. W. and KIPNIS, D. M. (1970): The measurement of cyclic nucleotides by radioimmunoassay. *J. clin. Invest., 49,* 93a, 296.

STEINER, D. F., CUNNINGHAM, D., SPIGELMAN, L. and ATE, B. (1967): Insulin biosynthesis: evidence for a precursor. *Science, 157,* 697.

STEINER, D. F. and OYER, P. E. (1967): The biosynthesis of insulin and a probable precursor of insulin by a human islet cell adenoma. *Proc. nat. Acad. Sci. (Wash.)*, *57*, 473.
UNGER, R. H., EISENTRAUT, A. M., MCCALL, M. S., KELLER, S., LANZ, H. C. and MADISON, L. L. (1959): Glucagon antibodies and their use for immunoassay for glucagon. *Proc. Soc. exp. Biol. (N.Y.)*, *102*, 621.
UTIGER, R. D., PARKER, M. L. and DAUGHADAY, W. H. (1962): Studies on human growth hormone. I. A radioimmunoassay for human growth hormone. *J. clin. Invest.*, *41*, 254.
WALSH, J. H., YALOW, R. S. and BERSON, S. A. (1970): Detection of Australia antigen and antibody by means of radioimmunoassay techniques. *J. infect Dis.*, *121*, 550.
YALOW, R. S. and BERSON, S. A. (1959): Assay of plasma insulin in human subjects by immunological methods. *Nature (Lond.)*, *184*, 1648.
YALOW, R. S. and BERSON, S. A. (1960): Immunoassay of endogenous plasma insulin in man. *J. clin. Invest.*, *39*, 1157.
YALOW, R. S. and BERSON, S. A. (1970*a*): Radioimmunoassay of gastrin. *Gastroenterology*, *58*, 1.
YALOW, R. S. and BERSON, S. A. (1970*b*): Size and charge distinctions between endogenous human plasma gastrin in peripheral blood and heptadecapeptide gastrins. *Gastroenterology*, *58*, 609.
YALOW, R. S. and BERSON, S. A. (1971): Further studies on the nature of immunoreactive gastrin in human plasma. *Gastroenterology, 60,* 203.

FACTORS AFFECTING THE EXCRETION OF CATECHOLAMINES AND RECENT METHODS FOR THEIR DETERMINATION*

H. WEIL-MALHERBE

Section on Neurochemistry, Laboratory of Clinical Psychopharmacology, Division of Special Mental Health Research, IRP, MH, Saint Elizabeth's Hospital, Washington, D.C., U.S.A.

Changes of catecholamine levels in tissues or body fluids are frequently measured and used as indicators of stress response. Basically, every interaction with the environment is a stress; therefore incidental stresses must be kept to a standardized minimum, especially when the stress under study is of marginal intensity. If, as is usually the case when we are dealing with human subjects, we are studying the urinary excretion of catecholamines and catecholamine metabolites, we have to pay attention to a number of factors which might influence our base line. These have been listed in Table I and will be considered in turn.

TABLE I

Factors affecting the excretion of catecholamines

1. Age, sex and body weight
2. Diurnal variation
3. Posture
4. Exercise
5. Emotional state
6. Ambient temperature
7. Diuresis
8. Urinary pH
9. Salt intake
10. Diet
11. Drugs

* *Abbreviations used in this paper:*

COMT	Catechol O-methyltransferase
Dopa	3,4-Dihydroxyphenylalanine
Dopac	3,4-Dihydroxyphenylacetic acid
Dopamine	3,4-Dihydroxyphenylethylamine
HVA	Homovanillic acid (3-methoxy-4-hydroxyphenylacetic acid)
MAO	Monoamine oxidase
MHPG	3-Methoxy-4-hydroxyphenylglycol
PNMT	Phenylethanolamine N-methyltransferase
SAM	S-Adenosylmethionine
VMA	Vanillyl mandelic acid (3-methoxy-4-hydroxymandelic acid)

1. Individual characteristics – such as age, sex, race, body weight, etc. – are of no particular concern as long as each subject serves as his own control by supplying a pre-stress base line, but these factors must be properly matched between groups in cross-sectional studies.

2. Diurnal variation – As shown by Von Euler *et al.* (1955) and many others (see Castrén (1963) for review of literature), the excretion of epinephrine and norepinephrine decreases during the hours of sleep and increases during the hours of waking. Similar changes have been demonstrated for several of the metabolites of catecholamines. The diurnal variation is reduced during continuous bed rest (Castrén, 1963; Januszewicz and Wocial, 1960), as one would expect; it is inverted in night workers (Januszewicz and Wocial, 1960), but it is not known how long it takes to establish the change of rhythm, a question which is also of interest when persons are transferred from one time zone to another. The diurnal variation has been reported to be absent in blind people (Januszewicz and Wocial, 1960), suggesting an effect transmitted by the eyes, presumably involving the pineal gland.

3., 4. and 5. Posture, exercise and emotional state – A change from supine to upright posture (Von Euler *et al.*, 1955; Sundin, 1958), increased muscular activity (Von Euler and Hellner, 1952), and the arousal of emotions (Levi, 1965) are part and parcel of the waking state and have each been shown to lead to increased catecholamine excretion. The highest increases in catecholamine excretion rates, apart from pheochromocytoma cases, which I have ever observed were those we found in racing car drivers (Table II). In spite of a dramatic

TABLE II

Excretion of catecholamines and metabolites in racing car drivers

	Time	Comment	Epinephrine	Norepinephrine	Dopamine	VMA	Metanephrine	Normetanephrine
			Sports car races					
			ng/min					
Subject: 1	9.40–10.40	Day before race	21.6	63.5	239	12,700	—	—
	8.00–10.40	Before race	5.8	30.4	107	1,540	—	—
	10.40–12.30	After race (winner)	106.0	143.0	376	4,720	—	—
Subject: 2	24.00–07.00		0	17.4	142	2286	90	129
	07.00–11.05		15.7	42.8	364	2340	116	129
	11.05–13.30	Before race	7.2	31.0	341	1032	66	88
	13.30–15.50	After race	95.5	287.0	625	1944	26	45
	15.50–19.50		12.2	32.9	171	3460	50	75

increase particularly in the excretion of epinephrine, there was no comparable effect on the excretion of metabolites during these short-term collections. The stress of motor car racing which demands tremendous concentration is predominantly psychological and I am mentioning these results mainly to show the importance which emotional factors can assume.

6. Ambient temperature – Cold stress as well as hot stress (Leduc, 1961; Hasselman *et al.*, 1960) can activate the sympathoadrenal system and lead to catecholamine discharge. When other stresses are studied, the temperature of the environment should be comfortable and constant. In experiments involving muscular activity, overheating should be avoided. The action of drugs may lead to changes of body temperature which should be corrected if necessary.

7. Diuresis – The question whether the excretion of catecholamines varies with the extent of diuresis has been debated for some time. Results have been contradictory: while some investigators (Von Euler *et al.*, 1955; Kärki, 1956; Overy *et al.*, 1967; Becker and Kreuzer, 1970; Graham *et al.*, 1967) found excretion rates to be independent of urine flow, others (De Schaepdryver and Leroy, 1961; Leroy and De Schaepdryver, 1961; Hathaway *et al.*, 1969; Baekeland *et al.*, 1969) found a positive correlation of urine flow with the excretion of both epinephrine and norepinephrine or only with that of epinephrine (Benfey *et al.*, 1958; Hollister and Moore, 1969) or norepinephrine (Dawson and Bone, 1963; Perman, 1961; Gawellek, 1969), possibly indicating a reduced rate of tubular re-uptake at high rates of flow. In the most systematic investigation so far, Hoeldtke and Martin (1970) exposed 5 volunteers to regimes of different fluid intake in a Latin-square design. Although the mean daily fluid output varied from less than 1000 to almost 4000 ml, the excretion of the free and conjugated fractions of epinephrine, norepinephrine and dopamine remained remarkably constant (Fig. 1).

8. pH of urine – It is of course well known that the stability of catecholamines decreases rapidly with increasing pH but the question which concerns us here is whether the excretion rate as such is affected by the pH of the urine.

The undissociated form of a weak base, especially if it is lipid-soluble, is subject to much more rapid tubular reabsorption than the cationic form; hence some amines have been shown to be excreted more rapidly in acid than in alkaline urine (Asatoor *et al.*, 1963; 1965). There is disagreement on the question whether the excretion of epinephrine is pH-dependent, one paper affirming it (Braun, 1964) and another one denying it (Overy *et al.*, 1967). In any case,

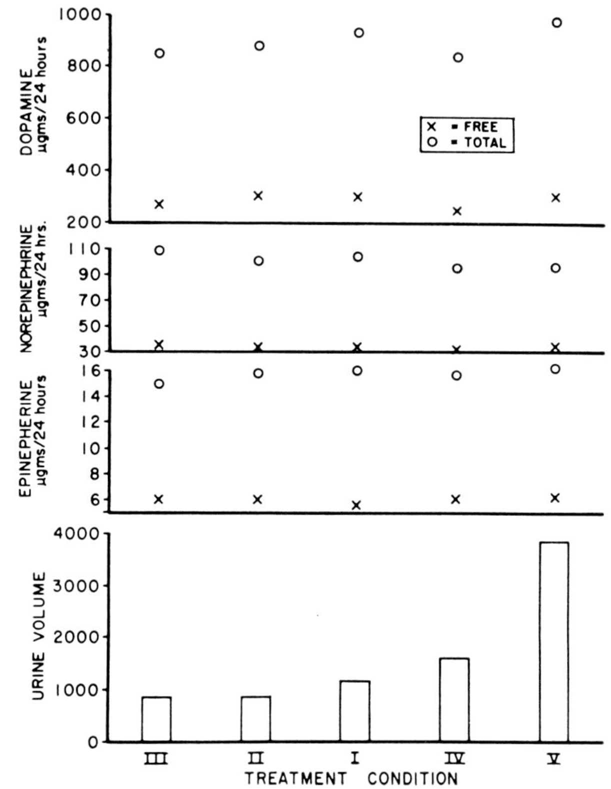

Fig. 1. Excretion of catecholamines with changing urine volumes (from Hoeldtke and Martin, 1970).

the excretion of an alkaline urine where this phenomenon would be noticeable should be avoided for a number of reasons.

9. Salt intake – Sodium loading has been shown to lead to increased catecholamine excretion in rats and men (Beauvallet, 1966; Ikoma, 1965), but these experiments probably amounted to a considerable stress. Conversely, a decrease of norepinephrine output has been observed during a sodium-restricted diet (Ikoma, 1965).

10. Dietary effects – This raises the more general problem of the effects of food components. Such effects may be due to sympathoadrenal discharge or to the fact that catecholamines or catecholamine precursors are ingested. A number of euphoriants, such as caffeine, nicotine or ethanol, belong to the first category. Some wines and beers, apart from their alcohol content, may raise catecholamine output by their content of tyramine which is known to elicit a release of norepinephrine. Some cheeses are also rich in tyramine. Citrus fruits contain octopamine and p-sympatol (Gjessing *et al.*, 1963; Stewart and Wheaton, 1964) which have a similar effect. Whether these natural amines are of much significance in the absence of MAO inhibitors is uncertain, but such a possibility should be kept in mind. As for the second category, the fact that bananas contain dopamine and norepinephrine is now well known (Crout and Sjoerdsma, 1959). Certain kinds of beans, especially *Vicia faba*, contain L-dopa, partly in the form of a glucoside (Andrews and Pridham, 1965). Some authors urge that vanilla should be prohibited when VMA or MHPG are to be determined; however, interference by small amounts is usually taken care of by the inclusion of an unoxidized blank in the analytical procedure.

We recently had occasion to study the effect of diet on the excretion of dopamine and two of its metabolites, HVA and dopac (Weil-Malherbe and Van Buren, 1969). I had noticed, as have others, that the excretion of dopamine is more variable than that of epinephrine or norepinephrine and I wondered whether these variations were of dietary origin. Our experiment was carried out on groups of patients with Parkinson's disease and normal controls who were studied for six consecutive days. During the first three days the subjects were on an unrestricted mixed diet; during the second three days they were limited to an infant formula preparation made from whole milk and hydrolyzed starch. The excretion of free and conjugated dopamine and of both metabolites decreased significantly during the milk diet in both groups (Fig. 2). The subjects found the diet not very appetizing and did not consume more than about 1500 calories per day. Their protein intake was thus reduced to about 60% of normal and we suggested that this reduction was mainly responsible for the decreased output of dopamine and dopamine metabolites, since less dopamine was presumably produced in surplus quantity.

The excretion of free dopamine was affected by the change in diet as much as, if not more than, that of the conjugated fraction. This does not support the claim that the free fraction is less susceptible to dietary effects than the conjugated fraction.

The only significant difference between patients and controls in our experiments was a lower excretion of free dopamine in the patients, and this difference persisted after the change of diet. If dopamine metabolism were generally impaired in Parkinson's disease, a similar decrease in the excretion of dopamine metabolites and particularly of conjugated dopamine would be anticipated. We suggested instead that the decrease in the excretion of free dopamine might be the result of more active conjugation processes in the patients which themselves might be an adaptive response to the chronic drug treatment to which these patients are subjected. Whatever the explanation, the example shows that, contrary to current practice, the conjugated fraction of catecholamines should not be overlooked.

11. Drugs – This brings us to the subject of drugs. Apart from the possibility just mentioned there are many ways in which drugs can affect the release or the metabolism of catecholamines. This is of course a vast subject which is beyond the scope of this discussion. Here I merely wish to stress that possible drug effects should be considered in the experimental design. To give you an example, I was recently asked to review a paper reporting an increased

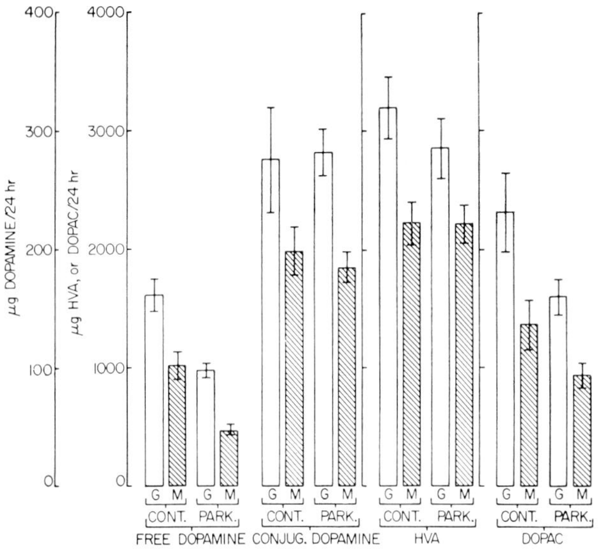

Fig. 2. Excretion of dopamine and metabolites.
G = general diet, M = 'milk' diet, Cont = Control group, Park = Parkinson's disease group.
The bars indicate the means ± SEM.

catecholamine output during labor. All the patients had received pre-delivery sedation with meperidine. In view of the well-known stimulation of catecholamine discharge by opiates the question should have been asked how much of the effect was due to the drug and how much, if any, to the stress of labor.

In the time that is left to me I should like to touch briefly upon some problems of analytical methodology. I mentioned the value of analyzing the conjugated fraction of catecholamines and I should therefore like to say a few words about its estimation. The sulfo-conjugates of catecholamines and 3-O-methyl catecholamines, which, in man, account for at least 80% of the conjugated fraction, are hydrolyzed either by boiling at pH 1.0–1.5 or enzymatically. Some compounds, such as VMA and MHPG, are destroyed by heating with acid which makes the use of an enzyme mandatory. The enzyme most frequently used, a commercial preparation called glusulase, is a crude extract from the hepatopancreas of *Helix pomatia* and contains both aryl sulfatase and glucuronidase. Owing to the lengthy incubation at 37° which is required, recoveries of catecholamines have usually been low. By carrying out the reaction in the presence of glycine buffer, antioxidants, and an atmosphere of nitrogen, we have been able to improve recoveries, but they are still somewhat erratic, especially in the case of epinephrine. Pending a further improvement, acid hydrolysis has still to be used. In our experience a pH of 1.5 is as efficient as a pH of 1.0. The boiling of the acidified urine results in alumina eluates which are yellow and highly quenching and which have a high blank. These complications are corrected by a further purification of the alumina eluate on a column of cation exchange resin. Table III shows a comparison of results obtained by applying the trihydroxyindole method to an alumina eluate and to the same eluate after the additional cation exchange purification. Although there are no significant differences in recoveries, the estimates of catecholamines are appreciably lower after purification, indicating the removal of interfering fluorescence.

Finally I should like to mention a recent development which has resulted in a great increase in analytical sensitivity. I am referring to the methods based on the incorporation of a labeled methyl group. Two enzymes have been used for this purpose, phenylethanolamine N-methyl-

TABLE III

Estimation of catecholamines in extracts of hydrolyzed urine prepared by (a) chromatography on alumina only and (b) successive chromatography on alumina and cation exchange resin (Weil-Malherbe, 1968).

	Alumina			Alumina + Amberlite CG 50		
	Epi-nephrine	Norepi-nephrine	Dop-amine	Epi-nephrine	Norepi-nephrine	Dop-amine
Mean excretion, μg/24 hr	27.0	67.3	226	9.6	29.1	132.3
± SEM, 24 experiments	± 5.45	±23.3	±45.9	±1.13	±4.28	±21.6
P[a]				0.006	0.1	0.1
Mean recoveries, %	105.2	75.6	69.9	85.8	81.4	54.5
± SEM, 12 experiments	±15.5	±10.8	±18.2	±6.13	±9.34	± 7.44
P[a]				0.3	0.7	0.5

[a] Significance of difference from corresponding value obtained after alumina purification.

transferase (PNMT), prepared from adrenal glands, and catechol-O-methyltransferase (COMT), usually prepared from rat liver. The same methyl donor, S-adenosylmethionine (SAM), acts with both enzymes (Fig. 3).

In the method of Kovacsics and Saelens (1968) an extract of 10 mg brain is incubated with PNMT and C^{14}-labeled SAM, resulting in the conversion of norepinephrine to epinephrine, labeled in the N-methyl group. This is followed by chromatography on cation exchange paper and counting. The method is stated to be sensitive to about 1 ng of norepinephrine. However, to avoid nonspecific methylation the reaction has to take place in concentrated solution, containing at least 100 ng norepinephrine/ml. Under these conditions only norepinephrine appears to be methylated. The method is of course not applicable to the estimation of dopamine or epinephrine.

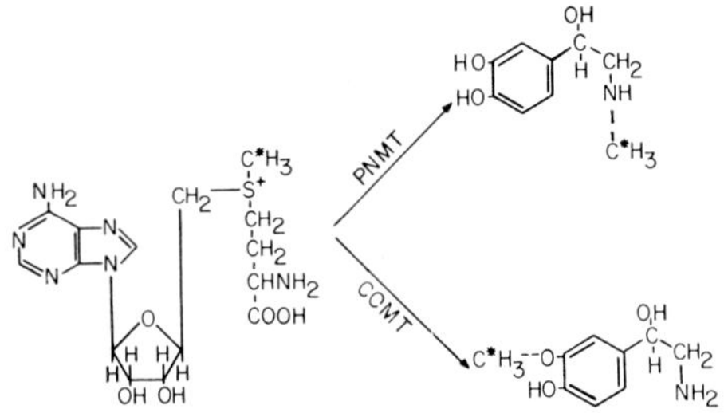

Fig. 3. Transfers of methyl group from S-adenosylmethionine to norepinephrine.

COMT has been used for the estimation of norepinephrine in heart extracts (Nikodijevic *et al.*, 1968) and for the estimation of epinephrine and norepinephrine in plasma (Engelman and Portnoy, 1970). In the first method an extract from 20 mg heart is incubated with the enzyme. Owing to the presence of an inhibitor the reaction proceeds only to 15–25% completion and an internal standard is therefore essential. Normetanephrine, the reaction product, is extracted at pH 10 with a mixture of isoamylalcohol and toluene and counted. The method can measure 0.3 ng of norepinephrine, but is subject to interference from other catechol compounds in the extract. When these are present, a thin-layer separation of the O-methylated products is necessary.

In the plasma method of Engelman and Portnoy (1970) the catecholamines are first isolated by cation exchange, then methylated with COMT. The reaction products are separated on silica gel thin-layer plates, the spots eluted and oxidized with periodate. The vanillin formed is extracted and counted. Recoveries are monitored by the addition of trace amounts of tritiated norepinephrine and epinephrine to plasma.

The disadvantages of these enzymatic isotope methods are, first, a relative lack of specificity which entails the need for elaborate separation procedures and, secondly, the high price of the counting equipment and the reagents required. On the other hand, they are unequalled in sensitivity and accuracy.

REFERENCES

ANDREWS, R. S. and PRIDHAM, J. B. (1965): Structure of a dopa glucoside from Vicia faba. *Nature (Lond.)*, *205*, 1213.

ASATOOR, A. M., GALMAN, B. R., JOHNSON, J. R. and MILNE, M. D. (1965): The excretion of dexamphetamine and its derivatives. *Brit. J. Pharmacol.*, *24*, 293.

ASATOOR, A. M., LOUDON, D. R., MILNE, M. D. and SIMENHOFF, M. L. (1963): The excretion of pethidine and its derivatives. *Brit. J. Pharmacol.*, *20*, 285.

BAEKELAND, F., SCHENKER, V. J., SCHENKER, A. C. and LASKY, R. (1969): Urinary excretion of epinephrine, norepinephrine, dopamine and tryptamine during sleep and wakefulness. Effects of pentobarbital, pentobarbital plus dextroamphetamine sulfate and placebo. *Psychopharmacologia (Berl.)*, *14*, 359.

BEAUVALLET, M., FUGAZZA, J. and GODEFROY, F. (1966): Influence d'une surcharge du régime en chlorure de sodium sur la teneur en catécholamines des surrénales et leur excrétion urinaire chez le rat. *C.R. Soc. Biol. (Paris)*, *160*, 1418.

BECKER, E. J. and KREUZER, F. (1970): Catecholamine excretion by the healthy adult human. *Pflügers Arch. ges. Physiol.*, *316*, 95.

BENFEY, B. G., MAZURKIEWICZ, I. and MELVILLE, K. I. (1958): Observations on the simultaneous urinary excretion of adrenaline and noradrenaline under various conditions. *Rev. canad. Biol.*, *17*, 312.

BRAUN, W. (1964): Zur Abhängigkeit der Adrenalinausscheidung vom Urin-pH. *Naunyn-Schmiedeberg's Arch. exp. Path. Pharmakol.*, *249*, 191.

CASTRÉN, O. (1963): Urinary excretion of noradrenaline and adrenaline in late normal and toxemic pregnancy. *Acta pharmacol. (Kbh.)*, *20, Suppl. 2.*

CROUT, J. R. and SJOERDSMA, A. (1959): The clinical and laboratory significance of serotonin and catecholamines in bananas. *New Engl. J. Med.*, *261*, 23.

DAWSON, J. and BONE, A. (1963): The relationship between urine volume and urinary adrenaline and noradrenaline excretion in a group of psychotic patients. *Brit. J. Psychiat.*, *109*, 629.

DE SCHAEPDRYVER, A. F. and LEROY, J. G. (1961): Urine volume and catecholamine excretion in man. *Acta cardiol. (Brux.)*, *16*, 631.

ENGELMAN, K. and PORTNOY, B. (1970): A sensitive double-isotope derivative assay for norepinephrine and epinephrine. Normal resting human plasma levels. *Circulat. Res.*, *26*, 53.

GAWELLEK, F. (1969): Die Veränderungen der Katecholaminausscheidung im Harn bei unterschiedlicher Diureserate. *Endokrinologie*, *55*, 199.

GJESSING, L. and ARMSTRONG, M. D. (1963): Occurrence of (–)-sympatol in oranges. *Proc. Soc. exp. Biol. (N.Y.)*, *114*, 226.

GRAHAM, L. A., COHEN, S. I., SHMAVONIAN, B. M. and KIRSHNER, N. (1967): Urinary catecholamine excretion during instrumental conditioning. *Psychosom. Med.*, *29*, 134.

HASSELMAN, M., SCHAFF, G. and METZ, B. (1960): Influences respectives du travail, de la température ambiante et de la privation de sommeil sur l'excrétion urinaire de catécholamines chez l'homme normal. *C.R. Soc. Biol. (Paris)*, *154*, 197.

HATHAWAY, P. W., BREHM, M. L., CHAPP, J. R. and BOGDONOFF, M. D. (1969): Urine flow, catecholamines and blood pressure. The variability of response of normal human subjects in a relaxed laboratory setting. *Psychosom. Med.*, *31*, 20.

HOELDTKE, R. D. and MARTIN, W. R. (1970): Urine volume and catecholamine excretion. *J. Lab. clin. Med.*, *75*, 166.

HOLLISTER, L. E. and MOORE, F. (1969): Urine flow and catecholamine excretion in man. *Pharmacol. Res. Commun.*, *1*, 36.

IKOMA, T. (1965): Studies on catechols with reference to hypertension. *Jap. Circulat. J. (Ni.), 29*, 1279.

JANUSZEWICZ, W. and WOCIAL, B. (1960): The influence of work, 24-hour rhythm and the visual impulse on the catecholamine excretion with urine. *Pol. Arch. Med. wewnet., 30*, 207.

KÄRKI, N. T. (1956): The urinary excretion of noradrenaline and adrenaline in different age groups, its diurnal variation and the effect of muscular work on it. *Acta physiol. scand., 39, Suppl. 132.*

KOVACSICS, G. B. and SAELENS, J. K. (1968): Measurement of the levels and turnover of norepinephrine in discrete areas of rat brain using an enzymatic assay. *Arch. int. Pharmacodyn., 174*, 481.

LEDUC, J. (1961): Catecholamine production and release in exposure and acclimation to cold. *Acta physiol. scand., 53, Suppl. 183.*

LEROY, J. G. and DE SCHAEPDRYVER, A. F. (1961): Urine and catecholamine output in normal and reserpinized dogs. *Arch. int. Pharmacodyn., 130*, 437.

LEVI, L. (1965): The urinary output of adrenaline and noradrenaline during pleasant and unpleasant emotional states. *Psychosom. Med., 27*, 80.

NIKODIJEVIC, B., DALY, J. and CREVELING, C. R. (1969): Catechol-O-methyltransferase. I. An enzymatic assay for cardiac norepinephrine. *Biochem. Pharmacol., 18*, 1577.

OVERY, H. R., PFISTER, R. and CHIDSEY, C. A. (1967): Studies on the renal excretion of norepinephrine. *J. clin. Invest., 46*, 482.

PERMAN, E. S. (1961): Effect of ethanol and hydration on the urinary excretion of adrenaline and noradrenaline and on the blood sugar of rats. *Acta physiol. scand., 51*, 68.

STEWART, I. and WHEATON, T. A. (1964): L-Octopamine in citrus: isolation and identification. *Science, 145*, 60.

SUNDIN, T. (1958): The effect of body posture on the urinary excretion of adrenaline and noradrenaline. *Acta med. scand., 161, Suppl.* 336.

VON EULER, U. S. and HELLNER, S. (1952): Excretion of noradrenaline and adrenaline in muscular work. *Acta physiol. scand., 26*, 183.

VON EULER, U. S., HELLNER-BJÖRKMAN, S. and ORWÉN, I. (1955): Diurnal variations in the excretion of free and conjugated noradrenaline and adrenaline in urine from healthy subjects. *Acta physiol. scand., 33, Suppl. 118*, 10.

VON EULER, U. S., LUFT, R. and SUNDIN, T. (1955): The urinary excretion of noradrenaline and adrenaline in healthy subjects during recumbency and standing. *Acta physiol. scand., 34*, 169.

WEIL-MALHERBE, H. (1968): The estimation of total (free + conjugated) catecholamines and some catecholamine metabolites in human urine. *Meth. biochem. Anal., 16*, 293.

WEIL-MALHERBE, H. and VAN BUREN, J. M. (1969): The excretion of dopamine and dopamine metabolites in Parkinson's disease and the effect of diet thereon. *J. Lab. clin. Med., 74*, 305.

RECENT ADVANCES IN THE INVESTIGATION OF CONTRACEPTIVE METHODS

JORGE MARTÍNEZ-MANAUTOU and JUAN GINER

Instituto Mexicano del Seguro Social, Apartado, 73-032,
Mexico, D.F., Mexico

Millions of people throughout the world are still in need of effective, safe and practical methods for fertility regulation. After more than 10 years of intensive research, oral and injectable formulations of hormonal steroids and various types of intrauterine devices have been developed, with an efficacy reaching virtually 100% against pregnancy. Nevertheless, their use is associated with important undesirable side effects which have received an unnecessary degree of publicity. This is threatening the development of research programs which would otherwise lead to a better basic and applied knowledge of human reproductive processes that may contribute to the discovery of safer methods of fertility regulation. In spite of these problems, scientists are continuing to do active research; each day new information is coming to light and undoubtedly will continue to do so, until the final goals are achieved.

LOW LEVEL PROGESTOGENS

Martínez-Manautou *et al.* (1965) reported on the contraceptive efficacy of the daily continuous administration of 500 μg of chlormadinone acetate in women. Based on these findings, other potent oral progestogens have been tested at lower dosages. DL-norgestrel at doses of 50 and 75 μg daily has shown an efficacy similar to that of 500 μg of chlormadinone acetate. The incidence of irregular bleeding and other side effects has also been very similar (Tyler, 1969).

More recently, the D-isomer of norgestrel has been tested by several investigators at the daily continuous dose of 30 μg. According to Correu (unpublished) in Mexico, no pregnancy has been reported in 734 women treated over a total of 6000 cycles, and Kesserü (unpublished) in Peru has observed only one pregnancy in 223 women over 1260 cycles, giving a pregnancy rate for both studies of 0.16 per 100 woman-years. This is clearly superior to other progestogens previously used, including DL-norgestrel at higher doses, and puts it at the same level of efficacy as the combined estrogen-progestogen contraceptive methods. The effect on the menstrual cycle and the frequency of breakthrough bleeding seems to be similar to that observed with other progestogens administered continuously. The mechanism of action of this therapy remains unexplained and more studies are needed.

ONCE-A-MONTH ORAL CONTRACEPTION

This technique was first described by Greenblatt *et al.* (1967). It employs a long-acting oral estrogen, administered on day 25 of the menstrual cycle, together with a short-acting progestogen. The estrogen suppresses ovulation, and the progestogen induces a withdrawal period within a few days so that the cyclic pattern of menstruation will not be disturbed. More recently, a variation of this technique has been reported using the 3-cyclo-pentyl-ether of ethinyl estradiol and a long-acting progestogen, the 3-cyclo-enol-ether of norethindrone acetate (Maqueo-Topete *et al.*, 1969; Larranaga and Berman, 1970). Two mg of the estrogen were given on the first day of menstrual bleeding and three weeks later a combination of 2 mg of the estrogen and 5 mg of the progestogen. In the following cycles, the estrogen-progestogen combination was given every four weeks, irrespective of the timing of withdrawal bleeding. Menstrual flow usually began 6 to 14 days after the administration of the monthly dose. The pregnancy rate of 2.0 per 100 woman-years in 2920 cycles of therapy and the effect on the endometrium found in this study are similar to that reported with sequential-type oral contraceptives. Side effects more often reported were nausea, mucorrhea, spotting and breakthrough bleeding. Missed menstrual periods were present in 0.4% of the cycles and the amount of menstrual flow was heavy in 22.7%.

POSTCOITAL ORAL CONTRACEPTION

Prevention of pregnancy in primates by the administration of estrogens after sexual exposure has been successful (Morris *et al.*, 1967). Limited clinical experience in women has shown that the administration of some estrogens such as stilbestrol and ethinyl estradiol at daily doses of 25 to 50 mg and 0.5 to 5 mg respectively, given during 4 to 5 days following intercourse, may curb pregnancy by preventing implantation of the fertilized ovum (Morris and Van Wagenen, 1968).

It is obvious that this contraceptive method has a practical use in those cases in which coitus is restricted to a few occasions during each menstrual cycle, otherwise its use will be associated with suppression of ovulation and many side effects will occur.

Postcoital contraceptives may achieve their objective by inhibiting fertilization, interfering with the transport of the fertilized ovum or with its implantation in the uterus.

Other steroids besides estrogens have been tested as postcoital contraceptives. Rubio *et al.* (1970) studied the 3-cyclopentyl-enol-ether of norethindrone given postcoitally in a single oral dose varying from 500 to 800 μg less than 24 hours after coitus with an average of 12 doses per menstrual cycle. Efficacy was good and the only important adverse effect noted was breakthrough bleeding.

Kesserü (unpublished) in Lima, Peru is also testing another progestogen, norgestrel, at the oral single dose of 250 μg given postcoitally with preliminary satisfactory results.

A great variety of compounds, steroidal and non-steroidal, have been tested by Emmens *et al.* (1970) and other investigators in rodents, rabbits and monkeys with variable results regarding postcoital efficacy; however, their efficacy in humans remains to be tested.

INJECTABLE HORMONAL CONTRACEPTIVES

One of the important drawbacks of oral contraceptives is the need for daily intake of medication. With the idea of avoiding this inconvenience, two methods using long-acting injectable steroids have been investigated.

1. Intramuscular administration of an estrogen and a progestogen of prolonged action, given at monthly intervals with the intention of producing artificial menstrual cycles. Estradiol enanthate, a long-acting estrogen at a dose of 10 mg and dihydroxyprogesterone acetophenide at a dose of 150 mg has been the combination more widely investigated and has proved the more satisfactory to insure regular cyclic bleeding (Reifenstein *et al.*, 1965). It is a very effective contraceptive method with a pregnancy rate comparable to that of the

classical combined oral preparations. Tyler (1969) reported that approximately 75 % of his patients have satisfactory cycles with acceptable bleeding patterns, while the remainder have cycles too short, too long or associated with profuse and irregular bleeding, making it necessary to interrupt therapy in some cases.

Other investigators (Plesner, 1969; Rutherford *et al.*, 1964; Rizkallah and Taymor, 1966) have found a tendency to shorter cycles, the mean cycle length being 20.4 days during treatment as compared with 28.2 days during the pre-treatment cycles.

2. Intramuscular administration of variable doses, from 100 to 300 mg, of a long-acting progestogen, usually medroxyprogesterone acetate or norethindrone enanthate, given at intervals of three months.

Medroxyprogesterone acetate at a dose of 150 mg every 3 months, has proved to be a very effective method of contraception. Schwallie in 14,239 patient-months of observation has found a failure rate of 0.51 per 100 woman-years of use (Schwallie, 1968).

The most common complaints reported with this method are tension in the breast, edema, irregular bleeding, amenorrhea and increased libido (Plesner, 1969). Three weeks or more following the first injection there is almost always marked regression and thinning of the endometrium with diffuse pre-decidual transformation with large, dilated vascular structures; and after two or more injections there is always a suppressed endometrium with rare and minimal signs of active secretion.

The mode of action of these injectable formulations is, in the majority of cases, inhibition of ovulation as demonstrated by basal body temperature curves, FSH and LH assays, pregnanediol determinations and endometrial biopsy studies.

The effects on steroid function tests, liver function and clotting mechanism are similar to those found with the oral estrogen-progestogen contraceptives.

Since resumption of spontaneous ovulation and regression of endometrial changes occur at prolonged and unpredictable intervals after stopping therapy, this method of contraception should probably be limited to those women who have decided not to bear any more children.

INTRAVAGINAL DEVICES

Absorption of progesterone through the vaginal mucosa is well documented (Greenblatt, 1954; Southam, 1954) and several reports have appeared recently in the medical literature on the contraceptive effect of continuous release of a progestogen contained or mixed in plastic rings which are placed in the vagina (Mishell *et al.*, 1970; Mishell and Lumkin, 1970). Medicated rings containing either 50, 100, 200 or 400 mg of medroxyprogesterone acetate, added to the silicone in its fluid state, were tested in women during one menstrual cycle. The estimated daily release of 550 to 1000 μg of medroxyprogesterone acetate was enough to inhibit ovulation, according to pregnanediol determination in all the cases tested. Breakthrough bleeding without relation to drug dosage was noted by 25 % of the subjects. After removal of the medicated rings, withdrawal bleeding of 2 to 5 days' duration occurred within 3 days in all subjects except one. Varying degrees of erosion and ulceration of the vaginal mucosa and submucosa were noted in the posterolateral fornices of approximately 68 % of the subjects. No expulsion of the rings were observed. Considerably more investigation is needed in this contraceptive method to evaluate its antifertility effect and tolerance.

SUBCUTANEOUS IMPLANTS

In 1965 we reported the contraceptive efficacy of the continuous daily administration of 500 μg of chlormadinone acetate given orally (Martínez-Manautou *et al.*, 1965), and Dziuk and Cook (1966) showed that physiologically active steroids encapsulated in silicone rubber were liberated at a slow and constant rate, which was dependent upon the thickness of the capsule wall and surface area. These two findings have been the basis for the use of subcutaneous implantation of silicone capsules containing pure progestogens for contraceptive purposes.

Croxatto *et al.* (1969) implanted in women 3 to 4 capsules of silastic-containing megestrol acetate with an *in vitro* release of 78 to 104 μg/24 hr, finding evidence of some contraceptive effectiveness and a definite dose/effect relationship. The mean length of the cycles was 30 days with a tendency toward longer cycles. Ovulation was present in 5% of the cycles and normal secretory endometrium in 30%. The mean complication observed with this method was the occurrence of spotting and breakthrough bleeding in approximately 25% of the treated cycles.

Tatum *et al.* (1969) implanted in the subcutaneous tissue the same type of plastic capsules filled with 18 mg of crystalline megestrol acetate with an *in vitro* release of 72 to 108 μg/24 hr. No woman conceived during 33 woman-months, using 6 of these implants. This approach to hormonal contraception needs a larger series of subjects and more prolonged observation to demonstrate its practicability.

INTRAUTERINE CONTRACEPTIVES

The effective, safe and practical use of intrauterine devices to prevent pregnancy has been pursued by a legion of scientists throughout the world during the past 150 years. Richter (1909) recommended the intrauterine insertion of silkworm gut, and later Gräfenberg (1931) reported his investigations with silkworm gut rings and later with a pliable coil of thin silver wire. These devices were followed by the Ota ring (1934) and some other types made with stainless steel wire (Hall and Stone, 1962).

Then during the early sixties a variety of devices made of plastic materials were described, among which are the Margulies spiral (1962); the Birnberg bow (Birnberg and Burnhill, 1964); the Lippes loop (1965) and others. They were made in various sizes to fit different uterine conditions. It has been stated that according to the experience accumulated, one of the more suitable intrauterine devices among those available at present is the large Lippes loop; however the designing and testing of new models has continued.

Among the devices which are undergoing trial at the present are the following: the Shamrock-shaped intrauterine device (Andersen and Burdick, 1969) made of a polyethylene poly-

TABLE I

Net cumulative rates of events per 100 users

	Type of contraceptive device				
	Shamrock 6 mth	M-211 6 mth	Majzlin spring 1 yr	Dalkon shield 1 yr	Lippes loop D 1 yr
Events					
Pregnancy	3.0	0.0	1.4	1.1	2.7
Expulsion					
First	10.0	1.0	1.6	2.3	9.5
Later	—	0.0	0.1	—	3.2
Removal					
Medical reasons	12.0	8.7	10.4	2.0	15.2
Planning pregnancy	—	0.2	1.5	—	0.9
Other personal reasons	—	0.3	3.7	0.6	2.2

mer; the M-211 (Bernard, 1969) constructed on non-reactive medical grade 314 stainless steel; the Majzlin spring (Solish and Majzlin, 1969) also constructed of stainless steel wire; and the Dalkon Shield (Davis, 1970) made of plastic. Net cumulative rates of events per 100 users with these devices are presented in Table 1.

Zipper *et al.* (1969) reported the combined use of a plastic 'T' device and copper wire. Their studies showed that the addition of 30 mm² of copper wire to the long arm of a T-shaped plastic device significantly decreases the rates of pregnancy and expulsion in comparison with the plastic 'T' alone.

The precise nature of the antifertility mechanism of copper has not yet been determined and it is probable that several mechanisms of action are involved, and a local rather than a systemic effect takes place. The rate of removal of this device is three times less, and the rate of accidental pregnancies is greater than that of the loop D during the same length of study. When the amount of copper added to the 'T' device was increased to 120 mm², the pregnancy rate was decreased from 18.3 per 100 woman-years of use to 1.5, and the expulsion rate from 5.9 to 4 (Zipper *et al.*, 1970). The efficacy of this type of IUD has been further improved by adding to the 'T' device zinc and copper wire, and no pregnancy has been reported after one year of study.

Tietze (1970) reports that in order to reduce calcium deposits and minimize bleeding, Dr. Lippes has blended 2% gum silicone with low-density polyethylene and molded it in identical shape and size with the loop D. After the first year of study of this silicone loop, pregnancy and expulsion rates for personal reasons have been similar to those of the classical loop D, but the rates of removal for bleeding and/or pain have been reduced. Another modification to the Lippes loop D is the Shell loop which is made of a co-polymer product of the Shell Oil Corporation, called Shell-526, blended with barium sulphate. This combination produces a very rigid loop which, after the first year of testing, has showed a smaller expulsion rate and, more important, a pregnancy rate of 0.5 per 100 users, which is quite favorable when compared with a pregnancy rate of 2.7 for the original Lippes device. The rate of removal for bleeding and/or pain or both remained the same and 2 perforations of the uterus have been reported.

More recently, and with the hope of further reducing removal for bleeding, Dr. Lippes has added 2% gum silicone to the Shell co-polymer. No data on the performance of this device are yet available.

Based on studies of the biologic effects of progesterone contained in silastic capsules attached to a Lippes loop and placed directly into the endometrial cavity of human volunteers (Scomegna *et al.*, 1970), plastic intrauterine devices containing different progestogens are being actively investigated with the hope of improving efficacy and reducing expulsion rates.

PROSTAGLANDINS

Finally, I would like to make some comments on a topic that is becoming fashionable in contraception. It has been shown by several investigators that the prostaglandin F2 alpha will induce luteal degeneration in both pseudopregnant rats and rabbits (Pharriss and Kirton, 1969; Pharriss and Wyngarden, 1969), and when injected to pregnant rats will terminate pregnancy any time between day 5 and day 15 (Gutknecht *et al.*, 1969). Another evidence that this prostaglandin has a luteolytic effect was presented by Pharriss (Pharriss and Kirton, 1969) who reported that in monkeys, within 12 to 24 hours of treatment, plasma progesterone was undetectable and menses followed shortly thereafter. These findings open a new and exciting approach to human contraception.

REFERENCES

ANDERSEN, M. V. and BURDICK, C. L. (1969): Preliminary experience with a shamrock-shaped IUD. In: *Advances in Planned Parenthood, 1st ed., Vol. V*, Chapter III, pp. 97–99. Editors: A. J. Sobrero and C. McKee. ICS No. 207, Excerpta Medica, Amsterdam.

BERNARD, R. P. (1969): The M-211 device – a possible turning point in approach (International IUD programme). In: *Advances in Planned Parenthood, 1st ed., Vol. V*, Chapter III, pp. 100–109. Editors: A. J. Sobrero and C. McKee. ICS No. 207, Excerpta Medica, Amsterdam.

BIRNBERG, C. H. and BURNHILL, M. S. (1964): A new intrauterine contraceptive device. *Amer. J. Obstet. Gynec.*, *89*, 137.

CROXATTO, H., DÍAZ, S., VERA, R., ETCHART, M. and ATRIA, P. (1969): Fertility control in women with a progestogen released in microquantities from subcutaneous capsules. *Amer. J. Obstet. Gynec.*, *105*, 1135.

DAVIS, H. J. (1970): The shield intrauterine device. A superior modern contraceptive. *Amer. J. Obstet. Gynec.*, *106*, 455.

DZIUK, P. J. and COOK, B. (1966): Passage of steroids through silicone ruber. *Endocrinology*, *78*, 208.

EMMENS, C. W. (1970): Postcoital contraception. *Brit. med. Bull.*, *26*, 45.

GRÄFENBERG, E. (1931): An intrauterine contraceptive method. In: *The Practice of Contraception, 1st. ed.*, pp. 38–45. Editors: M. Sanger and H. M. Stone. Williams & Wilkins, Baltimore, Md.

GREENBLATT, R. B. (1954): *J. clin. Endocr.*, *14*, 1564.

GREENBLATT, R. B. (1967): One-pill-a-month contraceptive. *Fertil. and Steril.*, *18*, 207.

GUTKNECHT, G. D., CORNETTE, J. A. and PHARRISS, B. B. (1969): Antifertility properties of prostaglandin F_2 alfa. *J. Biol. Reprod.*, *1*, 367.

HALL, H. H. and STONE, J. L. (1962): Observations on the use of the intrauterine pessary, with special reference to the Gräfenberg ring. *Amer. J. Obstet. Gynec.*, *83*, 683.

LARRANAGA, A. and BERMAN, E. (1970): Clinical study of a once-a-month oral contraceptive: quinestrol-quingestanol. *Contraception*, *1*, 137.

LIPPES, J. (1965): Contraception with intrauterine plastic loops. *Amer. J. Obstet. Gynec.*, *93*, 1024.

MAQUEO-TOPETE, M., BERMAN, E., SOBERÓN, J. and CALDERÓN, J. J. (1969): A pill-a-month contraceptive. *Fertil. and Steril.*, *20*, 884.

MARGULIES, L. C. (1962): Permanent reversible contraception with an intrauterine plastic spiral (perma spiral). In: *Intra-uterine Contraceptive Devices, 1st ed.*, pp. 61–68. Editors: C. Tietze and S. Lewit. ICS No. 54. Excerpta Medica, Amsterdam.

MARTÍNEZ-MANAUTOU, J., GINER-VELÁZQUEZ, J., CORTÉS-GALLEGOS, V., CASASOLA, J., AZNAR-RAMOS, R. and RUDEL, H. W. (1965): Fertility control with microdoses of progestogen. In: *Proceedings of the VI Pan-American Congress of Endocrinology*, pp. 157–165. Editor: C. Gual. ICS No. 112, Excerpta Medica, Amsterdam.

MISHELL, D. R., TALAS, M., PARLOW, A. F. and MOYER, D. L. (1970): Contraception by means of a silastic vaginal ring impregnated with medroxyprogesterone acetate. *Amer. J. Obstet. Gynec.*, *107*, 100.

MISHELL, D. R., JR and LUMKIN, M. E. (1970): Contraceptive effect of varying dosages of progestogen in silastic vaginal rings. *Fertil. and Steril.*, *21*, 99.

MORRIS, J. MCL. and VAN WAGENEN, G. (1968): Post-coital oral contraception. In: *Advances In Planned Parenthood, 1st ed., Vol. IV*, Chapter 6, pp. 125–128. Editors: A.J. Sobrero and S. Lewit. ICS No. 177, Excerpta Medica, Amsterdam.

MORRIS, J. MCL., VAN WAGENEN, G., MCCANN, T. and JACOBS, D. (1967): Compounds interfering with ovum implantation and development. II. Synthetic estrogens and antiestrogens. *Fertil. and Steril.*, *18*, 18.

OTA, T. (1943). In: *Jap. J. Obstet. Gynec.*, *17*, 210.

PHARRISS, B. B. and KIRTON, K. T. (1969): Prostaglandin F_2 alfa: A new contraceptive approach. In: *Advances in Planned Parenthood, 1st ed., Vol. V*, Chapter V, pp. 168–169. Editors: A. J. Sobrero and C. McKee. ICS No. 207, Excerpta Medica, Amsterdam.

PHARRISS, B. B. and WYNGARDEN, L. J. (1969): The effect of prostaglandin F_2 alfa on the progestogen content of ovaries from pseudopregnant rats. *Proc. Soc. exp. Biol. (N.Y.)*, *130*, 92.

PLESNER, R. (1969): Contraception by an injectable, long-acting oestrogen-progestogen agent. *Acta endocr.*, *61*, 494.

REIFENSTEIN, E. C. JR., PRATT, T. E., HARTZELL, K. A. and SHAFER, W. B. (1965): Artificial menstrual cycles induced in ovulating women by monthly injection of progestogen-estrogen. *Fertil. and Steril.*, *16*, 652.

RICHTER, R. (1909): Ein Mittel zur Verhütung der Konzeption. *Dtsch.med. Wschr.*, *35*, 1525.

RIZKALLAH, T. H. and TAYMOR, M. L. (1966): Ovulation inhibition with a long-acting injectable. *Amer. J. Obstet. Gynec.*, *94*, 161.

RUBIO, B., BERMAN, E., PLAINS, M., LARRANAGA, A. and GUILOFF, E. (1970): A new postcoital oral contraceptive. *Contraception*, *1*, 303.

RUTHERFORD, R. N., BANKS, A. L. and COBURN, W. A. (1964): Deladroxate for the prevention of ovulation. *Fertil. and Steril.*, *15*, 648.

SCHWALLIE, P. C. Cited in: MISHELL, D. R., EL-HABASHY, M. A., GOOD, R. G. and MOYER, D. L. (1968): Contraception with an injectable progestin. A study of its use in postpartum women *Amer. J. Obstet. Gynec.*, *101*, 1046.

SCOMMEGNA, A., PANDYA, G. N., CHRIST, M., LEE, A. W. and COHEN, M. R. (1970): Intrauterine administration of progesterone by a slow-releasing device. *Fertil. and Steril.*, *21*, 201.

SOLISH, G. I. and MAJZLIN, G. (1969): The Majzlin spring – study of over 1500 insertions. In: *Advances in Planned Parenthood, 1st ed., Vol. V*, Chapter III, pp. 117–122. Editors: A. J. Sobrero and C. McKee. ICS No. 207, Excerpta Medica, Amsterdam.

SOUTHAM, A. L. (1954): A comparative study of the effect of the progestational agents in human menstrual abnormalities. *Ann. N.Y. Acad. Sci.*, 71, 666.

TATUM, H. J., COUTINHO, E. M., FILHO, J. A. and SANT'ANNA, A. S. (1969): Acceptability of long-term contraceptive steroid administration in humans by subcutaneous silastic capsules. *Amer. J. Obstet. Gynec.*, *105*, 1139.

TIETZE, C. (1970): Experience with new IUDs. *Contraception*, *1*, 73.

TYLER, E. T. (1969): Current research in steroid contraception. *J. Reprod. Fertil.*, *20*, 319.

ZIPPER, J. A., TATUM, M., MEDEL, L., PASTENE, L. and RIVERA, M. (1970): Actividad anticonceptiva de metales intrauterinos. In: *Resúmenes de los Trabajos Presentados y Programa de Actividades*, IV Reunión de la Asociación Latino Americana de Investigaciones en Reproducción Humana (A.L.I.R.H.), p. 70. México, D. F.

ZIPPER, J. A., TATUM, H. J., PASTENE, L., MEDEL, M. and RIVERA, M. (1969): Metallic copper as an intrauterine contraceptive adjunct to the 'T' device. *Amer. J. Obstet. Gynec.*, *105*, 1274.

THYROID

CONTENTS

BIOSYNTHESIS OF THYROID HORMONE*

LESLIE J. DEGROOT, AKIO NAGASAKA, RATHA HATI,
MARIO BIGAZZI, BASIL RAPOPORT and SAMUEL REFETOFF

Thyroid Study Unit, University of Chicago, Chicago, Ill., U.S.A.

Iodide accumulated by the thyroid is bound within seconds to tyrosyl residues present in thyroglobulin, forming mono- and diiodotyrosine. These compounds appear within the briefest time measurable in the lumen of the follicle. Over a subsequent period of hours or days, iodotyrosines couple to form iodothyronines, again within thyroglobulin. This protein is stored within the colloid for days or weeks until taken into the cell by pinocytosis and hydrolyzed, and its constituent iodo-amino acids are then released. The present communication will attempt to analyze the present status of research on the mechanisms of some of these reactions.

IODIDE PEROXIDASE

By unanimous agreement of the investigators involved in this study over the past 30 years, the initial binding of iodide to tyrosyl groups in thyroglobulin is thought to be mediated by a peroxidase (DeGroot, 1965). This enzyme is located within the particulate fraction of the cell and sediments in particles that have neither the characteristics of heavy mitochondria or light microsomes (DeGroot and Dunn, 1964). Recent histochemical studies indicate that it is widespread within the cell, found at the Golgi area, at the apical cell membrane and on endoplasmic reticulum membranes (Strum and Karnovsky, 1970). The enzyme has been solubilized from the cell particles by trypsin and detergents in several laboratories, including those of this author (DeGroot and Davis, 1962; DeGroot *et al.*, 1965; Taurog (Coval and Taurog, 1967); Morrison (Hosoya and Morrison, 1967); Yip, 1965; Ljunggren and Akeson, 1968; Mahoney and Igo, 1966). While in its position in thyroid cell particles, iodination can be performed in the presence of oxygen alone, and is stimulated by NADPH and other reducing agents. After solubilization, the enzyme is dependent upon H_2O_2 for iodination. It mediates the peroxidation of several substances including iodide, pyrogallol, guaiacol, benzidine and orthodianisidine. Usually activity of the enzyme is measured by its ability to form iodotyrosine in a system involving either free tyrosine, or tyrosyl bound to protein as acceptor. The heme protein nature of the enzyme is attested in most studies by its absorbency peak at 409 mμ in the visible spectrum, formation of cyanide and CO complexes, and inhibition by cyanide and azide. Unfortunately the enzyme is labile, although it can be protected to some extent by keeping it in the presence of its substrates, iodide and tyrosine, during purification. Despite considerable effort to purify the enzyme in many laboratories through the use of salt fractionation and column chromatographic procedures, the highest reported RZ (that is the ratio of 409 mμ absorbency to that of the protein peak of 280) is 0.34 (Taurog *et al.*, 1970). This is in striking contrast to RZ values of 1–3 for other peroxidase enzymes.

* Supported in part by United States Public Health Service Grants AM 13,377 and AM 13,643.

The enzyme is not affected by perchlorate, is not inhibited by iodide (in contrast to the *in vivo* Wolff-Chaikoff effect), but is competitively inhibited by methimazole and propylthiouracil.

We have previously reported solubilization and partial purification of a thyroid iodide peroxidase-tyrosine-iodinase from calf thyroid tissue by treatment of the mitochondrial-microsomal fraction of homogenate with trypsin, deoxycholate and acetone. The enzyme was partially purified by sequential chromatography on Sephadex G-200 and DEAE cellulose (DeGroot and Davis, 1962; DeGroot *et al.*, 1965). We have now extended our studies on bulk fractionation of the enzyme, enzyme spectrum, the role of iodine in tyrosine iodination, polymeric structure and stabilization of the enzyme, and reconstruction of a defined *in vitro* iodinating system from thyroid enzymes. Iodination is routinely studied in our laboratory *in vitro* in a system containing phosphate buffer 10^{-5}M KI, I^{131}, 1 μ-mole glucose, 100 μg glucose oxidase and 1 μ-mole tyrosine. The iodinating enzyme used varies from 10 to 300 μg. Iodotyrosine formation is quantitated by absorption of labeled iodotyrosine to a cationic exchange resin.

Enzyme Fractionation

Soluble enzyme could be recovered by ammonium sulfate precipitation at 45% saturation. The procedure augments specific activity threefold.

Titration of enzyme to pH 4.8 causes precipitation of protein and enzyme activity, but enzyme can be brought back into solution from the precipitate by adjusting the pH to 7. Specific activity of the eluate is doubled, but there is much loss of activity. The cationic detergent hexadecyltrimethylammonium bromide when added to enzyme causes a precipitate to be formed and enzyme of increased specific activity is present in the supernatant (Table I). Considerable loss of total activity occurs.

TABLE I

Differential precipitation of enzyme by CTMB

	Specific activity (% MIT formation/mg protein)	
	Soluble fraction	Precipitated fraction
Original enzyme	2043	
+ CTMB, 0.7 mg/ml	2596	2000
+ CTMB, 0.85 mg/ml	2705	1718
+ CTMB, 1.2 mg/ml	3394	1459
+ CTMB, 1.35 mg/ml	3379	1121
+ CTMB, 3.0 mg/ml	2575	1208

Density gradient centrifugation in a linear 5 to 30% sucrose gradient resolves protein into two peaks and enzyme into one broad peak (Fig. 1). An increase in specific activity can be obtained, but the procedure is not applicable to bulk studies.

Recovery of enzyme in a typical preparation, carried through the preparative procedure including solubilization, pH fractionation, and ammonium sulfate fractionation, is about 0.1% of the protein and roughly 40% of the enzyme activity in the starting homogenate, and afforded a 3,000-fold increase in specific activity over the homogenate.

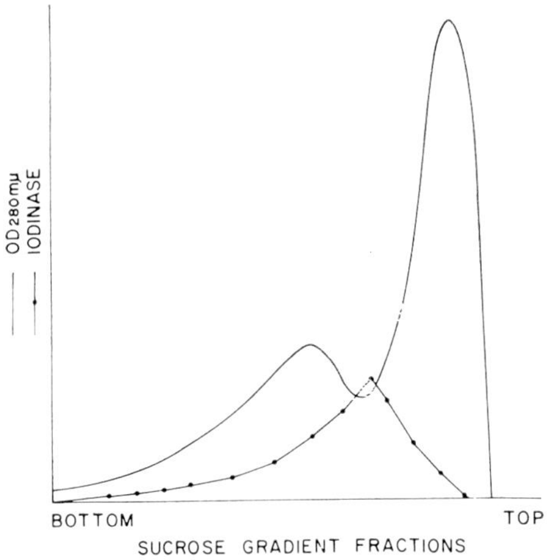

Fig. 1. Distribution of protein and iodinating activity after centrifugation of soluble enzyme in a 5–30% continuous sucrose gradient.

Enzyme Absorbency Spectrum

The starting mitochondrial-microsomal preparation has its major absorbency at 408 mμ in the oxidized state, shifting to 423 mμ in the reduced state, and smaller peaks are visible at 428, 446, 527, 560 and 605 mμ. Addition of KCN to the particulate preparation produces a broad peak at 427 mμ, and a carbon monoxide complex can be formed with a peak at 421 mμ. In preparations of the soluble enzyme, only the Soret band at 408 mμ is present. The Soret band moves to 423 mμ with reduction, and a very prominent band is present at 429 mμ in the difference spectrum (Fig. 2).

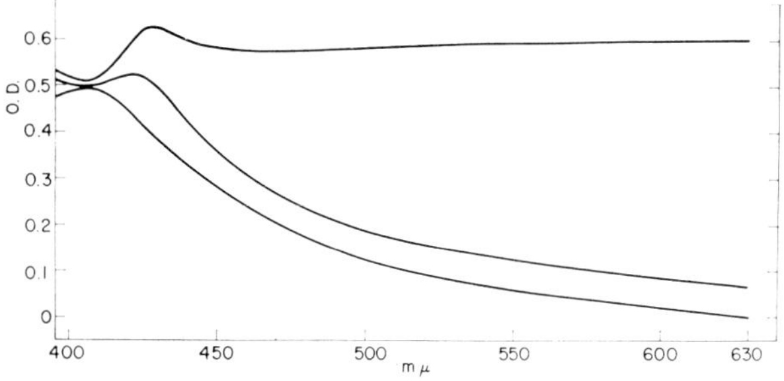

Fig. 2. Absorption spectrum of soluble enzyme.

Top: Reduced-oxidized difference spectrum.
Middle: Direct recording, dithionite reduced.
Bottom: Direct recording, air oxidized.

Compounds known to inhibit the iodinating enzyme were studied for their effect on the 408 mμ absorbency peak. Dicoumarol, sodium sulfite, cysteine, mercaptoethanol, sodium nitrite, penicillamine, dihydroxyfumarate, and dithionite all inhibit iodination when present at 10^{-3} molar, and at this concentration each causes a shift of the enzyme Soret absorbency band to 430 mμ. Parachloromercurobenzoate obliterates the 408 peak. These observations suggest that the reducing agents irreversibly inactivate the enzyme by altering the heme prosthetic group or its binding to apoenzyme. The enzyme was also inactivated by H_2O_2.

Absorbency in the 408 mμ region is lost. Dithionite does not return the H_2O_2 oxidized form back to the original spectral configuration.

Although much data suggests that the enzyme is a heme protein, up to this time we are unable to be certain of this relationship. During purification of the iodinating enzyme by solubilization, Sephadex and hydroxyl-apatite column chromatography, and ammonium sulfate fractionation, heme chromagen follows the enzyme, but there is no progressive augmentation in the ratio of optical density at 409 mμ to that at 280 mμ. Sephadex G-200 eluates with high enzyme activity have 409/280 ratios of as low as 0.05. Enzyme purified further by hydroxylapatite column chromatography has a 409/280 ratio of 0.2 to 0.3. Further, there is no direct correlation between the absorbency at 408 mμ and the peroxidase activity. Thus it is uncertain whether the 408 mμ band, which is due to a protoporphyrin IX group in the preparation, represents enzyme activity. Alternative possibilities are that it is a contaminant, that it represents a mixture of inactive and active heme proteins, or that the calf thyroid iodide peroxidase has spectral properties entirely different from those associated with other peroxidases.

Iodide Peroxidation

During incubation of the iodinating enzyme with iodide and H_2O_2, there is an increase in absorbency at 355 mμ due to generation of triiodide. After the reaction has plateaued, addition of tyrosine causes a prompt reduction in optical density, associated with formation of iodotyrosine. Iodotyrosine formation can be quantitated by addition of tracer quantities of radioactive I^{131} to the incubation medium. There is a mole for mole correlation between the optical density loss and the conversion of labeled iodide to iodotyrosine. Iodination is not accelerated by addition of fresh enzyme. These observations suggest that the iodide peroxidase leads to formation of I_2, and I^-_3 in equilibrium, and that iodination of tyrosine is not enzymatic and can be mediated, by I_2.

Stabilization of Enzyme

When soluble iodinating enzyme, prepared in 0.005 M phosphate buffer at pH 7, and with 10^{-5} molar KI, is stored at 37°F or 2°C, there is gradual loss of enzyme activity (Table II). Addition of phosphate buffer of 0.1 to 0.2 M causes some recovery of enzyme activity.

TABLE II

Stabilization of enzyme by phosphate

Enzyme incubated in listed concentrations of pH 7 phosphate buffer for one week at 4°C prior to assay.

Phosphate buffer concentration	% Iodotyrosine formation*
Basal (.005 M)	300
.009 M	378
.041 M	1,066
.081 M	1,132
.161 M	1,294

* Reported as % MIT formed per ml enzyme.

Storage in higher-strength phosphate buffer or several other solutes protects against inactivation, indicating that the effect is one of solute strength, and not a specific ion. Cysteine, glutathione, dithionite, penicillamine, dihydroxyfumarate, EDTA, manganese sulfate, albumin and glycerol do not protect the enzyme. Loss of enzyme activity is not due to loss of a prosthetic group, since added $FeCl_2$, hematin, FAD or $MnCl_2$ do not augment enzyme activity.

Polymeric Structure

During chromatography of the soluble iodinating enzyme in 0.1 molar sodium phosphate buffer through Sephadex G-200, enzyme is resolved into a small peak appearing at the void volume and a single major activity band. Recovery was from 70 to 85%. When chromatographed in 0.005 molar buffer, enzyme was resolved into a peak appearing at the void volume, a second peak conforming to the position of peak 2 in the 0.1 molar phosphate columns, and a third peak of smaller molecular size. When 0.01% Triton X-100 is added to the enzyme, a large portion of enzyme activity is displaced from peak 2 into peak 3. We have estimated the molecular weight of peak 2 to be approximately 90,000 and peak 3 to be 17,000 by co-chromatography with blue dextran, lactic dehydrogenase, ovalbumin and cytochrome-C. This indicates that the peroxidase exists as a tetramer (peak 2) and a monomer (peak 3). Peaks 1, 2 and 3 were recovered and concentrated by membrane filtration. Peaks 2 and 3 had increased enzyme activity with less hemachromogen absorbency (Table III), and had multiple

TABLE III

Absorption spectrum and activity of Sephadex column fractions

	O.D. 430–410	Protein mg/ml	Specific activity*
Original enzyme	.072	13.8	1,637
Column – Peak 1	.030	2.7	333
Peak 2	.041	3.5	3,028
Peak 3	.018	1.6	2,000

* = % MIT formed per mg protein.

bands on polyacrylamide gel electrophoresis. Activity of both peaks is stimulated by phosphate ion. Peak 3 was active when assayed under the conditions used for its preparation, indicating that both the monomer and tetramer probably have iodinating activity. We conclude that the iodinating enzyme exists as a tetramer and may dissociate readily into a monomer, suggesting that the units are not covalently bound. The monomer appears to have enzymatic activity. The monomer appears to be more labile to injury, probably by oxidation. Formation of the monomer is augmented by enzyme dilution, low ionic strength buffers, and the presence of detergents. Both tetramer and monomer preparations contain heme groups.

MECHANISM OF IODIDE OXIDATION AND BINDING

The intimate details of the peroxidation of iodide by the thyroidal enzyme are not well worked out. Nunez and Pommier (1969) have studied the peroxidation of iodide by horse radish peroxidase, and find that iodide binds to the enzyme in the presence of H_2O_2. The HRP-I complex then reacts with protein or tyrosine to form iodinated protein or iodotyrosine. HRP also reacts with thyroglobulin in the presence of H_2O_2 to form a bimolecular complex, and thyroglobulin competes with tyrosine for iodination. The interpretation of this data by

Nunez *et al.* is that the enzyme has two acceptor sites at which free radicals reformed involving iodide ion and tyrosyl group in a protein. After formation of these free radicals, a condensation occurs, liberating iodotyrosine. Similar studies using the thyroid enzyme have not been reported.

It has been suggested that iodination of tyrosine may involve a sulfenyl iodide group (Maloof and Soodak, 1963; Jirousek and Cunningham, 1968; Fawcett, 1968). Oxidation of cysteinyl residues in proteins by I_2 leads to the formation of cysteine residues or more highly oxidized radicals such as the cysteine sulfenic acid, cysteine sulfinic acid, or cysteine sulfonic acid. With low temperature, low I_2 concentrations, and at an appropriately low pH, fairly stable sulfenyl iodide residues can be formed in proteins (Trundle and Cunningham, 1969). These have been demonstrated clearly in albumin and lactoglobulin, and less certainly in thyroid proteins. Maloof and Soodak (1963) from studies involving the oxidation of thiocyanate and thiouracil by thyroid iodinating enzymes, came to the conclusion that these agents cleaved a disulfide bond to form a mixed disulfide addition product. He believes that, similarly, iodide could cleave a disulfide bond in the iodinating enzyme, leading to the formation of a reactive sulfenyl iodide group. Jirousek and Cunningham (1968) have found that I^-_3 stimulates thiouracil binding to thyroid microsomal protein and that this is inhibited less by thiols than by thioureylenes, a characteristic of sulfenyl iodide groups. Fawcett (1966; 1968) dialyzed thyroid cell particles against chlorine and found they then bound iodide and formed PBI^{131}. He suggested this involved intermediate formation of a sulfenyl chloride group which could be exchanged to a sulfenyl iodide group, and that this led to iodination. In this construction the sequence of the reaction involves splitting of a disulfide iodide group by iodide to form a sulfenyl iodide group which is the iodinating species. Peroxidase is necessary to reform a disulfide bond from two sulfhydryl groups. While this interesting possibility has not been disproven, it is apparent that as of this time there is no direct proof of this mechanism in iodination in the thyroid.

Tyrosine iodination can occur without the necessity of a specific tyrosine iodinase, following peroxidation of iodide. In fact there is no firm evidence for the presence of a tyrosine iodinase in the thyroid. The relative inspecificity of iodination for thyroglobulin may be occasioned more by the presence of high concentrations of non-iodinated thyroglobulin as acceptor protein, rather than by the presence of a specific enzyme mediating iodination or carrying the reactive iodine to thyroglobulin.

IODOTYROSINE COUPLING

Iodine can mediate formation of iodothyronines in proteins such as casein and thyroglobulin. It was long presumed that the coupling process, joining two iodotyrosyl residues together to form an iodothyronine residue, involved a molecular rearrangement within the thyroglobulin molecule, and possibly free radical formation. The coupling of free iodotyrosines and intrathyroglobulin iodotyrosyl groups can be mediated by the thyroid iodide peroxidase, as shown by Hosoya (1968), and Coval and Taurog (1967). An alternative coupling pathway has recently been documented through the work of Cahnmann *et al.* (Cahnmann and Funakoshi, 1969; Nishinaga *et al.*, 1968) and Blasi (Blasi, 1966; Blasi *et al.*, 1969). Cahnmann observed, using diiodotyrosine and diiodohydroxyphenylpyruvic acid *(in vitro)* that peroxidase and H_2O_2 would mediate formation of a DIHPPA-hydroperoxide. The hydroperoxide could then couple with thyroglobulin or DIT, probably by a mechanism involving a free radical, to form thyroxine. Blasi *et al.* demonstrated that such a process could occur in the thyroid. A transaminase present in the postmitochondrial supernatant can, in the presence of alpha-ketoglutarate and pyridoxal phosphate, mediate transamination of DIT with formation of DIHPPA. A second enzyme, a tautomerase, is present in the soluble fraction, and mediates exchange between the keto form of DIHPPA and the enol form of this same amino acid, and strongly favors the enol form. Through the mechanism previously indicated by Cahnmann, the DIHPPA-enol could lead to formation of thyroxine. Since DIHPPA is reputedly present in the thyroid, and the enzymes mediating all of these reactions occur in the gland, synthesis of thyroxine involving intrathyroglobulin iodotyrosine groups combining with free DIT derivatives seems possible. To date, however, no firm proof of this pathway has been established. Perhaps the most acceptable proof would be evidence that the carbon skeleton of free DIT can be joined during *in vitro* incubation of thyroid slices into thyroxine.

H_2O_2 SOURCE IN THE THYROID

The source of H_2O_2 within the thyroid, which is necessary for peroxidation of iodide and perhaps formation of the DIHPPA-hydroperoxide, is unknown, but some possibilities have been reported. Fischer *et al.* (1966; 1968*a*; *b*) found a monamine oxidase in the thyroid present in mitochondrial and microsomal fractions, which can support iodination in the presence of its preferred substrate, tyramine. The enzyme requires copper and free sulfhydryl groups. Tyrosine decarboxylase is present in the thyroid and could provide the necessary tyramine.

H_2O_2 Generation by NADPH cytochrome-C reductase

Because soluble enzyme preparations have always been found to contain NADPH cytochrome-C reductase, and because this enzyme has been considered a source of H_2O_2 in cells, we studied the role of NADPH cytochrome-C reductase activity in iodination by mitochondrial microsomal fractions. Heat inactivation (Fig. 3) causes a parallel loss of NADPH

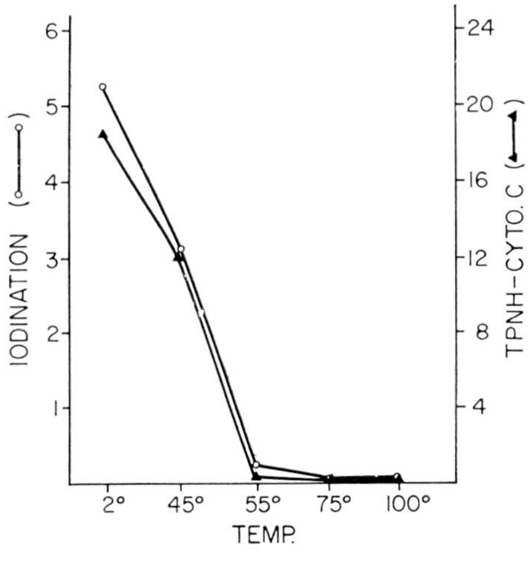

Fig. 3. Correlation of NADPH-suggested iodination and TPNH-cytochrome-C reductase activity in a thyroid mitochondrial-microsomal fraction. After heating for 5 minutes at 45–100°C.

cytochrome-C reductase activity and the ability of NADPH to stimulate iodination. Addition of PCMB also caused a parallel loss in these two enzyme activities. This indicates that the reductase might be active in endogenous iodination reactions supported by NADPH.

We purified NADPH cytochrome-C reductase from thyroid and reconstructed an iodinating system with this enzyme. Reductase was purified by lipase digestion of thyroid microsomes, ammonium sulfate fractionation, and hydroxylapatite chromatography. Twenty to forty-fold purification was achieved with recovery of 20% of original reductase activity. The reductase is specific for NADPH, but will transfer electrons to Vitamin K_3 or cytochrome-C.

In previous studies we have demonstrated that the soluble enzyme is dependent upon production of H_2O_2 by glucose and glucose oxidase for iodination of tyrosine. Addition of NADPH to the system containing glucose and glucose oxidase inhibits iodination, probably because NADPH is competitive with iodide for peroxidation. In the absence of glucose and glucose oxidase, NADPH cannot stimulate enzymatic iodination of tyrosine. However, addition of NADPH, NADPH cytochrome-C reductase, and Vitamin K_3 cause a marked stimulation of iodination activity, and the effect is dependent upon each of the factors named (Table IV). Cytochrome-C can replace Vitamin K_3. The stimulation of iodination by Vitamin

TABLE IV

Stimulation of ^{131}I incorporation by TPNH-cytochrome-C reductase

	% ^{131}I – Incorporation
Complete system*	27
– Vitamin K	4
– TPNH	1
– TPNH-Cytochrome-C Reductase	0.5
– Soluble Enzyme	0.3

* The complete iodinating system included 25 μg soluble enzyme, 0.1 μ-mole TPNH, 0.01 μ-mole Vitamin K, 0.011 μ-mole KI, 1 μ-mole tyrosine, 1 μC Na^{131}I and 0.7 ml K-R-P buffer, in 1 ml. Incubation was for 20 minutes at 37°C.

K_3 and cytochrome-C is catalase sensitive. The mechanism of action of Vitamin K_3 is presumably as a terminal electron acceptor which can be auto-oxidized to form H_2O_2. The role of cytochrome-C is less easily explained. It is possible that the preparation is partially auto-oxidizable. $FeCl_3$ does not replace cytochrome-C, but hematin can.

These studies indicate that NADPH-cytochrome-C reductase, a microsomal enzyme, may be involved in endogenous generation of H_2O_2, which is used by the peroxidase for the formation of iodotyrosine. This system may involve, in addition to the reductase and NADPH, a terminal electron acceptor such as Vitamin K_3 or another unkown factor (Fig. 4).

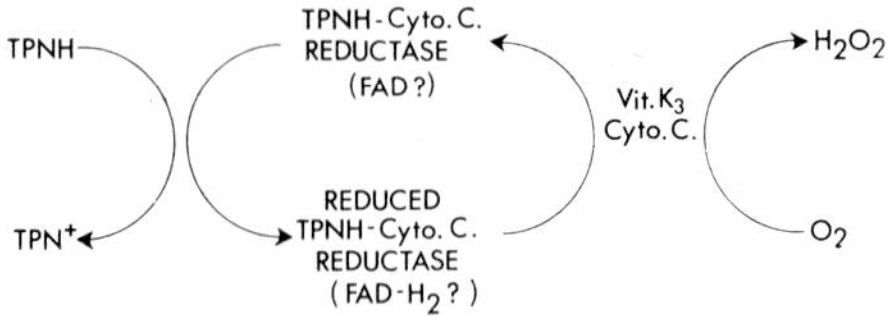

Fig. 4. Scheme indicating possible role of TPNH cytochrome-C reductase in H_2O_2 generation.

It is known that iodination reactions in the thyroid are stimulated by provision of NADPH and by augmentation of the hexose monophosphate shunt. This augmented iodinating activity may be related to increased provision of NADPH for the reductase. In addition TSH causes augmentation of the level of NADPH cytochrome-C reductase in the thyroid. Thus we may assume that control of iodination activity involves (1) the level of peroxidase, (2) reductase activity, and (3) reduced pyridine nucleotide supply.

CONTROL OF H_2O_2 SUPPLY

Formate, in the presence of H_2O_2 and a peroxidase, is oxidized with liberation of CO_2. This reaction has been used to study H_2O_2 production in thyroid slices and homogenates by Ahn and Rosenberg (1970) and by Benard and Brault (1970). Formate oxidation was found to be augmented by TSH, prostaglandin E_1, dibutyryl cyclic-AMP, and of course, by glucose and glucose oxidase. It is suggested that the mechanism involves stimulation by TSH or PGE_1 of adenyl cyclase, and production of increased intracellular concentrations of cyclic-AMP, which by some mechanism augments H_2O_2. After prolonged TSH stimulation, the iodide peroxidase in the thyroid is augmented (DeGroot and Dunn, 1964). However, acute stimulation by TSH does not augment the levels of iodide peroxidase, but does lead to elevated binding of iodide. This is probably an acute response mediated by augmented intracellular H_2O_2 production. It is tempting to speculate that H_2O_2 production may be somehow related to the process of TSH stimulated endocytosis, in analogy to the response known to occur following endocytosis by polymorphonuclear leukocytes. TSH-mediated increase in intracellular H_2O_2 may also be responsible for the accelerated oxidation of glucose via the hexose monophosphate shunt, since Benard and DeGroot (1969) found that catalase inhibited this response to TSH.

SUMMARY

Some details can be added to the reaction sequence stated in the introduction. Thus iodide peroxidation is probably mediated by a heme protein present in the cell particles. The enzyme is labile in low-ionic-strength buffer, and exists as a tetramer dissociable to a monomer. This enzyme is also involved in tyrosine iodination and in the coupling of iodotyrosine groups to form thyroxine as well. It has been suggested, though not proven, that thyroxine biosynthesis may proceed in a mechanism in which intrathyroglobulin iodotyrosine groups couple with free DIT after oxidation to a DIHPPA hydroperoxide. H_2O_2 supply for the reaction may be generated from NADPH via the microsomal enzyme NADPH cytochrome-C reductase. Minute to minute changes in the rate of iodide binding are probably mediated by changes in the production of H_2O_2, dependent in some way upon the action of TSH on membrane-bound adenyl cyclase. The marked increase in iodide peroxidase found in thyroid glands after prolonged TSH stimulation probably represents new protein synthesis.

REFERENCES

AHN, C. S. and ROSENBERG, I. N. (1970): Oxidation of ^{14}C-formate in thyroid slices: Effects of TSH, dibutyryl cyclic 3′, 5′-AMP (dbc-AMP) and prostaglandin E_1 (PGE_1). In: *Proceedings of the Sixth International Thyroid Conference*, p. 109.

BENARD, B. and BRAULT, J. (1970): Hydrogen peroxide production in thyrotropin-stimulated thyroid. In: *Proceedings of the Sixth International Thyroid Conference*, p. 101.

BENARD, B. and DEGROOT, L. J. (1969): The role of hydrogen peroxide and glutathione in glucose oxidation by the thyroid. *Biochim. biophys. Acta (Amst.)*, *184*, 48.

BLASI, F. (1966): The role of free radicals of 4-hydroxy-3,5-diiodophenylpyruvic acid in the synthesis of thyroxine. *Biochim. biophys. Acta (Amst.)*, *121*, 204.

BLASI, F., FRAGOMELE, F. and COVELLI, I. (1969): Enzymic pathway for thyroxine synthesis through p-hydroxy-3,5-diiodophenylpyruvic acid. *Endocrinology*, *85*, 542.

CAHNMANN, H. J. and FUNAKOSHI, K. (1969): Model reactions for the biosynthesis of thyroxine. Nonenzymic formation of 3,5,3′-triiodothyronine from 4-hydroxy-3-iodophenylpyruvic acid, 3,5-diiodotyrosine, and oxygen. *Biochemistry*, *9*, 90.

COVAL, M. L. and TAUROG, A. (1967): Purification and iodinating activity of hog thyroid peroxidase. *J. biol. Chem.*, *242*, 5510.

DEGROOT, L. J. (1965): Current views on formation of thyroid hormones. *New Engl. J. Med.*, *272*, 243.

DEGROOT, L. J. and DAVIS, A. M. (1962): Studies on the biosynthesis of iodotyrosines: a soluble thyroidal iodide-peroxidase tyrosine-iodinase system. *Endocrinology*, *70*, 492.

DeGroot, L. J. and Dunn, A. D. (1964): Electron-transport enzymes of calf thyroid. *Biochim. biophys. Acta (Amst.)*, *92*, 205.
DeGroot, L. J., Thompson, J. E. and Dunn, A. D. (1965): Studies on an iodinating enzyme from calf thyroid. *Endocrinology*, *76*, 632.
Fawcett, D. M. (1966): The binding of ^{131}iodide by cell-free thyroid homogenates measured by equilibrium dialysis. *Canad. J. Biochem.*, *44*, 1669.
Fawcett, D. M. (1968): The formation of sulfenyl iodides as intermediates during the *in vitro* iodination of tyrosine by calf thyroid homogenates. *Canad. J. Biochem.*, *46*, 1433.
Fischer, A. G., Schulz, A. R. and Oliner, L. (1966): The possible role of thyroid monoamine oxidase in iodothyronine synthesis. *Life Sci.*, *5*, 995.
Fischer, A. G., Schulz, A. R. and Oliner, L. (1968*a*): Distribution of monoamine oxidase in the thyroid gland. *Endocrinology*, *82*, 1098.
Fischer, A. G., Schulz, A. R. and Oliner, L. (1968*b*): Thyroidal biosynthesis of iodothyronines II. General characteristics and purification of mitochondrial monoamine oxidase. *Biochim. biophys. Acta (Amst.)*, *159*, 460.
Hosoya, T. (1968): The role of thyroid peroxidase in the synthesis of thyroxine residues in thyroglobulin. *Gunma Symp. Endocr.*, *5*, 219.
Hosoya, T. and Morrison, M. (1967): The isolation and purification of thyroid peroxidase. *J. biol. Chem.*, *242*, 2828.
Jirousek, L. and Cunningham, L. W. (1968): The reaction of thiouracil with β-lactoglobulin sulfenyl iodide. *Biochim. biophys. Acta (Amst.)*, *170*, 160.
Ljunggren, J. and Akeson, A. (1968): Solubilization, isolation and identification of a peroxidase from the microsomal fraction of beef thyroid. *Arch. Biochem.*, *127*, 346.
Mahoney, C. P. and Igo, R. P. (1966): Studies of the biosynthesis of thyroxine. II. Solubilization and characterization of an iodide peroxidase from thyroid tissue. *Biochim. biophys. Acta (Amst.)*, *113*, 507.
Maloof, F. and Soodak, M. (1963): Intermediary metabolism of thyroid tissue and the action of drugs. *Pharmacol. Rev.*, *15*, 43.
Nishinaga, A., Cahnmann, H. J., Kon, H. and Matsuura, T. (1968): Model reactions for the biosynthesis of thyroxine. XII. The nature of a thyroxine precursor formed in the synthesis of thyroxine from diiodotyrosine and its keto acid analog. *Biochemistry*, *7*, 388.
Nunez, J. and Pommier, J. (1969): Iodation des protéines par voie enzymatique. 3. Complexe intermédiaire enzyme-protéine et mécanisme de la réaction. *Europ. J. Biochem.*, *7*, 286.
Strum, J. M. and Karnovsky, M. J. (1970): Cytochemical localization of endogenous peroxidase in thyroid follicular cells. *J. Cell Biol.*, *44*, 665.
Taurog, A., Lothrop, M. L. and Estabrook, R. W. (1970): Improvements in the isolation procedure for thyroid peroxidase: nature of the heme prosthetic group. *Arch. Biochem. Biophys.*, *139/1*, 221.
Trundle, D. and Cunningham, L. W. (1969): Iodine oxidation of the sulfhydryl groups of creatine kinase. *Biochemistry*, *8*, 1919.
Yip, C. C. (1965): Column chromatographic separation of a peroxidase and an iodinase in solubilized beef thyroid preparations. *Biochim. biophys. Acta (Amst.)*, *96*, 75.

SIMULTANEOUS COMPARATIVE STUDIES OF THYROXINE (T4) AND TRIIODOTHYRONINE (T3) PRODUCTION RATES IN HEALTH AND DISEASE*

JOSEPH McCONNON, VAS V. ROW and ROBERT VOLPÉ

Department of Medicine, University of Toronto, and The Endocrinology Research Laboratory, The Wellesley Hospital, Toronto, Ontario, Canada

The kinetics of L-thyroxine (T4) in both health and disease in man have been carefully studied in the past 15 years. However, until recently, only scant data had accrued for triiodothyronine (T3) dynamics (Woeber *et al.*, 1970) and even those which have recently appeared have been subject to a variety of criticisms. The first of these problems has to do with the measurement of the total concentration of T3 in serum samples. Methods such as those of Nauman *et al.* (1967) (which we use) and of Sterling *et al.* (1969), both of which employ the steps of extraction, chromatography, and finally a protein displacement step using thyroxine binding globulin (TBG) as the protein, have been criticized by Hollander (personal communication) and by Fisher (personal communication) on the grounds that there is a systematic contribution of T4 by monodeiodination to T3 *in vitro* during the course of the analysis, so that some of the measured T3 actually derives from T4 within the plasma. As will be shown below, however, we were unable to show that this occurs during the T3 procedure, so that we do not accept this criticism as being a significant one. It should be further mentioned, however, that it is possible to raise anti-sera against T3 (Elkins *et al.*, 1970), so that an immunoassay for T3 may soon be practicable.

The second problem has been in the interpretation of disappearance curves for T3, particularly when a single bolus of T3 is injected, and a simple slope-intercept technique is employed. However, values of T3 disappearance obtained from such a single compartment model have been shown to be reasonably accurate (Woeber *et al.*, 1970) and correspond closely with values obtained by continuous infusion techniques (Woeber *et al.*, 1970; Nauman *et al.*, 1967). Another problem in the interpretation of T3 disappearance slopes has been the formation of iodoproteins derived from the injected labelled T3, as has been shown by Surks and Oppenheimer (1969). However, we rather belatedly recognized the importance of this contribution by iodoproteins to T3 disappearance slopes; consequently the slope values that are reported below will be those of serum samples precipitated by trichloracetic acid (TCA) to remove the iodide, but we unfortunately did not precipitate with butanol to additionally remove the iodoprotein, at least until only recently.

Despite these problems, and the few studies of T3 dynamics now available, it is evident that the production of T3 seems surprisingly great relative to that of T4, *i.e.*, in normal persons the T3 production rate is about half that for T4. This does not take into account *in vivo* conversion of T4 to T3 peripherally, which contributes a portion of the daily production of T3, although the degree of this remains unsettled (Braverman *et al.*, 1967; Pittman *et al.*, 1970). While studies of T3 production rates in hyperthyroidism and normal persons

* Supported by a grant from the Medical Research Council of Canada (MT 859).

have been published, these have not included observations of T4 productions in the same patients. It was thus felt that a systematic comparison of simultaneous T4 and T3 production rates in the same subjects was warranted, using a double isotope technique as previously suggested by Mirouze *et al.* (1967).

METHODS AND MATERIALS

The studies were carried out in several groups of subjects. The normal control group comprised 12 healthy volunteers drawn from hospital personnel. The hyperthyroid group was subdivided into two subgroups: (a) 5 patients with high serum T4 values (4 patients with Graves' disease, 1 with toxic adenoma), and (b) 3 patients with 'T3-toxicosis' who will be described separately later. The hypothyroid group likewise was divided into two subgroups: (a) 5 patients with primary thyroid deficiency, and (b) 3 patients with pituitary (secondary) hypothyroidism. In addition, 2 further patients with euthyroid goitrous Hashimoto's thyroiditis were similarly studied.

Each patient studied was given an intravenous dose of approximately 100 μC of ^{131}I-labelled T3, followed immediately by a similar dose of ^{125}I-labelled T4. Lugol's iodine was administered so as to prevent recycling of inorganic iodide. Blood samples were taken on the first, second, third, fourth and seventh days after the initial injection. Serum from these samples was precipitated with trichloracetic acid and the ^{131}I and ^{125}I counts were measured. The values for the daily counts after the initial injection were plotted on semilogarithmic graph paper as percentages of the injected dose.

From this single injection intercept technique using a one-compartment model, the volumes of distribution, half-times, fractional turnover rates and production rates were calculated using standard techniques (Woeber *et al.*, 1970). The production rate of either hormone was considered to be identical with the absolute disposal rate of the hormone, considering each patient to be in the steady state.

While the studies of T4 disappearance after distribution equilibrium has been attained have clearly shown it to be a single exponential, there have been difficulties in the assessment of T3 disappearance studies. These difficulties, as were mentioned earlier, include (a) the formation of labelled iodoproteins (Surks and Oppenheimer, 1969) from the degradation of T3, and (b) the question of whether distribution equilibrium has been attained during that period when accurate measurements of residual labelled T3 in the serum are still possible. In statistical analyses similar to those described by Woeber *et al.* (1970), we have found good concordance between 24–72 and 24–96 hour T3 slopes in at least the euthyroid and hypothyroid groups. Since Nicoloff and Dowling (1968) have shown that distribution equilibrium for T3 is reached before 24 hours, and since the contribution of labelled iodoprotein reached only 11% at 96 hours in our own studies, it was felt that the error introduced to an analysis of the data as a single-compartment model may be considered minimal. In the hyperthyroid group, however, the fourth day value was significantly above the regression line drawn through days 1–3, presumably due to the increased iodoprotein production, and thus the fourth day value was disregarded. It is recognized that the slope of days 1–3 in hyperthyroidism cannot be compared precisely to days 1–4 in the euthyroid and hypothyroid groups, but would nevertheless yield useful approximations.

Measurements of total T4 were performed by the method of Murphy (1965), with a normal range of 4 to 11 μg/100 ml. The total serum T3 was measured by modifications of the method of Nauman *et al.* (1967), with our current normal range of 0.15 to 0.27 μg/100 ml. In preliminary studies adding increasing amounts of stable T4 to aliquots of pooled normal serum failed to cause any increase in the total T3 value. In addition, when labelled T4 was added to serum samples, which were extracted and then chromatographed, no radioactivity appeared in the T3 spot. Thus there does not appear to be any significant *in vitro* conversion of T4 to T3 during the T3 analysis.

COMPARISON OF NORMAL GROUP, HYPERTHYROID GROUP, AND PRIMARY HYPOTHYROID GROUP

In Table I the values for both T4 and T3 are depicted for volumes of distribution in litres per kilogram, the fractional turnover rates, the serum hormone levels, and production rates in the three main groups, *i.e.*, the hyperthyroid group, the normal group and the primary hypothyroid group.

Volumes of distribution (Table I)

In all three groups, the volume of distribution in lit/kg for T3 is much greater than that for T4. In hyperthyroidism, the volume of distribution for T3 reaches very high levels averaging 1.21 lit/kg, obviously very significantly different from normal. The reason for this marked increase in T3 volume of distribution in hyperthyroidism is unclear, relating obviously to a difference in T3 concentration throughout its real volume of distribution. It has been suggested by Woeber *et al.* (1970) that this may be due to the saturation of TBG binding sites for T3. Conversely in hypothyroidism, the T3 volume of distribution is reduced significantly (0.506 lit/kg).

While there are the same trends in T4 volumes of distribution, these are not statistically significantly different between hyperthyroidism and euthyroidism, or between hypothyroidism and euthyroidism.

Fractional disappearance rates (Table I)

For both T4 and T3, the fractional disappearance rates increased in hyperthyroidism and decreased in hypothyroidism. For T3, however, these differences were not significant between the hyperthyroid and euthyroid group. For T4, conversely, the T4 turnover rate was significantly more rapid in hyperthyroidism as compared to normals, but the slowing of the T4 turnover rate in hypothyroidism was not significant.

TABLE I

*T4 and T3 kinetic studies (mean values) in normal group, hyperthyroid group and primary hypothyroid group**

oup		Serum hormone concentration µg/100 ml	Volume of distribution lit/kg	Fractional rate of disappearance %/day	Production rates µg/day	T4/T3 ratios serum concentration	T4/T3 ratios production rates
rmal = 12	T4	8.46 ±0.48	0.15 ±0.0113	10.5 ±0.526	95.42 ±5.53	42.30 ±4.77	2.25 ±0.46
	T3	0.20 ±0.046	0.69 ±0.042	45.66 ±7.27	42.44 ±4.30		
per-roid = 5	T4	21.50 ±2.48	0.285 ±0.023	18.4 ±3.98	523.46 ±102	39.76 ±2.86	3.05 ±0.45
	T3	0.534 ±0.0293	1.21 ±0.20	49.39 ±10.2	172.54 ±29.6		
mary xoedema 5	T4	1.2 ±0.671	0.152 ±0.014	10.31 ±0.37	13.98 ±4.19	12.0 ±6.12	0.91 ±0.44
	T3	0.12 ±0.393	0.506 ±0.0289	40.0 ±2.07	17.075 ±8.66		

Mean values ± standard error of the mean (SEM).

Serum T4 and T3 values (Table I)

It is apparent that both T4 and T3 values are markedly and significantly increased in hyperthyroidism, and to the same degree. As expected, the serum T4 value is very significantly reduced in hypothyroidism. The serum T3 value also is reduced in hypothyroidism but, surprisingly, not quite significantly. This then suggests a disproportionate decrease in serum T4 relative to T3 in primary hypothyroidism.

T4 and T3 production rates (Table I)

In hyperthyroidism, both T3 and T4 production rates are markedly increased to a mean of 523 μg/day for T4, and 172 μg/day for T3. In the normal control group, the T4 production rate averaged 95 μg/day, while the mean T3 production rate was 42 μg/day, yielding an approximately 2:1 ratio of T4/T3 for production rates in normal persons. In the primary myxoedema group, however, the mean T4 production rate was 13 μg/day, while the mean T3 production rate was 17 μg/day. That is, the T4 production in these cases of primary myxoedema is actually lower than T3 production, in marked contradistinction to the normal situation.

'T3-TOXICOSIS' VALUES (TABLE II)

The data from 4 patients with the peculiar syndrome of 'T3-toxicosis' in which the patients are clinically hyperthyroid, with normal serum thyroxines, high serum T3 values, and thyroid function which is non-suppressible with exogenous T3 are shown in Table II. Two of these patients had toxic adenoma of the thyroid gland and 2 were suffering from Graves' disease. Of the 2 patients with Graves' disease, 1 was recurrent following a subtotal thyroidectomy, while the other had concomitant Hashimoto's thyroiditis.

The patients showed normal T4 production rates, but increased rates of T3 production

TABLE II

Individual values for 4 patients with 'T3 toxicosis' – T4 and T3 kinetic studies

Patient	Type of disorder	T4 or T3	Serum hormone concentration μg/100 ml	Volume of distribution lit/kg	Fractional rates of disappearance %/day	Production rates μg/day	T4/T3 ratios (a) serum	T4/T3 ratios (b) production rates
		T4	8.0	0.209	14.14	90.56	23.9	1
1. F, age 63	Toxic adenoma							
		T3	0.33	0.996	69.3	87.95		
		T4	10.5	0.181	12.83	112.21		0.79
2. F, age 32	Recurrent Graves'						19	0.79
		T3	0.59	1.553	34.65	146.03		
		T4	12.5	0.136	9.24	92.4		
3. F, age 29	Toxic adenoma						36.9	1.17
		T3	0.34	0.678	57.75	78.54		
		T4	7.5	0.214	11.55	123.87		
4. F, age 34	Concomitant						11.3	0.77
	Graves' and Hashimoto's	T3	0.66	0.833	43.31	158.60		

ranging approximately from 2 to 4 times the normal range. One of these patients was reinvestigated three months after radioablation of her solitary toxic adenoma, at which time she was clinically euthyroid. Her T3 and T4 production rates were then within normal limits.

EUTHYROID GOITROUS HASHIMOTO'S THYROIDITIS (TABLE III)

Table III shows the data on 2 patients with euthyroid goitrous Hashimoto's thyroiditis. In these patients, the serum thyroxine was low, and the thyroxine production rates were likewise low. The serum T3 on the other hand, was within normal limits for these 2 patients, while their T3 production was only minimally reduced below normal. It would thus appear that these patients are producing enough T3 to sustain them in their apparent euthyroid clinical status.

TABLE III

Individual values for 2 patients with euthyroid Hashimoto's disease

Patient	T4 or T3	Serum hormone concentration μg/100 ml	Volume of distribution lit/kg	Fractional disappearance rate %/day	Production rate μg/day	T4/T3 ratios	
						serum concentration	production rates
1. F, age 80	T4	2.5	0.175	9.63	20.25	10	0.80
	T3	0.25	0.457	46.20	25.11		
2. F, age 52	T4	5.0	0.221	6.60	36.63	21.74	1.09
	T3	0.23	0.569	51.33	33.76		

VALUES FROM SECONDARY HYPOTHYROIDISM (TABLE IV)

Table IV shows data from 3 patients with secondary hypothyroidism due to hypopituitarism. In these patients, the T4 production rates were only minimally below the normal range. Contrary to the findings in primary myxoedema, however, the serum T3 and T3 production rates were reduced below normal, reversing the situation as seen in primary myxoedema.

TABLE IV

Individual values for 3 patients with secondary hypothyroidism due to hypopituitarism

Patient	T4 or T3	Serum hormone concentration μg/100 ml	Volume of distribution lit/kg	Fractional disappearance rate %/day	Production rate μg/day	T4/T3 ratios	
						serum concentration	production rates
1. M, age 26	T4	5.50	0.16	7.70	47.51	250	10.89
	T3	0.022	0.57	49.50	4.36		
2. F, age 48	T4	6.0	0.135	9.49	51.76	46.15	2.18
	T3	0.13	0.75	36.47	23.73		
3. M, age 34	T4	4.50	0.15	7.7	57.72	45.60	2.67
	T3	0.098	0.48	42.0	21.66		

T4/T3 RATIOS (FOR SERUM CONCENTRATIONS AND PRODUCTION RATES)

The normal T4/T3 ratio was 42:1 in the serum concentrations and approximately 2:1 in production rates (Table I). The T4/T3 ratios in hyperthyroidism were not significantly different from normal for either serum concentrations or production rates, indicating a proportionate increase in the secretion of these two hormones in hyperthyroidism. In primary myxoedema, however, there was a significant fall in T4/T3 ratios both in the serum and in production rates. This indicates that although both are lowered, T4 is more markedly reduced than T3. The same trend was detected in the 2 patients with euthyroid Hashimoto's disease, in which the T3 production rates were in the low normal range, and where T4 production was definitely reduced (Table III).

DISCUSSION

Thus it would appear that in primary thyroid disease there is an initial reduction in T4 production, while T3 may remain adequate to maintain a clinically euthyroid state. This circumstance may prevail until thyroid destruction is profound. These changes may result from increased endogenous TSH levels, as previously suggested (Volpé *et al.*, 1965).

On the other hand, in secondary hypothyroidism due to hypopituitarism, T3 is more markedly reduced than T4, just opposite to the state of affairs in primary myxoedema (Table IV).

CONCLUSION

In primary thyroid destruction, the synthesis of thyroxine fails first, followed only later by a failure of T3 production. The relatively increased T3 compared to T4 in primary thyroid damage probably results from an increased endogenous TSH.

REFERENCES

BRAVERMAN, L. E., INGBAR, S. H. and STERLING, K. (1969): *In vivo* conversion of thyroxine (T4) to triiodothyronine (T3) in man. In: *Abstracts, 51st meeting of the Endocrine Society*, p. 68.

CAVALIERI, R. R., STEINBERG, M. and SEARLE, G. L. (1970): Metabolism of T3 in Graves' disease. In: *Abstracts, VI International Thyroid Conference*, p. 48.

EKINS, R. P., BROWN, B. L., ELLIS, S. M. and REITH, W. S. (1970): The radioimmunoassay of serum triiodothyronine. In: *Abstracts, VI International Thyroid Conference*, p. 138.

MIROUZE, J., JAFFIOL, C., PASTORELLO, R. and BALDET, L. (1967): Nouvelle technique d'étude du métabolisme des hormones thyroïdiennes ($T4_{125}$-$T3_{131}$); données expérimentales et cliniques. *Ann. Endocr. (Paris)*, *28*, 445.

MURPHY, B. E. P. (1965): The determination of thyroxine by competitive protein binding analysis employing anion exchange resin and radiothyroxine. *J. Lab. clin. Med.*, *66*, 161.

NAUMAN, J. A., NAUMAN, A. and WERNER, S. C. (1967): Total and free triiodothyronine in human serum. *J. clin. Invest.*, *46*, 1346.

NICOLOFF, J. T. and DOWLING, J. T. (1968): Estimation of thyroxine distribution in man. *J. clin. Invest.*, *47*, 26.

PITTMAN, C. S., CHAMBERS, J. B. and READ, V. H. (1970): The extrathyroidal conversion rate of thyroxine (T4) to triiodothyronine (T3) in man. In: *Abstracts, VI International Thyroid Conference*, p. 36.

STERLING, K., BELLABARBA, D., NEWMAN, E. S. and BRENNER, M. A. (1969): Determination of triiodothyronine concentration in human serum. *J. clin. Invest.*, *48*, 1150.

SURKS, M. I. and OPPENHEIMER, J. H. (1969): Formation of iodoprotein during the peripheral metabolism of 3,5,3′-triiodo-L-thyronine-^{125}I in the euthyroid man and rat. *J. clin. Invest.*, *48*, 685.

VOLPÉ, R., ROW, V. V., WEBSTER, B. R., JOHNSTON, M. W. and EZRIN, C. (1965): Studies of iodine metabolism in Hashimoto's thyroiditis. *J. clin. Endocr.*, *25*, 593.

WOEBER, K. A., SOBEL, R. J., INGBAR, S. H. and STERLING, K. (1970): The peripheral metabolism of triiodothyronine in normal subjects and in patients with hyperthyroidism. *J. clin. Invest.*, *49*, 643.

PHYSIOLOGY OF THE THYROID FEEDBACK LOOP*

JAMES A. PITTMAN, JR. and JEROME M. HERSHMAN

Endocrinology and Metabolism Division and Division of Nuclear Medicine, Department of Medicine, UAB Medical Center, and Birmingham VA Hospital, Birmingham, Ala., U.S.A.

The first suggestion of a reciprocal relation between thyroid and pituitary activity was probably that of B. Niepce, who in 1851 noted the pituitary enlargement seen in some untreated cretins. Rogowitsch in 1889 also noted a reciprocal relation and described histological changes in rabbit pituitaries following thyroidectomy. However, it remained for the classic studies of P. E. Smith (1916; 1922) to demonstrate convincingly the presence of some substance in the pituitary capable of stimulating thyroid function. Other historical aspects of the development of current concepts of regulation of thyroid function have been well reviewed by Reichlin (1966). Some features of the system regulating thyroid function are shown in Figure 1.

This is the classic thyroid feedback loop or 'pituitary-thyroid axis'. It has 4 major units: (1) the hypothalamus (used here to designate only that portion of the hypothalamus which secretes TRF, thyrotropin-releasing factor**, in response to various stimuli); (2) the adeno-

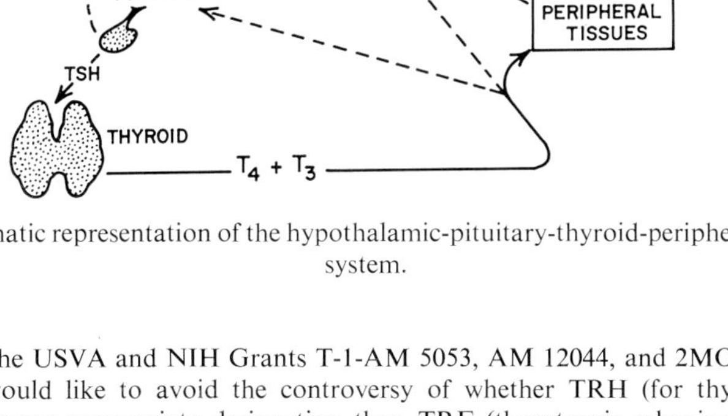

Fig. 1. Diagrammatic representation of the hypothalamic-pituitary-thyroid-peripheral tissue feedback system.

* Supported by the USVA and NIH Grants T-1-AM 5053, AM 12044, and 2MO1 FR32-09.

**The authors would like to avoid the controversy of whether TRH (for thyrotropin-releasing *hormone*) is a more appropriate designation than TRF (thyrotropin-releasing *factor*, the older designation). It has been suggested that TRF should stand for 'thyrotropin-regulating factor', to avoid choosing at this time between a stimulatory effect on release and one on synthesis (Meites, 1970). In this paper we shall use TRF for the simple reason that this term is more easily distinguished from TSH in writing and speaking.

hypophysis, or, more specifically, the thyrotroph cells of the adenohypophysis; (3) the thyroid gland; and (4) the 'periphery', a term used here to designate all tissues other than the above which may feed signals to the TRF-secreting portion of the hypothalamus to modulate the secretion of TRF. Thus, the 'periphery' in this sense might include temperature-sensitive portions of the hypothalamus. Though it seems unlikely, it is possible that the temperature-sensitive areas (Andersson, 1964; Reichlin, 1966) themselves release TRF in response to cooling. This problem might be approached by localization of TRF in the temperature-sensitive regions of the hypothalamus (Andersson, 1963; 1964) using antibody to TRF and some modification of the Coons' 'sandwich technique', now that synthetic TRF is available in relatively large quantities (Baugh *et al.*, 1970). Thus, this loop might be called the 'hypothalamic-pituitary-thyroid-periphery feedback loop'. However, it will be referred to here simply as the 'thyroid feedback loop' or 'the loop'. Its delicate balance is evident in the pretty oscillations which occur when the system is perturbed by administration of T_4 (Yamada *et al.*, 1971) or TSH (Einhorn, 1958).

The purpose of this paper is to point out some aspects of this loop which have been quantified recently or appear to be capable of quantification by methodology now developing. We do not propose to attempt even a primitive mathematical model for the loop, and, in particular, shall not dwell on iodine kinetics, for which several models have recently been proposed. Rather the aim is to achieve a clearer understanding of the physiology involved simply by trying to express some of the features of the loop quantitatively. The paper will thus be largely speculative, but, we hope, usefully so and of more interest than a simple recitation of published data. In addition, we shall comment on two related topics in which we have recently been interested – the action of TRF on the pituitary and placental thyrotropic factors. Unless otherwise stated, the speculations here will apply to man, though liberal use of animal data is necessary, with the usual assumptions in the use of such data.

The first quantification of a portion of this system was the measurement of basal metabolic rates, followed many years later by estimates of the function of the thyroid gland itself through measurements of circulating levels of thyroid hormones and turnover of iodine by the thyroid. Practical measurements of circulating thyrotropin (TSH, thyroid-stimulating hormone) levels awaited purification of pituitary thyrotropin. This was accomplished in 1963 (Condliffe) and radioimmunoassay of TSH sufficiently sensitive to measure levels in unextracted serum was developed several years later (Odell *et al.*, 1965; 1967; Utiger, 1965). Earlier bioassay techniques were not sufficiently sensitive to permit measurement of normal levels on reasonable quantities of blood (Condliffe and Robbins, 1967), and insensitivity of the immunoassay still restricts our perception of minor changes which may occur in normal man (*e.g.*, a possible circadian variation of serum TSH levels).

Table I shows some aspects of the feedback loop which have been quantified with apparently reasonable precision or appear to be susceptible to quantification in the near future. Several other terms are included for completeness, although their quantification seems more remote in the future. The first term is the threshold of the hypothalamus for secretion of TRF. This threshold is presumably related to the level of circulating thyroid hormone which reaches some sensitive center or centers. ('Hypothalamus' here might have to include some center other than that which actually synthesizes and releases TRF, since we are ignorant of whether the synthesis-release center is itself sensitive to thyroid hormone, and, indeed, whether synthesis and release both occur at the same site within the nervous system.) With the data available, one can only assume that the secretion of TRF may occur at the same serum level of thyroid hormone which triggers secretion of TSH by the pituitary, perhaps 2.5 ng/100 ml of free-T_4, excluding T_3 (Reichlin and Utiger, 1967). No immunoassay for TRF is yet available, but such might make it possible to measure the TRF level in hypophyseal portal blood at varying levels of thyroid hormones. The TRF threshold will be further discussed below in connection with TSH secretion.

One comment might be made, however, on the hypothalamic-pituitary 'threshold' ob-

TABLE I

Function	General definition	Quantitative definition	References
Hypothal. threshold T_4	Level of T_4 below which hypothalamus secretes TRF	2.5 ng/100 ml serum (as free T_4)	Reichlin and Utiger (1967)
Hypothal. threshold TSH	Level of TSH which suppresses TRF secretion via short feedback loop		
Pituitary threshold TRF	Level of TRF capable of eliciting TSH secretion	$< 10^{-11}$ moles of TRF	(see text)
Pituitary threshold T_4	Level of T_4 below which pituitary secretes TSH in absence of TRF		
T_4-Pit. blocking level	Level of T_4 which blocks effect of TRF on pituitary	2.6×10^{-10}M free T_4 ($+$ T_3)	(see text)
T_4-Eq (or simply T_4)	Total quantity of thyroactive substances expressed as that amount of T_4 which would cause an equal physiological effect		
(TRF) Hypoph. port.	Concentration of TRF in hypophyseal portal blood		
(TSH)	TSH concentration in peripheral blood	2.7 μU/ml	Odell *et al.* (1967*a*)
		3.9 μU/ml	(see text)
		4.4 μU/ml	Raud and Odell (1969)
		0.66 μU/ml	Adams *et al.* (1970)
Mult. fact. pituit.	Pituitary multiplier factor; number of molecules of TSH secreted in response to one molecule of TRF	7,000	Mittler *et al.* (1969)
Mult. fact. thyroid	Thyroid multiplier factor; number of molecules of iodothyronine (might preferably be expressed as T_4-Eq) secreted by thyroid in response to one molecule of TSH	2,000	(see text)
Calorig. independ.	Minimal calorigenesis independent of T_4 action		
Calorig. T_4-depend.	Calorigenic effect per unit T_4-Eq		
K-cortisol	Term for effect of glucocorticoids on system, expressed as moles of cortisol in circulation or acting at hypoth.-pituitary and possibly on thyroid.		

Thresholds are expressed in this paper in some places as concentrations in the perfusing medium and in others as quantities of stimulant or suppressant delivered to the target organ. The term 'level' in this table is used to include both. Unless otherwise specified, the term 'level' in the text is used as synonymous with concentration.

served by Reichlin and Utiger (1967). They found that the serum TSH level rose gradually at progressively lower levels of free T_4 (or, rather, fell gradually as they raised the free T_4 by thyroxine administration in hypothyroid subjects). Although they specify a free T_4 concentration of 2.5 ng/100 ml as the approximate inflection point of the curve (more properly called a shoulder than inflection point), the curve is in fact rather gently sloping without a clear break and with considerable scatter of the data. We have attempted to prepare a similar curve with data from our laboratories but have been frustrated by the scatter, and the data of others have shown a similar variability (Greenberg *et al.*, 1970). Although the curve may not be a rectangular hyperbola, its central portion might profitably be treated as such. This could then be solved for the vertex and would yield a single number, which might be more useful and constant as an expression of threshold, recognizing the great individual variations which must occur.

An interesting number which has been proposed in connection with the loop is the 'pituitary multiplier factor', suggested and calculated by Mettler *et al.*, (1969). Using *in vitro* results, they calculated that the number of TSH molecules released by the pituitary in response to the action of one molecule of TRF was 7,000. They have used this result as one point in their argument for the designation of this hypothalamic substance as a hormone – TRH – rather than a factor – TRF. This number, together with knowledge of the quantities of TSH capable of causing significant stimulation of thyroidal radioiodine uptake – 3 mU/kg given as a single intramuscular injection (Einhorn, 1958) – give some idea of the amplification in this portion of the loop.

One might reasonably assume that pure human TSH has a specific activity of 30 international units per mg. Figures of 60–80 U/mg have been reported for bovine TSH (Condliffe, 1963; Morris, 1963; Odell *et al.*, 1967; Utiger *et al.*, 1963). The 60 U/mg may be correct for native TSH, but preparations generally stabilize around 25 U/mg (Condliffe, 1963; Odell *et al.*, 1967). If TSH has an activity of 30 U/mg and a molecular weight of 25,000, then 3 mU would represent 0.1 μg or 4×10^{-12} moles. Thus, $(4 \times 10^{-12}) \times (6.02 \times 10^{23})$ or 2.4×10^{12} molecules, or about 1.7×10^{14} TSH molecules/man, are capable of stimulating the thyroid, and this amount of TSH might result from the action of 2.4×10^{10} molecules (or $4 \times 10^{\ 14}$ moles) of TRF. In order to label this number of molecules with 1 mC of ^{14}C, one-third of the molecules would have to contain a radioactive carbon atom (1 mC of ^{14}C equals 10^{13} molecules), which approaches a carrier-free preparation.

A similar thyroid multiplier factor relating the secretion of the thyroid to stimulation by TSH has not been calculated. This might be approached from *in vitro* studies, as was done for the pituitary multiplier factor, but a physiologically more valid number might be obtained by measuring the arteriovenous gradient of TSH across the thyroid. We have calculated a 'thyroid multiplier factor' making the following assumptions, some of which, though not strictly true, seem necessary to allow even a guess: (1) all thyroxine secretion is secondary to TSH stimulation; (2) the thyroid extracts a tenth of the TSH perfusing it; (3) thyroid blood flow is 5 ml/g/min, or about 80 ml/min; (4) the thyroid secretes 100 μg of thyroxine/day (including triiodothyronine, T_3). Using a normal TSH level of 4 μU/ml of plasma, the thyroid multiplier factor comes to about 2,000. Thyroxine might better be expressed as T_4-Eq, since the loop is more likely to protect the latter rather than the number of molecules of iodothyronine secreted.

The pituitary threshold for response to TRF (the smallest quantity of TRF capable of eliciting TSH secretion) is probably considerably less than 10^{-10} moles of TRF, expressed as total TRF reaching the pituitary rather than concentration of TRF. Doses of TRF as low as 50–60 μg given into a peripheral vein in adult humans can bring about a rise in serum TSH concentration (Hall *et al.*, 1970; Hershman and Pittman, 1970). Other assumptions made to calculate this number of moles of TRF include the following: (1) the TRF is instantaneously distributed throughout a plasma volume of 2.5 l; (2) the human pituitary plasma flow is 0.5 ml/min (Porter *et al.*, 1970); (3) no TRF is inactivated by the plasma during the period under consideration and (4) action occurs within 3 minutes. Although the first assumption is obviously inaccurate, we have shown that a large dose of TRF, 1000 μg, gives the same response whether given as a single intravenous 'push' over 1–3 minutes or as an infusion given over 30 minutes (Hershman and Pittman, 1970). Infusion of small quantities over prolonged periods would be necessary to obtain a better estimate of the quantities reaching the pituitary. The third assumption is conservative, since TRF inactivation in blood is known to be very rapid. Redding and Schally (1969) found that rat plasma had to be diluted 1 : 8 to permit study of inactivation and that even at this dilution the plasma inactivated 60–70% of added TRF in 30 minutes. Bowers *et al.* (1966; 1970) found that human serum inactivated all added TRF in 15 minutes. Therefore, the average concentration of TRF in plasma over even a brief period would be substantially less than the initial concentration. The fourth assumption is also conservative. Bowers *et al.* found a rise in serum TSH 6 minutes after TRF injection in man, and the rise was probably present at 3 minutes as well (1968); it may occur at 2 minutes or earlier (1970). Thus, the threshold quantity of TRF required for TSH release in man is probably considerably less than 10^{-10} moles. The minimal stimulatory concentration *in vitro* is about 10 pg for a rat pituitary fragment that might weigh as much as 5 mg (Schally and Redding, 1967). So for a human pituitary of 500 mg, 1 ng should be stimulatory – or around 3×10^{-12} moles.

Curiously, the other result obtained above for this value using the TSH dose which was minimally effective in man is an even smaller number, 4×10^{-14} moles. This value for the pituitary threshold for the minimal amount of TRF (4×10^{-14} moles) which will release TSH was calculated starting from a thyroidal response in short-term radioiodine uptake (Einhorn, 1958), yet we found no response in thyroid function in patients given much larger doses of TRF (Hershman and Pittman, 1970). Administration of 500 μg of TRF may release 64 mU of TSH, which approaches the 210 mU found to give the thyroidal response (3 mU/kg $\times$ 70). This suggests the possibility that changes in thyroid function may be detected using current methodology if the correct indices of thyroid function are chosen, if several doses of TRF are given, and if the TSH response to consecutive doses is not greatly diminished.

The foregoing considerations raise another question regarding the best expression for thresholds in the loop. It is probably less meaningful to express them as concentrations than in terms of delivery rates or total number of moles reaching a target as a pulse, as just illustrated for TRF. Also, since hormonal systems, unlike some portions of the nervous system, respond in a graded manner rather than an all-or-none fashion, it might be preferable to relate the quantity delivered to the midportion of the dose-response curve (the quantity of stimulus needed to elicit a response 50% of the maximum). This function would then be an 'RD-50' rather than a threshold.

The thyroid feedback loop is complicated by the fact that thyroid hormones exert a negative influence on TSH secretion at the pituitary as well as at the hypothalamus. (See Reichlin (1960) for discussion.) This is listed in Table I as 'T_4 Pituitary Blocking Level.' There is as yet little data on which to speculate about the quantities involved. The doses of thyroxine used by Mittler *et al.* (1969) to inhibit TRF action *in vitro* were relatively large (100 μg/ml), and lower doses must be explored before physiologic action can be further evaluated. However, the fact that administration of thyroxine or T_3 prior to TRF blocks the response to the latter *in vivo* (Bowers *et al.*, 1967; 1970; Bowers and Schally, 1970; Redding and Schally, 1967) indicates that this action must be considered in regulation of pituitary TSH secretion. Since the response to TRF is either blocked or almost completely blocked in hyperthyroid patients (Fleischer *et al.*, 1970; Hershman and Pittman, 1970) in whom the free T_4 concentration is 13 ng/100 ml, or 2.6×10^{-10}M, (Sterling and Brenner, 1966), this level of T_4 may approximate the 'T_4 Pituitary Blocking Level' (but does not take into account the T_3 level or turnover in such patients).

The mechanism by which T_4 blocks TSH secretion is of interest. The suggestion has been made (Bakke, 1966; Bakke and Lawrence, 1965; Bowers and Schally, 1970) that T_4 (or T_3)

stimulates formation of an intrapituitary protein inhibitor, based on the finding that actinomycin-D inhibits the blockade (Bowers and Schally, 1970). The suggestion has also been made that T_4 may increase cyclic AMP degradation by increasing phosphodiesterase activity (Geschwind, 1970).

The possibility of one or more 'short feedback loops' for TSH must be considered, though quantitative data for the concentrations or amounts delivered are not available. There may be one such loop in which TSH acts on the hypothalamus to diminish TRF secretion, and there may be an even shorter one, conceptually, in which TSH limits its own secretion by an action directly on the adenohypophysis. The suggestion that exogenously administered TSH increases hypothalamic and pituitary TSH content (Bakke, 1963; 1966; Bakke and Lawrence, 1962*a*) is consistent with this idea. While it is difficult to rationalize the existence or function of such loops, perhaps their development is related in some way to similar short loops for prolactin and growth hormone. In the latter cases they seem to make more sense, since there is no known target product for the inhibitory arm of the feedback loop from the periphery. There is probably not a short feedback loop for T_4 on the thyroid gland itself (Yamada *et al.*, 1961).

The pituitary threshold below which the adenohypophysis secretes TSH in the absence of TRF is not only speculative, but one can cite a clinical suggestion that it does not occur. Some patients with 'isolated TSH deficiency' have had associated evidence of cerebrovascular disease, leading to the suggestion that the basic deficiency in such individuals was TRF lack (Lohrenz *et al.*, 1964). The question of *in vivo* TSH secretion in the absence of TRF, as well as the possibility that all the adenohypophyseal hormones have inhibiting factors as well as releasing factors (Meites, 1970), remains to be investigated.

The problem of expressing thyroid hormone activity as a single term requires assigning some number to the moles of T_4 equalled by one mole of T_3 and perhaps acetic acid analogue metabolites of T_4 (Pittman *et al.*, 1970*a*). The total of T_4 plus the equivalent number from T_3 might be designated the 'T_4-Eq' – thyroxine equivalents. This problem is at once becoming simpler in some ways and more complex in others. Multiplying the plasma concentration of T_3 by 4 does not take into account the total turnover, which may be more important. The probable conversion of a fraction of secreted T_4 to T_3 by peripheral tissues (Braverman *et al.*, 1970) further complicates it. On the other hand, current methodology probably gives a reasonably accurate estimate of circulating T_3. In one study the value found was 200 ng/100 ml (Sterling *et al.*, 1966) which, together with the newer half-life of slightly more than 1 day (Pittman *et al.*, 1970*a*), gives a T_3 turnover of 40 μg/day as opposed to perhaps 77 μg/day for T_4. Values for T_3 of 273 ng/100 ml and 60 μg/day, which would give 240 μg T_4-Eq and make T_3 account for some 80% of the total T_4-Eq, have also been reported (Wilber and Utiger, 1969). Unfortunately this gives us no idea of the proportions of T_4 and T_3 degraded by tissues of particular interest – the hypothalamus and the pituitary, and this problem may be compounded by selective concentration and special metabolism in these areas. Perhaps *in vitro* approaches, together with measurements of circulating levels, offer the only means of estimating the effects of the two hormones together as they occur *in vivo*. Because of these difficulties, no guesses are made in Table I as to a T_4-Eq for the whole man or for any component of the system.

TRF has apparently been found in rat portal blood (Porter *et al.*, 1970) and in peripheral blood of hypothyroid rats exposed to cold (Redding and Schally, 1969). Quantification was not reported, and whether this can be accomplished with current methodology is doubtful, but rough estimates may be possible.

For the last three terms listed in Table I we have not even guessed at the quantities involved. They are listed because they seem pertinent. In fact the maintenance of calorigenesis at some optimal level is the function, or 'purpose', of the whole system, the left side of the equation the studies are presumably aiming for as a quantitative description of the thyroid feedback loop.

Minimal calorigenesis as used here refers to the possibility that there may be some level of heat production by the body independent of T_4 action. (It is not the 'minimum metabolic rate' of Kleiber, which does not take T_4 into consideration.) Aside from the possibility that such T_4-independent heat production may not occur, it is likely to prove unmeasurable because total absence of T_4 throughout the organism may result in such an unsteady state as to preclude determination or simply result in death. A suggestion that this is so is the infrequency with which T_4 levels approach zero even in severe clinical myxedema with coma.

The necessity for various correction factors complicates expression of calorigenesis in a simple fashion. These include rate of heat loss (including terms for ambient temperature, humidity, body insulation etc. (Kleiber, 1961), body size, and age. Metabolic rate should be related to body size by the 3/4 power of weight rather than surface area, as is the custom clinically (Kleiber, 1961), despite Kleiber's disparaging remarks on allometric corrections (Sturtevant, 1955). Age is known to decrease metabolic rate as customarily expressed (Pittman, 1962), but it is not known whether this reduction depends on diminution of some T_4-independent metabolic rate, a reduced secretion of thyroid hormone (Oddie *et al.*, 1966), diminished effect of T_4 on the periphery, or reduction in quantity of 'metabolic body size' (Shock, 1960). Some data indicate that older rats are more sensitive to T_4 rather than less sensitive (Grad and Hoffman, 1955).

In any case, although knowledge of minimal (T_4-independent) calorigenesis might be useful in some situations, it is not necessarily required for determination of calorigenesis due to T_4. Curiously, recent preoccupation with other aspects of thyroid function have left the metabolic rate relatively unstudied, and because of the multiplicity of factors just mentioned which affect it no simple expression can be given here.

Some effect of T_4 in addition to the level of the hormone itself may be important in regulating the thyroid feedback loop. This possibility has been pointed out in the past (Goldberg, 1954; Goldberg *et al.*, 1955), but the findings in those studies are now interpretable as due in part to changes in free T_4 (Larsen *et al.*, 1970), and the possibility of such a component in the loop seems less likely (Bakke, 1966; Bakke and Lawrence, 1962*b*).

Glucocorticoids suppress thyroid function at least partly by inhibiting pituitary TSH secretion (Wilber and Utiger, 1969). The fact that electrical stimulation of the mid- and posterior-median eminence results in increased thyroid activity only after adrenalectomy (Harris, 1964; Harris and Woods, 1958) also suggests that endogenous glucocorticoids may exert some regulatory influence on the systems (Nicoloff *et al.*, 1970).

Temperature alterations are known to affect the loop, but the mechanisms are not clear. While local cooling of the hypothalamus causes thyroid activation (Andersson, 1964; Reichlin, 1964), it seems possible that peripheral receptors may be involved when the ambient temperature is manipulated. Lowered body temperature can elevate serum TSH and activate thyroid function in man, but the effect is marked only in early infancy perhaps persisting to the age of 1½ years (Fisher and Odell, 1969; Wilber and Baum, 1970). The effect is readily apparent in adult rats (Hershman *et al.*, 1970). The effect of temperature is discussed further below.

The component of the loop which has received most attention the past few years has been TSH, owing to development of radioimmunoassay methods for human (Odell *et al.*, 1965; 1967; Utiger, 1965; Utiger *et al.*, 1963) and now rat (Wilber and Utiger, 1967) TSH applicable to biological samples. Using this method, Odell *et al.* (1967) made some fundamental observations on TSH metabolism in man. They found the half-life in blood to be 54 minutes, the volume of distribution 5.8% of body weight, the mean plasma concentration 2.7 μU/ml, the total pool aside from the pituitary 8.7 mU, and the daily turnover rate 165 mU. In three hypothyroid subjects the mean half-life was 85 minutes, the pool 87 mU, and the secretion rate 1,033 mU/day. Assuming a normal distribution volume and similar half-life the secretion in some hypothyroid patients may be as high as 23,000 mU/day. This is an extremely high value – more than 140 times normal. If one takes a value of 800 μU/ml (see below), the rate might be more than twice this, or perhaps 300 times normal. This suggests that any short feedback loops which may exist are of minor importance in man. Elevated serum levels thus result from both increased secretion and reduced disposal of TSH.

These data are interesting in connection with the serum TSH response to TRF discussed below. If the serum TSH rises by 16 μU/ml and the distribution space is 4,000 ml, the total increase of 64 mU represents a 39% increase in the total daily turnover rate of 165 mU. The actual increase is more, since the elevated serum TSH level persists over the better part of an hour.

The serum TSH level in 173 euthyroid individuals determined in our laboratories was 3.9 ± 2.0 (SD) μU/ml, based on the International Research Standard A. (Since an International Bovine TSH Standard used in many previous bioassay studies was shown to have a significantly greater slope than the human standard in the McKenzie bioassay (Hershman, 1970), and since bioassay gives higher values than immunoassay (Hershman, 1969; Miyai *et al.*, 1969), the results of these prior studies may not be entirely comparable with those done later with the human standard.) The TSH level in 'pituitary blood' has been estimated at 220 μU/ml (Conway *et al.*, 1969).

An outstanding characteristic of circulating TSH levels, at least in man, is their relative constancy and stability in the face of various manipulations and stresses which cause major alterations in the circulating levels of other hormones. In the human adult in a region outside an endemic goiter area there is really only one change which results in substantial elevation of serum TSH levels: hypothyroidism. Subjects residing in areas of goiter endemia may apparently have elevations of serum TSH without being overtly hypothyroid (Adams *et al.*, 1968; Buttfield *et al.*, 1968; De Lange *et al.*, 1970). The exact mechanism for this TSH elevation is not clear, but the possibility exists that application of more precise measures of thyroid function than have been possible might reveal mild hypothyroidism. Levels in the hypothyroid patients in our series are shown in Figure 2 and rise as high as 800 μU/ml. Various other

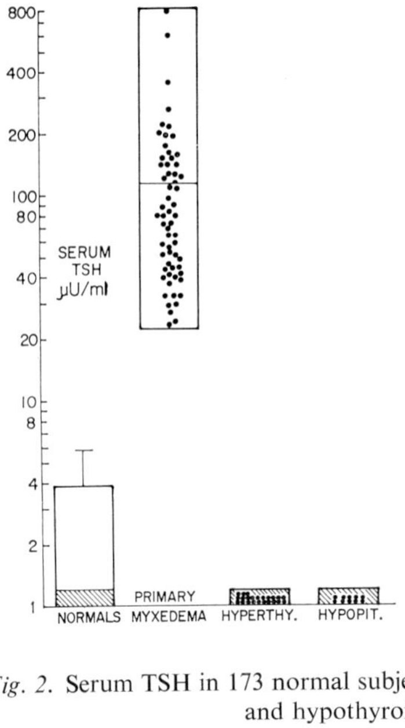

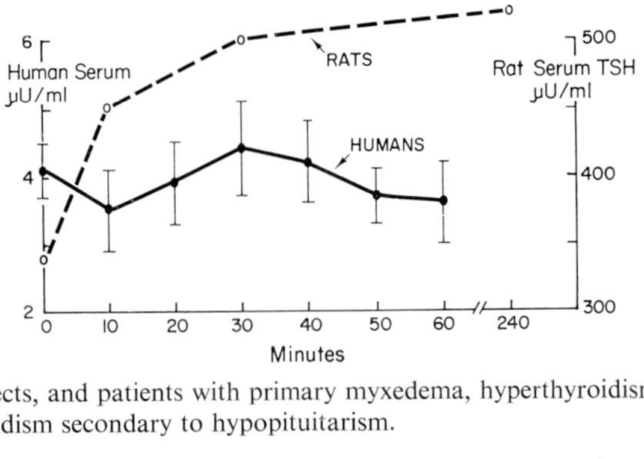

Fig. 2. Serum TSH in 173 normal subjects, and patients with primary myxedema, hyperthyroidism, and hypothyroidism secondary to hypopituitarism.

Fig. 3. Serum TSH during cold exposure of 2–4°C in 14 euthyroid male subjects and in male rats on a low iodine diet, 5 rats/point. Vertical bars show ± SE (Hershman *et al.*, 1970).

TABLE II

Factors Affecting Circulating TSH

Manipulation or change	Species and comments	References
Increase TSH:		
Hypothyroidism	All studied, including man, rat, etc.	Odell *et al.* (1967*a*; *b*); (see text)
Birth	Man	Fisher and Odell (1969)
Cold	Rat	Hershman *et al.* (1970*b*)
	Human infant	Fisher and Odell (1969); Wilber and Baum (1970)
Hypothalamic cooling	Goat (measured $PB^{131}I$ and thyroidal ^{131}I uptake)	Andersson (1964)
Decrease TSH:		
Glucocorticoid	Man	Wilber and Utiger (1970)
Stress	Rat	Ducommun *et al.* (1966)
Heat, ambient	Rat (measured PBI, RAI, and thyroid morphology)	Goldberg (1954)
No effect:		
Hypoglycemia	Man	Odell *et al.* (1967*b*)
Pyrogen (bacterial endotoxin)	Man	Odell *et al.* (1967*b*)
Arginine	Man	Odell *et al.* (1967*b*)
Electroshock	Man	Ryan *et al.* (1970)
Androgen	Man	Hershman *et al.* (1970*b*); Odell *et al.* (1967*b*)
Glucagon	Man	Sawin *et al.* (1970)
Vasopressin	Man	Read *et al.* (1969)

alterations examined for an effect on serum TSH are listed in Table II and discussed below. This resistance to elevation on the part of serum TSH makes it *the* most valuable test clinically for confirmation of the diagnosis of primary hypothyroidism (*i.e.*, that due to disease of the thyroid gland itself).

As mentioned above, the problem of determining the circulating concentration of TSH is complicated by the fact that bioassays (McKenzie) give consistently higher values than immunoassays on the same samples (Hershman, 1969; Miyai *et al.*, 1969). Furthermore, the biological activity of TSH can be markedly diminished or destroyed by heavy iodination with ^{127}I despite retention of immunologic activity (Hershman, 1969). Similar problems exist with other peptide hormone assays (Besser *et al.*, 1969). It would seem reasonable that bioassays more accurately reflect intact TSH, but immunoassays seem satisfactory in most situations.

The question of whether or not there is a circadian rhythm for serum TSH concentration also reflects partly a limitation in the methodology. Euthyroid individuals have values which are undetectable in about 13% of the cases in our institution, and normal values are thus just above the 'noise range' of the assay. This makes it difficult to evaluate small changes in concentrations of TSH unless these follow a very consistent pattern. Our values for 21 patients without endocrine disorders showed no diurnal variation when sampled at 4-hour intervals for 24 hours. Odell *et al.* (1967) have reported similar findings. However, Nicoloff (1969) has found a diurnal variation of small magnitude, and Blum *et al.* (1968) and Bakke and Lawrence (1965; 1966) have found larger changes. The latter studies were in rats, and it seems likely that a circadian rhythm may be more prominent in that species. Nicoloff (1969) has ascribed the variations in TSH concentration to reciprocal variations in plasma cortisol levels. Further studies are necessary to clarify this problem, but it already seems clear that the variations in circulating TSH concentration, if they occur consistently, are not of great magnitude on an absolute scale.

Birth, in addition to hypothyroidism, is the only situation in which large increases in serum TSH occur. The increase is probably already occurring at time of birth – or exists previously in utero, since TSH levels on cord blood are higher than maternal blood (Fisher and Odell, 1969; Hershman *et al.*, 1969; Robin *et al.*, 1969). Fisher and Odell (1969) found cord and maternal levels of 9.5 and 3.9 μU/ml, respectively, and Robin *et al.* (1969) found 11.9 and 7.2 μU/ml. The major rise occurred within the first half-hour of life, the level rising from 9.5 to 60 μU/ml at 10 minutes of age, then 86 μU/ml at 30 minutes of age (Fisher and Odell, 1969). This high level fell rapidly between 30 minutes and 4 hours, then more gradually to 13 μU/ml at 48 hours, the half-life being 77 minutes during the period of rapid fall, suggesting cessation of most of the increased secretion after 30 minutes of age. The early rise was not prevented by warming the newborns, but the later relatively high levels were augmented by cooling at 3 hours of age. Thus, the physiological hyperthyroidism known to occur neonatally (Van Middlesworth, 1954) is TSH-dependent. The mechanisms for these rises and any functions they may serve are unknown but may hold clues to basic aspects of thyroid function in other situations.

Cold exposure, though effective to a small degree in human infants shortly after birth and perhaps up to the age of 1 year (Fisher and Odell, 1969; Wilber and Baum, 1970), is ineffective in raising TSH in adults to any large degree (Hershman *et al.*, 1970*b*). In 11 euthyroid human volunteers there was no rise in serum TSH on cold exposure for 1 hour despite a fall in rectal temperature of 1.4°F. In contrast, rats exposed to cold had a significant increase in serum immunoassayable TSH within 30 minutes (Fig. 3). Even the hypothermia used for cardiac surgery, which resulted in a fall in temperature to 87°F, did not increase TSH, though drugs were used in these procedures which might alter the response (Hershman *et al.*, 1970*b*). Wilber and Baum (1970) found acute rises in 6 of 7 children subjected to hypothermia during cardiac surgery during which the rectal temperatures fell to a mean nadir of 63°F. This response appeared as late as 1½ years of age. Odell and co-workers have found a small rise in TSH in 12 human adults exposed to 7 days of arctic temperature (1968; Raud and Odell, 1969). This change was of very small magnitude as compared with the changes observed, for example, in rats. Nevertheless, the observation points up the possible importance of such temperature-induced alterations in man, despite the smallness of the change on an absolute

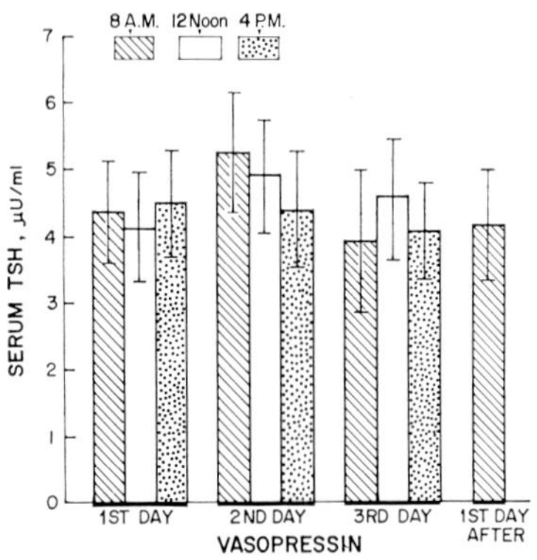

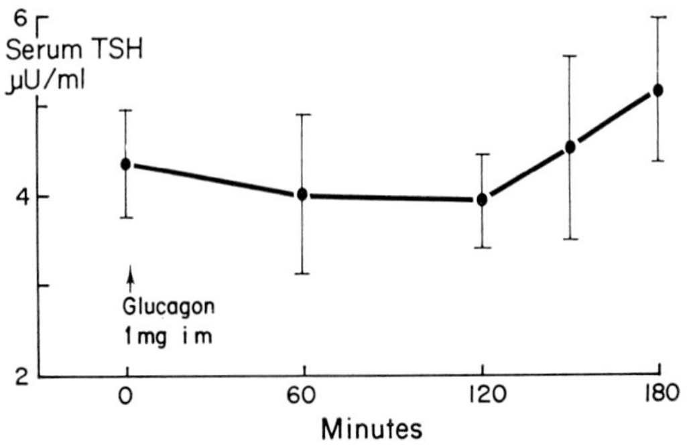

Fig. 4. Serum TSH in 10 subjects before and during 8-hr infusion of vasopressin (5 U) beginning at 8.00 a.m. Vertical lines show SE (Read *et al.*, 1969).

Fig. 5. Serum TSH in 5 euthyroid subjects given 1 mg glucagon i.m. after withdrawal of the 0 time sample; vertical bars show ± SE (Sawin *et al.*, 1970).

scale. Such small changes may be responsible for the seasonal variations in PBI which have been reported (De Ruisseau, 1965).

Other studies also generally attest the remarkable stability of the serum TSH concentration, as noted in Table II. Vasopressin has been reported to stimulate thyroid function in the rabbit (Harris, 1964), estrogen-treated rat (Harris *et al.*, 1964), and man (Gilbert-Dreyfus *et al.*, 1964). In the first two studies (Harris, 1964; Harris *et al.*, 1964) the vasopressin appeared to stimulate the thyroid directly. We have repeated the last mentioned study with measurements of serum TSH as well as other indices of thyroid function (Read *et al.*, 1969). As shown in Figure 4, there was no rise in serum TSH following intravenous administration of 5 units of vasopressin. In other studies intramuscular administration of 10 units failed to raise TSH (Odell *et al.*, 1967; Sawin *et al.*, 1970). It seems clear that in man vasopressin is not a potent stimulus, and probably not a stimulus at all. Whether or not it is in other animals remains to be seen; the observed effects may have been the result of a direct action on the thyroid.

Similarly, administration of 1 mg of glucagon intramuscularly caused no rise in TSH in 5 euthyroid subjects (Sawin *et al.*, 1970) (Fig. 5), nor did electroshock therapy (Hershman *et al.*, 1970; Ryan *et al.*, 1970). Administration of the glucocorticoid dexamethasone in large doses gave an acute fall in serum TSH in hypothyroid subjects to about half the control values with a rebound to 156% of control levels (Wilber and Utiger, 1969). The reduction could be seen within 8 hours after oral or intravenous cortisol or dexamethasone. Similar

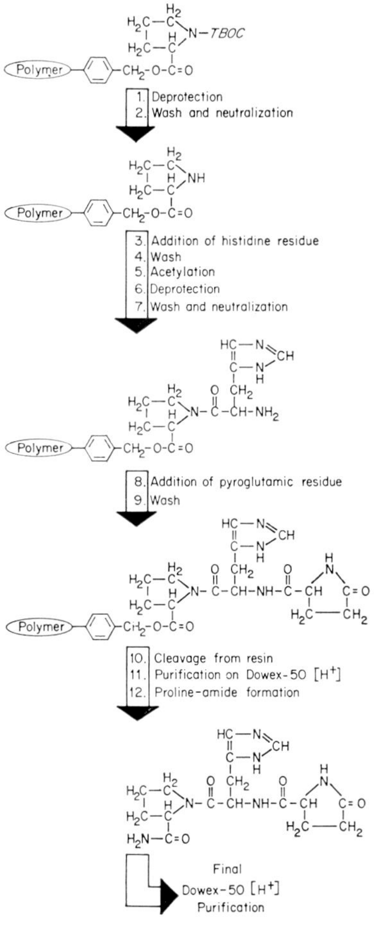

Fig. 6. Schematic outline for solid phase synthesis of TRF (Baugh *et al.*, 1970).

changes of smaller magnitude were found in normal subjects. In our patient with Cushing's disease the TSH response to TRF was not blocked (Hershman and Pittman, 1970), suggesting that glucocorticoids may act at the hypothalamic level in man, as has been proposed for the rat (Wilber and Utiger, 1969). Stress tended to reduce TSH secretion in rats (Ducommun *et al.*, 1966). Hypoglycemia had no effect (Odell *et al.*, 1967). Data for estrogens are conflicting, with reports of increase (Adams and Maloof, 1970) and decrease (Nicoloff *et al.*, 1970).

The recent discovery of the tripeptide structure of TRF (Boler *et al.*, 1969; Bowers *et al.*, 1965; 1969; Burgus *et al.*, 1969; 1970; Folkers *et al.*, 1969; Vale *et al.*, 1970) was a major advance in this field. The apparent lack of species specificity (Bowers *et al.*, 1965; 1970; Burgus *et al.*, 1970) and the preparation of relatively large quantities synthetically (Baugh *et al.*, 1970) make possible direct manipulation of the pituitary secretion of TSH for the first time and thus provide a readily utilizable test for pituitary TSH reserve. An outline of one such synthesis is shown in Figure 6.

Using a preparation synthesized with this procedure by Baugh *et al.* (1970), we have administered the material intravenously to normal subjects and patients with various diseases. Some results are presented in Table III and Figures 7–10. In confirmation of previous findings (Bowers *et al.*, 1970*a*; *b*; Fleischer *et al.*, 1970) it is apparent that elevation of serum TSH occurs in normal subjects after administration of 500 or 1000 μg of TRF intravenously (Fig. 7). Administration of 1000 μg i.v. as an infusion given over a period of 30 minutes did

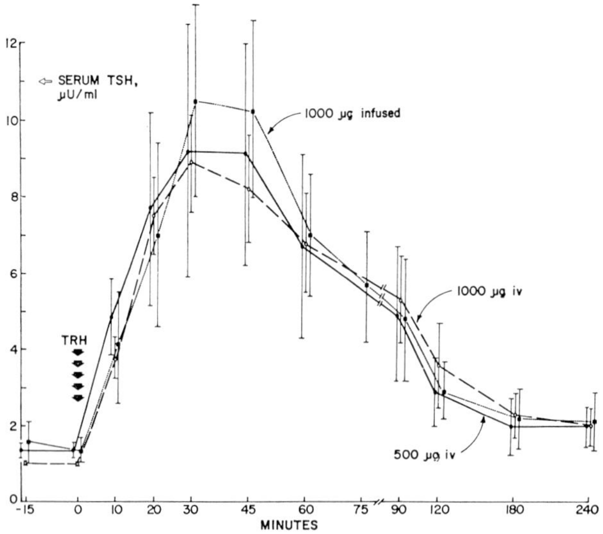

Fig. 7. Serum TSH in 6 euthyroid subjects given TRF; vertical bars show ± SE (Hershman and Pittman, 1970).

not enhance the response. This response is specific in that it is limited to TSH; other pituitary hormones (FSH, LH, GH) do not increase in man (Bowers *et al.* 1970*a*; *b*; Fleischer *et al.*, 1970). Small rises in growth hormone concentration to about 6 ng/ml were observed in 2 of 7 subjects by Fleischer *et al.* (1970), and occasional rises in plasma cortisol levels were ascribed to nonspecific stress effects of the tests (Bowers *et al.*, 1970*b*; Fleischer *et al.*, 1970). Such stress is minimal, however, consisting chiefly of a slight abdominal queasy feeling or vague discomfort and occasionally mild nausea. We have not observed serious side effects in more than 50 tests nor have any been reported.

The dose-response curve appears to extend from somewhat less than 50 μg to about 500

TABLE III

*Response of serum TSH concentration to TRF**

No.	Diagnosis	Sex, Age	Serum T_4-I μg/100 ml	Minutes after TRH given: 0	10	20	30	45	60	90	120	180	240
				Serum TSH μU/ml									
1.	Hypothyroidism	M, 48	5.4	15	42	84	95	89	98	71	55	35	21
2.	Chromophobe adenoma	M, 51	4.7	$<$ 1.2	2.5	5.0	10.0	10.2	11.2	9.0	6.2	4.0	4.4
	Post-hypophysectomy		3.3	$<$ 1.2	$<$ 1.2	$<$ 1.2	$<$ 1.2	$<$ 1.2	$<$ 1.2	$<$ 1.2	$<$ 1.2	$<$ 1.2	$<$ 1.2
3.	Hypopituitarism	M, 54	1.3	$<$ 1.2	$<$ 1.2	$<$ 1.2	$<$ 1.2	$<$ 1.2	$<$ 1.2	$<$ 1.2	$<$ 1.2	$<$ 1.2	$<$ 1.2
4.	Enlarged sella turcica	F, 26	6.1	$<$ 1.2	9.3	20.0	18.7	18.3	10.4	8.0	5.8	$<$ 1.2	$<$ 1.2
5.	Enlarged sella turcica	F, 46	5.2	$<$ 1.2	28.0	32.5	30.5	21.5	12.3	8.5	5.5	2.8	2.5
6.	Hyperthyroidism	M, 48	20.2	$<$ 1.2	$<$ 1.2	$<$ 1.2	$<$ 1.2	$<$ 1.2	$<$ 1.2	$<$ 1.2	$<$ 1.2	$<$ 1.2	$<$ 1.2
7.	Hyperthyroidism	F, 46	11.8	$<$ 1.2	$<$ 1.2	$<$ 1.2	$<$ 1.2	$<$ 1.2	$<$ 1.2	$<$ 1.2	$<$ 1.2	$<$ 1.2	$<$ 1.2
8.	Hyperthyroidism	F, 13	20.0	$<$ 1.2	$<$ 1.2	4.5	4.4	3.2	$<$ 1.2	$<$ 1.2	$<$ 1.2	$<$ 1.2	$<$ 1.2
9.	Cushing's disease	M, 46	4.6	$<$ 1.2	3.0	4.7	10.6	7.5	7.3	5.3	5.6	3.3	1.9
10.	Euthyroid, i.v.	M, 43	4.2	3.4	9.5	20.0	21.0	20.7	19.2	12.2	10.8	6.5	3.4
	oral*			5.8	4.0	5.6	12.7	10.6	23.2	18.0	22.3	22.0	16.8
11.	Euthyroid, i.v.	M, 42	5.4	$<$ 1.2	6.6	8.0	13.3	7.9	5.1	4.7	4.4	$<$ 1.2	$<$ 1.2
	oral*			$<$ 1.2	$<$ 1.2	2.3	4.1	5.3	5.5	5.7	4.5	4.5	3.5

* The TRH dose was 1000 μg i.v. push in all instances except the two (*) who received 10 mg orally.

or 750 μg, given as a single i.v. dose over several minutes to average-size adult subjects. We have observed consistent responses to 62.5 μg, and responses to 50 μg have been reported (Hall *et al.*, 1970). Hopefully the data will not show large individual variability, possibly due to variations in disposal rates, because knowledge of this dose-response relation will be important in assessing the effects of various manipulations and diseases on the system, particularly if these exert small influences.

As shown in Table III, mildly hypothyroid patients display an exaggerated response, while hyperthyroid patients are resistant to TRF stimulation. This is to be expected, in view of the prior finding that the TRF effect could be blocked by thyroid hormone (Bowers *et al.*, 1967; 1970*a*; *b*; Fleischer *et al.*, 1970; Mittler *et al.*, 1969; Schally and Redding, 1967; Vale *et al.*, 1970). The response appropriately disappears after hypophysectomy (Table III), and such disappearance can be used to assess the completeness of hypophysectomy clinically before other evidence of secondary hypothyroidism appears.

The TSH response to TRF administered in this manner is extremely fast, and rises in the TSH concentration in peripheral blood are readily observable in less than 5 minutes – possibly from the first circulation of the administered TRF past the pituitary and the first circulation of pituitary blood to the sampling needle, an almost instantaneous effect (Fig. 7) (Bowers and Schally 1970; *et al.*, 1968; Fleischer *et al.* 1970; Hall *et al.*, 1970; Hershman and Pittman, 1970). The rapidity of this response is interesting in view of the general tendency to view the thyroid loop as a very sluggish one compared with the pituitary-adreno-cortical loop, for example. As noted in the foregoing discussion, some of the other responses also occur fairly quickly, and thyroidal responses to TSH may be observed in a few minutes (release of $PB^{131}I$ (Ackerman and Arons, 1958)), less than 5 minutes (stimulation of glucose oxidation

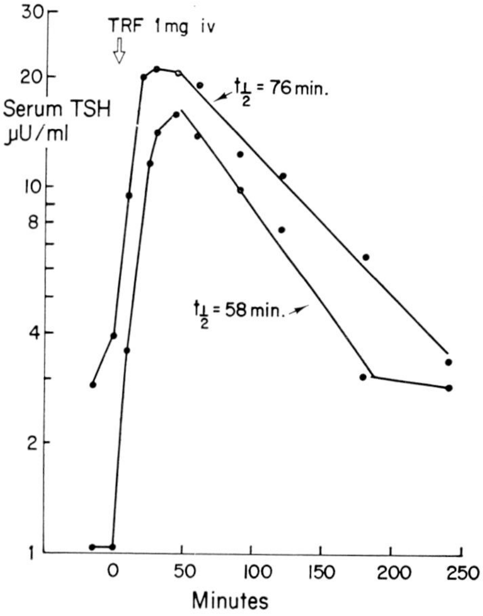

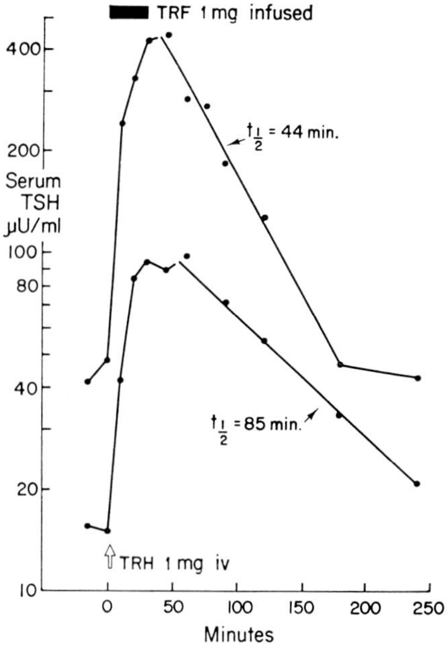

Fig. 8. Serum TSH in 2 normal subjects given 1 mg TRF i.v. The descending portion of the semilogarithmic decay curve was drawn from calculation of the line of best fit and the half-time of disappearance (t 1/2) was computed from it.

Fig. 9. Serum TSH in 2 hypothyroid patients given 1 mg TRF i.v. (in 3 min in lower curve and infused over 30 min in upper curve). See legend for Figure 8.

(Field, 1968), lipid ^{32}P uptake (Vilkki, 1961), or sodium transport (Solomon, 1960)), or even a few seconds (alteration of electrical potential *in vivo* (Krüskemper and Reichertz, 1959)). It is not known whether these rapid changes simply reflect relatively good methodology for detecting early biochemical and biophysical effects in the chain of events in the system or are clues to some more important physiological significance which we are currently failing to perceive.

The disappearance of endogenous TSH from the high serum levels generated by TRF administration occurs with half-lives approximating those observed in other situations (Odell *et al.*, 1970*a*; *b*) (Figs. 8 and 9).

Interestingly, this tripeptide is active after oral administration (Vale *et al.*, 1970) (Fig. 10).

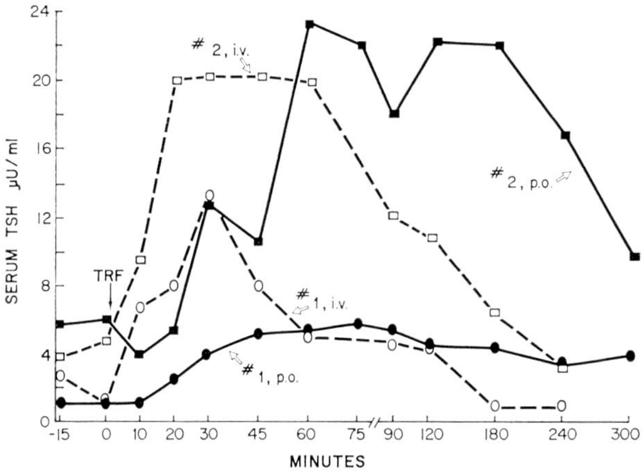

Fig. 10. Serum TSH in 2 normal subjects after being given 10 mg TRF orally followed by 1 mg TRF i.v. the next day (Hershman and Pittman, 1970).

The response is slower and the effect longer lasting than that seen after i.v. administration. Bowers *et al.* (1970*a*) have reported even larger responses using a dose of 20 mg p.o. Such prolonged responses together with ease of administration of TRF when given orally may make it practical to use indirect estimates of the response for clinical purposes (e.g., PBI or thyroidal ^{131}I uptake) when serum TSH measurements are not readily available.

One patient with Cushing's disease and a cortisol secretion rate of 55 mg/day showed a clear response (Table III), as might be expected from the previous studies mentioned above (Wilber and Utiger, 1969).

One problem in using TRF to test the integrity of the thyroid feedback loop is that as a positive signal its effect is dissipated on the one or two components of the loop immediately downstream from the point of input, the pituitary, and little effect is evident as a change in function of the thyroid gland (Hershman and Pittman, 1970), unless perhaps the stimulus can be continued over a period of hours or days as mentioned above. In the latter case a signal of large strength and duration might give increases as far downstream as the metabolic rate. However, it would not test the hypothalamus. For this a negative signal is required unless some signal akin to cold or a direct electrical discharge can be found. The impeded estrogen clomiphene apparently provides such a signal for gonadotropin secretion (Baier and Taubert, 1969). Prior attempts to use thyroidal blockade with antithyroid drugs and measure rebound in thyroid activity to test the hypothalamic-pituitary unit have not met with general success (Jensen, 1969; Powell and Blizzard, 1966; Studer *et al.*, 1964). We have attempted to provide a negative signal using antithyroxine analogues of T_4 (Pittman *et al.*, 1969) but have not been successful to date. One can visualize other points in the loop at which a negative signal might be applied, *e.g.*, prolonged administration of acetylated TSH (Sonnenberg *et al.*, 1957), use of antibodies to TSH, or use of TRF analogues with anti-TRF activity. However, the most physiologic signal would seem to be reduction of the effective T_4 action at the hypothalamic-pituitary receptor sites, such as might be provided by antithyroxine compounds or acute reduction of effective circulating T_4 concentration. Infusion of concentrated TBG (thyroxine-binding globulin) has been suggested for this (Pittman, 1971) and exchange transfusions in rats substituting a dextran solution for plasma have activated thyroid function (Langer, 1970).

The mechanism by which TRF exerts its effect on the pituitary to enhance secretion is unknown and little studied to date. Because of the rapidity of the response, it is generally assumed that acute 'release' is effected by TRF independent of synthesis of new TSH. Synthesis may be coupled to release or stimulated separately by TRF. Recent data indicate that the latter is the case (Wilber, 1970). In pituitaries incubated for up to 24 hours, synthesis of new TSH was blocked by cycloheximide without blocking release, while addition of T_4 to, or omission of calcium from, the medium blocked release without blocking synthesis (Wilber, 1970). It is known that enhanced secretion resulting from TRF is energy requiring (Geschwind, 1970), and in this connection it is of interest that TRF can stimulate pituitary glucose oxidation (Pittman *et al.*) (Fig. 11), an effect which may reflect TRF-enhancement of adenyl cyclase in the pituitary (Steiner *et al.*, 1970). Attempts to elucidate the mechanism of action of TRF by electron microscopy at our institution and by others (Guillemin, 1970) have thus far not met with success.

The mechanisms by which TSH stimulates the thyroid gland have received considerable attention and have been well reviewed by Field (1968). This subject will therefore not be considered further here.

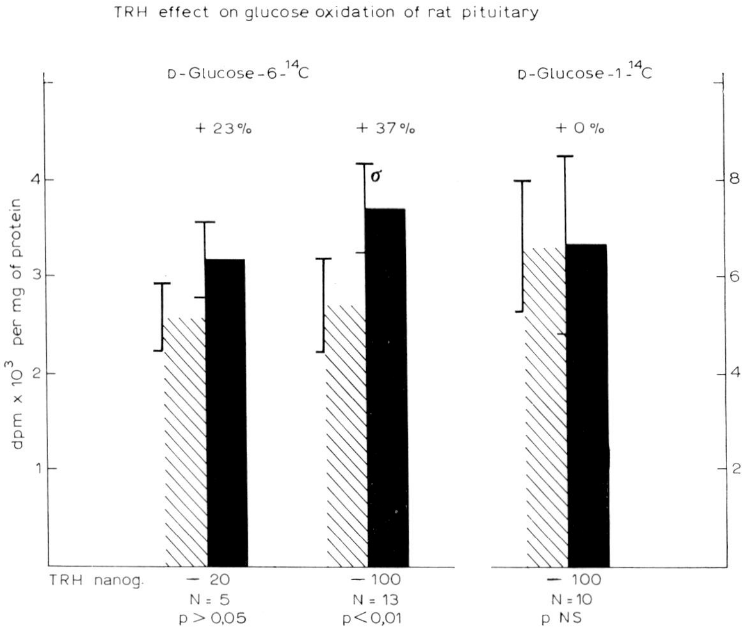

Fig. 11. Pituitary oxidation of glucose-6-^{14}C (first two pairs of bars) or glucose-1-^{14}C (bars on right) expressed as dpm of $^{14}CO_2$ trapped at end of incubation. Shaded bars represent control hemipituitaries and solid bars those incubated in medium to which TRF was added in quantities shown at the bottom (Pittman *et al.*, 1970*b*).

A final aspect of this subject is the possible role of the placenta in thyroid physiology. TSH levels in pregnancy, measured by radioimmunoassay, appear to lie within the normal range. Both our group and that of Hennen (1969) have been studying another thyrotropin found in normal placentas in man. Such a substance has not yet been found in placentas from other species. This substance, human chorionic thyrotropin (HCT), has a molecular size similar to that of pituitary TSH and a similar duration of action in the McKenzie bioassay. However, it differs from human pituitary TSH immunologically. Recent studies showed a very marked variation in the HCT content of individual placentas. The most potent HCT isolated, 1 U/mg, is about 1/25 as potent as highly purified human TSH. Preliminary data on blood levels of this material suggest that its concentration is highest early in pregnancy. In contrast to the recent report of Hennen *et al.* (1969), we have not yet detected high concentrations of HCT in pregnancy blood measured by either immunoassay or bioassay.

The relation of HCT to a thyrotropic substance found in hydatidiform moles and choriocarcinomas is uncertain at present. Molar pregnancies and choriocarcinomas have been associated with increased thyroid function or frank hyperthyroidism (Cohen and Utiger, 1970; Hershman *et al.*, 1970*a*; Odell *et al.*, 1963). 'Molar TSH' from one patient (Hershman *et al.*, 1970*a*) had different immunologic activity, a larger molecular weight, and longer duration of action than HCT. The molar thyrotropin appeared to be identical with the thyrotropin activity found in impure preparations of chorionic gonadotropin, a material isolated from the urine of presumably normal women. The possible importance of these substances in the regulation of thyroid function during pregnancy remains to be clarified.

REFERENCES

ACKERMAN, N. B. and ARONS, W. L. (1958): The effects of epinephrine and norepinephrine on the acute thyroid release of thyroid hormones. *Endocrinology, 62*, 723.

ADAMS, D. D., KENNEDY, T. H., CHOUFOER, J. C. and QUERIDO, A. (1968): Endemic goiter in Western New Guinea. 3. Thyroid-stimulating activity of serum from severely iodine-deficient people. *J. clin. Endocr. 28*, 685.

ADAMS, D. D., KENNEDY, T. H. and UTIGER, R. D. (1970): Serum thyrotropin (TSH) concentrations: measurements by bioassay and immunoassay in iodine-deficiency and other states. In: *Abstracts of the Sixth International Thyroid Conference*, p. 131. Gistel, Vienna, Austria.

ADAMS, L. and MALOOF, F. (1970): The effect of estrogens on the serum level of thyrotropic hormone in humans. *J. clin. Invest., 49*, la.

ANDERSON, B. (1964): Hypothalamic temperature and thyroid activity. In: *Ciba Foundation Study Group No. 18. Brain-Thyroid Relationships*, pp. 35–59. Editors: M. P. Cameron and M. O'Connor. Little, Brown, Boston, Mass.

ANDERSSON, B., EKMAN, L. and GALE, C. C. (1963): Control of thyrotrophic hormone (TSH) secretion by the 'heat loss center'. *Acta physiol. scand., 59*, 12.

BAIER, H. and TAUBERT, H. D. (1969): Effect of clomiphene upon plasma FSH-activity and hypothalamic FSH-RF content in ovariectomized estrogen-progesterone blocked rats. *Endocrinology, 84*, 946.

BAKKE, J. L. (1963): The distribution and metabolic fate of thyrotropin. In: *Thyrotropin*, Chapter VI, pp. 95–128. Editor: S. C. Werner. Charles C. Thomas, Springfield, Ill.

BAKKE, J. L. (1966): Some factors affecting thyroid stimulating hormone (TSH) synthesis, secretion, serum titers, and effects. In: *Endemic Goiter and Allied Diseases*, pp. 283–289. Editors: K. Silink and K. Cerny. Slovak Academy of Sciences, Bratislava, Czechoslovakia.

BAKKE, J. L. and LAWRENCE, N. L. (1962): Disappearance rate and distribution of exogenous thyrotropin in the rat. *Endocrinology, 71*, 43.

BAKKE, J. L. and LAWRENCE, N. (1965*a*): Circadian periodicity in thyroid stimulating hormone titer in rat hypophysis and serum. *Metabolism, 14*, 841.

BAKKE, J. L. and LAWRENCE, N. (1965*b*): Effect of dinitrophenol on pituitary-thyroid activity in the rat. *Endocrinology, 77*, 382.

BAUGH, C. M., KRUMDIECK, C. L., HERSHMAN, J. M. and PITTMAN, J. A. (1970): Synthesis and biological activity of thyrotropin-releasing hormone. *Endocrinology*, *87*, 1015.

BESSER, G. M., ORTH, D. N., NICHOLSON, W. E. and ABE, K. (1969): Dissociation of biological and radioimmunological disappearance rates and concentrations of plasma ACTH in man. *Clin. Res.*, *17*, 280.

BLUM, A. S., GREENSPAN, F. S. and MAGNUM, J. (1968): Circadian rhythm of serum TSH in normal human subjects. In: *Third International Congress of Endocrinology*, p. 14. Editor: C. Gual. ICS No. 157. Excerpta Medica, Amsterdam.

BOLER, J., ENZMANN, F., FOLKERS, K., BOWERS, C. Y. and SCHALLY, A. V. (1969): The identity of chemical and hormonal properties of the thyrotropin releasing hormone and pyroglutamyl-histidyl-proline amide. *Biochem. biophys. Res. Commun.*, *37*, 705.

BOWERS, C. Y., REDDING, T. W. and HAWLEY, W. D. (1966): The effect of thyrotrophin-releasing factor (TRF) in animals and man. In: *Program of the Forty-Eighth Meeting of the Endocrine Society*, p. 48.

BOWERS, C. Y., REDDING, T. W. and SCHALLY, A. V. (1965): Effect of thyrotropin releasing factor (TRF) of ovine, bovine, porcine and human origin on thyrotropin release *in vitro* and *in vivo*. *Endocrinology*, *77*, 609.

BOWERS, C. Y. and SCHALLY, A. V. (1970): Assay of thyrotropin-releasing hormone. In: *Hypophysiotropic Hormone of the Hypothalamus: Assay and Chemistry*, Chapter 6, pp. 74–89. Editor: J. Meites. Williams and Wilkins, Baltimore, Md.

BOWERS, C. Y., SCHALLY, A. V., ENZMANN, F., BOLER, J. and FOLKERS, K. (1969): Discovery of hormonal activity of synthetic tripeptides structurally related to thyrotropic releasing hormone. In: *Program of the Forty-Fifth Meeting of the American Thyroid Association, Inc.*, p. 15.

BOWERS, C. Y., SCHALLY, A. V., HAWLEY, W. D., GUAL, C. and PARLOW, A. (1968): Effect of thyrotropin-releasing factor in man. *J. clin. Endocr.*, *28*, 978.

BOWERS, C. Y., SCHALLY, A. V., REYNOLDS, G. A. and HAWLEY, W. D. (1967): Interactions of L-thyroxine or L-triiodothyronine and thyrotropin-releasing factor on the release and synthesis of thyrotropin from the anterior pituitary gland of mice. *Endocrinology*, *81*, 741.

BOWERS, C. Y., SCHALLY, A. V., SCHALCH, D. C., GUAL, C., KASTIN, A. J., CASTANEDA, E. and FOLKERS, K. (1970*a*): Synthetic thyrotropin releasing hormone (TRH): effect in man. In: *Program of the Fifty-Second Meeting of the Encodrine Society*, p. 41.

BOWERS, C. Y., SCHALLY, A. V., SCHALCH, D. S., GUAL, C., KASTIN, A. J. and FOLKERS, K. (1970*b*): Activity and specificity of synthetic thyrotropin-releasing hormone in man. *Biochem. biophys. Res. Commun.*, *39*, 352.

BOWERS, C. Y., SCHALLY, A. V., WEIL, A., REYNOLDS, G. A. and FOLKERS, K. (1970): Chemical and biological identity of thyrotropin releasing hormone (TRH) of bovine and human origin. In: *Abstracts of the Sixth International Thyroid Conference*, p. 129. G. Gistel, Vienna, Austria.

BRAVERMAN, L. E., INGBAR, S. H. and STERLING, K. (1970): Conversion of thyroxine (T_4) to triiodothyronine (T_3) in athyreotic human subjects. *J. clin. Invest.*, *49*, 855.

BURGUS, R., DUNN, T. F., DESIDERIO, S. and GUILLEMIN, R. (1969): Structure moléculaire du facteur hypothalamique hypophysiotrope TRF d'origine ovine: mise en évidence par spectrométrie de masse de la séquence PCA-His-Pro-NH_2. *C.R. Acad. Sci. D: Sciences Naturelles*, *269*, 1870.

BURGUS, R., DUNN, T. F., DESIDERIO, D., WARD, D. N., VALE, W. and GUILLEMIN, R. (1970): Characterization of ovine hypothalamic hypophysiotropic TSH-releasing factor. *Nature (Lond.)*, *226*, 321.

BURR, I. M., SIZONENKO, P. C., KAPLAN, S. L. and GRUMBACK, M. M. (1969): Observations on the binding of human TSH by antisera to human chorionic gonadotropin. *J. clin. Endocr.*, *29*, 691.

BUTTFIELD, I. H., HETZEL, B. S. and ODELL, W. D. (1968): Effect of iodized oil on serum TSH determined by immunoassay in endemic goiter subjects. *J. clin. Endocr.*, *28*, 1664.

COHEN, J. D. and UTIGER, R. D. (1970): Metastatic choriocarcinoma associated with hyperthyroidism. *J. clin. Endocr.*, *30*, 423.

CONDLIFFE, P. G. (1963*a*): In: *Thyrotropin*, Chapter XIII, p. 237. Editor: S. C. Werner. Charles C. Thomas, Springfield, Ill.

CONDLIFFE, P. G. (1963*b*): Purification of human thyrotrophin. *Endocrinology*, *72*, 893.

CONFLIFFE, P. G. and ROBBINS, J. (1967): Pituitary thyroid-stimulating hormone and other thyroid-stimulating substances. In: *Hormones in Blood, 2nd ed.*, Vol. I, Chapter XIV, pp. 333–381. Editors: C. H. Gray and A. L. Bacharach. Academic Press, New York.

CONWAY, L. W., SCHALCH, D. S., UTIGER, R. D. and REICHLIN, S. (1969): Hormones in human pituitary sinusoid blood: concentration of LH, GH, and TSH. *J. clin. Endocr.*, *29*, 446.

DeLange, F., Hershman, J. M. and Ermans, A. M. (1970): Blood TSH level Idjwi Island; modification related to the regional prevalence of goiter and not to individual thyroid size and function. In: *Proceedings of the Sixth International Thyroid Congress*, p. 7.

Ducommun, P., Sakiz, E. and Guillemin, R. (1966): Dissociation of the acute secretions of thyrotropin and adrenocorticotropin. *Amer. J. Physiol.*, *210*, 1257.

DuRuisseau, D. P. (1965): Seasonal variation of PBI in healthy Montrealers. *J. clin. Endocr.*, *25*, 1513.

Einhorn, J. (1958): Studies on the effect of thyrotropic hormone on the thyroid function. *Acta radiol., Suppl.*, *160*, 1.

Field, J. B. (1968): Studies on the mechanism of action of thyroid-stimulating hormone. *Metabolism*, *17*, 226.

Fisher, D. A. and Odell, W. D. (1969): Acute release of thyrotropin in the newborn. *J. clin. Invest.*, *48*, 1670.

Fleischer, N., Burgus, R., Vale, W., Dunn, T. and Guillemin, R. (1970): Preliminary observations of the effect of synthetic thyrotropin releasing factor on plasma thyrotropin levels in man. *J. clin. Endocr.*, *31*, 109.

Folkers, K., Enzmann, F., Boler, J., Bowers, C. Y. and Schally, A. V. (1969): Discovery of modification of the synthetic tripeptide-sequence of the thyrotropin releasing hormone having activity. *Biochem. biophys. Res. Commun.*, *37*, 123.

Geschwind, I. I. (1970): Mechanism of action of hypothalamic adenohypophysiotropic factors. In: *Hypophysiotropic Hormones of the Hypothalamus: Assay and Chemistry*, Chapter 20, pp. 298–319. Editor: J. Meites. Williams and Wilkins, Baltimore, Md.

Gilbert-Dreyfus, Sebaoun, J., Delzant, G., Outzekhovsky, G. and Gali, P. (1964): Exploration de la fonction thyroidienne dans les panhypopituitarismes, les tumeurs hypophysaires et chez les hypophysectomisés (à la lumière de 30 cas personnels). *Ann. Endocr. (Paris)*, *25*, *Suppl.*, 699.

Goldberg, R. C. (1954): Thyroid pituitary relationships as affected by pyrogenic agents. *Fed. Proc.*, *13*, 56.

Goldberg, R. C., Wolff, J. and Greep, R. O. (1955): Mechanism of depression of plasma protein bound iodine by 2, 4 dinitrophenol. *Endocrinology*, *56*, 560.

Grad, B., and Hoffman M. M. (1955): Thyroxine secretion rates and plasma cholesterol levels of young and old rats. *Amer. J. Physiol.*, *182*, 497.

Greenberg, A. H., Czernichow, P., Hung, W., Schelley, W., Winship, T. and Blizzard, R. M. (1970): Juvenile chronic lymphocytic thyroiditis: clinical, laboratory and histological correlations. *J. clin. Endocr.*, *30*, 293.

Guillemin, R. (1970): In: *Hypophysiotropic Hormones of the Hypothalamus: Assay and Chemistry*, Chapter 20, pp. 315. Editor: J. Meites. Williams and Wilkins, Baltimore, Md.

Hall, R., Amos, J., Garry, R. and Buxton, R. L. (1970): Thyroid-stimulating hormone response to synthetic thyrotrophin releasing hormone in man. *Brit. med. J.*, *2*, 274.

Harris, G. W. (1964): A summary of some recent research on brain-thyroid relationships. In: *Ciba Foundation Study Group No. 18 Brain-Thyroid Relationships*, pp. 3–16. Editors: M. P. Cameron and M. O'Connor. Little, Brown, Boston, Mass.

Harris, G. W., Levine, S. and Schindler, W. J. (1964): Vasopressin and thyroid function in the rat: the effect of oestrogens. *J. Physiol.*, *170*, 516.

Harris, G. W. and Woods, J. W. (1958): The effect of electrical stimulation of the hypothalamus or pituitary gland on thyroid activity. *J. Physiol.*, *143*, 246.

Hennen, G., Pierce, J. G. and Freychet, P. (1969): Human chorionic thyrotropin: further characterization and study of its secretion during pregnancy. *J. clin. Endocr.*, *29*, 581.

Hershman, J. M. (1970): Different slopes of the dose-response curves of human and bovine TSH in the McKenzie bioassay. *Endocrinology*, *86*, 1004.

Hershman, J. M. (1969): Molecular heterogeneity of human TSH. *Program of the Forty-fifth Meeting, American Thyroid Association, Inc.*, p. 31.

Hershman, J. M., Higgins, H. P. and Starnes, W. R. (1970*a*): Differences between thyroid stimulator in hydatiform mole and human chorionic thyrotropin. *Metabolism*, *19*, 735.

Hershman, J. M. and Pittman, J. A., Jr. (1970): Response to synthetic thyrotropin-releasing hormone in man. *J. clin. Endocr.*, *31*, 457.

Hershman, J. M., Read, D. G., Bailey, A. L., Norman, V. D. and Gibson, T. B. (1970*b*): Effect of cold exposure on serum thyrotropin. *J. clin. Endocr.*, *30*, 430.

Hershman, J. M., Read, D. G., Gibson, T. B. and Bailey, A. L. (1969): Utility of the radioimmunoassay of serum thyrotropin. *Ann. intern. Med.*, *70*, 1062.

HERSHMAN, J. M. and STARNES, W. R. (1969): Extraction and characterization of a thyrotropic material from the human placenta. *J. clin. Invest.*, *48*, 923.

JENSEN, S. E. (1969): A new way of measuring thyrotropin (TSH) reserve. *J. clin. Endocr.*, *29*, 409.

KLEIBER, M. (1961*a*): *The Fire of Life: An Introduction to Animal Energetics*, pp. 166–216. Wiley, New York.

KLEIBER, M. (1961*b*): Death from starvation. In: *The Fire of Life: An Introduction to Animal Experiments*, Chapter 13, pp. 238–249. Wiley, New York.

KRÜSKEMPER, H. L. and REICHERTZ, P. (1959): Elektrographischer Nachweis der Wirkung von thyreotropem Hormon an Meerschweinchen. *Klin. Wschr.*, *37/12*, 717.

LANG, S. and REICHLIN, S. (1961): Time course of thyroid response to rising and to falling blood levels of thyroxine. *Proc. Soc. exp. Biol. (N.Y.)*, *108*, 789.

LANGER, P. (1970): Change in thyroidal radioiodine following exchange transfusion in rats. In: *Proceedings of the International Thyroid Conference*, Smolenice, Czechoslovakia.

LARSEN, P. R., ATKINSON, A. J., JR., WELLMAN, H. N. and GOLDSMITH, R. E. (1970): The effect of diphenylhydantoin on thyroxine metabolism in man. *J. clin. Invest.*, *49*, 1266.

LEMARCHAND-BERAUD, T. and VANNOTTI, A. (1969): Relationships between blood thyrotrophin level, protein bound iodine and free thyroxine concentration in man under normal physiological conditions. *Acta endocr. (Kbh.)*, *60*, 315.

LOHRENZ, F. N., FERNANDEZ, R. and DOE, R. P. (1964): Isolated thyrotropin deficiency: review and report of three cases. *Ann. intern. Med.*, *60*, 990.

MARTIN, J. B. and REICHLIN, S. (1970): Thyrotropin secretion in rats after hypothalamic electrical stimulation or injection of synthetic TSH-releasing factor. *Science*, *168*, 1366.

MEITES, J. (1970): Direct studies of the secretion of the hypothalamic hypophysiotropic hormones (HHH). In: *Hypophysiotropic Hormones of the Hypothalamus: Assay and Chemistry*, Chapter 18, pp. 261–281. Editor: J. Meites. Williams and Wilkins, Baltimore, Md.

MITTLER, J. C., REDDING, T. W. and SCHALLY, A. V. (1969): Stimulation of thyrotropin (TSH) secretion by TSH-releasing factor (TRF) in organ cultures of anterior pituitary. *Proc. Soc. exp. Biol. (N.Y.)*, *130*, 406.

MIYAI, K., FUKUCHI, M. and KUMAHARA, Y. (1969): Correlation between biological and immunological potencies of human serum and pituitary thyrotropin. *J. clin. Endocr.*, *29*, 1438.

MORRIS, C. J. O. R. (1963): In: *Thyrotropin*, Chapter XIII, p. 234. Editor: S. C. Werner. Thomas, Springfield, Ill.

NICOLOFF, J. T., FISHER, D. A. and APPLEMAN, M. D. (1969): Glucocorticoid (G) regulation of thyroidal release (TR). In: *Program of Fifty-First Meeting of the Endocrine Society*, p. 72.

NICOLOFF, J. T., GROSS, H. A. and APPLEMAN, M. D. (1970): Inhibition of thyroid release (TR) by estradiol. In: *Abstracts of the Sixth International Thyroid Conference*, p. 144, G. Gistel, Vienna, Austria.

NIEPCE, B. (1851): *Traité du goitre et du crétinisme, suivi de la statistique des goitreux et des crétins dans le basin de l'Isère en Savoie, dans les départements de l'Isère, des Hautes-Alpes et des Basses-Alpes*. Paris, France.

ODDIE, T. H., MEADE, J. H., JR. and FISHER, D. A. (1966): An analysis of published data on thyroxine turnover in human subjects. *J. clin. Endocr.*, *26*, 425.

ODELL, W. D., BATES, R. W., RIVLIN, R. S., LIPSETT, M. B. and HERTZ, R. (1963): Increased thyroid function without clinical hyperthyroidism in patients with choriocarcinoma. *J. clin. Endocr.*, *23*, 658.

ODELL, W. D., UTIGER, R. D., WILBER, J. F. and CONDLIFFE, P. G. (1967*a*): Estimation of the secretion rate of thyrotropin in man. *J. clin. Invest.*, *46*, 959.

ODELL, W. D., VANSLAGER, L. and BATES, R. (1968): In: *Radioisotopes in Medicine: In Vitro Studies*, p. 185. Editors: R. L. Hayes, F. H. Goswitz and B. E. P. Murphy. U.S. Atomic Energy Commission, Oak Ridge, Tenn.

ODELL, W. D., WILBER, J. F. and PAUL, W. E. (1965): Radioimmunoassay of human thyrotropin in serum. *Metabolism*, *14*, 465.

ODELL, W. D., WILBER, J. F. and UTIGER, R. D. (1967*b*): Studies of thyrotropin physiology by means of radioimmunoassay. *Rec. Progr. Hormone Res.*, *23*, 47.

PITTMAN, C. S., CHAMBERS, J. B., JR. and READ, V. H. (1970*a*): The rate of extrathyroidal conversion of thyroxine to triiodothyronine in man. *J. clin. Invest.*, *49*, 75a.

PITTMAN, J. A., JR.: Hypopituitarism. In: *The Thyroid*, 3rd Edition. Editors: S. C. Werner and S. H. Ingbar. Harper and Row.

PITTMAN, J. A. JR. (1962): The thyroid and aging. *J. Amer. geriat. Soc.*, *10*, 10.

PITTMAN, J. A., JR., BESCHI, R. J., GIBBS, L. L. and BLOCK, P., JR. (1969): Studies with 3,3′, 5-trichloro-DL-thyronine and a hypothesis for a test of physical TSH reserve. *Endocrinology*, *84*, 976.

PITTMAN, J. A., DUBOVSKY, E. and BESCHI, R. J. (1970*b*): Stimulation of pituitary glucose oxidation by thyrotropin-releasing hormone. *Biochem. biophys. Res. Commun.*, *40*, 1246.

PORTER, J. C., GOLDMAN, B. D. and WILBER, J. F. (1970): Hypophysiotropic hormones in portal vessel blood. In: *Hypophysiotropic Hormones of the Hypothalamus*, Chapter 19, pp. 282–297. Editor: J. Meites. Williams and Wilkins, Baltimore, Md.

POWELL, G. F. and BLIZZARD, R. M. (1966): An attempt to establish a test for thyrotropin (TSH) reserve. *J. clin. Endocr.*, *26*, 1389.

RAUD, H. R. and ODELL, W. D. (1969): The radioimmunoassay of human thyrotropin. *Brit. J. Hosp. Med.*, *2*, 1366.

READ, D. G., HERSHMAN, J. M. and PITTMAN, J. A., JR. (1969): Effect of vasopressin infusions on thyroidal radioiodine uptake and serum TSH concentration. *J. clin. Endocr.*, *29*, 1496.

REDDING, T. W. and SCHALLY, A. V. (1967): Depletion of pituitary thyrotropic hormone by thyrotropin releasing factor. *Endocrinology*, *81*, 918.

REDDING, T. W. and SCHALLY, A. V. (1969*a*): Studies on the inactivation of thyrotropin-releasing hormone (TRH). *Proc. Soc. exp. Biol. (N.Y.)*, *131*, 415.

REDDING, T. W. and SCHALLY, A. V. (1969*b*): Studies on the thyrotropin-releasing hormone (TRH) activity in peripheral blood. *Proc. Soc. exp. Biol. (N.Y.)*, *131*, 420.

REICHLIN, S. (1966): Control of thyrotropin hormone secretion. In: *Neuroendocrinology*, Vol. I, Chapter 12, pp. 445–536. Editors: L. Martini and W. F. Ganong. Academic Press, New York.

REICHLIN, S. (1964): Function of the hypothalamus in regulation of pituitary-thyroid activity. In: *Ciba Foundation Study Group No. 18 Brain-Thyroid Relationships*, pp. 17–34. Editors: M. P. Cameron and M. O'Connor. Little, Brown, Boston, Mass.

REICHLIN, S. and UTIGER, R. D. (1967): Regulation of the pituitary-thyroid axis in man: relationship of TSH concentration to concentration of free and total thyroxine in plasma. *J. clin. Endocr.*, *27*, 251.

ROBIN, N. I., REFOTOFF, S., FAN, V. and SELENKOW, H. A. (1969): Parameters of thyroid function in maternal and cord serum at term pregnancy. *J. clin. Endocr.*, *29*, 1276.

ROGOWITSCH, N. (1889): Die Veränderungen der Hypophyse nach Entfernung der Schilddrüse. *Beitr. path. Anat.*, *4*, 453.

RYAN, R. J., SWANSON, D. W., FAIMAR, C., MAYBERRY, W. E. and SPADONI, A. J. (1970): Effects of convulsive electroshock on serum concentrations of follicle stimulating hormone, luteinizing hormones, thyroid stimulating hormone and growth hormone in man. *J. clin. Endocr.*, *30*, 51.

SAWIN, C. T., HERSHMAN, J. M., HANDLER, S. D. and UTIGER, R. D. (1970): Attempts to augment thyrotropin secretion: effects of methimazole, methimazole-iodide, vasopressin, and glucagon. *Metabolism*, *19*, 488.

SCHALLY, A. V., AVIMURA, A., BOWERS, C. Y., KASTIN, A. J., SAWANO, S. and REDDING, T. W. (1968): Hypothalamic neurohormones regulating anterior pituitary function. *Rec. Progr. Hormone Res.*, *24*, 497.

SCHALLY, A. V., BOWERS, C. Y. and REDDING, T. W. (1966): Purification of thyrotropic hormone-releasing factor from bovine hypothalamus. *Endocrinology*, *78*, 726.

SCHALLY, A. V. and REDDING, T. W. (1967): *In vitro* studies with thyrotropin releasing factor. *Proc. Soc. exp. Biol. (N.J.)*, *126*, 320.

SHOCK, N. W. (1960): In: *The Biology of Aging*, p. 258. Editor: B. L. Strehler. American Institute of Biological Sciences, Washington, D.C.

SMITH, P. E. (1916): Experimental ablation of the hypophysis in the frog embryo. *Science*, *16*, 280.

SMITH, P. E. and SMITH, I. P. (1922): Repair and activation of thyroid in hypophysectomized tadpole by parenteral administration of fresh anterior lobe of bovine hypophysis. *J. med. Res.*, *43*, 267.

SOLOMON, D. H. (1963): The effects of thyrotropin on thyroidal transfers of water and electrolytes. In: *Thyrotropin*, Chapter X, pp. 178–194. Editor: S. C. Werner. Thomas, Springfield, Ill.

SOLOMON, D. H. (1960): Enhancement of thyroidal water content and uptake of ^{24}Na after TSH administration. *Biochim. biophys. Acta (Amst.)*, *43*, 346.

SONENBERG, M., MONEY, W. L., BERMAN, M., BRENER, J. and RAWSON, R. W. (1957): Inhibition of thyrotrophic activity with chemically modified thyrotrophin preparations. *Trans. Ass. Amer. Phycns*, *70*, 192.

STEINER, A. L., PEAKE, G. T., UTIGER, R. D., KARL, I. E. and KIPNIS, D. M. (1970): Hypothalamic stimulation of growth hormone and thyrotropin release *in vitro* and pituitary 3′ 5′-adenosine cyclic monophosphate. *Endocrinology*, *86*, 1354.

STERLING, K. (1970): The significance of circulating triiodothyronine. *Rec. Progr. Hormone Res.*, *26*, 249.

STERLING, K., BELLABARBA, D., NEWMAN, E. S. and BRENNER, M. A. (1969): Determination of triiodothyronine concentration in human serum. *J. clin. Invest.*, *48*, 1150.

STERLING, K. and BRENNER, M. A. (1966): Free thyroxine in human serum: simplified measurement with the aid of magnesium precipitation. *J. clin. Invest.*, *45*, 155.

STUDER, H., WYSS, F. and JFF, H. W. (1964): A TSH reserve test for detection of mild secondary hypothyroidism. *J. clin. Endocr.*, *24*, 964.

STURTEVANT, F. M. (1955): Effect of 2 steroid analysis on organ weights of intact and hypophysectomized rats. *Endocrinology*, *56*, 256.

UTIGER, R. D. (1965): Radioimmunoassay of human plasma thyrotropin. *J. clin. Invest.*, *44*, 1277.

UTIGER, R. D., ODELL, W. D. and CONDLIFFE, P. G. (1963): Immunologic studies of purified human and bovine thyrotropin. *Endocrinology*, *73*, 359.

VALE, W., BURGES, R., DUNN, T. F. and GUILLEMIN, R. (1970): Release of TSH by oral administration of a synthetic peptide derivative of TRF activity. *J. clin. Endocr.*, *30*, 148.

VANMIDDLESWORTH, L. (1954): Radioactive iodide uptake of normal newborn infants. *Amer. J. Dis. Child.*, *88*, 439.

VILKKI, P. (1961): *In vitro* studies on phospholipid metabolism of the thyroid. In: *Advances in Thyroid Research*, p. 231. Editor: R. Pitt-Rivers. Pergamon Press, New York.

WILBER, J. F. (1970): Stimulation of thyrotropin (TSH) synthesis by thyrotropin releasing factor (TRF) and 59 mM K. In: *The Fifty-Second Meeting of the Endocrine Society*, p. 42.

WILBER, J. F. and BAUM, D. (1970): Elevation of plasma TSH during surgical hypothermia. *J. clin. Endocr.*, *31*, 372.

WILBER, J. F. and UTIGER, R. D. (1967): Immunoassay studies of thyrotropin in rat pituitary glands and serum. *Endocrinology*, *81*, 145.

WILBER, J. F. and UTIGER, R. D. (1970): The effect of glucocorticoids on thyrotropin secretion. *J. clin. Invest.*, *48*, 2096.

WOEBER, K. A., SOBEL, R. J., INGBAR, S. H. and STERLING, K. (1970): The peripheral metabolism of triiodothyronine in normal subjects and in patients with hyperthyroidism. *J. clin. Invest.*, *49*, 643.

YAMADA, T., IINO, S. and GREER, M. A. (1961): Comparison of the effect of hypophysectomy and thyroxine administration in thyroid function in the rat. *Endocrinology*, *69*, 1.

LATS AND GRAVES' DISEASE: CLINICAL AND RADIOIMMUNOLOGICAL STUDIES*

A. PINCHERA, L. ROVIS, C. DAVOLI, L. GRASSO and L. BASCHIERI

Istituto di Medicina del Lavoro, University of Pisa, Pisa, Italy, and II Clinica Medica, University of Rome, Rome, Italy

About 14 years ago Adams and Purves first described the presence in some patients with Graves' disease of a thyroid-stimulating substance which differed from thyrotropin (TSH) in the time course of its effects on the thyroid. Since then, it has been clearly established that this substance, now known as the long-acting thyroid stimulator (LATS), is a separate entity having the properties of an immunoglobulin G (IgG) (McKenzie, 1968).

The object of the present paper is to report some recent data on the LATS changes occurring during antithyroid drug therapy and the results of a radioimmunological study on the interaction between LATS and thyroid tissue. Before describing these investigations, however, we would like to comment briefly on current concepts of the clinical role and the nature of LATS.

CLINICAL ROLE AND NATURE OF LATS

The discovery of LATS and the availability of sensitive radioimmunological methods for the measurement of TSH in the blood have led to the development of new concepts of the pathogenesis of Graves' disease. As shown by Utiger (1965) and by Odell *et al.* (1965), active hyperthyroidism is associated with low or, at most, normal levels of circulating TSH. Furthermore, clinical (Adams and Kennedy, 1965) and histochemical (Ezrin and Murray, 1963) evidence for a normally functioning TSH secretion mechanism has been obtained in patients with Graves' disease. These and other data seem to exclude the possibility that, in this condition, hyperthyroidism is sustained by an excessive and unregulated secretion of thyrotropin.

While its pathogenetic role in the infiltrative ophthalmopathy and the pretibial myxedema remains to be clarified, considerable evidence has been accumulated to suggest that LATS may be responsible for the maintainance, if not for the onset, of the thyroid hyperfunction of Graves' disease (McKenzie, 1968). This hypothesis has been recently questioned by Chopra *et al.* (1970), on the basis of their finding of a dissociation of serum LATS content and thyroid suppressibility. These results, however, have not been confirmed in a similar study carried out by other workers (Harden *et al.*, 1970). Clearly further investigations are required to elucidate this problem. Most of the other objections to the causative role of LATS have been extensively discussed by McKenzie (1968).

The demonstration that the biological activity of LATS is an inherent property of an IgG structure (Kriss *et al.*, 1964; Meek *et al.*, 1964) has led to the hypothesis that LATS is an anti-

* This work was supported by the USPHS (Grants AM-11030 and TW-00184) and by the Consiglio Nazionale delle Ricerche (Contract No. 69.01750).

body. The following data suggest that its postulated antigen may be localized in the thyroid and possibly in the plasma membrane of the follicular cells. Thyroid subcellular fractions have been shown to inhibit LATS (Kriss *et al.*, 1964) and their inhibitory activity seems to be correlated with the presence of 5′-nucleotidase (Beall *et al.*, 1969), which is considered an enzyme marker for plasma membrane. Partial recovery of the LATS activity inhibited by the thyroid may be obtained by the use of an elution procedure, known to disrupt antigen-antibody complexes (Beall and Solomon, 1966). A transient rise in the level of circulating LATS has been observed after radioiodine therapy of Graves' disease (Kriss *et al.*; Pinchera *et al.*, 1969). The time course of these changes is consistent with the viewpoint that the radiation damage leads to an anamnestic LATS response by temporarily increasing the availability of the antigen to the immune system. As shown in our laboratory (Pinchera *et al.*, 1965) and confirmed by other workers (McKenzie, 1967; Beall and Solomon, 1968), sera from rabbits immunized with human thyroid tissue may elicit LATS-like responses in McKenzie's bioassay. Solomon *et al.* (1970) have recently demonstrated that these responses are due, at least in part, to the release of thyroidal iodine indicating a real thyroid-stimulating effect.

The concept that an antithyroid antibody activates rather than inhibits the function of its target organ should not be regarded as surprising, since several antibody molecules have been found to augment rather than decrease enzyme activity. This has been reported for antibodies directed against such enzymes as amylase, penicillinase and ribonuclease (Suzuki *et al.*, 1969). As far as LATS is concerned, a number of studies have provided clear evidence that this substance has a true stimulatory action on the thyroid gland, involving the adenyl cyclase-cyclic AMP system (McKenzie, 1968). Furthermore, morphological studies have failed so far to demonstrate any damaging effect of LATS on the thyroid (Sharard, 1969). As described by Ochi and DeGroot (1969), this is also true when chronic rather than acute effects are considered. Electron microscopic evidence for the thyroid-stimulating property of LATS has been obtained in our laboratory (Tonietti *et al.*, 1968). As illustrated in Figure 1, the injection of LATS to thyroxine-treated mice was followed by the formation of pseudopods projecting into the follicular cavity and the appearance of large colloid droplets and of cytosegregosomes resulting from the fusion of colloid droplets with lysosomes. These changes were virtually indistinguishable from those produced by TSH, with the exception that the effects of LATS occurred later and lasted for a longer period of time. This finding is in agreement with other data suggesting that the two substances act on the same receptor site (Burke, 1969).

EFFECTS OF ANTITHYROID DRUGS ON LATS

The question whether treatment of toxic diffuse goiter influences the level of LATS has been the object of several studies. We have previously observed that during the administration of methimazole or propylthiouracil circulating LATS tends to decrease if initially present and to remain undetectable in the subjects with negative assays prior to therapy (Pinchera *et al.*, 1969). Similar results have been recently reported by at least two other laboratories (Chopra *et al.*, 1970; Harden *et al.*, 1970). Since spontaneous fluctuations in LATS activity may also occur, these data do not necessarily indicate that the drug therapy is responsible for the LATS changes. In this respect, more indicative may be the different behavior observed between a group of patients with toxic diffuse goiter submitted to a combined therapy with ^{131}I and methimazole and a comparable group treated with radioiodine alone. As illustrated in Figure 2, the addition of methimazole 7–10 days after the administration of a therapeutic dose of ^{131}I seemed to prevent the rise of LATS which was noted in several patients treated only with radioiodine.

On the basis of these observations, it was considered of interest to study the effects of methimazole on euthyroid subjects with positive LATS assays. So far two such patients have been investigated. Both of them had a past history of thyrotoxicosis and clinical and labora-

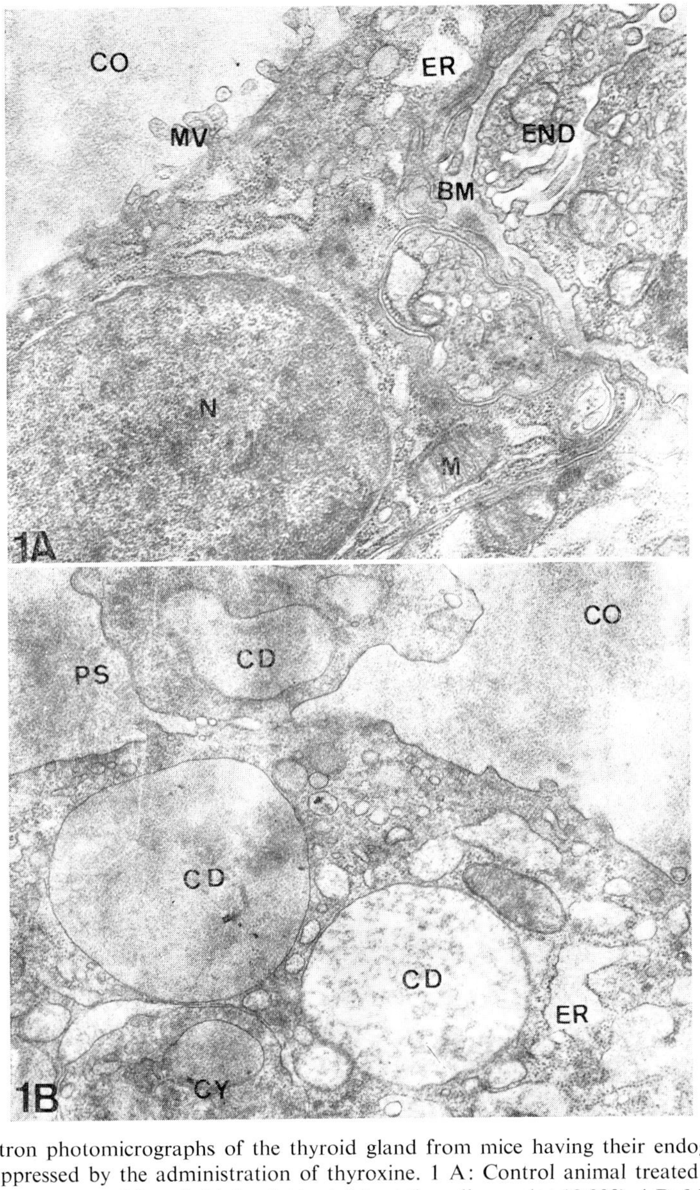

Fig. 1. Electron photomicrographs of the thyroid gland from mice having their endogenous TSH secretion suppressed by the administration of thyroxine. 1 A: Control animal treated with 0.5 ml of normal human serum. No colloid droplet is visible at the cell apex (× 18,000). 1 B: Mouse treated with 0.5 ml of a potent LATS serum (72 hr after the injection). Note the presence of a pseudopod and of large colloid droplets. A cytosegregosome is also visible (× 27,500). Figures were reduced 20% for reproduction.

Key: BM = follicular basement membrane; CD = colloid droplet; CO = follicular cavity; CY = cytosegregosome; END = endothelium of perifollicular capillary; ER = endoplasmic reticulum; M = mitochondrion; MV = microvilli; N = nucleus; PS = pseudopod. (From Tonietti *et al.*, 1968).

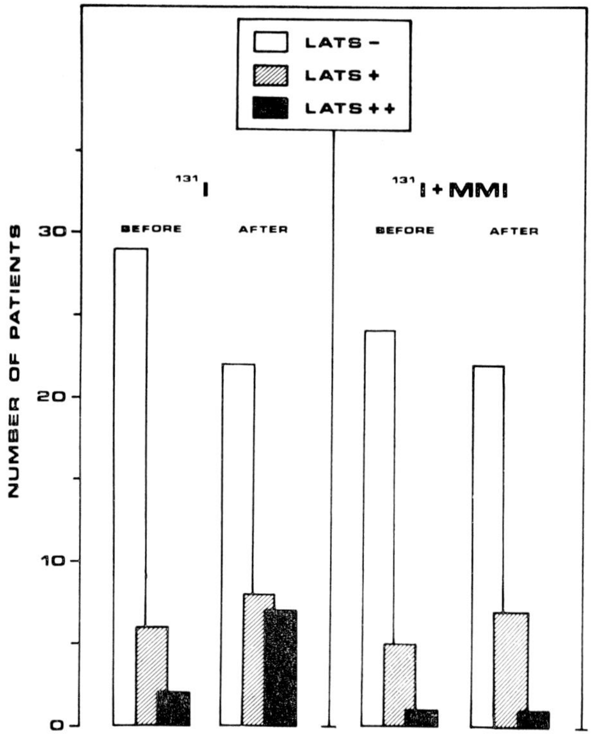

Fig. 2. Serum LATS activity before and after treatment of toxic diffuse goiter with either radioiodine alone (^{131}I) or radioiodine supplemented with methimazole (^{131}I + MMI). The mean doses of ^{131}I given to the 2 groups of patients were similar: 10.3 and 11.2 mCi, respectively. Methimazole was added 7-10 days after the administration of ^{131}I at the daily dose of 30 mg for 3 weeks and of 5–15 mg for 2–4 months. Post-treatment samples were drawn 46–180 days after radioiodine therapy. An increase in the number of patients with detectable LATS and particularly of those with high LATS activity (LATS ++) was observed in the group treated with radioiodine alone. No such increase was noted in the other group. Further details on this study will be presented elsewhere (Martino *et al.*, in press).

tory evidence of euthyroidism. Other pertinent data are given under Figures 3 and 4. LATS assays were performed before, during and after administration of methimazole. Triiodothyronine was added to maintain the euthyroid state. In order to avoid fluctuations in the response of different batches of animals, samples of the same subject were tested in a single bioassay. Serial assays showed that in both patients LATS activity was stable for at least two months prior to treatment, whereas a significant fall occurred during the course of the drug therapy. These data provide further support to the view that antithyroid drugs, such as methimazole, interfere with the production of LATS. If this is the case, the following explanations may be considered: 1. Antithyroid drugs have a direct action on the antibody-forming system. This is not consistent with the negative data provided by a screening test for the detection of immunosuppressive agents, which showed no evidence that methimazole decreases the immune response of mice immunized with sheep red-blood cells (Pinchera *et al.*, 1969). 2. Antithyroid drugs act on the antibody-forming system by reducing the level of the thyroid hormone. This explanation did not receive support from the observation reported here that a fall of LATS may also occur in euthyroid patients receiving methimazole and

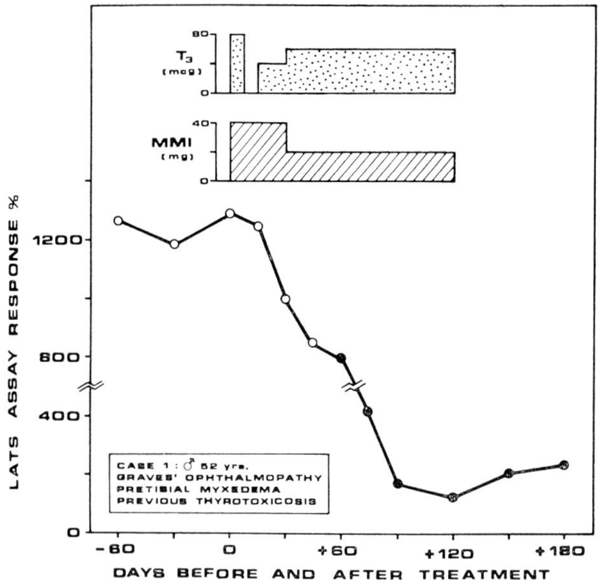

Fig. 3. Changes in the LATS level in a patient with a past history of thyrotoxicosis treated with methimazole (MMI) and triiodothyronine (T3). This subject had severe infiltrative ophthalmopathy and active pretibial myxedema and was euthyroid 2 years after radioiodine therapy. Both the eye signs and the skin changes improved during the treatment. All samples were tested in a single bioassay. Closed circles indicate values differing significantly ($p < 0.05$) from the pre-treatment level.

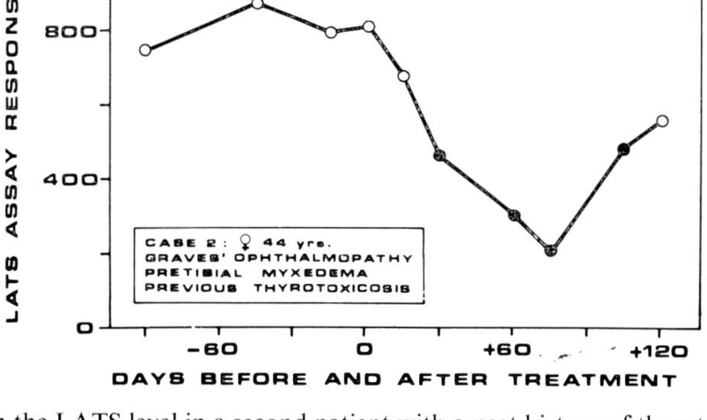

Fig. 4. Changes in the LATS level in a second patient with a past history of thyrotoxicosis treated as described under Fig. 3. This subject had severe infiltrative ophthalmopathy and pretibial myxedema and was euthyroid 5 years after radioiodine therapy. Improvement of the skin changes but not of the eye signs was noted during treatment. All samples were tested in a single bioassay. Symbols as in Fig. 3.

triiodothyronine. 3. Antithyroid drugs interfere with the production of LATS by reducing the antigen availability to the immune system or by modifying its antigenic properties. This possibility is at present conjectural and further investigations are required to establish its validity.

RADIOIMMUNOLOGICAL STUDIES ON THE INTERACTION BETWEEN LATS AND THYROID TISSUE

The inhibition of LATS activity by the thyroid has been interpreted as evidence for binding of LATS to its antigen. The possibility of using this binding reaction as a model for an *in vitro* LATS assay has been explored by an application of the paired label radioantibody technique. Details of the methods have been reported elsewhere (Pinchera *et al.*, 1970). Briefly, IgG from sera eliciting high LATS responses ($> 1000\%$) and from normal human serum were labeled with ^{125}I and ^{131}I, respectively, and then mixed together. Prior to use, the radioactive mixture was supplemented with normal rabbit serum as protein carrier, and preincubated with an excess of purified human thyroglobulin in order to avoid the interference of antithyroglobulin antibodies. After removal of the insoluble material, aliquots of the preincubated mixture were added to thyroid or control sediments. These were prepared from homogenates by centrifugation for 1 hour at 30,000 or 105,000 *g*. Preliminary experiments showed that thyroid sediments fixed greater amounts of radiolabeled LATS IgG than of normal radioimmunoglobulins, but the difference was rather small. Therefore, in subsequent studies the following procedures were used to concentrate thyroid-reacting components from LATS IgG:1.5 M potassium thiocyanate, an eluting agent known to disrupt antigen-antibody complexes, was added to thyroid sediments which had been previously incubated with the mixture of radiolabeled LATS IgG and normal IgG and then washed with buffered saline. After separation by centrifugation, the eluate was fractionated by filtration through Sephadex G-200 and subsequent ammonium sulfate precipitation, to separate the IgG fraction from other eluted material. As shown in Figure 5, 3 main radioactive peaks were obtained by gel-filtration. It is of interest that the second peak, corresponding to the fraction enriched in 7 S proteins, has a higher concentration of radiolabeled components deriving from LATS IgG than from normal IgG, as indicated by the increase in the $^{125}I/^{131}I$ ratio. The major constituent of the material which could be precipitated from this fraction by treatment with 1.65 M ammonium sulfate exhibited immunoelectrophoretic properties of IgG (Fig. 6). This material was incubated with thyroid or control sediments and tested for its tissue reactivity. Results were evaluated by an uptake index, given by the ratio between the percentage of ^{125}I and ^{131}I fixed on the tissue specimen. Two separate experiments showed that, with respect to the value observed with the original mixture (1.20), a 4-fold increase in the thyroid uptake index could be obtained by the adsorption-elution procedure. Similar experiments carried out with placenta, liver and lung sediments showed no difference in the reactivity to these tissues between ^{125}I-labeled and ^{131}I-labeled components.

Since the yield of radioactivity in the active eluate fraction was rather low, further studies were carried out on LATS IgG which was labeled with ^{125}I *after* adsorption on and elution from thyroid microsomes and subsequent fractionation by gel-filtration and DEAE chromatography. Assays performed prior to iodination showed that this preparation of 'eluted' LATS IgG elicited high LATS responses, with a purification ratio of 32.8 in terms of LATS activity per mg of IgG. Aliquots of radiolabeled 'eluted' LATS IgG were submitted to a second adsorption-elution procedure. As shown in Figure 7, a high degree of reactivity to the thyroid was exhibited by these preparations of 'eluted' LATS IgG. The concentration of the thyroid-reacting components was greatly enhanced by the use of the double elution procedure. Most of these components could be removed by preincubation with thyroid tissue, whereas little change was produced by liver or lung sediments. The specificity of the interaction between radiolabeled 'eluted' LATS IgG and the thyroid was further supported by other experiments

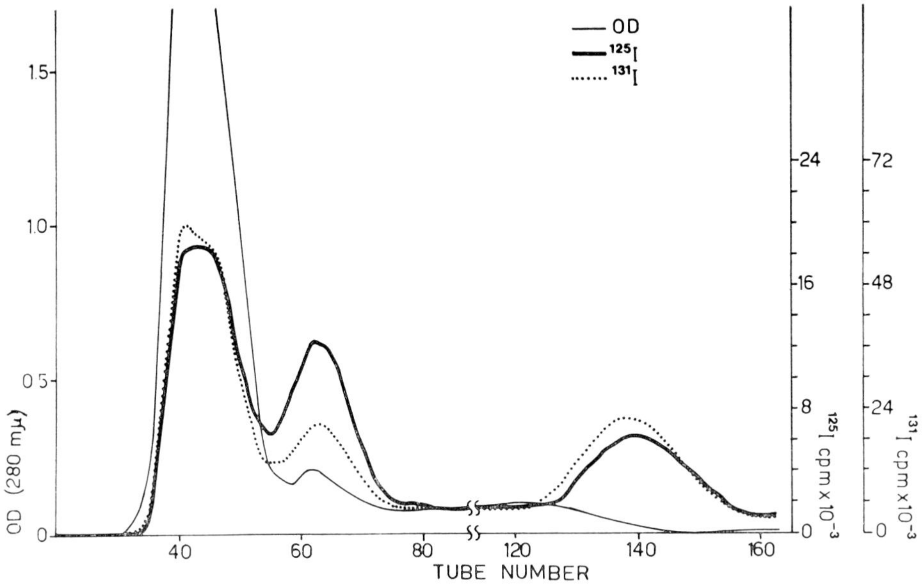

Fig. 5. Sephadex G-200 column chromatography of the radioactive material eluted by 1.5 M potassium thiocyanate (KSCN) from a thyroid sediment which was preincubated with a mixture of ^{125}I-labeled LATS IgG and ^{131}I-labeled normal IgG. Unlabeled purified thyroglobulin and normal IgG were added to the column as protein carrier. Gel-filtration was made with 1.5 M KSCN.

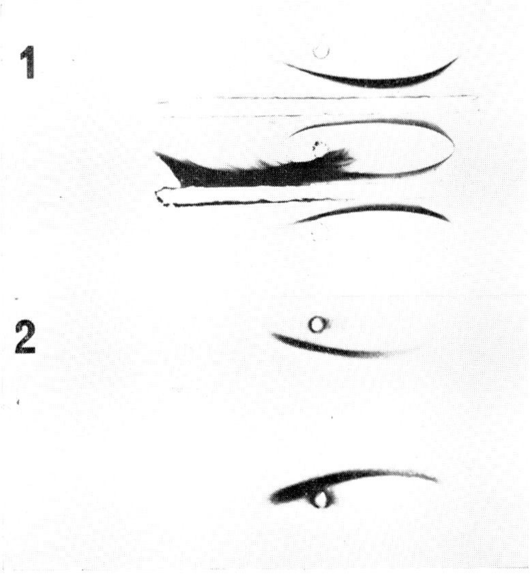

Fig. 6. Immunoelectrophoresis (1) and corresponding autoradiograph (2) of the ammonium sulfate precipitate obtained from the second Sephadex G-200 fraction of the eluate described under Fig. 5. Upper and lower well: fractionated eluate supplemented with unlabeled normal IgG. Center well: control serum. Upper trough: anti-human IgG serum. Lower trough: anti-whole serum. The anode is at the left.

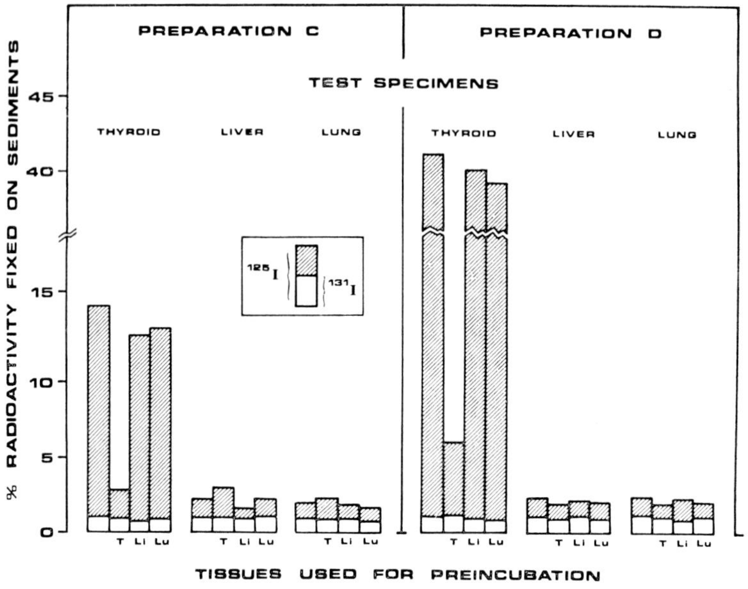

Fig. 7. Tissue reactivity of preparations of 'eluted' LATS IgG labeled with ^{125}I after adsorption on and elution from thyroid microsomes and subsequent fractionation of the eluate. A single and a double adsorption-elution procedure was used for preparations C and D, respectively. Both preparations of ^{125}I-labeled 'eluted' LATS IgG were mixed with ^{131}I-labeled normal IgG and then incubated for 1 hr at 37°C with sediments of thyroid and control tissues containing 1.5 mg of protein. The radioactivity fixed on test specimens was determined after extensive washing with buffered saline. Tests were performed before and after preincubation of the radioactive mixtures with sediments of thyroid (T), liver (Li), and lung (Lu). All values represent the mean of closely agreeing duplicates.

which showed that the addition of graded amounts of the original LATS serum resulted in a dose-dependent inhibition of the binding reaction, whereas normal human serum was not effective. Thus, in agreement with Wong and Litman (1969), a high degree of specific reactivity to the thyroid was found in preparations of LATS IgG, which were labeled with ^{125}I either before or after adsorption on and elution from thyroid sediments.

In order to ascertain whether the binding reaction described above could be attributed to LATS itself, further experiments on its inhibition were performed on LATS-positive and LATS-negative sera other than those used for the adsorption-elution procedure. While no effect was observed with any of the 15 samples from euthyroid subjects, a dose-dependent inhibition was obtained with each of the 15 sera from patients with active Graves' disease. However, no correlation was found between the degree of inhibition and the degree of LATS activity, as assessed by McKenzie's bioassay. Furthermore, a dose-dependent inhibition was also observed with each of the 6 LATS-negative but TSH-positive sera from patients with primary idiopathic myxedema and serological evidence of thyroid autoimmunity. The possibility that the inhibitory effects elicited by these sera could be attributed to the presence of TSH is not supported by the negative results obtained in 5 patients with congenital hypothyroidism due to thyroid aplasia or hypoplasia. From the data reported in Figure 8, it is apparent that the inhibition curves obtained with the sera from patients with either Graves' disease or primary idiopathic myxedema were virtually parellel. These results are consistent with the interpretation that these patients had circulating antithyroid antibodies competing for the same binding sites, and differing from LATS. Similar conclusions have been drawn

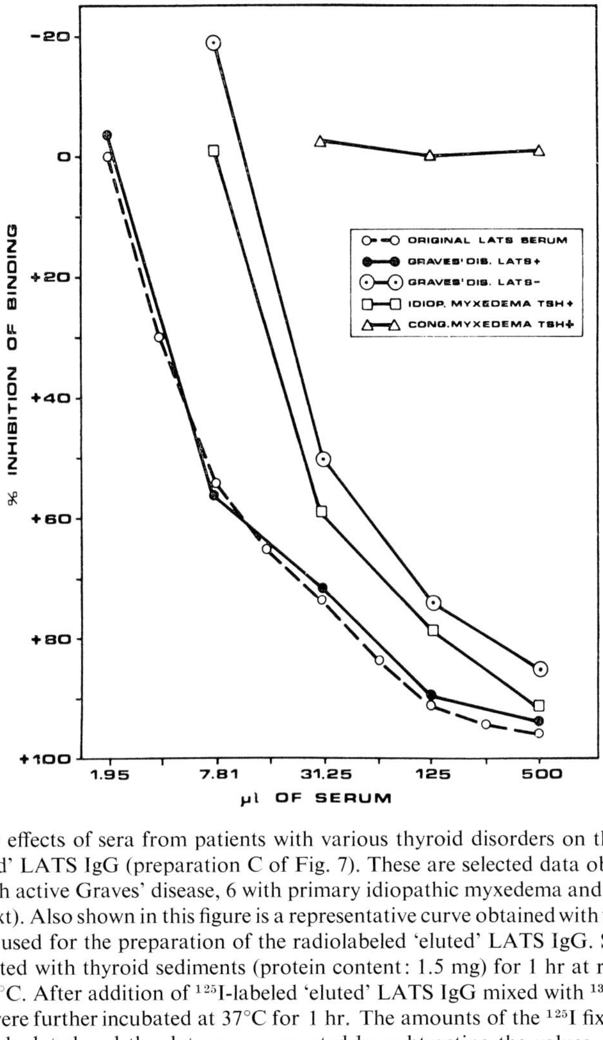

Fig. 8. Inhibitory effects of sera from patients with various thyroid disorders on thyroid fixation of ^{125}I-labeled 'eluted' LATS IgG (preparation C of Fig. 7). These are selected data obtained in a study on 15 patients with active Graves' disease, 6 with primary idiopathic myxedema and 5 with congenital myxedema (see text). Also shown in this figure is a representative curve obtained with the original LATS serum which was used for the preparation of the radiolabeled 'eluted' LATS IgG. Serial serum dilutions were incubated with thyroid sediments (protein content: 1.5 mg) for 1 hr at room temperature and for 48 hr at 4°C. After addition of ^{125}I-labeled 'eluted' LATS IgG mixed with ^{131}I-labeled normal IgG the samples were further incubated at 37°C for 1 hr. The amounts of the ^{125}I fixed on the washed sediments were calculated and the data were corrected by subtracting the values of the nonspecific ^{131}I fixation. The results are the mean of duplicates and are expressed as % inhibition of the corrected ^{125}I fixation with respect to a control specimen which was preincubated with pooled normal human serum.

by Mori *et al.* (1970) from a study carried out with different radioimmunological techniques.

The fact that a high level of LATS activity was found in the preparation of 'eluted' LATS IgG, which after radioiodination exhibited a high degree of specific reactivity to the thyroid, suggests that LATS contributed to some extent to the binding reaction. On the basis of the inhibition studies, however, it appears that this contribution should be very small and that LATS accounts only for a minute portion of the thyroid-reacting immunoglobulins which are present in Graves' disease. The question whether the binding of LATS to the thyroid could be used for the development of an *in vitro* LATS-assay remains to be established.

REFERENCES

ADAMS, D. D. and KENNEDY, T. H. (1965): Evidence of a normally functioning pituitary TSH secretion mechanism in a patient with a high blood level of long-acting thyroid stimulator. *J. clin. Endocr.*, *25*, 571.

ADAMS, D. D. and PURVES, H. D. (1956): Abnormal responses in the assay of thyrotropin. *Proc. Univ. Otago med. Sch.*, *34*, 11.

BEALL, G. N., DONIACH, D., ROITT, I. and EL KABIR, D. (1969): Inhibition of the long-acting thyroid stimulator (LATS) by soluble thyroid fractions. *J. Lab. clin. Med.*, *73*, 988.

BEALL, G. N. and SOLOMON, D. H. (1966): Inhibition of long-acting thyroid stimulator by thyroid particulate fractions. *J. clin. Invest.*, *45*, 552.

BEALL, G. N. and SOLOMON, D. H. (1968): Thyroid-stimulating activity in the serum of rabbits immunized with thyroid microsomes. *J. clin. Endocr.*, *28*, 503.

BURKE, G. (1969): The cell membrane: a common site of action of thyrotropin (TSH) and long-acting thyroid stimulator (LATS). *Metabolism*, *18*, 720.

CHOPRA, I. J., SOLOMON, D. H., JOHNSON, D. E., CHOPRA, U. and FISHER, D. (1970): Dissociation of serum LATS content and thyroid suppressibility during treatment of hyperthyroidism. *J. clin. Endocr.*, *30*, 524.

EZRIN, C. and MURRAY, S. (1963): The cell of the human adenohypophysis in pregnancy, thyroid disease and adrenal cortical disorders. In: *Cytologie de l'Adénohypophyse*, pp. 183–199. Editors: J. Benoit and C. Dallage. Editions du C.N.R.S., Paris.

HARDEN, R. McG., McKENZIE, J. M., McLARTY, D. and ALEXANDER, W. (1970): Thyroid suppressibility and serum LATS in patients treated with antithyroid drugs for thyrotoxicosis. (Abstract). In: *Program, VI International Thyroid Conference, Vienna*, p. 84.

KRISS, J. P., PLESHAKOV, V. and CHIEN, J. R. (1964): Isolation and identification of long-acting thyroid stimulator and its relation to hyperthyroidism and circumscribed pretibial myxedema. *J. clin. Endocr.*, *24*, 1005.

KRISS, J. P., PLESHAKOV, V., ROSENBLUM, A. L., HOLDERNESS, M., SHARP, G. and Utiger, R. (1967): Studies on the pathogenesis of the ophthalmopathy of Graves' disease. *J. clin. Endocr.*, *27*, 582.

MARTINO, E., FENZI, G. F., LIBERTI, P., GRASSO, L., ROVIS, L., PINCHERA, A. and BASCHIERI, L. (1971): Observations on the LATS changes after combined therapy of thyrotoxicosis with radioiodine and antithyroid drugs. To be published.

McKENZIE, J. M. (1967): The long-acting thyroid stimulator: its role in Graves' disease. *Recent Progr. Hormone Res.*, *23*, 1.

McKENZIE, J. M. (1968): Humoral factors in the pathogenesis of Graves' disease. *Physiol. Rev.*, *48*, 252.

MEEK, J. C., JONES, A. E., LEWIS, U. J. and VANDERLAAN, W. P. (1964): Characterisation of the long-acting thyroid stimulator of Graves' disease. *Proc. nat. Acad. Sci. USA*, *52*, 342.

MORI, T., FISHER, J. and KRISS, J. P. (1970): Studies of an *in vitro* binding reaction between thyroid microsomes and long-acting thyroid stimulator globulin (LATS): I. Development of solid-state competitive binding radio-assay methods for measurement of antimicrosomal and antithyroglobulin antibodies. *J. clin. Endocr.*, *31*, 119.

OCHI, Y. and DEGROOT, L. J. (1969): Stimulation of thyroid hyperplasia and protein synthesis by LATS. *Endocrinology*, *85*, 344.

ODELL, W., WILBER, J. and PAUL, W. (1965): Radioimmunoassay of thyrotropin in human serum. *J. clin. Endocr.*, *25*, 1179.

PINCHERA, A., LIBERTI, P. and BADALAMENTI, G. (1965): Attività tireostimolante ad azione prolungata nel siero di conigli immunizzati con tiroide umana. *Folia endocr. (Roma)*, *18*, 522.

PINCHERA, A., LIBERTI, P., MARTINO, E., FENZI, G. F., GRASSO, L., ROVIS, L., BASCHIERI, L. and DORIA, G. (1969): Effects of antithyroid therapy on the long-acting thyroid stimulator and the antithyroglobulin antibodies. *J. clin. Endocr.*, *29*, 231.

PINCHERA, A., ROVIS, L., GRASSO, L., LIBERTI, P., MARTINO, E., FENZI, G. F. and BASCHIERI, L. (1970): Radioimmunological studies on the long-acting thyroid stimulator. *Endocrinology*, *87*, 217.

SHARARD, A. (1969): Thyroid histology in neonatal mice injected with LATS-containing serum from patients with Graves' disease. *Proc. Univ. Otago med. Sch.*, *47*, 30.

SOLOMON, D. H., BEALL, G. N. and CHOPRA, I. J. (1970): Mobilization of tissue thyroxine in mice by thyroxine-binding proteins: studies with a double-isotope McKenzie assay. (Abstract). In: *Program, VI International Thyroid Conference, Vienna*, p. 74.

SUZUKI, T., PELICHOVA, H. and CINADER, B. (1969): Enzyme activation by antibody. I. Fractionation of immune sera in search for an enzyme-activating antibody. *J. Immunol.*, *103*, 1366.
TONIETTI, G., LIBERTI, P., GRASSO, L. and PINCHERA, A. (1968): A comparative study on the mouse thyroid ultrastructure after stimulation with TSH and LATS. In: *Pharmacology of Hormonal Polypeptides and Proteins*, pp. 263–270. Editors: N. Black, L. Martini and R. Paoletti. Plenum Press, New York.
UTIGER, R. D. (1965): Radioimmunoassay of human plasma thyrotropin. *J. clin. Invest.*, *44*, 1277.
WONG, E. T. and LITMAN, G. W. (1969): Interaction of purified long-acting thyroid stimulator (LATS) and thyroid microsomes *in vitro*. *J. clin. Endocr.*, *29*, 72.

BIOCHEMICAL AND PATHOPHYSIOLOGICAL OBSERVATIONS IN ACTIVE THYROID IMMUNITY*

B. N. PREMACHANDRA**

Veterans Administration Hospital, Jefferson Barracks and Washington University, St. Louis, Mo., U.S.A.

In our laboratory extensive investigations have been carried out on biochemical and pathophysiological aspects in induced thyroid (thyroglobulin) immunity on the premise that some of the observations may typify those occurring in autoimmune states or at least may provide a basis for an intelligent interpretation of events occurring in such states. The primary objectives have been to study (a) the physico-chemical and immunological characteristics of antibodies in naturally occurring and in actively induced thyroid immunity, and their ability and avidity to interact with thyroid hormones, (b) the intimate details of the dynamics of iodine metabolism in animals of various species subjected to thyroid iso- and heteroimmunization, (c) the effect of experimental thyroid immunity on immuno-pathophysiology of other organs and tissues. Several aspects involving these objectives have been dealt with in various publications from this laboratory (Premachandra *et al.*, 1963*a*; *b*; 1965; Premachandra, 1967). Some of these observations which aid in the focusing of certain unsolved problems of current interest will be reviewed briefly in this communication, along with certain other recent findings.

EXPERIMENTAL

Active immunization in rabbits and rats was carried out by subcutaneous or intramuscular injections of 1 % bovine thyroglobulin once weekly for 3 weeks. Maximum antibody response as determined by hemagglutination techniques was attained generally at 6–8 weeks after immunization, and blood samples were drawn at various intervals 4 weeks after initial antigen administration. The measurement of hapten inhibition of thyroid antibody was carried out by serological and radioimmunological techniques (Margherita and Premachandra, 1969). In the former procedure, antigen-antibody precipitates formed in the presence or absence of test inhibitor were assayed for N content by the micro-Kjeldahl method (Margherita and Premachandra, 1969). In the radioimmunologic method, compounds whose serologic similarity to thyroxine were to be studied were equilibrated with antithyroglobulin sera prior to the addition of labeled T_4; displacement of the label from gammaglobulin to the albumin region as seen in the electrophoretogram would then indicate immunologic similarity (Fig. 1).

* Throughout this communication the use of the expression 'active immunity' signifies artificial immunization, *i.e.*, exogenous inoculation followed by antibody synthesis *de novo*. Active thyroid immunity, therefore, implies injection of an animal with thyroglobulin or other components of the thyroid tissue.

** Investigations aided in part by N.I.H. grant AM07676.

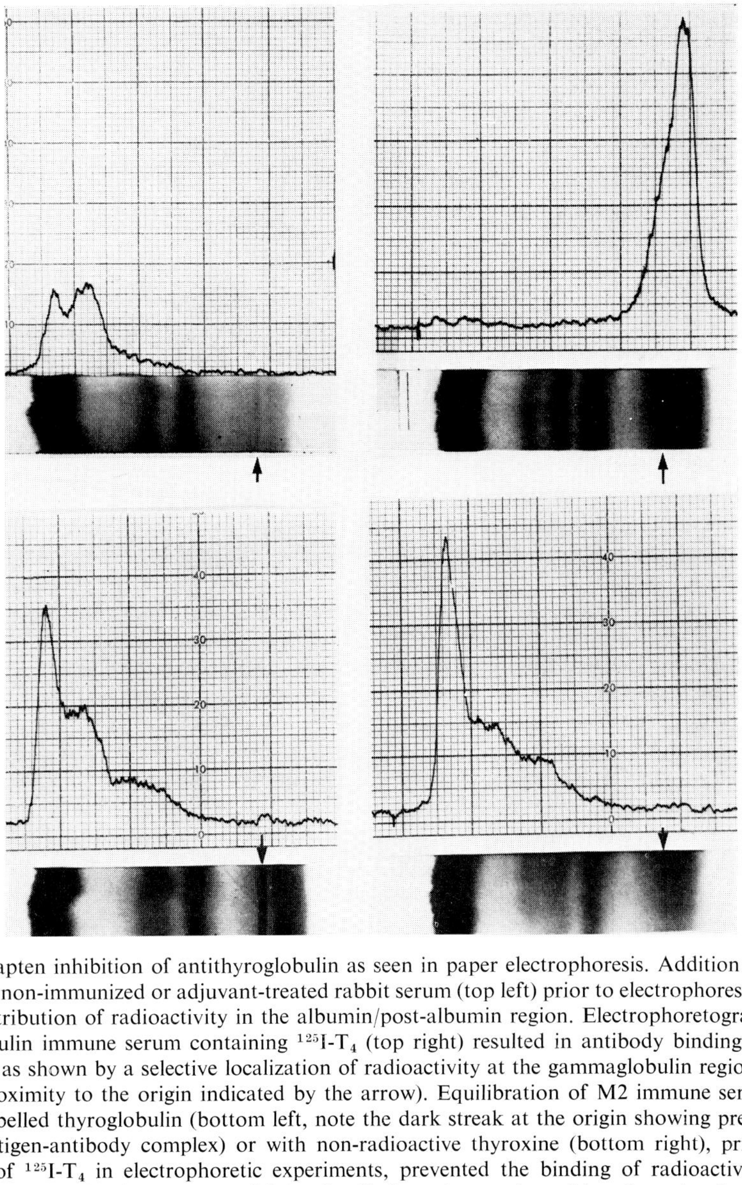

Fig. 1. Hapten inhibition of antithyroglobulin as seen in paper electrophoresis. Addition of $^{125}I\text{-}T_4$ *in vitro* to non-immunized or adjuvant-treated rabbit serum (top left) prior to electrophoresis resulted in the distribution of radioactivity in the albumin/post-albumin region. Electrophoretogram of M2 thyroglobulin immune serum containing $^{125}I\text{-}T_4$ (top right) resulted in antibody binding of radiothyroxine as shown by a selective localization of radioactivity at the gammaglobulin region (area at and in proximity to the origin indicated by the arrow). Equilibration of M2 immune serum either with unlabelled thyroglobulin (bottom left, note the dark streak at the origin showing precipitation of the antigen-antibody complex) or with non-radioactive thyroxine (bottom right), prior to the addition of $^{125}I\text{-}T_4$ in electrophoretic experiments, prevented the binding of radioactivity at the gammaglobulin region (compare top right) and radiothyroxine was bound largely at the albumin/post-albumin area; these experiments show the serologic similarity of T_4 and thyroglobulin in inhibition of antithyroglobulin, thus pointing to the role of T_4 as a hapten in active thyroid immunity.

By this method, and by quantitation, information concerning the structural configurations participating in thyroglobulin specificity could be determined. Kinetic parameters of thyroid function and thyroxine metabolism as well as serum thyroxine transport were investigated by procedures described previously (Premachandra *et al.* 1963*a*; *b*; 1965). Hepatic clearance of thyroxine in normal and thyroglobulin-immune rats was determined utilizing $^{131}I\text{-}T_4$. Eighteen hours after $^{131}I\text{-}T_4$ injection the common bile ducts were cannulated and bile samples collected each hour for 4 hours. Blood was drawn halfway between each bile collection. Organic and inorganic radioactivity in plasma and bile was determined and the bile radioactivity was subjected to thin-layer chromatography. Hepatic clearance was obtained by dividing total biliary radioactivity secreted in an hour by plasma radioactivity;

$$\frac{\text{c/m}}{\text{hr secretion}} \; \frac{.}{.} \; \frac{\text{c/m}}{\text{ml}} = \text{ml/hr}$$

Serum insulin was measured by radioimmunoassay utilizing commercially available kits (Amersham/Searle). Tissue sections for light and fluorescent microscopy were prepared by conventional techniques (Premachandra *et al.*, 1965).

RESULTS AND COMMENTS

BIOCHEMICAL STUDIES

Thyroid antibody binding of thyroxine in active thyroid immunity

Structural aspects of thyroxine-containing determinants:

One of the characteristics of active thyroid (thyroglobulin) immunization is the formation, invariably, of antibodies to determinants containing thyroxine residues (Fig. 1). This immunological reaction has been demonstrated in the sera of various animals immunized against thyroid components by radio-electrophoretic as well as by hapten inhibition techniques (Margherita and Premachandra, 1969); antibody binding of thyroid hormone is not a matter of adsorption of thyroxine to antigen-antibody complex since the binding can be demonstrated long after the disappearance of immune complexes from circulation and various other specificity studies detailed elsewhere (Premachandra *et al.*, 1963*b*; Premachandra and Blumenthal, 1967) strongly suggest a true haptenic role for thyroxine. While on the surface, thyroxine antibody formation consequent on thyroglobulin immunization might appear unusual, a more careful consideration of the chemical composition of thyroglobulin (approximately 2 residues of thyroxine/molecule of thyroglobulin) along with the well-known ability of iodoamino acids to function as determinants, suggests that this unusual phenomenon is not altogether unexpected. In order to understand the nature of thyroxine-binding antibodies in induced thyroglobulin immunity, the inhibiting activity of various compounds (as listed in Table I) was tested with rabbit antibovine thyroglobulin sera to determine the extent of their serologic similarity to thyroxine. The main conclusions from these investigations are: (1) Position of iodine substitution is important for inhibition as judged by the results obtained with 3:5 diiodothyronine (3:5 T_2) and 3:3′ diiodothyronine (3:3′ T_2); only 3% inhibition was obtained with 3:5 T_2 in comparison to 68% inhibition with 3:3′ T_2. (2) The degree of iodine substitution in the nonphenolic ring is not as important as the presence of iodine in the phenolic ring (*cf.* inhibition obtained by 3-monoiodothyronine and 3:5 diiodothyronine (Table I)). (3) Diphenyl ether linkage is essential, as shown by an absence of antibody inhibition with various compounds lacking this linkage. (4) Unsubstituted thyronine which lacks iodine is totally ineffective. (5) Tyrosine in peptide linkage is not as effective as thyronines substituted with iodine in the phenolic ring.

In summary, therefore, it would appear that a combination of aromatic ether linkage and iodine substitution in the phenolic ring is essential for most effective inhibition (Fig. 2). The requirement for iodine substituted in the phenolic ring to elicit antibody inhibition as shown by the radioelectrophoretic experiments, raises a question as to the function of iodine in this position. The iodine could make a direct contribution relating to fit or it could affect the dissociation of the hydroxyl group present on this ring. Nevertheless, the observation that raising the pH of the buffer (from 8.6 to 11.0) above the pK′ of the hydroxyl group in thyronine did not impart inhibitory activity to the latter, suggests that charge is not the main consideration.

TABLE I

Hapten inhibition of antithyroglobulin detected by the radioimmunologic method*

Compounds	Molar concentration added	Serum			
		AS-1	SM-8	R-4	M-6
Tetraiodothyroacetic acid	2.6×10^{-4} M	100		100	100
Triiodothyropropionic acid	3.1×10^{-4} M	89		90	91
Thyroxine	2.5×10^{-4} M	100	100	100	100
Triiodothyronine	3.0×10^{-4} M	97	85	82	93
3,5-Diiodothyropropionic acid	3.9×10^{-4} M	25	0	22	14
3,5-Diiodothyronine	3.8×10^{-4} M		3	10	13
3,3′-Diiodothyronine	3.8×10^{-4} M	76	68	70	66
3-Monoiodothyronine	5.0×10^{-4} M	30	9	13	14
l-Thyronine	7.4×10^{-4} M	0	0	1	9
Glycyl-l-leucyl-l-tyrosine	5.6×10^{-4} M	0	0	8	26
3,5 Diiodotyrosine	4.6×10^{-4} M	8	0	49	55
3-Iodotyrosine	6.5×10^{-4} M	0	0	4	0
Phenylalanine	12.1×10^{-4} M	2	0	0	0
Iodophenol	9.0×10^{-4} M	0	1	2	0
Tyrosine	11.0×10^{-4} M	0	0	0	0

* Expressed as % inhibition by comparison with the reference controls. Values below 10% are not considered significant. (Data from Margherita and Premachandra (1969): *J. Immunol.*, *102*, 1511.)

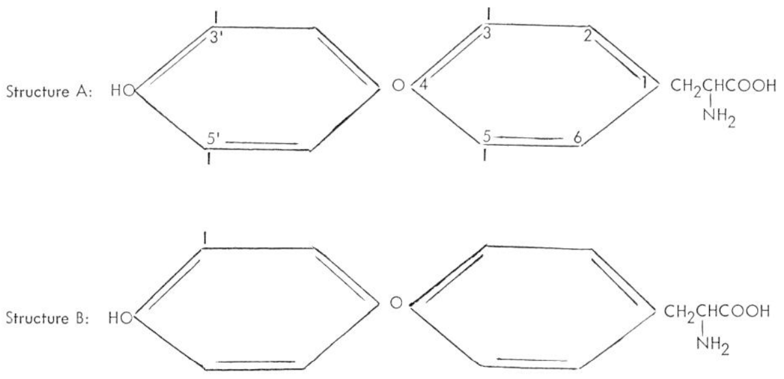

Fig. 2.

Structure A: Thyroxine

Structure B: Proposed minimum structural configuration for effective inhibition of antibody binding of thyroxine in active thyroglobulin immunity. The structure represents 3′ monoiodothyronine. While we have not tested diphenyl ether derivatives without side chain, it may be that diphenyl ether alone with hydroxy and iodine substitution may elicit significant inhibition.

Specificity considerations:

The assigning of importance to phenolic iodothyronines as determinants has been challenged by Metzger *et al.* (1962) on the grounds that the specificity of iodoamino acids fail to explain the specificity of thyroglobulin from different animal species. It is possible that the use of techniques more sensitive than gel precipitation may permit detection of minor hapten inhibition reactions in heterologous thyroglobulin-antithyroglobulin systems; it is also possible that only a portion of the specificity of thyroglobulin is directed against iodoamino acids and that the remainder of the specificity could involve combinations of noniodinated amino acids in peptide linkage or of peptide linked iodoamino acids in a folded state. The rat peptide maps of tryptic peptides of thyroglobulin (equilibrated with labeled iodine) have shown that 40% of radioactivity could be consistently accounted for in the 19 peptide fragments containing the iodoamino acids (Alexander, 1968). It is probable that more than one determinant site exists (Godal, 1967) and those which do not involve iodoamino acids may be concerned with species specificity.

In line with some of the above considerations are also the differential aspects in regard to thyroid hetero-, iso- and autoantibody interaction of thyroxine as examined by electrophoretic and other serologic procedures. The situation can be summarized as follows: heterologously-produced thyroglobulin antibodies invariably react with those determinants containing thyroxine residues, followed by a somewhat less widespread interaction between thyroxine and thyroid antibodies in isoimmunization. Thyroid autoantibodies do not generally bind thyroxine although sporadic interactions in certain pathological states have been reported in the literature (Premachandra and Blumenthal, 1967).

How do we account for the failure of antibody-thyroxine interaction despite the presence of elevated serum thyroglobulin autoantibody titer in various pathological states? In other words, why does the T_4 determinant which asserts itself in hetero- and isoimmunization fail to do so in the autoimmune state? The reason is not known. One of the more obvious possibilities is that in the natural state an adjuvant-like action may be lacking which may then result in formation of incomplete antibodies (see below). While the precise role of the adjuvant is not clear, recent investigations (Weigle *et al.* 1969) seem to indicate that it indirectly facilitates *in vivo* antigenic alteration and/or enhancement of the immune response, and establishment of cellular sensitivity. Whether this heightened macrophage activity is translated into a more intense scrutiny and processing of the antigen, thereby unlocking otherwise buried determinants, is not clear. It is known, however, that artificial processing of rabbit or human IgG by various enzymes has revealed otherwise buried fragments which are detected by appropriate agglutinating reactions (Mandy *et al.*, 1965; Richie *et al.*, 1970).

On the other hand, the conclusions from an elegant series of investigations by Shulman and his co-workers (Mates and Shulman, 1967; 1968; Shulman, 1968) while not necessarily at variance with the views expressed above, seem to indicate the exclusive nature of some of the determinants in the thyroglobulin molecule, *i.e.*, there are some determinants which participate only in the heteroimmune system and are totally ineffective in the autoimmune state. These investigators, based on their findings on the differences in precipitation reactions between thyroglobulin-autoantibody and thyroglobulin-heteroantibody, proposed that only a fraction of the antigenic sites active in heteroimmunization are also active in autoimmunization (Shulman and Witebsky, 1960), and similar suggestions were also made by Roitt *et al.* (1958; 1968). Evidence for this hypothesis was obtained by splitting thyroglobulin (enzymatically or nonenzymatically) into various fragments as characterized in the ultracentrifuge, and immunologic activity of these fragments was examined by gel precipitation reactions by allowing them to react with appropriate hetero- and autoimmune sera. The reaction of the fragments with heteroantibodies always predominated over the autoantibody interaction. In more recent investigations (Shulman and Ghayasuddin, 1971) enzymatically-derived thyroglobulin fragments were further purified on Sephadex G-200 column and resulting fractions tested against auto- and heteroantibodies. The number of precipitin lines developed in the heteroimmune system was always greater than in the autoimmune system, indicating an actual reduction in the number of determinants participating in the autoimmune state fFig. 3). When one of the major fractions obtained through Sephadex G-200 run was further (ractionated on Sephadex G-100, none of the resultant fractions precipitated with the autoantibodies whereas some of these same fractions reacted with the heteroantibodies. Supporting evidence bearing on some of these observations has also been obtained by Stylos and Rose (1969). These investigations, therefore, point to the success in obtaining enzymatically-

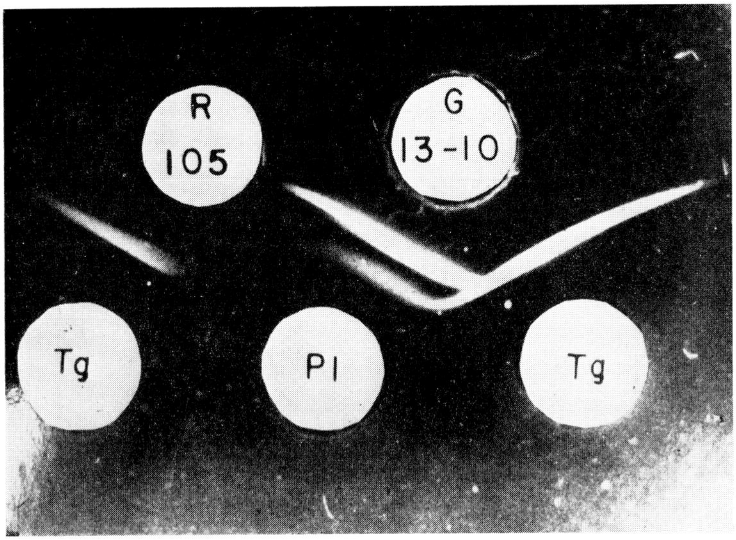

Fig. 3. Gel precipitation reactions of native and fractionated rabbit thyroglobulin with thyroid auto- and heteroantibodies.

Pl – G200 fraction from trypsin digested thyroglobulin
TG – Rabbit thyroglobulin
R105 – Autoantibodies
G 13-10 – Heteroantibodies

(Data from Shulman and Ghayasuddin, 1971.)

derived fragments which carry antigenic sites active only in heteroimmunization but not in autoimmunization.

Despite these carefully carried out studies by Shulman and co-workers, one would wonder whether the conclusions drawn from *in vitro* enzymatic thyroglobulin degradation studies would obtain *in vivo*. While this question cannot be answered at the present time, our repeated observations of the lack of antigenicity of thyroxine residues in the autoimmune system, while at the same time exhibiting a strong determinant character in heteroimmune system, provides some evidence that conclusions derived from *in vitro* enzymatic studies may indeed pertain *in vivo*. The manner in which differences in antigenic specificity of some determinants (*e.g.*, thyroxine residues) are brought to bear in autoimmune and heteroimmune states is not known. Whether this is a reflection of differences in molecular mechanisms by which macrophages process the antigen in hetero- and autoimmune states, or whether this is related to the differences in physico-chemical characteristics of the antigen as presented to antibody-forming cells, or whether genetic and other factors are also involved in this process, are questions future investigations should resolve.

PHYSIOLOGICAL INVESTIGATIONS

Thyroid function studies in experimental thyroiditis

Once it became known that thyroid lesions similar to those seen in Hashimoto's disease could be readily elicited experimentally, various parameters of thyroid function in experimentally-induced thyroid immunity have been studied by several investigators (Hung *et al.*, 1962;

Torizuka *et al.*, 1964; Biassoni *et al.*, 1965; Flax and Bilote, 1965; Smith and Adams, 1966; Anderson *et al.*, 1969; Gorman *et al.*, 1969) in the hope they may contribute to a further and better understanding of the intimate details of iodine metabolism in human disease. Thyroid-function studies carried out in this laboratory in thyroglobulin-immunized guinea pigs have been reviewed elsewhere (Premachandra *et al.*, 1965). Because of the antibody binding of T_4, one of the cardinal effects in induced thyroglobulin immunity is the delayed degradation of thyroxine, *i.e.*, increase in t½ (Fig. 4). Elevation in t½ by 200–400% is not uncommon.

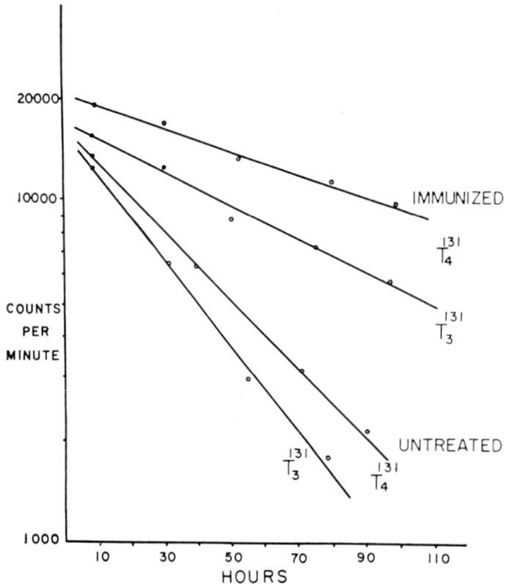

Fig. 4. Disappearance of ^{131}I-labeled thyroxine and ^{131}I-labeled triiodothyronine from the blood in untreated and thyroglobulin-immunized guinea pigs is shown in representative individual animals. In the groups of immunized animals, the mean half-times ($t^1/_2$) were 61 hr for triiodothyronine and 71 hr for thyroxine. These half-time values are strikingly prolonged as compared with results in the untreated control animals, which had mean values of 30 hr for triiodothyronine and 33 hr for thyroxine.

(Data from Premachandra *et al.*, 1963*a*.)

Because of the augmented peripheral binding of thyroxine, the extrathyroidal organic iodine (EOI) pool is significantly elevated. The increase in EOI coupled with a markedly diminished fractional turnover of T4 results in near normal thyroxine degradation rate.

Some of the other thyroid parameters investigated by various workers include thyroid iodine uptake, organification of iodine and synthesis of thyroxine, thyroid to serum iodine ratio, detailed chromatographic analysis of iodine in the thyroid and serum, ability of the thyroid to respond to exogenous TSH, and free thyroxine levels in plasma. When one reviews the results of various workers on thyroid function in thyroid-immunized animals, one becomes impressed by the discordant findings. That these conflicting claims are more apparent than real becomes evident when one examines these results under the framework of two basic findings, one of which was recently discovered. The two basic aspects are:

(1) The degree of the thyroid lesion at the time of measurement of thyroid function is of the utmost importance. In thyroid immune animals hypofunction, hyperfunction or no change in the functioning of the thyroid has been described. If the lesions are mild, it is possible that there may not be a significant impairment of thyroid function at all, and yet plasma organic iodine may be high if there is formation of thyroxine-binding antibodies; with moderate lesions, one may encounter hypo- or hyperthyroid state. It is possible that the high level of circulating organic iodine, due probably to a combination of release of abnormal iodinated compounds from the thyroid as well as to the appearance of thyroxine-binding antibodies, may inhibit pituitary. On the other hand, with persistent moderate lesions, the colloid stores may gradually get depleted due to basement membrane damage and/or its removal and disposal by the wandering phagocytosing macrophages, with a resultant loss

in total plasma PBI. The low level of organic iodine may then stimulate TSH secretion and cause hyperplasia of the undamaged thyroid follicles; with advanced lesions, there is virtual loss of parenchyma with accompanying fibrotic changes contributing to a frank hypothyroid state. On the basis of the severity of the lesions as detailed above, one could also bridge the apparent discrepancies noted with regard to the ability of the thyroid to respond to exogenous TSH in active thyroid immunity.

(2) In animals subjected to hetero- or isoimmunization against thyroid components, antibodies to determinants containing thyroxine residues are invariably formed. The importance of this observation resides in the fact that antibody-thyroxine interaction phenomenon has been shown to cause spuriously low turnover of thyroxine (*i.e.*, elevation in t½ of radiothyroxine) as mentioned previously, elevate PBI and affect various other aspects of thyroxine kinetics (Premachandra *et al.*, 1965). The discordant PBI values reported in immune animals with comparable thyroid lesions may perhaps be resolved partially, if the contribution of thyroxine-binding antibodies on circulating thyroid hormones is taken into account.

The nature of organic iodine in experimental thyroiditis deserves comment. If thyroid immunization elicits only humoral antibodies but does not result in the formation of thyroid lesions, there will be an elevation in butanol extractable PBI. On the other hand, if the immunization results in extensive lymphocytic embarrassment to the thyroid, nonhormonal iodinated compounds from the thyroid would be released into the circulation and these butanol-insoluble iodinated components have been characterized as iodinated albumin. Torizuka *et al.* (1964) analyzed this iodoalbumin material in induced allergic thyroiditis and have shown that the peptide-linked labeled amino acid in this component comprises largely monoiodotyrosine. DeGroot *et al.* (1962) suggested that the enhanced circulating levels of iodinated albumin in Hashimoto's thyroiditis may be due to iodination of albumin or other proteins consequent on the loss of colloid from the thyroid.

The effect of experimental thyroiditis on circulating free thyroxine is not clear because of very limited studies in this regard. In thyroid-immunized animals, no real convincing evidence has been presented to indicate deviation from normal free thyroxine levels.

On balance it must be said that some of the thyroid function parameters and other observations made in thyroid-immunized animals parallel those noted in lymphocytic thyroiditis in the human so that the credibility of certain observations and interpretations in the human disease is fortified. On the other hand, it must be recognized that certain other observations in human disease, *e.g.*, defect in organification of iodine (Morgans and Trotter, 1957), have not been confirmed in animal investigations. It may be that certain thyroidal deficiencies occur in conjunction with Hashimoto's disease without necessarily being causally related.

Hepatic clearance of thyroxine in active thyroglobulin immunity

As indicated previously the peripheral metabolism of thyroxine is markedly affected in thyroglobulin-immune animals. In consonance with these observations it was of interest to determine the hepatic clearance of thyroxine in thyroid-immune animals since the liver is one of the main centers involved in the peripheral metabolism of thyroxine. The hepatic clearance experiments were carried out in normal and thyroglobulin-immune rats by techniques described under methods, utilizing ^{131}I-labeled T_4. In thyroglobulin-immune animals hepatic clearance of thyroxine was markedly reduced and in animals with a high antibody titer there was a 4-fold reduction (Table II). The marked reduction in hepatic clearance of thyroxine was accompanied by a corresponding elevation in t½ of thyroxine in these animals as determined by whole body counting (unpublished observations). Chromatographic experiments did not reveal qualitative differences in the nature of biliary radioactivity secreted in control and thyroglobulin-immune animals (Fig. 5). There was also no difference in the biliary volume between control and thyroglobulin-immune rats (Table II).

TABLE II

Hepatic clearance of radiothyroxine (^{131}I-T_4) in normal and thyroglobulin immune rats

Treatment	No. of rats	Hepatic clearance of ^{131}I-T_4* (ml/hr)	Biliary volume (ml/hr)
Control rats (a)	6	1.04 ±0.06**	0.89 ±0.08
Thyroglobulin immune rats (b)	6	0.26 ±0.04	0.85 ±0.10

* Chromatographic analysis showed that the bulk of the radioactivity cleared by the liver was not ^{131}I-T_4. It would be more appropriate, therefore, to refer to biliary radioactivity as radioiodine derived from administered ^{131}I-T_4.

** Standard error.

(a) Animals injected with complete adjuvant alone once weekly for 3 weeks.

(b) Animals immunized against 1% bovine thyroglobulin in complete adjuvant once weekly for 3 weeks.

In order to determine whether or not passive transfer of thyroglobulin-immune serum would also affect hepatic clearance of thyroxine as described in active immunity, rabbit antibovine thyroglobulin serum was administered in rats (2 ml/animal in divided doses) followed by ^{131}I-T_4 administration. Hepatic clearance was reduced 50% in animals which received thyroglobulin immune serum by passive transfer, as compared to the clearance in animals which received either saline or normal human serum.

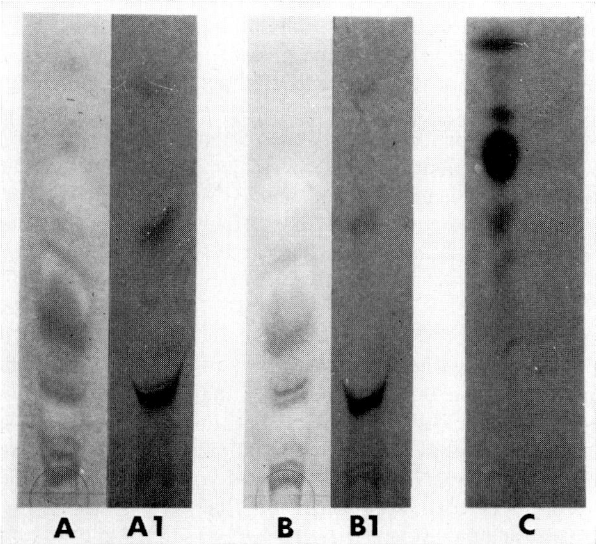

Fig. 5. Representative illustration of TLC chromatograms of bile from a control (A) and a thyroglobulin-immunized rat (B) along with their radioautographs (A1) and (B1) respectively. The intense dark band in the radioautograph at the extreme right (C) represents radiothyroxine used for reference. It is evident there was no difference in the nature of radioactivity secreted in the bile from control and thyroglobulin-immunized rats administered radiothyroxine. Little or no thyroxine was secreted in the bile of either normal or actively immunized rats.

PATHOPHYSIOLOGICAL ASPECTS IN INDUCED THYROID IMMUNITY

Long-acting thyroid stimulator (LATS) in induced thyroid immunity

The manner in which induced thyroid immunity may affect various thyroid parameters is of interest in other areas as well, *e.g.*, in the experimental production of long-acting thyroid stimulator. Historically, Adams (1958) first described in the sera of thyrotoxic patients the presence of an abnormal thyroid stimulator which differed from TSH in the duration of its action on the thyroid to elicit maximal response. To signify the delayed time course of action the abnormal thyroid stimulator has been referred to as long-acting thyroid stimulator (LATS). Kriss *et al.* (1964) showed LATS to be an IgG antibody and Beall and Solomon (1966) reported that incubation of LATS sera with thyroid microsomes resulted in the loss of thyroid-stimulating activity (the implication in these observations being that LATS interaction with a thyroid component may bring about augmented thyroid hormone release *in vivo*). These and other recent observations on the antibody nature of LATS (McKenzie, 1968) have prompted investigators to test the converse possibility, *i.e.* whether LATS could indeed be produced experimentally by immunization with a thyroid preparation. The experience of practically all the investigators in this area has been that only limited success is attained in the experimental production of LATS.

One of the consistent findings in rabbits immunized against a heterologous thyroid antigen (human thyroid microsomes or homogenate) is the formation of antibodies which bind thyroxine thus contributing to an increase in total T_4 or PBI (as discussed previously). Furthermore, as indicated earlier, even the passive transfer of experimentally-induced thyroglobulin immune serum affects the hepatic clearance of thyroxine as well as other thyroid parameters in the recipient. In experimental production of LATS* the blood of animals showing a positive LATS response invariably contains high T_4 and also shows thyroxine antibody binding activity. These observations have raised the possibility that sustained increase in blood ^{131}I of mice injected with antithyroid rabbit serum might merely represent delayed degradation of labeled thyroxine and really not represent true stimulation at all (Burke, 1968). To further complicate matters, thyroxine binding antibodies have been shown to affect *net* transfer of tissue thyroxine into the circulation (Solomon *et al.*, 1971; Florsheim, 1971). To demarcate the contribution of T_4 binding antibody from that of the thyroid stimulator to blood radioactivity, a double-isotope technique was devised by Solomon *et al.* (1971) who labeled mouse thyroid with ^{131}I and administered ^{125}I-T_4 one day prior to assay as a marker for peripheral thyroxine turnover. Any increase in difference between plasma ^{131}I (as percentage of 0-hr count) and ^{125}I activity (also as percentage of 0-hr count) after test injection, was interpreted to indicate true thyroid stimulation.

Notwithstanding these ingenious attempts to clearly establish the production of LATS experimentally, thyrotoxic symptoms in thyroid-immunized rabbits have not been observed by any of the investigators. The inherent limitations of the McKenzie TSH assay itself, together with the complexities involved in the proper interpretation of kinetic parameters of thyroid function in animals subjected to passive transfer of thyroid immune serum, coupled with a lack of biological evidence of thyrotoxicosis, would compel one to conclude that much further research is necessary before the validity of experimental LATS production can be established conclusively.

---

* LATS measurement is obtained by the administration of serum to be assayed into suitably prepared mice injected initially with labeled iodine, and subsequently with thyroxine to block endogenous TSH. The radioactivity in blood is then measured, generally at 2 and 9 hours, and the presence of LATS is usually inferred if greater response is obtained at 9 hours.

Pathological Aspects

The characteristic lymphocytic infiltration of the thyroid in thyroglobulin-immune animals (Fig. 6) and certain other aspects and similarities of this lesion with that seen in Hashimoto's disease are well known and will not be discussed further in this article. What is less well known is the occurrence of a variety of lesions in various other tissues of thyroid-immunized animals (kidney, pancreas, brain, heart, muscle, spleen, etc.). These have been discussed in some detail in our previous publication (Premachandra, 1967), and, in brief, the three main types of lesions are as follows:

(*a*) Proliferative vascular lesions: These were characterized by hyperplasia and hypertrophy of the lining endothelial cells accompanied by a deposition of PAS positive basement membrane-like material generally as a thickened structure (Fig. 7). Mostly these lesions occurred in the small intraparenchymal vessels of several organs (in arteries less than 150 μ in diameter, in arterioles, and occasionally in venules). Specific antibody binding of antigen has been demonstrated in these vascular lesions. In some instances antigen binding has been

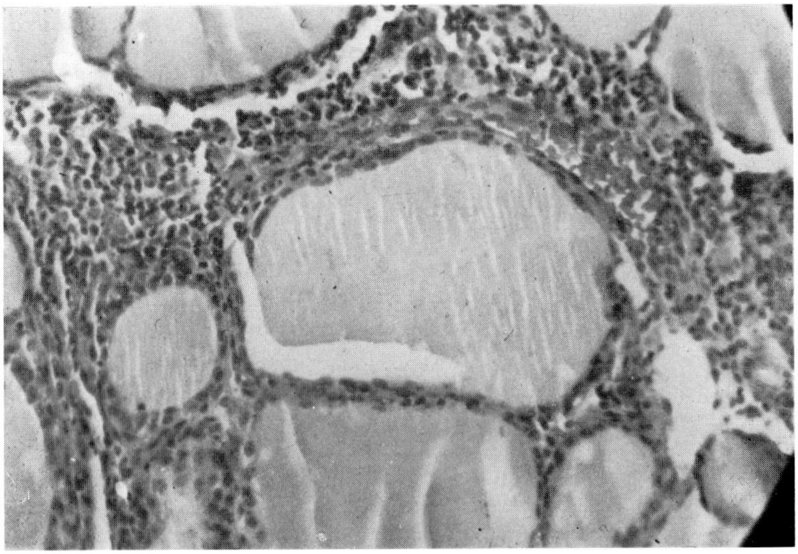

Fig. 6. Section of thyroid from a thyroglobulin-immunized guinea pig 15 weeks after immunization. Hematoxylin-eosin stain, mag. approx. 450 ×. Replacement of thyroid follicles by a confluent interstitial reaction at the center can be seen.

shown to occur in endothelial cells (thus raising the possibility that these cells may also be immunologically competent), and in others, only in basement membrane structures. The significance of these observations resides in the fact that if these lesions are sufficiently widely disseminated they may constitute a cause of peripheral resistance to blood flow and thus, among other things, affect TSH secretion, thyroid hormone transport and other metabolic processes. The various types of lesions observed in the kidneys (to be discussed below) of thyroid-immune rabbits may also impair iodine metabolism significantly to contribute to abnormal thyroid function in such animals. The increase in $t\frac{1}{2}$ of thyroid hormone, *i.e.*, inhibition of extravascular diffusion, in thyroglobulin-immunized animals referred to previously, may also originate, in part, due to the binding of thyroxine by the immune globulin in the vessels of muscle and subcutaneous fat as well as at the capillary endothelial barrier in various tissues.

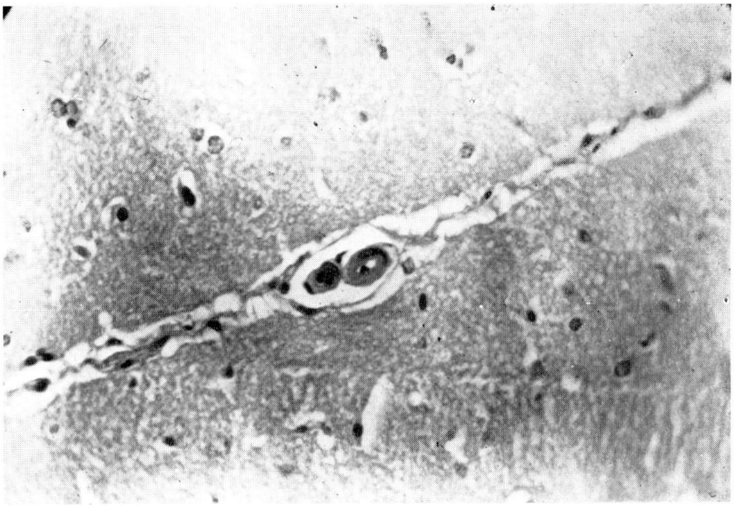

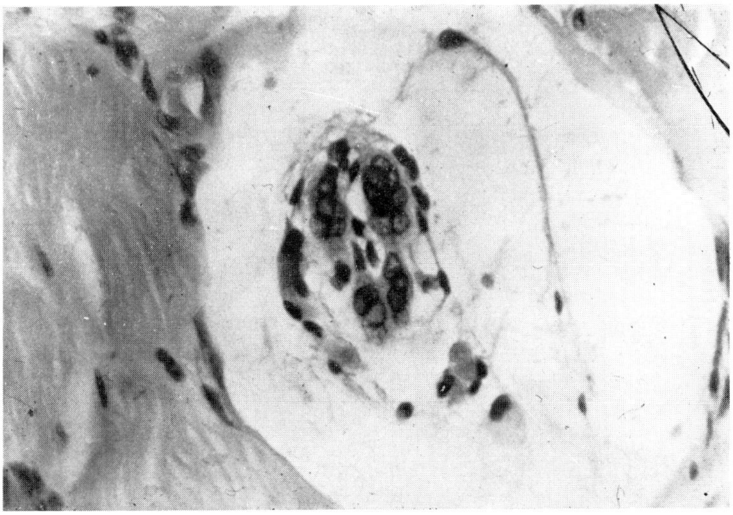

Fig. 7.

Top: Section of the brain from a thyroglobulin-immunized rabbit. Hyaline thickening of a small artery and a proliferation of endothelial cells (almost to the point of occlusion of another) can be seen.
Bottom: Hematoxylin-eosin stained muscle section from an immunized animal. In the interstitial adipose tissue there is a capillary showing proliferation of endothelial cells.

(*b*) Interstitial and perivascular infiltration: These lesions involving infiltration by lymphocytes and histiocytes (Figs. 6 and 8) are well known and commonly noted in various immune states. Depending on the severity of the lesions, typical inflammatory reactions around vesicles and other vascular components may be noted, and in advanced cases the follicles or the parenchyma can be replaced by the formation of active germinal centers. These inter-

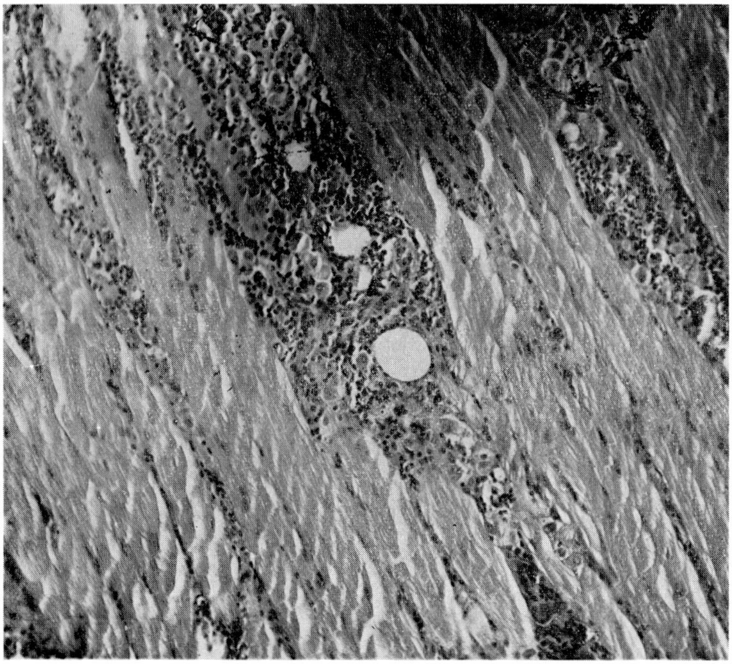

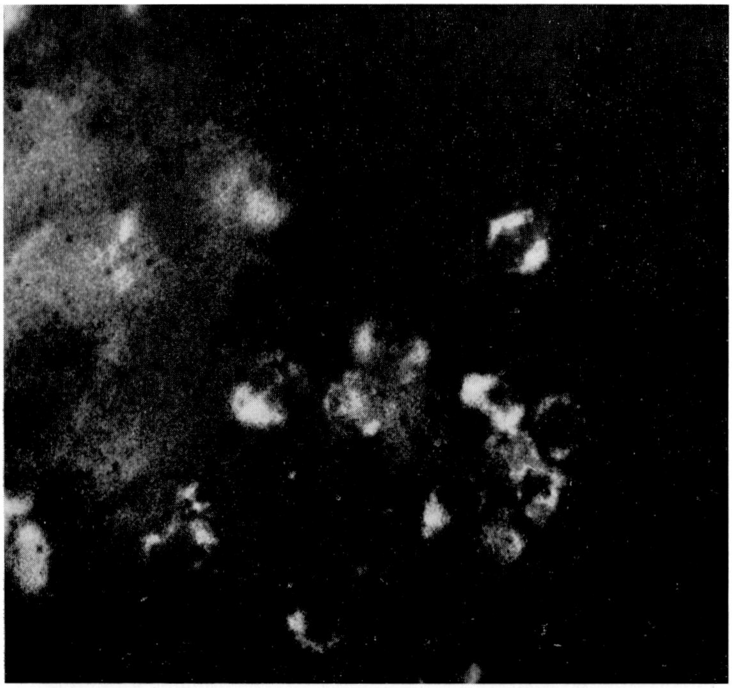

Fig. 8.

Top: Hematoxylin-eosin stained muscle section from an immunized animal showing extensive infiltration of lymphocytes and histiocytes.
Bottom: Muscle section stained with fluorescein-conjugated thyroglobulin. Uptake of fluorescence by cells of the interstitial infiltrate in an immunized animal can be seen clearly.

stitial and perivascular infiltrating cells also bind antigen (thyroglobulin) as demonstrated by fluorescent microscopic techniques (Premachandra *et al.*, 1965). It must be stressed that both the lesions described in (*a*) and (*b*) are not specific to any particular immune state. They occur in a variety of immune states and even in apparently normal individuals particularly after the age of 50.

(*c*) Nodular glomerular lesion: This lesion originally described by Kimmelstiel and Wilson in 1936 is generally considered to be specific for diabetes and has not been noted in other disease states. Further discussion on this lesion will be presented along with studies on serum insulin in active thyroglobulin immunity.

Nodular glomerulosclerosis and serum insulin in active thyroid immunity

The discussion on serum insulin and nephropathy in thyroid immune animals was reserved until this time to treat these aspects concomitantly to suggest the possibility that there may be an interrelationship between thyroid immunity and insulin immunity and diabetes. This interrelation hypothesis will be developed in more detail after reviewing the experimental observations made in our laboratories (see Section A below); some of the supporting observations from other laboratories are cited in Section B.

A. *Experimental observations*

A variety of glomerular lesions in thyroid-immunized animals were seen often in the same kidney. Of all the various lesions (diffuse glomerulosclerosis, proliferative glomerulitis, hyaline thickening of capillary loops, etc.) the appearance of hyaline nodules in the glomeruli of approximately 30% of immunized animals was significant. These hyaline nodules appeared to be similar to those in the human diabetic kidney (Kimmelstiel-Wilson nodules) and were usually situated at the periphery of the glomerulus, and contained a few cells presumably of mesangial origin (Fig. 9). The nodules gave a variable PAS reaction (periodic acid Schiff reagent) sometimes indicating the glycoprotein nature. Comparable glomerular nodular lesions were seen only in insulin-immunized rabbits (Blumenthal, personal communication) but not in animals treated with Freund's adjuvant, cortisone or alloxan. In some animals treated with Freund's adjuvant alone, proliferative glomerular lesions were seen (not nodular) and a significant number of cortisone-injected rabbits showed exudative (droplet) lesions in the glomeruli. Of interest in this connection are the observations of Blumenthal (personal communication) who reported the requirement of repeated antigen challenge to elicit nodular glomerular lesions in insulin-immunized animals, while, in our investigations with thyroglobulin, no such frequent antigen administration was essential to induce nodular lesions. These differences may probably be related to the differences in $t\frac{1}{2}$ of insulin and thyroglobulin as well as due to differences in physico-chemical characteristics of these antigen-antibody complexes, and to other unknown factors.

The finding of glomerular nodular lesions in both thyroid- and insulin-immunized animals as noted above, prompted investigations on serum insulin in active thyroid immunity. In the investigations carried out so far, the dramatic increase in serum immunoreactive insulin in thyroglobulin-immunized animals is particularly noteworthy. The preimmune serum-insulin level in a group of rabbits fasted 18 hr was 17 μU/ml, and at 2, 3, 4, 6 and 12 weeks after immunization the increases (over the preimmune value) were 98, 388, 425, 441, and 425% respectively (Fig. 10). The maximum insulin response at 6 weeks after immunization paralleled maximum TRC antibody titer. The specificity of elevated insulin response consequent on thyroglobulin immunization was shown by (*a*) lack of increase in serum insulin in adjuvant-injected animals, albumin-immunized rabbits or in patients with markedly elevated serum gamma globulin or other organ-specific antibodies, and by (*b*) *in vitro* specificity studies (Premachandra *et al.*, 1970).

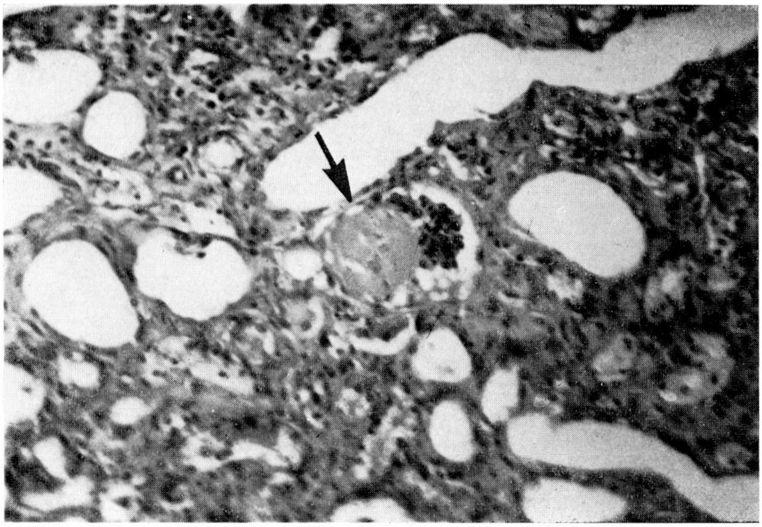

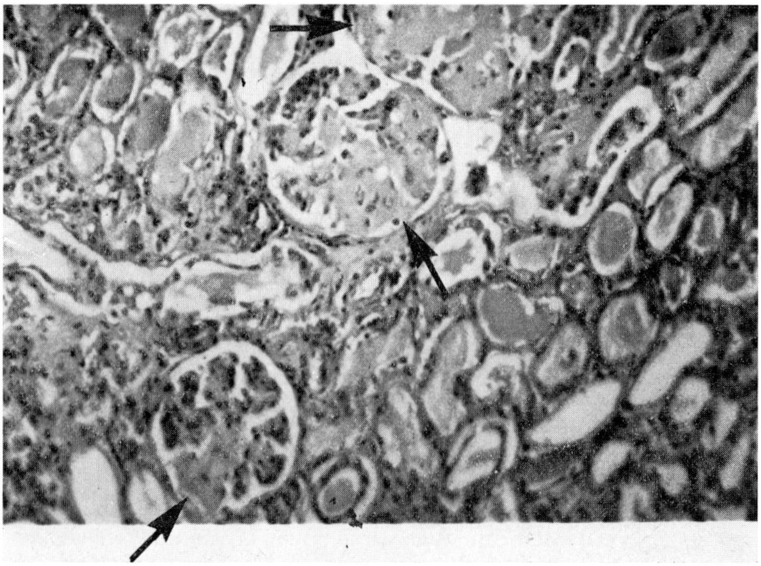

Fig. 9. Sections of kidneys from thyroglobulin-immunized rabbits.

Top: In the center of the figure is a single large hyaline nodule compressing the remainder of the glomerulus. Note the absence of basement membrane thickening in the compressed portion.
Bottom: This figure shows three glomeruli with the nodular lesion in various stages. At the lower margin is a single peripheral nodule containing a few mesangial nuclei. In the center several nodules coalesce, and at the upper edge is a portion of a glomerulus in which glomerular capillaries have been completely replaced by coalescent nodules.

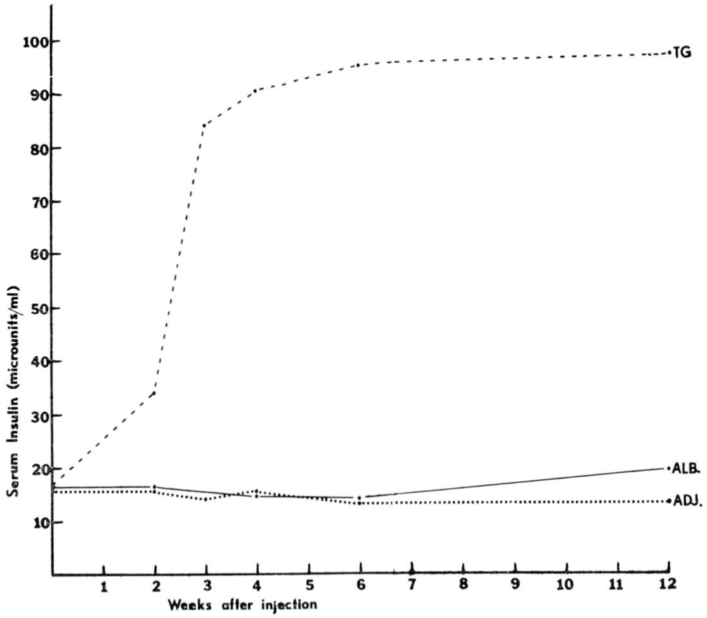

Fig. 10. Serum immunoreactive insulin levels in rabbits at various intervals after thyroglobulin, albumin or adjuvant administration. Each point represents the mean value for 6 animals.

B. *Other observations*

A majority of investigations from many laboratories have shown a greater than chance association of humoral and cell-bound thyroid autoantibodies in human diabetes (Irvine *et al.*, 1970; Landing *et al.*, 1963; Simkins, 1968).

C. *Implications of patho-physiological observations*

The observations reviewed in Sections A and B above signify many interesting implications and permit a speculative hypothesis relating thyroid immunity to certain pathophysiological changes in diabetes. First of all, is the nodular glomerular lesion really pathognomonic of diabetes mellitus in view of the duplication of similar lesions in insulin-immune and thyroglobulin-immune animals? This question can be answered in either of two ways assuming human and animal lesions are otherwise similar. It can be ascertained that the nodular lesions are really not specific for diabetes; or it can be hypothesized that thyroid immunity in some way induces elaboration of altered insulin which then evokes antibody response, similar to the elaboration of thyroid antibodies in response to altered thyroglobulin (Weigle, 1965). Nodular lesions may then arise as a result of glomerular trapping of circulating insulin-antibody complexes (it should also be pointed out that the possibility of antibody formation to another pancreatic antigen and its entry into this dynamic interplay of the proposed events is not excluded).

On the other hand, in non-insulin-treated human diabetics (who may or may not demonstrate thyroid autoimmunity) the inability to readily demonstrate insulin autoantibodies may argue against the proposed immunity hypothesis to explain the pathogenesis of glomerular and other vascular alterations. However, more recently, suggestive evidence for autoimmune processes involving pancreas in human diabetics (receiving no insulin) has begun to accrue; thus, lymphocytic infiltration around β-cells of the islets of Langerhans has been described by Gepts (1965) whereas sera from untreated diabetics were shown to interact with β-cells in immunofluorescent studies (Mancini *et al.*, 1965) as well as to fix complement in the presence of insulin (Chetty and Watson, 1965; Pav *et al.*, 1963). Furthermore, Penchev *et al.* (1968) have reported the detection of insulin-precipitating antibodies in untreated diabetic patients.

Preliminary investigations have indicated that blood sugar levels in animals with high immunoreactive serum insulin are not markedly different from the controls. It is possible that the elaborated insulin in induced thyroglobulin immunity is not biologically active, or this may also be an expression of the interplay of various homeostatic mechanisms in maintaining normal blood sugar. Should the latter be the case, it is conceivable that only when the immuno-patho-physiological embarrassment (altered insulin and antibody formation, glomerular nodular lesion, and other vascular complications) becomes severe that this will override the compensatory blood sugar regulatory mechanisms. Clinical symptoms of diabetes may then ensue. The hypothesis relating thyroglobulin immunity to insulin immunity and diabetes is not entirely new and derives support from the following: (*a*) many instances of concurrent autoimmune phenomena have been described by various investigators (Anderson *et al.*, 1967; Mackay and Macfarlane Burnet, 1963) and are generally well known; (*b*) Fialkow (1966) has even suggested that thyroid immunity may trigger various other immunities. It should be pointed out, however, that thyroid autoantibodies are present only in a certain proportion of diabetic population, and conservative estimates maintain the occurrence of nodular glomerular lesions in diabetes to be no greater than 20%. The interrelation hypothesis is probably applicable only in such cases, and in the remaining instances diabetes may result from other unknown causes.

SUMMARY

Some of the recent biochemical and immuno-pathophysiological investigations in experimentally-induced thyroid immunity are reviewed. Based on the inhibiting activity of various compounds as examined by a radioimmunological method, minimum structural configuration for haptenic inhibition of thyroxine-binding thyroid antibodies has been proposed. Data from this and other laboratories on antigenic specificity of thyroglobulin are reviewed and seem to suggest a decrease in the number of determinants participating in the autoimmune system. The effect of induced thyroid immunity on thyroid function and thyroxine metabolism are briefly reviewed; it is suggested that cognizance of antibody effects on circulating thyroxine as well as the stage of the thyroid lesion at the time of investigation, together may resolve apparent discrepancies evident in thyroid function studies in experimental thyroiditis. The various ways by which thyroxine-binding antibodies in thyroid-immune serum may affect thyroxine metabolism in mice, and hence the validity of LATS, are briefly reviewed. In addition to lymphocytic infiltration of the thyroid, vascular and perivascular lesions are also described in thyroglobulin-immunized animals. Of significance is the finding of nodular glomerular lesions similar to the human diabetic nodular lesion (K-W lesion), accompanied by elevated immunoreactive serum insulin levels in a significant proportion of thyroglobulin-immunized rabbits. Based on these and other observations, an interrelated hypothesis has been proposed linking thyroglobulin immunity, nodular glomerular lesion and diabetes.

ACKNOWLEDGMENT

Grateful acknowledgment is made of the assistance of Dr. H. T. Blumenthal in pathological investigations.

REFERENCES

ADAMS, D. D. (1958): The presence of an abnormal thyroid-stimulating hormone in the serum of some thyrotoxic patients. *J. clin. Endocr. 18*, 699.

ALEXANDER, N. M. (1968): Iodopeptides from rat thyroglobulin. *Endocrinology*, *82*, 925.

ANDERSON, J. R., BUCHANAN, W. W. and GOUDIE, R. B. (1967): *Autoimmunity, Clinical and Experimental.* Charles C. Thomas, Springfield, Ill.

ANDERSON, J. W., WAKIM, K. G. and MCCONAHEY, W. M. (1969): The influence of experimental thyroiditis on thyroid function. *Mayo Clin. Proc.*, *44*, 711.

BEALL, G. N. and SOLOMON, D. H. (1966): Inhibition of long-acting thyroid stimulator by thyroid particulate fractions. *J. clin. Invest. 45*, 552.

BIASSONI, P., INDIVERI, F. and FRESCO, G. (1965): Stude di funzionelità tiroidea in corso di tireopatia immunitaria sperimentale. II. Effetto del TSH sull'attivita proteolitica dell'omogenato tiroideo. *Pathologica*, *57*, 187.

BURKE, G. (1968): Experimental production of long-acting thyroid stimulator *in vivo*. *J. Lab. clin. Med.*, *72*, 17.

CHETTY, M. P. and WATSON, K. C. (1965): Antibody-like activity in diabetic and normal serum, measured by complement consumption. *Lancet*, *I*, 67.

DEGROOT, L. J., HALL, R., MCDERMOTT, W. V., JR and DAVIS, A. M. (1962): Hashimoto's thyroiditis. A genetically conditioned disease. *New. Engl. J. Med.*, *267*, 267.

FIALKOW, P. J. (1966): Autoimmunity and chromosomal aberrations. *Amer. J. hum. Genet.*, *18*, 93.

FLAX, M. H. and BILOTE, J. B. (1965): Experimental allergic thyroiditis in the guinea pig. III. Correlation of morphologic and functional changes in early lesions. *Ann. N.Y. Acad. Sci. 124*, 234.

FLORSHEIM, W. H. (1971): On several mechanisms determining LATS responses in the McKenzie assay. In: *Further Advances in Thyroid Research. Proceedings, VI International Thyroid Conference.* Editors: K. Fellinger and R. Hofer.

GEPTS, W. (1965): Pathologic anatomy of the pancreas in juvenile diabetes mellitus. *Diabetes 14*, 619.

GODAL, T. (1967): On the specificity of human thyroglobulin auto-antibodies. *Acta path. microbiol. scand.*, *69*, 205.

GORMAN, C. A., ANDERSON, J. W., FLOCK, E. V., OWEN, C. A., JR. and WAKIM, K. G. (1969): Effect of experimentally induced thyroiditis on biosynthesis of thyroxine in rats. *Acta endocr. (Kbh.) 62*, 11.

HUNG, W., CHANDLER, R. W., KYLE, M. A. and BLIZZARD, R. M. (1962): Studies of thyroid hormone synthesis in experimental autoimmune thyroiditis. *Acta endocr. (Kbh.)*, *40*, 297.

IRVINE, W. J., SCARTH, L., CLARKE, B. F., CULLEN, D. R. and DUNCAN, L. J. P. (1970): Thyroid and gastric autoimmunity in patients with diabetes mellitus. *Lancet*, *II*, 163.

KIMMELSTIEL, P. and WILSON, C. (1936): Intercapillary lesions in the glomeruli of the kidney. *Amer. J. Path.*, *12*, 83.

KRISS, J. P., PLESHAKOV, V. and CHIEN, J. R. (1964): Isolation and identification of the long-acting thyroid stimulator and its relation to hyperthyroidism and circumscribed pretibial myxedema. *J. clin. Endocr.*, *24*, 1005.

LANDING, B. H., PETTIT, M. D., WIENS, R. L., KNOWLES, H. and GUEST, G. M. (1963): Antithyroid antibody and chronic thyroiditis in diabetes. *J. clin. Endocr.*, *23*, 119.

MACKAY, I. R. and BURNET, F. M. (1963): *Autoimmune Diseases.* Charles C. Thomas, Springfield, Ill.

MCKENZIE, J. M. (1968): Humoral factors in the pathogenesis of Graves' disease. *Physiol. Rev.*, *48*, 252.

MANCINI, A. M., ZAMPA, G. A., VECCHI, A. and COSTANZI, G. (1965): Histoimmunological techniques for detecting anti-insulin antibodies in human sera. *Lancet*, *I*, 1189.

MANDY, W. J., FUDENBERG, H. H. and LEWIS, F. B. (1965): A new serum factor in normal rabbits. I. Identification and characterization. *J. Immunol.*, *95*, 501.

MARGHERITA, S. S. and PREMACHANDRA, B. N. (1969): Studies on thyroglobulin immunity. VI. Thyroid hormones and thyroglobulin specificity. *J. Immunol.*, *102*, 1511.

MATES, G. P. and SHULMAN, S. (1967): Studies on thyroid proteins. III. Precipitating activity of autoimmune and heteroimmune antisera with human thyroglobulin. *Immunochemistry*, *4*, 319.

MATES, G. P. and SHULMAN, S. (1968): Studies on thyroid proteins. IV. Haemagglutinating activity of molecular fragments of human thyroid proteins. *Immunology*, *14*, 89.

METZGER, H., SHARP, G. C. and EDELHOCH, H. (1962): The properties of thyroglobulin. VII. The immunologic activity of thyroglobulin fragments. *Biochemistry*, *1*, 205.

MORGANS, M. E. and TROTTER, W. R. (1957): Defective organic binding of iodine by the thyroid in Hashimoto's thyroiditis. *Lancet, I*, 553.

PAV, J., JEZKOVA, Z. and SKRHA, F. (1963): Insulin antibodies. *Lancet, II*, 221.

PENCHEV, I., ANDREEV, D. and DITZOV, S. (1968): Insulin-precipitating antibodies in insulin treated and untreated diabetic patients. *Diabetologia, 4*, 164.

PREMACHANDRA, B. N. (1967): Thyroglobulin immunity: Recent physiological and histological observations. In: *Proceedings, III Asia and Oceania Congress of Endocrinology*, p. 89. Editor: A. D. Litonjua.

PREMACHANDRA, B. N., BERNS, A. W. and BLUMENTHAL, H. T. (1965): Physiological aspects of thyroglobulin immunity. III. Studies of localization of antibodies in vascular tissue and abnormal plasma thyroxine binding in the guinea pig. *J. Lab. clin. Med., 66*, 893.

PREMACHANDRA, B. N. and BLUMENTHAL, H. T. (1967): Abnormal binding of thyroid hormone in sera from patients with Hashimoto's disease. *J. clin. Endocr., 27*, 931.

PREMACHANDRA, B. N., IBRAHIM, I. I. and BLUMENTHAL, H. T. (1970): Nodular glomerulosclerosis and serum insulin in active thyroglobulin immunity. In: *Abstracts, VII Congress International Diabetes Federation*, p. 135. Editors: R. R. Rodriguez, F. J. G. Ebling, I. Henderson and R. Assan. ICS No. 209. Excerpta Medica, Amsterdam.

PREMACHANDRA, B. N., RAY, A. K. and BLUMENTHAL, H. T. (1963*a*): Effect of thyroglobulin immunization on thyroid function and morphology in the guinea pig. *Endocrinology, 73*, 145.

PREMACHANDRA, B. N., RAY, A. K., HIRATA, Y. and BLUMENTHAL, H. T. (1963*b*): Electrophoretic studies of thyroxine and triiodothyronine binding by the sera of guinea pigs immunized against thyroglobulin. *Endocrinology, 73*, 135.

RICHIE, E. R., WOOLSEY, M. E. and MANDY, W. J. (1970): A new serum factor in normal rabbits. VI. Reaction with buried determinants of IgG exposed sequentially with CNBr, pepsin and papain. *J. Immunol., 104*, 984.

ROITT, I. M., CAMPBELL, P. N. and DONIACH, D. (1958): The nature of the thyroid auto-antibodies present in patients with Hashimoto's thyroiditis (lymphadenoid goitre). *Biochem. J., 69*, 248.

ROITT, I. M., TORRIGIANI, G. and DONIACH, D. (1968): Immunochemical studies on the thyroglobulin autoantibody system in human thyroiditis. *Immunology, 15*, 681.

SHULMAN, S. (1968): Tissue specificity and autosensitization: The thyroid model. In: *International Convocation on Immunology*, p. 313. Editors: N. R. Rose and F. Milgrom. Karger, Basel.

SHULMAN, S. and GHAYASUDDIN, M. (1971): Isolation and antigenic characterization of thyroglobulin fragments. In: *Further Advances in Thyroid Research. Proceedings, VI International Thyroid Conference.* Editors: K. Fellinger and R. Hofer.

SHULMAN, S. and WITEBSKY, E. (1960): Studies on organ specificity. IX. Biophysical and immunochemical studies on human thyroid autoantibody. *J. Immunol., 85*, 559.

SIMKINS, S. (1968): Antithyroglobulin antibodies in diabetes mellitus. *Diabetes, 17*, 136.

SMITH, D. W. E. and ADAMS, W. R. (1966): Alterations in the values for tests of thyroid function in rabbits with immunologically produced thyroiditis. *Lab. Invest., 15*, 885.

SOLOMON, D. H., BEALL, G. N. and CHOPRA, I. J. (1971): Mobilization of tissue thyroxine in mice by thyroxine-binding proteins: studies with a double-isotope McKenzie assay. In: *Further Advances in Thyroid Research. Proceedings, VI International Thyroid Conference.* Editors: K. Fellinger and R. Hofer.

STYLOS, W. A. and ROSE, N. R. (1969): Splitting of human thyroglobulin. II. Enzymatic digestion. *Clin. exp. Immunol., 5*, 285.

TORIZUKA, K., FLAX, M. H. and STANBURY, J. B. (1964): Metabolic studies on experimental allergic thyroiditis. *Endocrinology, 74*, 746.

WEIGLE, W. O. (1965): The production of thyroiditis and antibody following injection of unaltered thyroglobulin without adjuvant into rabbits previously stimulated with altered thyroglobulin. *J. exp. Med., 122*, 1049.

WEIGLE, W. O., HIGH, G. J. and NAKAMURA, R. M. (1969): The role of mycobacteria and the effect of proteolytic degradation of thyroglobulin on the production of autoimmune thyroiditis. *J. exp. Med., 130*, 243.

NEWER ASPECTS OF THYROID CANCER

BORIS CATZ

University of Southern California School of Medicine, Los Angeles, Calif., U.S.A.

The newer aspects of thyroid cancer are the following:

A high incidence of anaplastic thyroid cancer has been observed in endemic goiter areas. A personal report given to me by Dr. Jaime Cortázar from the Instituto Nacional de Cancerologia in Bogota, Colombia shows this clearly (Table I).

These data suggest that a thyroid-suppressive medication should be used at an early stage of the development of the goiter. This treatment will facilitate the inhibition of thyroid-stimulating hormone release from the pituitary, thus avoiding the stimulation of the goiter.

The rare occurrence of cancer in Graves' disease has been emphasized by many authors (Beahrs *et al.*, 1951; Sokal, 1954; Olen and Klinck, 1966). They report an incidence range from 0.5% to 2.5%. In all these reports, subtotal thyroidectomy was the surgical procedure. We have found an incidence of 9% of cancer of the thyroid in 172 consecutive thyroidectomies for Graves' disease (Shapiro *et al.*, 1970). Fifty per cent of the cases with carcinoma had multicentricity or intrathyroidal metastases. As seen in Table II, 20 of the 172 cases received previous treatment with radioactive iodine for Graves' disease. Three of them had carcinoma of the thyroid, a suggested incidence of 15%.

This high incidence of thyroid carcinoma in hyperthyroidism would indicate that surgery should be given greater consideration in the selection of a modality for the management of Graves' disease and that a total thyroidectomy should be performed.

Medullary carcinoma of the thyroid has ceased to be a rare occurrence (Table III). It has

TABLE I

Total # of cases	Anaplastic cancer	%
362	114	31.5

(Data from Dr. Jaime Cortázar, Instituto Nacional de Cancerologia, Bogota, Colombia, S. A.)

TABLE II

		Cancer	%
Total no. of cases	172	15	9
Previous treatment with I^{131}	20	3	15
No previous treatment with I^{131}	152	12	8

TABLE III

Medullary carcinoma
High levels of calcitonin

Clinical manifestations	Associated tumors
Multiple mucocutaneous neuromas	
(eyelids, tongue, buccal mucosae)	Pheochromocytoma
Ganglioneuromatosis of the large intestines	
Hyperpigmentation	Parathyroid adenoma or hyperplasia
Diarrhea	
Myopathy	
Marfan features	

been recognized as a dangerous disease, with a potential for multiglandular involvement and multiple manifestations (Cunliffe *et al.*, 1968; 1970; Hill, 1969; Tashjian and Melvin, 1968).

A high level of calcitonin is characteristic of this disease (Tashjian and Melvin, 1968).

Patients with medullary carcinoma should be followed closely, in order to be able to uncover the presence of pheochromocytoma and/or parathyroid pathology.

The rarity of reports of metastatic thyroid carcinoma producing hyperthyroidism may be misleading. Its occurrence may not be as rare (Leiter *et al.*, 1946; McLaughlin *et al.*, 1970; Ginsberg *et al.*, 1963; Valenta *et al.*, 1970). Recent reports seem to confirm that with the presently available techniques, the diagnosis can be established promptly and with ease (McLaughlin *et al.*, 1970; Valenta *et al.*, 1970).

As we suggested previously (Ginsberg *et al.*, 1963) by following our program of treatment

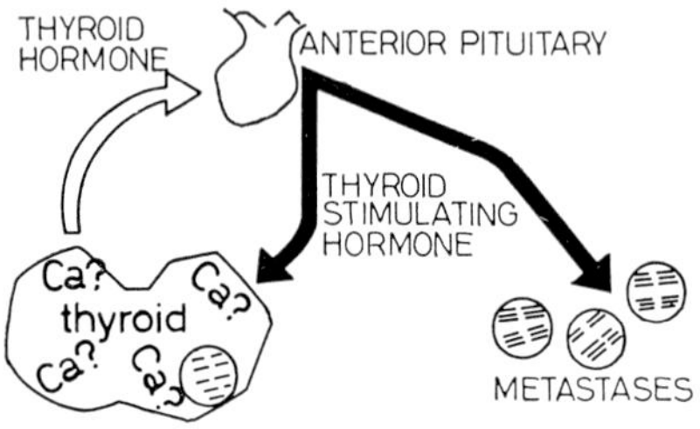

Fig. 1. Thyroid cancer (pre-operational).

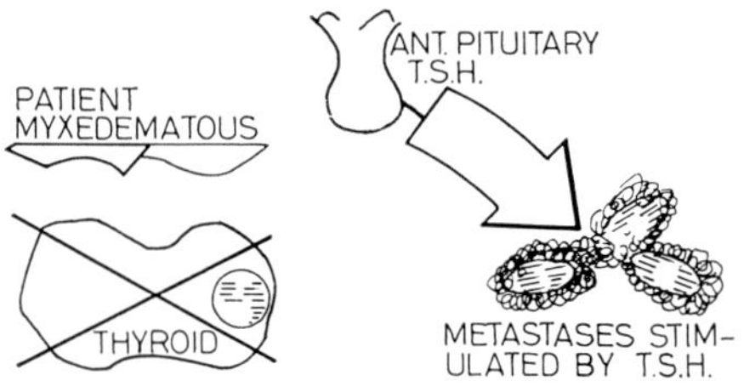

Fig. 2. Total thyroidectomy.

for cancer of the thyroid, this occurrence can be avoided. In all cases reported, less than a total thyroidectomy was done.

Cancer of the thyroid kills, even though slowly.

Our program of treatment for thyroid carcinoma consists of the following (Figs. 1–4):

1. Total thyroidectomy.
2. Thyroid medication to tolerance for life.
3. Periodic treatment with I^{131} in cancerocidal amounts after previous preparation with bovine TSH. This treatment will eliminate remnant thyroid and/or metastatic tissue. Scanning is done as early as 48 hours after the treatment dose of I^{131}.

This program we consider to be a complete treatment for thyroid cancer (Catz *et al.*, 1959*a*; *b*; Ginsberg *et al.*, 1963).

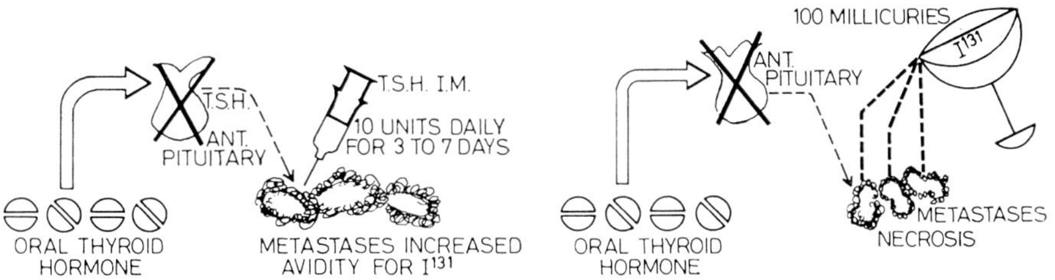

Fig. 3. Periodic use of exogenous thyrotropic hormone – before treatment with I^{131}.

Fig. 4. After bovine TSH therapeutic dose of I^{131} shows positive collection in 78%.

REFERENCES

BEAHRS, O. H., PEMBERTON, J. DE J. and BLACK, B. M. (1951): Nodular goiter and malignant lesion of the thyroid gland. *J. clin. Endocr.*, *11*, 1157.

CATZ, B., PETIT, D. W., SCHWARTZ, H., DAVIS, F., MCCANNON, C. and STARR, P. (1959): Treatment of cancer of the thyroid postoperatively with suppressive thyroid medication, radioactive iodine and thyroid nonstimulating hormone. *Cancer*, *12*, 371.

CATZ, B., PETIT, D. and STARR, P. (1959): The diagnostic and therapeutic value of thyrotropic hormone and heavy dosage scintigrams for the demonstration of thyroid cancer metastases. *Amer. J. med. Sci.*, *237*, 158.

CORTÁZAR, J.: Personal communication.

CUNLIFFE, W. J., *et al.* (1968): A calcitonin-secreting thyroid carcinoma. *Lancet*, *1*, 63.

CUNLIFFE, W. J., *et al.* (1970): A calcitonin-secreting medullary thyroid carcinoma associated with mucosal neuromas, marfanoid features, myopathy and pigmentation. *Amer. J. Med.*, *48*. 120.

GINSBURG, E., CATZ, B., NELSON, C. L., KOZIKOWSKI, B. M. and Chesne, E. L. (1963): Hyperthyroidism secondary to metastatic functioning thyroid carcinoma. *Ann. intern. Med.*, *58*, 684.

HILL, C. S., JR. (1969): *The 'Bad' Thyroid Cancer*. G. P. Press.

LEITER, L., SEIDLIN, S. M., MARINELLI, L. D. and BAUMANN, E. J. (1946): Adenocarcinoma of the thyroid with hyperthyroidism and functional metastases. Studies with thiouracil and radio-iodine. *J. clin. Endocr.*, *6*, 247.

MCLAUGHLIN, R. P., SCHOLZ, D. A., MCCONAHEY, W. M. and CHILDS, D. S., JR. (1970): Metastatic thyroid carcinoma with hyperthyroidism: Two cases with functioning metastatic follicular thyroid carcinoma. *Mayo Clin. Proc.*, *45*, 328

OLEN, E. and KLINCK, G. H. (1966): Hyperthyroidism and thyroid cancer. *Arch. Path. 81*, 531.

SHAPIRO, S. J., FRIEDMAN, N.B., PERZIK, S. L. and CATZ, B. (1970): Incidence of thyroid carcinoma in Graves' disease. *Cancer*, in press.

SOKAL, J. E. (1954): Incidence of malignancy in toxic and nontoxic nodular goiter. *J. Amer. med. Ass.*, *154*, 1321.

TASHJIAN, A. H., JR. and MELVIN, K. E. W. (1968): Medullary carcinoma of the thyroid gland: Studies of thyrocalcitonin in plasma and tumor extracts. *New Engl. J. Med.*, *279*, 279.

VALENTA, L., LEMARCHAND-BÉRAUD, T., NEMES, J., GRIESSEN, M. and BEDNAR, J. (1970): Metastatic thyroid carcinoma provoking hyperthyroidism with elevated circulating thyrostimulators. *Amer. J. Med.*, *48*, 72.

PATHOGENESIS AND VARIABILITY OF ENDEMIC GOITER

JOSÉ BARZELATTO*

School of Medicine, University of Chile, Santiago, Chile

I have been asked to present a review for this congress on the pathogenesis and variability of endemic goiter. However, it did not seem advisable to me to attempt to write a complete review of the medical literature and I have chosen to limit myself to presenting my personal view of the problem, emphasizing especially those aspects which I believe require further research.

I. ETIOLOGY

a. *Iodine intake*

For more than a century, evidence has been accumulated relating a low iodine intake to endemic goiter (Langer, 1960). Iodine deficiency was generally accepted to be the main or only etiological factor, after the work of Marine and Kimball demonstrating the effectiveness of iodide prophylaxis in preventing endemic goiter (Kimball, 1961). Finally, Stanbury and co-workers in Argentina, using modern research tools, demonstrated that iodine lack could be the cause of endemic goiter (Stanbury *et al.*, 1954).

From a practical standpoint we could end this review here. Endemic goiter is a public health concept and not a disease in a strictly nosological sense. It is accepted that endemic goiter exists when an 'important' percentage of the population shows a 'definite' enlargement of the thyroid gland. An epidemiological definition is arrived at by arbitrary conventions expressing what percentage is required to define endemia, size and selection of the sample of the population that should be examined, criteria to establish and classify an enlargement of the gland, etc. Nowhere in such a definition is the etiology mentioned, although implicitly a common cause is assumed. Experience has shown almost always, that when a significant goitrous endemia is present, the population has a low iodine intake, usually less than 50 mg daily. Furthermore, when iodine supplementation of the diet is provided, epidemiological indices show spectacular improvements. To the public health administrator what has been said might be enough for practical purposes, but for the endocrinologist such an oversimplified view ignores the most interesting aspects of the problem.

During the last decade, increasing examples of goiter endemias have been demonstrated, where iodine intake is 'normal' or 'increased' (Costa and Cottino, 1963; Peltola, 1960; Suzuki *et al.*, 1965; Clements *et al.*, 1968, Gaitán *et al.*, 1969; Balan *et al.*, 1969; London *et al.*, 1965; Vought *et al.*, 1967). On the other hand, the observation that iodine deficiency does not always produce a goiter (Barzelatto *et al.*, 1954; Barzelatto *et al.*, 1955; Roche, 1959) has been confirmed in several parts of the world (Demarchi *et al.*, Buzina *et al.*, 1959; Lamberg *et al.*, 1962; Campos *et al.*, 1962; Sunderland and Cartwright, 1968; Malvaux *et al.*, (1969) including those endemic areas where the deficiency is most extreme, as in New Guinea

* Present address: Organization of American States, 1735 Eye Street, N.W. Washington, D.C., 20006, U.S.A.

(Choufoer *et al.*, 1963; Buttfield *et al.*, 1966). Repeatedly, it has been shown that individuals without goiter, living in endemic goiter areas, show no difference in iodine metabolism in relation to those persons with goiter (Malamos *et al.*, 1966; Gandra, 1967; Barzelatto *et al.*, 1967; Beckers *et al.*, 1967; Gray *et al.*, 1969; Greig *et al.*, 1970).

Such facts pose, as a first problem, the need to define what is a 'normal' iodine intake. It could be said that it is the amount required by the thyroid to maintain euthyroidism, without developing endemic goiter. Such a definition is obviously inadequate.

In New Guinea (Choufoer *et al.*, 1963) the inhabitants of Tiom do not have endemic goiter with a daily iodine intake of about 20 μg, while their neighbors in Mulia, with a similar intake, demonstrate one of the most severe endemias present in our time. In Hokkaido, on the northern coast of Japan, among children eating more than 20 mg of iodine daily, about one of every four develop a goiter while the other three do not (Suzuki *et al.*, 1965). Between these two extreme cases, the medical literature reveals practically every intermediary situation.

From a different point of view, it is of interest to point out that in areas considered free of endemic goiter, iodine intake as judged by urinary iodine excretion, is usually of the order of 100 to 300 μg daily. In the United States, where endemic goiter does not exist in general, recent surveys estimate iodine intake as varying from 240 to 700 μg daily and over most of the country the range is 240 to 400 μg (Oddie *et al.*, 1970). These figures are higher than some previously recorded and attributable to a more widespread use of iodized salt. It will be of interest to observe if the prevalence of goiter increases in the areas with the highest intakes.

It thus seems preferable, rather than to define a normal intake, to try to establish both a minimal and a maximal level of intake that could be recommended. For this purpose one should remember that the daily obligatory loss of iodine by the human body seems to be of the order of 10 μg and the people of Tiom seem to show that normal thyroid function without goiter can be maintained with little more than that (Choufoer *et al.*, 1963). Nevertheless, several empirical criteria, based on the minimal effective prophylactic dose, coincide with kinetic data in suggesting a minimal daily requirement of 70 to 120 μg (Wayne *et al.*, 1964). It is even more difficult to look for an acceptable maximal level.

It is well known that excessive iodine intake temporarily blocks thyroid function and that this block may persist in 'susceptible' persons and initiate goiter and hyperthyroidism. Such persons presumably have another coadjuvant factor, genetic or environmental, that does not manifest itself *per se* (Wolff, 1969). It is of interest that there are chemical compounds that act synergistically to produce 'iodide goiter' as is the case with phenazone (Pasternak *et al.*, 1969). The study of goiter endemias with high iodine intake such as those of Japan (Suzuki *et al.*, 1965) and Colombia (Gaitán *et al.*, 1969) might be considered with these facts in mind. Let me also mention that Stewart and Murray (1967) demonstrated in normal subjects that in order to obtain an acute block of organification, 750 μg corresponding to a PII (Plasma Inorganic Iodide) of 30 to 38 μg/l, were necessary. After TSH stimulation, the same effect was obtained with 350 μg, equivalent to a PII of 15 μg/l. In Colombia (Wahner and Gaitán, 1969) PII levels of 12 to 18 μg/l and a daily urinary excretion of 568 μg have been demonstrated. In Hokkaido (Suzuki *et al.*, 1965) the PII levels observed ranged from 140 to 500 μg/l.

In summary, a 'normal' daily iodine intake, the goal of any good prophylaxis, should probably be between a minimum of 100 to 150 and a maximum of 300 to 400 μg. It is unnecessary to say that there is a great need for improving such estimates, since it seems quite possible that either lack or excess of iodine intake may contribute to the pathogenesis of endemic goiter.

b. *Other environmental factors*

The existence of endemic goiter with such different levels of iodine intake and the fact that goiter is present only in a percentage of the population forces one to look for other factors which might be involved in the etiopathogenesis of endemic goiter.

It would be a formidable task to classify the great number of natural compounds that have been demonstrated experimentally to be goitrogenic. Nevertheless, until recently, very few of them had been thought to be involved in the etiology of goiter endemias (Podoba and Langer, 1964) probably because most investigators did not look into the possibility of a goitrogen being involved once they had found iodine deficiency and no block of thyroid radioiodine metabolism. This reasoning was no longer acceptable once Peltola and his co-workers (Peltola, 1965; Krusius and Peltola, 1966) demonstrated experimentally that the dose of a compound with goitrogenic activity was 1000 times smaller than the one needed to show its effect upon radioiodine metabolism, as had been previously suggested (Mitchell *et al.*, 1961; Mulvey and Slingerland, 1962; Yamada and Scichijo, 1962). Furthermore, goitrogenic foods frequently contain a combination of active compounds that can act upon the thyroid by different mechanisms and that can potentiate each other (Langer, 1966). Goitrogens can also act by influencing the peripheral metabolism of thyroid hormones (Herrera *et al.*, 1968).

Natural goitrogens are present in cow's milk in Finland in a concentration sufficient to produce goiter in man (Arstila *et al.*, 1969). Clements in Australia has evidence for the role of plant natural goitrogens transmitted through milk in the pathogenesis of human endemic goiter (Clements *et al.*, 1968). In Navarra, in the north of Spain, goiter prevalence has been related to the ingestion of turnips by cattle (Muñoz-Rodriguez, 1964). In Nigeria, Ekpechi (1967) explains the different prevalence of a goiter endemia from one village to another by the amount of cassava ingested, a very popular foodstuff that he has shown experimentally to be goitrogenic (Ekpechi *et al.*, 1966). Langer in Czechoslovakia (cited in Greig *et al.*, 1970) and Ermans in the Congo (Ermans *et al.*, 1969) have found elevated blood levels of thiocyanate among subjects living in endemic goiter areas that could reflect an increased intake of goitrogenic foods.

In Turkey (Kologlu and Kologlu, 1968) a study showed no change in endemic goiter prevalence among people who ate 100 to 400 g daily of 'kale' in relation to those who did not eat this vegetable, which is known to be goitrogenic and which has been linked to differences in prevalence in another endemia with iodine deficiency (Podoba and Langer, 1964). In Chile (Barzelatto and Covarrubias, 1969) we were able to demonstrate a relation between prevalence and size of goiter and the amount of 'piñón' ingested, a nut that is experimentally goitrogenic in rats (Tellez *et al.*, 1969). In Spain, the ingestion of chestnuts has been related to a goiter endemia and their goitrogenic effect has also been demonstrated in rats (Linazasoro *et al.*, 1970).

Greer (Podoba and Langer, 1964) has written an excellent review of the different types of natural goitrogens. Let me merely point out that most of them are in the form of glycosides and that the active principle has to be liberated by enzymatic hydrolysis. The enzymes necessary are present in the same foods, but are destroyed by boiling, and are also present in the bowel as a bacterial product.

It is of interest that Sedlak (1961) was able to grow cabbage with or without goitrogenic activity by changing the supply of sulphur in the liquid used as nutrient. This experiment correlated well with the old observation that the amount of rain is proportional to the goitrogenic capacity of some plants and their sulfyhydryl content (Podoba and Langer, 1964; Jirousek, 1959). Recently in Ceylon (*Nutrition Reviews*, 1968) the clinical correlation between rain and endemic goiter has again been made. Zak, in an area with iodine deficiency, has related the presence of goiter to a high sulphate content of drinking water which is not present in areas without goiter (Zak, 1967). Allcroft and Salt had demonstrated that the goitrogenic activity of a species of cabbage could be increased by fertilizing the plant with chilean nitrate instead of ammonium sulphate (Allcroft and Salt, 1960). This type of information may allow us to explain the geographical correlation of endemic goiter and certain types of soil (World Health Organization, 1960) that are related to iodine content (Merke, 1965; 1967) but could also influence the goitrogenic activity of local food (Ermans *et al.*, 1969).

Various mineral salts are able to influence the experimental production of goiter. Sodium chloride favors the renal loss of iodide (Yamada and Scichijo, 1962; Isler, 1961; Boatman *et al.*, 1960) but this effect apparently is not present in man (Stanbury, 1960). Many metallic cations interfere with thyroid iodide uptake (Verzhikovskaya and Shvaiki, 1959) and some with the goitrogenic activity of some compounds (Samofal, 1959). Magnesium deficiency could be goitrogenic (Corradino and Parker, 1962) but in man it has been reported that high doses of magnesium are antigoitrogenic (Naguib, 1963). Patients have developed goiter when receiving lithium (Schou *et al.*, 1968), fluoride and cobalt (Kriss, 1955; Klinck, 1955; Paley *et al.*, 1958; Chamberlain, 1961; Sederholm *et al.*, 1968). Nevertheless, experimental and epidemiological evidence are strongly against a goitrogenic role for fluoride (Knizhnikov, 1959; Siddiqui, 1960; Henning, 1961; Leone *et al.*, 1964; Saka *et al.*, 1965; Frada *et al.*, 1969; Costa *et al.*, 1967). Cobalt does not seem to be important as a goitrogen in endemic goiter areas; on the contrary an inverse correlation with its concentration in food has been reported (Oparin, 1969). Foods in endemic goiter areas could have a higher proportion of zinc; nevertheless, goiters may have a lower content than normal glands in endemic areas (Kovalev, 1960). Goiters in endemic goiter areas would also have a higher bromine content (Turetskaya, 1961) which has been shown in rats to interfere with thyroid iodide uptake (Clode *et al.*, 1960). With respect to calcium, experimental evidence is contradictory (Gandra and Coniglio, 1961; Braham *et al.*, 1962; Boyle *et al.*, 1966; Harrison *et al.*, 1967), but the epidemiological data only exceptionally point towards a possible role of an excess of calcium in endemic goiter areas (Sunderland and Cartwright, 1968).

Research also continues on the possible role of vitamins in the development of goiter. Experimental evidence has been reported for goitrogenic activity of both excess and lack of vitamin A (Benedek, 1962; Shimoda and Shichijo, 1963) and a deficiency of this vitamin has been related to an endemic (Horvat and Maver, 1958) where iodine deficiency was also present (Buzina *et al.*, 1959), but its administration had no effect upon the goiters of another similar endemia (Scrimshaw, 1958). It is important to point out that Benedek (1962) has reported a patient who developed a goiter when given vitamin A and phenylbutazone, but did not do so when administered these two substances separately at the same dose. The goitrogenic activity of vitamin C has been experimentally demonstrated (Cruz-Coke and Plaza de los Reyes, 1947; Andreas and Andreas, 1962) but it has also been reported that its deficiency potentiates the goitrogenic effect of methylthiouracil (Byshevskii, 1960). In endemic goiter the vitamin C content of the gland is proportional to the amount of colloid, while in Graves' disease both colloid and epithelium are rich in this vitamin (Kasabian and Chernyavskaya, 1957). It has been claimed that the administration of an excess of vitamins C and B in iodine-deficient goiters enhances the ability to accumulate iodine (Turetskaya, 1960).

Many papers have pointed out the higher frequency of endemic goiter in rural areas and its correlation with the standard of living (Kelly and Snedden, 1960). Lai observed an increase of goiter prevalence in Formosa by the end of the Second World War that declined later to increase again in 1958 and '59, the changes being greater in mountainous and rural communities than in industrial cities and correlated with price indices, nutritional status and availability of potable water (Lai, 1960).

Similar increases have been reported in other parts of the world (Clements, 1960; Costa and Mortara, 1960). Lowenstein followed in Brazil (Lowenstein, 1959) a group of 75 families among whom the prevalence of goiter correlated with their degree of poverty and diminished as their standard of living increased. This author reviews early medical literature that would seem to suggest that the quality of food in general is important for the production of goiter, an observation that is in agreement with accumulated evidence in experimental research on goiter production (Tellez, 1966).

In summary, there is enough evidence to accept that food, including drinking water (Gaitan, 1969), may contain goitrogenic factors that in various proportions can play a role in the pathogenesis of endemic goiter. These goitrogenic factors can potentiate each other but, what is probably more important, can also enhance the effect upon the thyroid of a lack or excess of iodine.

c. *Genetic factors*

The common clinical observation of families with many goitrous members has suggested the presence of hereditary factors in the etiopathogenesis of goiter, either sporadic or endemic. Research in this direction has been stimulated during the last decade by the demonstration of hereditary enzymatic defects, causing sporadic cretinism, and of iodine metabolism abnormalities in families with euthyroid goiters in non-endemic areas. Nevertheless, the presence of hereditary enzymatic defects in the pathogenesis of endemic goiter has not been demonstrated.

Koutras, in the Greek endemic (Koutras *et al.*, 1967; 1968) has indirect evidence suggesting that the difference between goitrous and non-goitrous subjects could be explained by a greater efficiency of the normal-size glands to trap and utilize iodine. Thiocyanate and perchlorate tests have repeatedly shown no radioiodine discharge from the thyroid in many different endemias. Roche *et al.* (1957) demonstrated in Venezuela a very moderate discharge shortly after administering the radioisotope. Only in the Hokkaido endemic has a definite block been demonstrated with positive discharge tests, as seen in sporadic goiter due to excessive iodine intake (Suzuki *et al.*, 1965). Needless to say, demonstrating a trap impairment or an organification block does not explain whether such a defect is genetic or environmental in origin.

In the same fashion, abnormal iodinated compounds have been looked for in the blood and urine of people living in endemic goiter areas. A frequent finding in iodine-deficient areas, is an increase in the serum of non-butanol-extractable radioiodine, especially among subjects with nodular goiters.

Such findings could be explained by a diminished intrathyroidal exchangeable radioiodine pool (Barzelatto and Covarrubias, 1968), but stable iodine determinations also show an increase in the fraction not extractable by butanol (Parker and Beierwaltes, 1962). The thyroid output of non-hormonal iodine, as iodide, iodotyrosines, polypeptides or thyroglobulin, directly into the blood or indirectly through lymphatics (Daniel *et al.*, 1966; 1967), increases with TSH stimulation and such a mechanism could explain these findings in endemic goiter (Sunderland and Cartwright, 1968; Rhodes, 1968; Wellby and O'Halloran, 1969). Furthermore, non-butanol-extractable iodinated compounds can originate outside the thyroid, as in the case of the peripheral metabolism of triiodothyronine (Surks and Oppenheimer, 1969), or can be serum albumin-iodinated by the thyroid (Lissitzky *et al.*, 1968). In other words, such findings also are not easy to interpret as being related to genetic defects.

The ability to deiodinate iodotyrosines has also been studied in many endemics, usually with negative results. Our finding in Pedregoso (Barzelatto *et al.*, 1967) of a very moderate impairment correlated with goiter size, could be explained as a result of the increased amount of circulating iodotyrosines, or a goitrogen could be postulated. Again this is *per se* another unsatisfactory approach to the study of genetic factors involved in endemic goiter.

The search for an association of genetic markers and endemic goiter has proved fruitful in the case of the tasting ability for phenylthiocarbamide (PTC). Non-tasters have a higher prevalence of nodular goiter (Azevedo *et al.*, 1965). We were unable to study such a relationship in Pedregoso, due to the very low percentage of non-tasters among the American Indians (Covarrubias *et al.*, 1965), but we could demonstrate that those with nodular goiters had higher tasting thresholds than those having diffuse goiters (Covarrubias *et al.*, 1969). On the other hand, numerous studies in different endemias have shown no relationship between goiter prevalence and PTC, with very few exceptions (Sunderland and Cartwright, 1968).

In agreement with these findings, family distribution studies for the presence of goiter in endemic areas have shown contradictory and in general negative results, when looking for simple Mendelian mechanisms (Covarrubias *et al.*, 1969; Malamos *et al.*, 1966). Instead we demonstrated a significant family relationship for nodularity (Covarrubias *et al.*, 1969): when both parents had nodular goiters 20.3% of their offspring also had it, while this was true for 9.3% of those where only one parent presented a nodular goiter and for 5.9% of the offspring of parents without nodular goiter. We also found that consanguinity seemed to favor the precocity of the appearance of goiter as well as the prevalence of nodularity.

Of special interest from a genetic point of view are studies of twins. Among 379 pairs studied in Greece, in an endemic goiter area, the discrepancy for the presence or absence of goiter was significantly lower for the monozygotes than for the heterozygotes, the figures also suggesting that the hereditary factor was much less important than the environmental (Malamos *et al.*, 1967). In Glasgow, a study of 120 pairs suggested a genetic factor among women, the study not being possible among men due to the low prevalence of goiter among them (Greig *et al.*, 1967). It would be of great interest to look in studies of this type not only for prevalence of goiter but also for the clinical presence of nodules.

In summary, the influence of genetic factors in endemic goiter has not been well documented. We believe that present evidence allows us to accept them as probably influencing goiter prevalence, but in a much less important way than environmental factors. On the other hand, genetic factors could be of much greater importance in the tendency of goiters to become nodular.

II. PATHOGENESIS

Among all the etiological factors previously mentioned iodine lack is the one which is best studied as to the mechanisms involved in its goitrogenic activity. The excellent monograph by Studer and Greer (1968) shows that experimental studies in rats provide an adequate model for such a study. The iodide trap has a greater capacity than the organification mechanism and hence it is not a limiting step for thyroid hormone synthesis. Iodine lack limits synthesis only when the amount offered is below a certain level or if the transport mechanism is altered, due either to an enzymatic defect or to goitrogen action. The thyroid-stimulating hormone influences all thyroid cell activities and its presence is necessary for normal thyroid hormone production, but the organification process is much more dependent on TSH action than the trapping mechanism. Goiter appears only as a result of increased TSH as a response to diminished thyroid hormone circulating in the blood. Iodine lack stimulates trapping more than organification and its effect is in part independent of TSH. An intrathyroidal control mechanism would be triggered by a decrease of the thyroid organic iodine concentration diminishing thyroid hormone secretion, which tends to be a fixed percentage of the iodine content of the gland, thus inducing an early increase of TSH secretion, much earlier than the one resulting from decreased thyroid secretion due to depletion of the thyroid hormone content. This is why in the first stage of experimental iodine deficiency, as also happens in most endemic goiters, there is an increase in size of the gland with significant diminution of its iodine concentration, but with a total content that is only subnormal and a normal circulating PBI. Colloid accumulation would be the result of increases in iodide supply, even if transitory, which would inhibit TSH production. This also explains why single very small doses of iodine block organification in an iodine-deficient animal. The key to this intrathyroidal control mechanism, sensitive to fluctuations in iodine supply, would be the histological and functional heterogeneity of the thyroid: a small functional pool located in the colloid-cell interphase would be rapidly affected by changes in iodide supply, while the rest of the thyroid iodine pool would respond only to TSH. This is why the specific activity of the thyroid secretion diminishes after injecting TSH. Finally, Studer and Greer (1968) point out that the increased MIT/DIT ratio observed in iodine deficiency is a very early finding, while the increase in the T3/T4 ratio appears much later and in the long run is quantitatively much larger. Hence the final increased ratio of T3/T4 secretion is not the result of a predominant formation of MIT in iodine-deficient thyroglobulin. The predominant secretion of T3 that allows a euthyroid animal to maintain a very low PBI (Pineda *et al.*, 1970), would be the result of chronic TSH overstimulation since T3 synthesis is more TSH dependent than T4. There could even be present a preferential secretion of T3 (Emrich *et al.*, 1966; Greer *et al.*, 1968). Nevertheless, it is possible that both iodine deficiency and pituitary overstimulation need to be present together in order to give a clear increase of T3 over T4 secretion. The observation made by our group that the same effect is seen when Graves' disease co-exists with iodine deficiency points in this same direction (Pineda *et al.*, 1970).

In Studer and Greer's model there would be an initial period of iodine deficiency with goiter, increased TSH and normal PBI, and a more advanced phase with bigger goiter, maximal TSH production and diminished PBI. This model is not totally in agreement with clinical experience in endemic goiter. In New Guinea, subjects with and without goiter, in extreme deficiency were clinically euthyroid, with low PBI and increased TSH, although not maximally increased since the TSH values were below those observed among athyreotic individuals in non-endemic areas (Buttfield *et al.*, 1966; Adams *et al.*, 1968; Buttfield *et al.*, 1968). High normal values of TSH have been observed in a much less severe endemic in Argentina (Pisarev *et al.*, 1970). Furthermore, it would be necessary to accept that goitrous individuals as opposed to non-goitrous would have been exposed to fluctuations in iodine supply, due to variations in intake that seem unlikely in New Guinea, or due to changes in the amount of goitrogens ingested, which seems to me more likely.

Of special interest are the observations of Ermans and co-workers (Ermans *et al.*, 1968) in sporadic goiter suggesting that when thyroglobulin iodination diminishes below a certain critical level (around 0.1%), coupling is impaired. A vicious circle could be thus started: iodine lack stimulating TSH and goiter growth further diluting the iodine content of the gland. Other experimental evidence (Inoue and Taurog, 1968) also points in this direction. It could thus be explained why iodine is sequestered in hormone precursors which are never utilized and why the thyroid iodine content is rather high but its concentration low, a common characteristic of iodine-deficient endemic goiter.

In summary, it seems we are beginning to understand the mechanisms involved in the pathogenesis of endemic goiter and to explain some findings that appeared as contradictory. Nevertheless, we are far from understanding why some individuals in endemic areas develop goiter and others do not, despite being apparently exposed to similar conditions.

Purposely I have omitted from this discussion immunological factors since their meaning is not clear to me in general and particularly in relation to endemic goiter. With the exception of one or two endemias (Soto *et al.*, 1967) the search for thyroid antibodies has given negative results, including histochemical techniques (Asamer *et al.*, 1968). Furthermore, diminished lymphocytic infiltration is a characteristic of endemic goiter and a low prevalence of Hashimoto's thyroiditis has been repeatedly reported in endemic goiter areas (Asamer *et al.*, 1968; Headington and Tantajumroon, 1967).

III. VARIABILITY

Variability is one of the least studied aspects of endemic goiter despite the fact that it is one of the most striking characteristics to the physician. Apart from the fact that in endemic areas there is always a percentage of the population that does not develop goiter, the goitrous subjects vary from those with slightly enlarged glands to monstrous sizes, and goiters range from very soft and diffuse to very hard and nodular.

It is generally accepted that when iodine lack persists, prevalence, size and nodularity tend to increase with age and that these three aspects are more intense in women. Nevertheless, we have observed in the Pedregoso endemia that women do have a greater prevalence and larger goiters, but sex does not seem to affect nodularity, while age increases the size of the goiters and the presence of nodularity, but goiter prevalence seems to stabilize after the third decade of life (Barzelatto *et al.*, 1967).

This initial observation suggested to us that these four aspects of endemic goiter: variability, prevalence, size and nodularity, could be influenced separately. Further studies showed that environmental factors like iodine lack and goitrogen ingestion (piñón), seem to influence goiter size but not nodularity, while genetic factors, like PTC, family distribution and consanguinity, seemed to be related to nodularity and not to goiter size (Covarrubias *et al.*, 1969). The very high prevalence of goiter in this population did not allow us to analyze these factors in relation to prevalence.

We are aware of the statistical and methodological problems of this type of analysis. Nevertheless, we believe that such studies could help to define the role of the different factors involved in the etiology and pathogenesis of goiter, better than if prevalence only is taken into consideration. If our observations are confirmed, we could reach a better understanding as to why in endemic areas one can find young men with small and hard multinodular goiters and old women with small and soft diffuse goiters, which are exceptions to the findings in most of the population.

For Studer and Greer (Studer and Greer, 1968) a nodular goiter would be the extreme variant of the functional and morphologic heterogeneity that is characteristic of the thyroid gland. They suggest that colloid accumulation could induce an increase in connective tissue by areas, which would later retract and impair blood circulation and thus accentuate the functional heterogeneity of the gland. When analyzing the adaptation of rats to iodine deficiency they point out the great variability observed experimentally and that it is not related to the ability to secrete thyroid hormones. The variability in goiter size would be the expression of the variability in functional heterogeneity of the different glands. Functional heterogeneity has been demonstrated in human endemias (Riccabona *et al.*, 1968) and even within one gland, either normal (Ermans *et al.*, 1968) or goitrous, and is particularly accentuated in nodules (Podoba *et al.*, 1967).

CONCLUSIONS

In the pathogenesis of endemic goiter three main types of factor seem to influence its development: (1) Iodine supply, usually acting because of being insufficient, but which can play a role when in excess. (2) Natural goitrogens in food, which can potentiate each other as well as the effect of an abnormal iodine supply. (3) Genetic factors that could be more important in goiter variability than in goiter prevalence.

It has been pointed out that these factors do not exclude each other (Stanbury, 1968) but on the contrary it seems reasonable to assume that they combine in different proportions in the various endemias (Barzelatto and Covarrubias, 1968). The importance of iodine supply and its interaction with the other factors have been referred to as 'permissive action' (Ermans *et al.*, 1969; Delange *et al.*, 1968) or as 'necessary but not sufficient cause' (Roche, 1961) in most endemias. Such a way of thinking could possibly also explain the variability of the results observed in experimental production of iodine-deficient goiter (Gaitán and Wahner, 1969).

It seems reasonable to postulate that in order to develop endemic goiter, the interaction is required of two and maybe of the three types of factors already mentioned. It is possible that goiter is developed only by those subjects in whom one or more environmental factors interact with a genetic factor that limits the ability to adapt to changes in iodine supply.

Finally, it seems possible that endemic goiter variability reflects the proportion in which these factors act in a given individual. Environmental factors would appear to have a greater relation to goiter size while genetic factors could be linked more to nodularity.

REFERENCES

ADAMS, D. D., KENNEDY, T. H., CHOUFOER, J. C. and QUERIDO, A. (1968): Endemic goiter in Western New Guinea. III. Thyroid-stimulating activity of serum from severely iodine deficient people. *J. clin. Endocr.*, *28*, 685.

ALLCROFT, R. and SALT, F. J. (1960): Goitrogenic factors in kale (Brassica oleracea). In: *Abstracts, IV International Goitre Conference, Section 1, p* 2. ICS No 26. Excerpta Medica, Amsterdam.

ANBAR, M. and INBAR, M. (1964): The effect of certain metallic cations on the iodide uptake in the thyroid gland of mice. *Acta endocr. (Kbh.)*, *46*, 643.

ANDREAS, J. and ANDREAS, J. (1962): Experimente über die strumigene Wirkung von Flavonfarbstoffen. *J. Hyg. Epidemiol. (Praha)*, *6*, 100.

ARSTILA, A., KRUSIUS, F. and PELTOLA, P. (1969): Studies on the transfer of thiooxazolidone type goitrogens into cow's milk in goitre endemic districts of Finland and in experimental conditions. *Acta endocr. (Kbh.)*, *60*, 712.

ASAMER, H., RICCABONA, G. and HOLTHAUS, N. (1968): Immunohistologic findings in thyroid disease in an endemic goiter area. *Arch. klin. Med.*, *215*, 270.

AZEVEDO, E., KRIEGER, H., MI, M. P. and MORTON, N. E. (1965): P.T.C. taste sensitivity and endemic goiter in Brazil. *Amer. J. hum. Genet.*, *17*, 87.

BALAN, M., STANCOU, H., CONSTANTINESCO, A., VOICULET, N. and MUSETEANU, P. (1969): Le goitre endémique par régime hyperiode. *Rev. roum. Endocr.*, *6*, 55.

BARZELATTO, J., ATRIA, A. and ACEVEDO, H. (1954): El yodo radioactivo en el diagnóstico del estado funcional tiroideo. *Rev. méd. Chile*, *82*, 519.

BARZELATTO, J., BECKERS, C., STEVENSON, C., COVARRUBIAS, E., GIANETTI, A., BOBADILLA, E., PARDO, A., DONOSO, H. and ATRIA, A. (1967): Endemic goiter in Pedregoso (Chile). I. Description and function studies. *Acta endocr. (Kbh.) 54*, 577.

BARZELATTO, J. and COVARRUBIAS, E. (1968): Study of endemic goiter in the American Indian. In: *Biomedical Challenges presented by the American Indian*, pp. 124–132. Scientific Pub. No. 165. Pan-American Health Organization-World Health Organization, Washington, D.C.

BARZELATTO, J. and COVARRUBIAS, E. (1969): Study of endemic goiter in the American Indian. In: *Endemic Goiter*, pp. 233–244. Editor: J. B. Stanbury. Scientific Pub. No. 193. Pan-American Health Organization-World Health Organization, Washington, D.C.

BARZELATTO, J., STEVENSON, C. and ATRIA, A. (1955): Uso clinico del yodo radioactivo en las enfermedades del tiroides. II. El yodo radioactivo y su valor diagnóstico. *Rev. méd. Chile*, *83*, 735.

BECKERS, C., BARZELATTO, J., STEVENSON, C., GIANETTI, A., PARDO, A., BOBADILLA, E. and DE VISSCHER, M. (1967): Endemic goitre in Pedregoso (Chile). II. Dynamic studies on iodine metabolism. *Acta endocr. (Kbh.) 54*, 591.

BENEDEK, T. C. (1962): Goiter formation as the result of therapy with phenylbutazone and Vitamin A. *J. clin. Endocr.*, *22*, 959.

BOATMAN, J. B., RABINOVITZ, M. J. and WALSH, J. M. (1960): Effect of salt feeding on thyroid metabolism of I^{131} in the dog. *Amer. J. Physiol. 198*, 1251.

BOYLE, J. A., GREIG, W. R., FULTON, S. and DALAKOS, T. G. (1966): Excess dietary calcium and human thyroid function. *J. Endocr.*, *34*, 531.

BRAHAM, J. E., TEJADA, C., BRESSANI, R. and GUZMAN, M. A. (1962): Effect of calcium and iodine on the experimental production of goiter in the rat. *Fed. Proc. 21*, 308.

BUTTFIELD, I. H., BLACK, M. L., HOFFMANN, M. J., MASON, E. K., WELLBY, M. L., GOOD, B. F. and HETZEL, B. S. (1966): Studies of the control of the thyroid function in endemic goiter in Eastern New Guinea. *J. clin. Endocr.*, *26*, 1201.

BUTTFIELD, I. H., HETZEL, B. S. and ODELL, W. D. (1968): Effect of iodized oil on serum TSH determined by immunoassay in endemic goiter subjects. *J. clin. Endocr.*, *28*, 1664.

BUZINA, R., MILUTINOVIC, P., VIDOVIC, V., MAVER, H. and HORVAT, A. (1959): Endemic goitre in the Island of Krk studied with I^{131}. *J. Nutr. 68*, 465.

BYSHEVSKII, A. S. (1960): The effect of Vitamin C deficiency on iodine metabolism in guinea-pigs. *Probl. Endokr. Gormonoter.*, *6*, 32.

CAMPOS, P. C., BALTASAR, B. S., GARABATO, N., MOYA, L. T. and CLEMENTE, A. O. (1962): The use of radioiodine in endemic goitre investigations. In: *Radioisotopes in Tropical Medicine*, pp. 151–171. International Atomic Energy Agency, Vienna.

CHAMBERLAIN, J. L. (1961): Thyroid enlargement probably induced by cobalt. *J. Pediat. 59*, 81.

CHOUFOER, J. C., VAN RHIJN, M., KASSENAAR, A. A. H. and QUERIDO, A. (1963): Endemic goiter in

Western New Guinea: Iodine metabolisms in goitrous and nongoitrous subjects. *J. clin. Endocr.* *23*, 1203.

Clements, F. W. (1960): Health significance of endemic goitre and related conditions. In: *Endemic Goitre*, pp. 255–260. Monograph Series No. 44. World Health Organization, Geneva.

Clements, F. W., Gibson, H. B. and Howeler-Coy, J. F. (1968): Goiter studies in Tasmania. 16 years prophylaxis with iodide. *Bull. Wld Hlth Org.*, *38*, 297.

Clode, W., Sobral, J. M. and Baptista, A. M. (1960): Bromine interference in iodine metabolism and its goitrogenic action. *In: Abstracts, IV International Goitre Conference*, Section 1a, p. 11. ICS No. 26. Excerpta Medica, Amsterdam.

Corradino, R. A. and Parker, H. E. (1962): Magnesium and thyroid function in the rat. *J. Nutr.*, *77*, 455.

Costa, A. and Cottino, F. (1963): Research on iodine metabolism in endemic goiter in Piedmont. *Metabolism*, *12*, 35.

Costa, A., Ferro-Luzzi, G., Marocco, E., Cottino, F., Gianti, S., Patrito, G., Zopetti, G., Magro, E., Buccini, G. and Balsamo, A. (1967): An investigation of endemic goitre in some piedmontese valleys. *Panminerva med.*, *9*, 55.

Costa, A. and Mortara, M. (1960): A review of recent studies of goitre in Italy. *Bull. Wld Hlth Org.*, *22*, 493.

Covarrubias, E., Barzelatto, J. and Guiloff, R. (1969): Genetic questions related to the goiter endemic of Pedregoso (Chile). In: *Endemic Goiter*, pp. 252–264. Editor: J. B. Stanbury. Scientific Pub. No. 193. Pan-American Health Organization-World Health Organization Washington, D.C.

Covarrubias, E., Barzelatto, J., Stevenson, C., Bobadilla, E., Pardo, A. and Beckers, C. (1965): Taste sensitivity to phenyl-thio-carbamide and endemic goitre among Pewenche Indians. *Nature (Lond.)*, *205*, 1036.

Cruz-Coke, E. and Plaza de los Reyes, M. (1947): Quercétine et fonction thyroïdienne. *Bull. Soc. Chim. biol.*, *29*, 573.

Daniel, P. M., Plaskett, L. G. and Pratt, O. E. (1966): Radioactive iodoprotein in thyroid lymph and blood. *Biochem. J.*, *100*, 622.

Daniel, P. M., Pratt, O. E., Roitt, I. M. and Torrigiani, G. (1967): The release of thyroglobulin from the thyroid gland into thyroid lymphatics; the identification of thyroglobulin in the thyroid lymph and in the blood of monkeys by physical and immunology methods and its estimation by radioimmunology. *Immunology*, *12*, 489.

Davis, P. J. (1966): Fluoride therapy and the thyroid gland. *J. Amer. med. Ass.*, *196*, 1159.

Delange, F., Thilly, D. and Ermans, A. M. (1968): Iodine deficiency, a permissive condition in the development of endemic goiter. *J. clin. Endocr.*, *28*, 114.

Demarchi, M., Al-Hindawi, A., Abdulnabi, M. and Taj El-Din, H. (1969): Prevalence of etiology of goiter in Iraq. *Amer. J. clin. Nutr.*, *22*, 1160.

Ekpechi, O. L. (1967): Pathogenesis of endemic goiter in Eastern Nigeria. *Brit. J. Nutr.* *21*, 537.

Ekpechi, O. L., Dimitriadou, A. and Fraser, R. (1966): Goitrogenic activity of cassava. *Nature (Lond.)*, *210*, 1137.

Emrich, D., Pfannenstiel, P., Hoffmann, G. and Keiderling, W. (1966): Significance of triiodothyronine for thyroid hormone supply during stimulation. *Acta endocr. (Kbh.)*, *53*, 151.

Ermans, A. M., Kinthaert, J. and Camus, M. (1968): Defective intrathyroidal iodine metabolism in nontoxic goiter; inadequate iodination of thyroglobulin. *J. clin. Endocr.*, *28*, 1307.

Ermans, A. M., Kinthaert, J., Delacroix, C. and Collard, J. (1968): Metabolism of intrathyroidal iodine in normal man. *J. clin. Endocr.*, *28*, 169.

Ermans, A. M., Thilly, C., Vis, H. L. and Delange, F. (1969): Permissive nature of iodine deficiency in the development of endemic goiter. In: *Endemic Goiter*, pp. 101–117. Editor: J. B. Stanbury. Scientific Pub. No. 193. Pan American Health Organization-World Health Organization, Washington, D.C.

Frada, G., Mentesana, G. and Guajana, U. (1969): Thyroid function in fluorotic subjects from a large endemic centre in Sicily. *Minerva med.*, *60*, 545.

Gaitán, E. (1969): Identification of a naturally occurring goitrogen in water. *Trans. Ass. Amer. Phycns.* *82*, 141.

Gaitán, E. and Wahner, H. W. (1969): Studies on the pathogenesis of endemic goiter in the Cauca Valley, Colombia, South America. In: *Endemic Goiter, Chapter 24*, pp. 267–290. Editor: J. B. Stanbury. Scientific Pub. No. 193. Pan-American Health Organization-World Health Organization, Washington, D.C.

GAITÁN, E., WAHNER, H. W., CUELLO, C., CORREA, P., JUBIZ, W. and GAITÁN, J. E. (1969): Endemic goiter in the Cauca Valley. I. Results and limitations of 12 years of iodine prophylaxis. *J. clin. Endocr.*, *29*, 675.

GANDRA, Y. R. (1967): O bócio endêmico e o suprimento e excreção urinária de iodo no estado de São Paulo. *Arch. lat.-amer. Nutr.*, *17*, 129.

GANDRA, Y. R. and CONIGLIO, J. G. (1961): Calcium and metabolism of I^{131} in rats and homogenates of rat thyroid. *Amer. J. Physiol.*, *200*, 1023.

GRAY, H. W., MURPHY, A. V., LOGAN, R. W., GREIG, W. R. and MCGIRR, E. M. (1969): Investigation of Nithsdale goitre. *Scot. med. J.*, *14*, 48.

GREER, M. A., GRIMM, Y. and STUDER, H. (1968): Quantitative changes in the secretion of the thyroid hormones induced by iodine deficiency. *Endocrinology*, *83*, 1193.

GREIG, W. R., BOYLE, J. A., DUNCAN, A., NICOL, J., GRAY, M. J. B., BUCHANAN, W. W. and MCGIRR, E. (1967): Genetic and non-genetic factors in simple goiter formation. Evidence from a twin study. *Quart. J. Med.*, *36*, 175.

GREIG, W. R., GRAY, H. W., MCGIRR, E. M., KAMBAL, A. and RAHMAN, I. A. (1970): Investigation of endemic goitre in Sudan. *Brit. J. Surg.*, *57*, 11.

HARRISON, M. T., HARDEN, R. M. and ALEXANDER, W. D. (1967): Effect of calcium on iodine metabolism in man. *Metabolism*, *16*, 84.

HEADINGTON, J. T. and TANTAJUMROON, T. T. (1967): Surgical thyroid disease in northern Thailand. *Arch. Surg.*, *95*, 157.

HENNING, K. and STRAHLENKLIN, F. H. (1961): Fluorine and the thyroid gland. *Schweiz. med. Wschr.*, *91*, 79.

HERRERA, E., ESCOBAR DEL REY, F. and MONRREALE DE ESCOBAR, G. (1968): Mechanism of goitrogenesis by very low doses of propylthiouracil and the role of iodine intake. *Acta endocr. (Kbh.)*, *59*, 529.

HORVAT, A. and MAVER, H. (1958): The role of vitamin A in the occurrence of goitre in the island of Krk, Yugoslavia. *J. Nutr.*, *66*, 189.

INOUE, D. and TAUROG, A. (1968): Acute and chronic effects of iodide on thyroid radioiodine metabolism in iodine-deficient rats. *Endocrinology*, *83*, 279.

ISLER, H. (1961): Effect of sodium chloride on the thyroid gland and on iodine metabolism. *Amer. J. Cardiol.*, *8*, 688.

JIROUSEK, L., REISENAUER, R. and HOVORKA, J. (1959): Polarographische Bestimmung von Sulphydrylsubstanzen in biologischem Material. IV. Uber die Möglichkeit einer Beziehung zwischen Sulphhydryl Substanzen und Strumaendemia. *Endokrinologie*, *37*, 269.

KASABIAN, S. S. and CHERNYAVSKAYA, G. L. (1957): Histochemical characteristics of the ascorbic acid distribution in the thyroid gland in endemic goiter. *Probl. Endokr. Gormonoter.*, *3*, 89.

KELLY, F. C. and SNEDDEN, W. W. (1960): Prevalence and geographical distribution of endemic goitre. In: *Endemic Goitre*, pp. 27–233. Monograph Series No. 44. World Health Organization, Geneva.

KIMBALL, O. P. (1961): Prevention of endemic goiter in man. *Arch. intern. Med.*, *107*, 290.

KLINCK, G. H. (1955): Thyroid hyperplasia in young children. *J. Amer. med. Ass.*, *158*, 1347.

KNIZHNIKOV, V. A. (1959): The effect of drinking water with high content of fluorine on thyroid gland function. *Gig. i San.*, *1*, 20.

KOLOGLU, S. and KOLOGLU, K. Y. M. (1968): A study on the role of naturally occurring goitrogens in the etiology of Eastern Black Sea goiter endemic in Turkey. *Ankara Univ. Tip Fak. Mec.*, *21*, 420.

KOUTRAS, D. A., PAPADOPOULOS, S. N., SFONTOURIS, J., RIGOPOULOS, G. A., PHARMAKIOTIS, A. D. and MALAMOS, B. (1968): Endemic goiter in Greece. Clinical and metabolic effects of iodized salt. *J. clin. Endocr.*, *28*, 1651.

KOUTRAS, D. A., TASSOPOULOS, C. N. and MARKETOS, S. (1967): Endemic goiter in Greece: Salivary iodide clearance in goitrous and nongoitrous persons. *J. clin. Endocr.*, *27*, 783.

KOVALEV, M. M. (1960): Zinc content in some substances in external environment in normal thyroid and in thyroids with pathological changes. *Probl. Endokr. Gormonoter.*, *6*, 52.

KRISS, J. P., CARNES, W. H. and GROSS, R. T. (1955): Hypothyroidism and thyroid hyperplasia in patients treated with cobalt. *J. Amer. med. Ass.*, *157*, 117.

KRUSIUS, F. E. and PELTOLA, P. (1966): The goitrogenic effect of naturally occurring L5-vinyl and L5-phenyl-2-thiooxazolidone in rats. *Acta endocr. (Kbh.)*, *53*, 342.

LAI, C. L. (1960): Studies on changes of the prevalence of simple goiter. *J. Osaka Cy med. Cent.*, *9*, 3445.

LAMBERG, B. A., HONKAPOHJA, H., HAIKONEN, M., JUSSILA, R., HINTZE, G., AXELSON, E. and CHOUFOER, J. C. (1962): Iodine metabolism in endemic goitre in the east of Finland with a survey of recent data on iodine metabolism in Finland. *Acta med. scand.*, *172*, 237.
LANGER, P. (1960): History of goitre. In: *Endemic Goitre*, pp. 9–25. Monograph Series No. 44. World Health Organization, Geneva.
LANGER, P. (1964): Serum thiocyanate level in large section of the population as an index of the presence of naturally occurring goitrogens in the organism. In: *Naturally Occurring Goitrogens and Thyroid Function, Vol. 1*, Topic 3, pp. 281–295. Editors: J. Podoba and P. Langer. Publishing House of the Slovak Academy of Sciences, Bratislava.
LANGER, P. (1966): Antithyroid action in rats of small doses of some naturally occurring compounds. *Endocrinology*, *79*, 1117.
LEONE, N. C., LEATHERWOOD, E. C., PETRIC, I. M. and LIEVERMAN, L. (1964): Effect of fluoride on thyroid gland: clinical study. *J. Amer. dent. Ass.*, *69*, 179.
LINAZASORO, J. M., SANCHEZ-MARTIN, J. A. and JIMENEZ-DIAZ, C. (1970): Goitrogenic effect of walnut and its action on thyroxine excretion. *Endocrinology*, *86*, 696.
LISSITZKY, S., BISMUTH, J., CODACCIONI, J. and CARTOUZON, G. (1968): Congenital goiter with iodoalbumin replacing thyroglobulin and defect of deiodination of iodotyrosines. Serum origin of the thyroid iodoalbumin. *J. clin. Endocr.*, *28*, 1797.
LONDON, W. T., KOUTRAS, D. A., PRESSMAN, A. and VOUGHT, R. L. (1965): Epidemiologic and metabolic studies of a goiter endemic in Eastern Kentucky. *J. clin. Endocr.* *25*, 1091.
LOWENSTEIN, F. W. (1959): Endemic goiter and nutrition. II. A follow-up study of 75 families in a Brazilian Amazon community. *Amer. J. clin. Nutr.*, *7*, 339.
MALAMOS, B., KOUTRAS, D. A., KOSTAMIS, P., RIGOPOULOS, G. A., ZEREFROS, N. S. and KRALIOS, A. C. (1966): Endemic goiter in Greece. Epidemiologic and genetic studies. *J. clin. Endocr.* *26*, 688.
MALAMOS, B., KOUTRAS, D. A., KOSTAMIS, P., RIGOPOULOS, G. A., ZEREFROS, N. S. and YATAGANAS, X. A. (1967): Endemic goitre in Greece. A study of 379 twin pairs. *J. med. Genet.*, *4*, 16.
MALAMOS, B., MIRAS, K., KOUTRAS, D. A., KOSTAMIS, P., BINOPOULOS, D., MANTZOS, J., LEVIS, G., RIGOPOULOS, G., ZEREFROS, N. and TASSOPOULOS, C. N. (1966): Endemic goiter in Greece. Metabolic studies. *J. clin. Endocr.*, *26*, 696.
MALVAUX, P., BECKERS, C. and DE VISSCHER, M. (1969): Iodine balance studies in nongoitrous children and adolescents on low iodine intake. *J. clin. Endocr.*, *29*, 79.
MERKE, F. (1965): Die Eiszeit als primordiale Ursache des endemischen Kropfes. *Schweiz. med. Wschr.*, *95*, 1183.
MERKE, F. (1967): Weitere Belege für die Eiszeit als primordiale Ursache des endemischen Kropfes: Eiszeit und Kropf im Wallis. *Schweiz. med. Wschr.*, *97*, 131.
MITCHELL, M. L., SANCHEZ-MARTIN, J. A., HARDEN, A. B. and O'ROURKE, M. E. (1961): Failure of thiourea to prevent hormone synthesis by the thyroid gland of man and animals treated with thyrotropin. *J. clin. Endocr.*, *21*, 157.
MULVEY, P. F. and SLINGERLAND, D. W. (1962): The *in vitro* stimulation of thyroidal activity by propylthiouracil. *Endocrinology*, *70*, 7.
MUÑOZ-RODRIGUEZ, M. (1964): Importancia de la alimentación del ganado vacuno en la bociogénesis humana. *Rev. med. Navarra*, *8*, 149.
NAGUIB, M. A. (1963): Effect of magnesium on the thyroid. *Lancet*, *1*, 1405.
NUTRITION REVIEWS (1968): Goiter among Ceylonese and Nigerians. *Nutr. Rev.*, *26*, 77.
ODDIE, T. H., FISCHER, D. A., MCCONAHEY, W. M. and THOMPSON, C. S. (1970): Iodine in the United States: A reassessment. *J. clin. Endocr.*, *30*, 659.
OPARIN, I. A. (1969): Role of natural cobalt content in food stuffs in the etiology of endemic goiter. *Probl. Endokr. Gormonoter.* *15*, 26.
PALEY, K. R., SOBEL, E. S. and YALOW, R. S. (1958): Effect of oral and intravenous cobaltous chloride on thyroid function. *J. clin. Endocr.*, *18*, 850.
PARKER, R. H. and BEIERWALTES, W. H. (1962): Elevated serum protein-bound iodine values with dietary iodine deficiency. *J. clin. Endocr.*, *22*, 19.
PASTERNAK, D. P., SOCOLOW, E. L. and INGBAR, S. H. (1969): Synergistic interaction of phenazone and iodide on thyroid hormone biosynthesis in the rat. *Endocrinology*, *84*, 769.
PELTOLA, P. (1960): Goitrogenic effect of cow's milk from the goitre district of Finland. *Acta endocr. (Kbh.)*, *34*, 121.
PELTOLA, P. (1965): The role of 1–5 vinyl-2-thio-oxazolidone in the genesis of endemic goiter in Finland. In: *Current Topics in Thyroid Research*, pp. 872–876. Editors: C. Cassano and M. Andreoli.

Academic Press, New York.
PINEDA, G., SILVA, E., GIANETTI, A., STEVENSON, C. and BARZELATTO, J. (1970): Influence of iodine deficiency upon PBI in hyperthyroidism. *J. clin. Endocr. 30*, 120.
PISAREV, M. A., UTIGER, R. D., SALVANESCHI, J. P., ALTSCHULLER, N. and DEGROOT, L. J. (1970): Serum TSH and thyroxine in goitrous subjects in Argentina. *J. clin. Endocr. 30*, 680.
PODOBA, J. and LANGER, P. (1964): *Naturally Occurring Goitrogens and Thyroid Function, Vol. 1.* Editors: J. Podoba and P. Langer. Publishing House of the Slovak Academy of Sciences, Bratislava.
PODOBA, J., KNOPP, J. and MITRO, A. (1967): On the etiology and prevention of endemic goiter. *Bratisl. lek. Listy, 48*, 719.
RHODES, B. A. (1968): The circulating iodotyrosines. *Acta endocr. (Kbh.), 57, Suppl., 127*, 5.
RICCABONA, G., HESS, P. and HUBER, P. (1968): The histotopography of the iodine metabolism in endemic goiter and in healthy thyroids. *Acta endocr. (Kbh.), 59*, 564.
ROCHE, M., DEVENANZI, F., VERA, J., COLL, E., SPINETTI-BERTI, M., MENDEZ-MARTINEZ, J., GERARDI, A. and FORERO, J. (1957): Endemic goiter in Venezuela studied with I^{131}. *J. clin. Endocr., 17*, 99.
ROCHE, M. (1959): Elevated thyroidal I^{131} uptake in the absence of goiter in isolated Venezuelan Indians. *J. clin. Endocr., 19*, 1440.
ROCHE, M. (1961): Endemic goitre. In: *Coloquio sobre a Tireoide*, pp. 427–442. Editors: C. Chagas and L. E. G. Lobo. Universidade do Brasil, Rio de Janeiro.
SAKA, O., HALLAC, P. and URGANCIOGLU, I. (1965): The effect of fluoride on the thyroid of the rat. *New Istambul Contr. clin. Sci., 8*, 87.
SAMOFAL, T. S. (1959): The effect of manganese on the development of experimental goiter caused by 6-methylthiouracil. *Probl. Endokr. Gormonoter., 5*, 7.
SCHOU, M., AMDISEN, A., JENSEN, S. E. and OLSEN, T. (1968): Occurrence of goitre during lithium treatment. *Brit. med. J., 3*, 710.
SCRIMSHAW, N. S. (1958): Endemic goiter. Introduction. *Fed. Proc., 17, Suppl., 2*, 57.
SEDERHOLM, T., KOUVALAINEN, K. and LAMBERG, B. A. (1968): Cobalt-induced hypothyroidism and polycythemia in lipoid nephrosis. *Acta med. scand., 184*, 301.
SEDLAK, J. (1961): Cultivation of goitrogenous and non-goitrogenous cabbage. *Nature (Lond.), 192*, 377.
SHIMODA, S. and SHICHIJO, K. (1963): Hypothyroidism due to Vitamin A administration. *Endocr. Metab. (Tokyo), 4*, 297.
SIDDIQUI, A. M. (1960): Incidence of simple goiter in areas of endemic fluorosis. *J. Endocr., 20*, 101.
SOTO, R. J., IMAS, B., BRUNENGO, A. M. and GOLDBERG, D. (1967): Endemic goiter in Misiones, Argentina: Pathophysiology related to immunology phenomena. *J. clin. Endocr., 27*, 1581.
STANBURY, J. (1968): Endemic goiter. In: *Clinical Endocrinology II*, pp. 195–209. Editors: E. B. Astwood and C. E. Cassidy. Grune & Stratton, New York.
STANBURY, J., BROWNELL, G. L., RIGGS, D. S., PERINETTI, H., ITOIZ, J. and DEL CASTILLO, E. (1954): *Endemic goiter. The Adaptation of Man to Iodine Deficiency.* Harvard University Press, Cambridge, Mass.
STANBURY, J. B. (1960): Physiology of endemic goitre. In: *Endemic Goitre*, pp. 261–277. Monograph Series No. 44. World Health Organization, Geneva.
STEWART, R. D. H. and MURRAY, I. P. C. (1967): Effect of small doses of carrier iodide upon organic binding of radioactive iodine by the human thyroid gland. *J. clin. Endocr., 27*, 500.
STUDER, H. and GREER, M. A. (1968): *The Regulation of Thyroid Function in Iodine Deficiency.* Huber, Berne.
SUNDERLAND, E. and CARTWRIGHT, R. A. (1968): Iodine estimations, endemic goiter and phenylthiocarbamide (PTC) tasting ability. *Acta genet. (Basel), 18*, 593.
SURKS, M. I. and OPPENHEIMER, J. H. (1969): Formation of iodoprotein during the peripheral metabolism of 3,5,3′ triodo-1-thyronine in the euthyroid man and rat. *J. clin. Invest., 48*, 685.
SUZUKI, H., HIGUCHI, T., SAWA, K., OHTAKI, S. and HORIUCHI, Y. (1965): 'Endemic coast goiter' in Hokkaido, Japan, *Acta endocr. (Kbh.), 50*, 161.
TELLEZ, M. (1966): *Actividad Bocígena Experimental del Piñon.* Thesis, School of Medicine, University of Chile, Santiago de Chile.
TELLEZ, M., GIANETTI, A., COVARRUBIAS, E. and BARZELATTO, J. (1969): Endemic goiter in Pedregoso (Chile). Experimental goitrogenic activity of 'Piñon'. In: *Endemic Goiter*, pp. 245–251. Editor: J. B. Stanbury. Scientific Pub. No. 193. Pan-American Health Organization-World Health Organization, Washington, D.C.
TURETSKAYA, E. S. (1960): Content of iodine and bromine in the thyroid glands of albino rats de-

pending on the vitamins in the food. *Ukr. biokhim. Zh.*, *32*, 578.
TURETSKAYA, E. S. (1961): Studies of the iodine and bromine content in goitrous thyroids. *Probl. Endokr. Gormonoter.*, *7*, 75.
VERZHIKOVSKAYA, N. V. and SHVAIKO, I. I. (1959): Dietary excess of manganese and function of the thyroid gland under conditions of iodine deficiency. *Probl. Endokr. Gormonoter.*, *5*, 90.
VOUGHT, R. L., LONDON, W. T. and STEBBIG, G. E. T. (1967): Endemic goiter in northern Virginia. *J. clin. Endocr.*, *27*, 1381.
WAHNER, H. W. and GAITÁN, E. (1969): Thyroid function in adolescents from the goiter endemic of the Cauca Valley, Colombia, South America. In: *Endemic Goiter*, Chapter 25, pp. 291–303. Editor: J. B. Stanbury. Scientific Pub. No. 193. Pan-American Health Organization-World Health Organization, Washington, D.C.
WAYNE, E. J., KOUTRAS, D. A. and ALEXANDER, W. D. (1964): *Clinical Aspects of Iodine Metabolism*, pp. 93–98. Blackwell, Oxford.
WELLBY, M. L. and O'HALLORAN, M. W. (1969): The iodotyrosine content of normal human serum. *Biochem. J.* *112*, 543.
WOLFF, J. (1969): Iodide goiter and the pharmacologic effects of excess iodide. *Amer. J. Med.*, *47*, 101.
YAMADA, T. and SCICHIJO, K. (1962): Role of iodine, sodium chloride and antithyroid drugs in the development of goiter in the rat. *Endocrinology*, *70*, 314.
ZAK, V. I. (1967): Sulfates in the drinking water of goiter foci in Orenburg region. *Probl. Endokr. Gormonoter.*, *13*, 41.

DYNAMIC ASPECTS OF ENDEMIC GOITER*

ENRIQUE TOVAR, JORGE A. MAISTERRENA and LAURA NIETO

Thyroid Clinic, National Institute of Nutrition, Mexico, D.F., Mexico

Studies in endemic goiter continue to play a relevant role in modern medicine and indeed this disease is still considered to be a major health problem in some countries.

When faced with goiter as an endemic problem the investigator must also consider other conditions which may be related to abnormal growth of the thyroid gland. These may include insufficient iodine in the diet, the presence of goitrogenic agents in the diet, hereditary, immunologic and bacteriologic factors and others which have been accorded varying degrees of importance over the years. Nonetheless, it frequently turns out that our efforts to explain the endemic state, either on the basis of one or a series of causes, meet with complete failure, and the endemic condition of the disease persists, for reasons we cannot discover.

Therefore the identification of goiter in an endemic state which is undergoing changes would present us with the opportunity to evaluate the capacity of the human organism to adapt to an iodine-deficiency state, either at the nutritional level or at that of a thyroid barrier. Thus we could obtain a quantitative approximation of the degree of absolute or relative deficiency necessary to bring about goiter.

The Mexican Institute of Nutrition has been engaged in studies in endemic goiter in several rural communities and especially in one closely controlled area near Mexico City for about the last ten years. In the course of this study, which was concentrated on schoolchildren and in which iodine nutritional requirements were being established, we noted an important change in the prevalence of the endemic state.

Our studies have shown that endemic goiter continues to be an important problem in our country and that the endemic zones are the same as those identified in previous years (Maisterrena *et al.*, 1969). At the same time we have been able to record an inverse relationship between the extent of the goiter problem and the socio-economic growth of the country (Maisterrena and Tovar, 1969).

In this paper we present our results obtained during the last two years of study in the principal area of observation near Mexico City.

During this time there was a clear increase in the incidence of goiter and we will compare this finding with those of previous years when the prevalence and incidence of goiter were in frank retreat, both in this special area and in other zones under study (Tovar *et al.*, 1968).

CROSS-SECTION STUDIES IN ENDEMIC GOITER

In order to set up long-range studies of endemic goiter we chose rural communities with 5–10,000 inhabitants, easily reached from Mexico City and in which the civil authorities offered their cooperation. We decided to limit our studies to schoolchildren since they are subject to few environmental changes, can easily be located in their school, and since it may

* This work was supported in part by United States Public Health Service Grant AM – 08428.

be supposed that the process which brings about goiter in them is in a developing state. Thus, on studying them we can expect to obtain information on the dynamic aspects of the disease.

The town of Tepetlixpa was an ideal site for our study according to the criteria mentioned above. The characteristics of its inhabitants and of the endemic goiter found there have been presented in previous publications (Maisterrena *et al.*, 1964; 1968; 1969). These children have been found to be euthyroid, and in 1962 92% of them had goiter. Their average uptake of radioactive iodine was 85% and their daily urinary iodine excretion was 11 μg. The only apparent cause for their endemic state was a deficient ingestion of iodine. From the first it was evident that iodine intake varied seasonally in accord with the available foodstuffs. When local food products predominated, iodine ingestion was low, but when local stores of foods were exhausted and the town had to import products from other parts of the country, iodine ingestion increased. This factor became frankly evident in the iodine balance studies which we carried out (Maisterrena and Tovar, 1969). In addition to these seasonal changes we also noted a slow increase in the average iodine intake which showed an inverse relationship with the gradually decreasing incidence of goiter and a similar decrease in the uptake of radioactive iodine in the thyroid gland (Fig. 1).

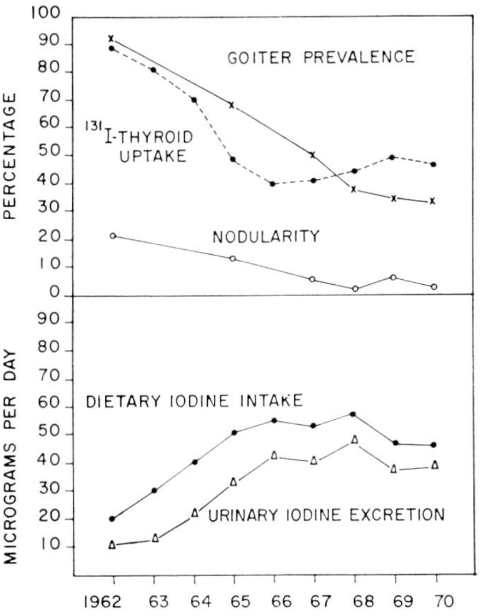

Fig. 1. Increase in iodine intake and urinary iodine excretion showing an inverse relationship with the decreasing incidence of goiter and uptake of radioactive iodine by the thyroid gland.

On the other hand, a study of the content of the schoolchildren's diet showed that it was the increasing variety of the foodstuffs and not an increased consumption which accounted for the increase in iodine intake. This finding was compatible with the theory that the change in the origin of the foodstuffs accounted for their increased iodine content (Maisterrena *et al.*, 1968).

These studies concerning iodine intake in schoolchildren with endemic goiter have been well worth while. In the first place they provided a basis from which to reach the valid conclusion that goiter was the result of deficient iodine ingestion only, and secondly, our observations during the period of decrease in goiter incidence have provided us with an approximate idea of minimum iodine requirements in these schoolchildren (Maisterrena and Tovar, 1969).

In similar studies on other groups of schoolchildren in Mexico, essentially the same results have been reported (Tovar *et al.*, 1968). Goiter prevalence varied from 0% to 65%, with iodine intake being significantly different only in the groups represented in the extremes of this range. Endemic goiter tends to disappear in the various areas under study in our country. There is a good correlation between thyroid uptake of radioactive iodine and the levels of urinary iodine excretion. Our findings suggest that within the rather arbitrary limits of normality the majority of schoolchildren would need 30–40 μg of iodine daily (Maisterrena and Tovar, 1969; Tovar *et al.*, 1968).

On studying the changes in the prevalence of goiter as related to age of the children one observes that there is less goiter in younger children. This may be explained on the basis of a diminished basic requirement for iodine or a smaller depletion of iodine based on a shorter lifetime in surroundings providing deficient iodine intake.

During the last two years of this study we noted that iodine intake, which had risen at first and had then been maintained at an almost constant level, showed a moderate fall. This change was not statistically significant at the level of the total population of schoolchildren, but could be related to other factors in the overall study. Thus, the prevalence of goiter in the general population remained about the same and thyroid uptake of radioactive iodine showed a slight increase.

On investigating the possible causes of this modification we found that during the last two years the foodstuffs used were practically all of local origin since the harvests had been exceptionally good. The level of iodine ingestion did not descend to those reported in the first investigation, but was maintained during the two-year period.

LONGITUDINAL STUDIES OF ENDEMIC GOITER

Up to this point the data we have presented in this paper, although drawn from observations over a long-time interval, have been based on a comparison of several pertinent factors in a cross-sectional pattern at one given instant using average values as a guide. This method ignores the individual condition of any one of the children under study as regards the absence of goiter or its appearance or disappearance. Although the present study was not designed to investigate the longitudinal aspects of the problem a review of all the information obtained permits us to at least approximate that type of study. In Figure 2 is shown the incidence of goiter in schoolchildren as compared with their age and the time phase of the study. One can see that the decrease in prevalence is more marked in children of the same age during the most recent years and that there was a marked increase in goiter incidence during the last two years in the very young children. This example illustrates the necessity of carrying out long-term studies in individual patients in order to better understand the dynamics of endemic goiter and arrive at valid conclusions concerning its etiology.

In all of our studies we have confirmed that low iodine ingestion is related to a high thyroid

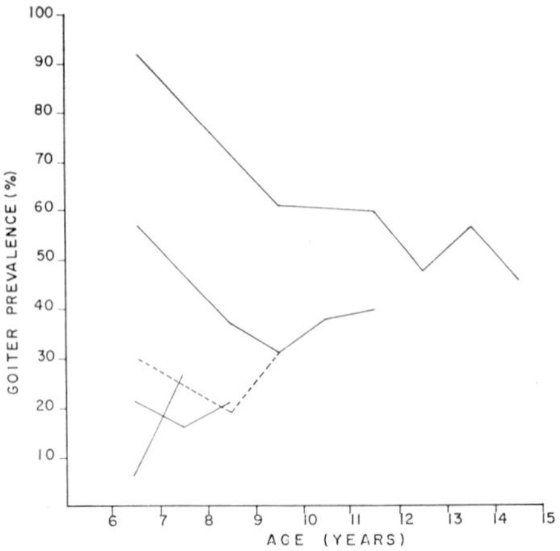

Fig. 2. Changes in goiter prevalence in relation with the children's age showing a clear increase in goiter incidence during the last years of observation.

uptake of radioactive iodine, and this relationship suggests, at least indirectly, that no goitrogenic factors unrelated to a deficient iodine ingestion are involved. On comparing these two measurements with the children's age in 1969 and 1970 we found a statistically significant difference between two age-groups.

Children with lower iodine intake had a higher incidence of goiter. At the same time, on studying similar data from another endemic zone in which recently there had been a marked decrease in the incidence of goiter, we found approximately the same levels of iodine ingestion and thyroid uptake with no evident relation to age, as shown in Figure 3.

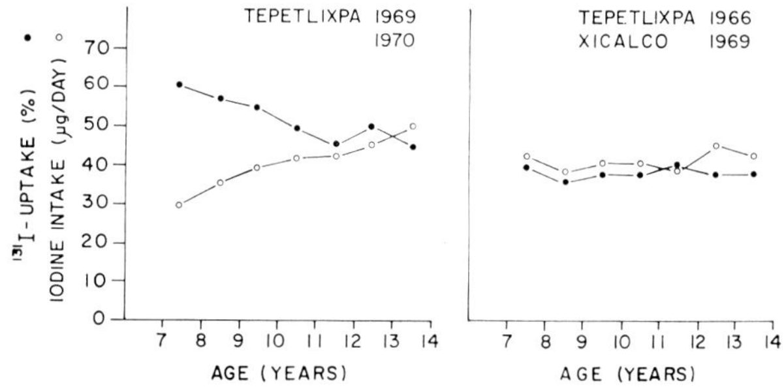

Fig. 3. Slight difference in iodine intake and radioiodine thyroid uptake in Tepetlixpa 1969–70 when the goiter incidence increased, in comparison with no difference in Tepetlixpa 1966 and Xicalco 1969 when there was a marked decrease in the incidence of goiter.

The opposite case, that is a decrease in the prevalence of goiter in persons who were control cases living with patients who were receiving iodinated oil, has also been observed. This has been attributed to a re-circulation of environmental iodine in undetectable amounts (Delange *et al.*, 1969).

We do not contend that these are conclusive data, but we do feel that they clearly show the importance of small changes in iodine ingestion and may offer a hypothetical explanation of the absence of goiter in the presence of a minimal but constant iodine intake or even of the occurrence of goiter in the presence of adequate iodine ingestion, at least for the majority of the group under study. These changes, when considered in the light of previous iodine depletion or repletion, of eating habits and the intake of substances which to a greater or lesser degree interfere with the use of iodine for the production of thyroid hormones, provide us with a new outlook when considering investigations of possible pathologic states in human patients as a result of nutritional deficiencies.

REFERENCES

Delange, F., Thilly, C., Pourbaix, P. and Emans, A. M. (1969): Treatment of Idjwi Island endemic goiter by iodized oil. In: *Endemic Goiter*, p. 118. Editor: J. B. Stanbury. WHO Scientific Publications No. 193.

Maisterrena, J. A. and Tovar, E. (1969): Iodine nutrition in endemic goiter. In: *Progress in Endocrinology*, p. 675. Editor: C. Gual. ICS 184. Excerpta Medica, Amsterdam.

Maisterrena, J. A., Tovar, E., Cancino, A. and Serrano, O. (1964): Nutrition and endemic goiter in Mexico. *J. clin. Endocr.*, *24*, 166.

Maisterrena, J. A., Tovar, E. and Chávez, A. (1968): Daily iodine intake in goiter endemic. *J. clin. Endocr.*, *28*, 919.

Maisterrena, J. A., Tovar, E. and Chávez, A. (1969): Endemic goiter in Mexico and its changing pattern in rural countries. In: *Endemic Goiter*, p. 397. Editor: J. B. Stanbury. WHO Scientific Publications No. 193.

Tovar, E., Maisterrena, J. A. and Chávez, A. (1968): Iodine nutrition levels of school children in rural Mexico. In: *Endemic Goiter*, p. 411. Editor: J. B. Stanbury. WHO Scientific Publications No. 193.

ROLE OF L-TRI-IODOTHYRONINE IN ENDEMIC GOITER*

R. CARLOS STEVENSON, V. GUSTAVO PINEDA and S. ENRIQUE SILVA

Departamento de Endocrinología y Metabolismo, Hospital Salvador, Universidad de Chile
Santiago, Chile

The thyroid gland secretes two hormones of biological significance: thyroxine (T_4) and 3-5-3′-tri-iodothyronine (T_3). Both are iodoamino acids which can be found in the thyroid gland, in the blood and in the tissues. In the gland they are integral units of the peptide chain of thyroglobulin; in the blood they are found free, or bound to certain serum proteins (Robbins and Rall, 1967).

Through the use of *isotopic displacement* techniques (Nobel and Barnhart, 1969; Sterling *et al.*, 1969) it is possible to prove that in humans, as in experimental animals, T_4 accounts for 96.9 to 98.5% of circulating hormonal iodine, only 1.5 to 3.1% being T_3.

The partial deiodination of T_4 to T_3 in the tissues, shown by *in vivo* (Pitt-Rivers *et al.*, 1955) as well as *in vitro* (Larson *et al.*, 1955; Tata *et al.*, 1957) experiments, is probably not metabolically significant (Pitt-Rivers and Rall, 1961), and so plasma T_3 can be considered to arise exclusively as the result of thyroid gland secretion.

Both in human and experimental animals, other iodinated compounds have been found. Roche *et al.* (1956) have demonstrated the presence of 3–3′di-iodothyronine (DIT) and 3-5′-3′tri-iodothyronine. Mono- and especially di-iodothyronine can be detected in man under normal conditions (Weinert *et al.*, 1967; Werner and Nauman, 1968; Row *et al.*, 1967). Circulating DIT may be a more common finding in endemic goiter. We (Barzelatto *et al.*, 1967) have found endogenous labeled DIT in the serum of 6 out of 58 patients studied in Pedregoso.

The glandular secretion can be studied qualitatively and quantitatively in the thyroid vein or it can be estimated through kinetic analysis of the peripheral metabolism of thyroid hormones. Matsuda and Greer (1965) have used the first mentioned method and have shown a greater concentration of T_4 and T_3 in the vein than in the thyroid artery. This gradient is augmented by TSH administration, which also considerably increases serum T_3 concentration (Taurog *et al.*, 1964).

It is a well-known fact that T_3 has a rapid turnover which has been attributed to its weak binding to TBG and entire lack of binding to thyroxine-binding pre-albumin. However, T_3 binding to thyroxine-binding globulin is now doubtful (Zaninovich *et al.*, 1966).

Since Gross and Pitt-Rivers, in 1952, demonstrated the presence of T_3 in human serum its metabolic role has been studied intensively. The biological significance of this hormone as an adaptive mechanism to iodine deficiency is currently under discussion (Querido *et al.*, 1951; De Visscher *et al.*, 1961; Ramalingasmani *et al.*, 1961; Parra-Jimenez *et al.*, 1962; Choufoer *et al.*, 1963; Buttfield *et al.*, 1966; Heninger and Albright, 1966; Beckers *et al.*, 1967; Greer *et al.*, 1968; Pineda *et al.*, 1970).

* Partially supported by the Chilean National Council for Scientific and Technological Research.

It is possible to speculate, in view of the common finding of a low protein-bound iodine (PBI) in euthyroid subjects, or from the kinetic analysis of the peripheral metabolism of T_4 and the determination of the AIU, which have revealed an iodine leak in the gland, or from the high number of hyperthyroid subjects with normal PBI, found in iodine deficient areas (Pineda *et al.*, 1970), that there might exist a calorigenic hormone, not detectable in the PBI, which might be 3-5-3′-triiodothyronine. This supposition is also supported by the experimental evidence, showing a higher MIT/DIT and T_3/T_4 ratio in iodine deficient glands (Querido *et al.*, 1957; Heninger and Albright, 1966), as well as a relatively higher secretion of T_3 (Greer *et al.*, 1968) and a greater concentration of T_3 in the blood and tissues, in these conditions. In spite of the small contribution of T_3 to the total blood hormone level, this hormone represents approximately 20% of hormonal iodine secretion. As T_3 has approximately 4 times the biological potency of T_4, it represents about half of the biologically effective hormones secreted, as Robbins and Rall have stated (1967), so it could play an adaptive role in iodine deficiency.

The relative metabolic efficiency of T_3 is well shown by Feldman's data (1957).

TABLE I

Comparative calorigenic efficiency of T_4 and T_3 in humans and in rats

		Replacement dose (24 hr)		QO_2	QO_2/QI_2	
		µg hormone	µg iodine	µl/g x min	ml/ng	T_3/T_4*
MAN (70 kg)	T_4	200	130	3.1	2.4	
						2.9
	T_3	75	45		7.0	
RAT (200 g)	T_4	3.66	2.36		1.86	
				15.2		2.4
	T_3	1.66	0.96		4.5	

* QO_2/QI_2T_3 QO_2/QI_2T_4.

This author has pointed out that to maintain thyroidectomized rats euthyroid, one has to administer 3.66 µg of T_4 per 200 g body weight per day or 1.66 µg of T_3 per 200 g body weight per day. This is an iodine consumption of 2.36 and 0.96 µg per 200 g body weight per day, respectively. Since a rat's oxygen consumption is 15.2 µl/g per min, the ratio oxygen consumption/iodine consumption for T_4 is 1.86 ml of oxygen per ng of iodine, and for T_3 this ratio is 4.5 (ml of oxygen per ng of iodine), demonstrating quantitatively the greater calorigenic efficiency of T_3.

In man, oxygen consumption is approximately 3.1 µl/g per minute and to maintain a man weighing 70 kg in a euthyroid state requires 75 µg of T_3 (45 µg of I) or 200 µg of T_4 (130 µg of I), so the relation of oxygen consumption to iodine consumption for T_4 is 2.4 ml/ng of I_2 and for T_3 is 7 ml/ng of I_2.

It is of some interest to point out that the relative calorigenic effect of these hormones is similar in man and rat, *i.e.*, T_3 is 2.4 and 2.9 more active than T_4. This gives a molar ratio of 3.2 to 3.9, which is in agreement with the ratio of 3.7 given by Braasch *et al.* (1955). These calculations are also of interest because they show the possibility of extrapolating from data obtained in rats to human studies.

In most studies in which T_4 secretion in iodine deficient subjects has been calculated, the thyroxine distribution space (TDS), the fractional rate of turnover (k), and the PBI have been determined.

Our studies in Pedregoso led us to the conclusion that there would be a significant spillage of iodine (as iodide and/or iodinated tyrosines) by the goitrous gland (Beckers *et al.*, 1965). This iodine leak has also been postulated by Ermans *et al.* (1963) based on the following facts:

When interference from I^{131} could be avoided, in most of his patients the specific activity of iodide in urine was found to be higher than the specific activity of the plasma PBI; the amount of endogenous iodide-I^{131} appearing in the extra-thyroidal space was about 6 times higher than the estimated amount of organic I^{131} broken down during the same time; the amounts of I^{127} and I^{131} taken up by the gland were 3 times higher than those released as hormonal iodine. All these facts suggest that part of the tracer is incorporated into a compound not detectable as PBI^{131}. This could be relevant to the pathogenesis of endemic goiter.

Since the calculations have been based on the degradation of T_4 (assuming PBI is all T_4), without considering the iodine derived from T_3, one can speculate that this apparent loss of iodine is in fact T_3 secretion.

More evidence for this, which we will discuss later on, is the finding which we have recently communicated (Pineda *et al.*, 1970) of a significant number of thyrotoxic patients, from iodine deficient areas, with normal PBI and 6 to 87% of endogenous labeled tri-iodothyronine, two hours after administration of I^{131}.

Though direct data on T_3 concentration in the blood with varying levels of iodide intake are not available, one can calculate its relative concentration from the information we have.

From our studies in Pedregoso (Barzelatto, 1967) on the peripheral metabolism of T_3 and those we are currently making in Peumo (unpublished observations), an area of endemic goiter in the Central Valley of Chile, we have obtained the following results:

TABLE II

L-triiodothyronine turnover data in two areas of endemic goiter and in normal subjects

	Pedregoso	Peumo	Fischer and Oddie (1964)
T_3DS 1/70 kg	30.19	25.9	30
KT_3% day	38.26	46.8	50
T_3 μg/100 ml			0.22*
M μg/day			33

* = Sterling *et al.* (1969)
T_3 DS = l-triiodothyronine distribution space
KT_3 = l-triiodothyronine fractional rate of turnover
T_3 = serum concentration of l-triiodothyronine
M = hormonal disposal rate

From this we can calculate the disposal rate, using the T_3 concentration of .22 μg% found by Sterling *et al.* (1969) as 25.4 μg/day in Pedregoso, and 26.5 μg/day in Peumo. These are normal values, compatible with those obtained by Fischer and Oddie (1964) who estimated the T_3 DS in normal subjects by total body counting to be 30 l, and the fractional turnover rate constant to be 50% per day. Thus the disposal rate turns out to be 33 μg/day. If the T_3 concentration in the subjects living in the above-mentioned iodine-deficient areas is greater than normal, then the values of the disposal rates would be as well.

Assuming a normal thyroid T_3/T_4 ratio of 1:4 in the subjects studied in Peumo, and using their T_3 DS and K values, we could expect a blood concentration ratio of 1:49. That is, 2% of T_3 and 98% of T_4. However, based on the data of Ermans and Decostre (1968),

Heninger and Albright (1966), Greer *et al.* (1968) and Silva and Stevenson (1970), we can state that in thyroid glands with low iodine content, the T_3/T_4 ratio is greater and therefore the blood T_3/T_4 ratio would be the same. Let us assume that the thyroid T_3/T_4 ratio in Peumo is 1, a rather conservative figure compared with 3.3 obtained by us in rats on a low iodine diet (less than 0.2 μg/day) (unpublished observations) and with the value of 1.7 obtained by Inoue and Taurog (1968) in rats on a daily iodine intake of 0.3 μg/day. With a thyroid T_3/T_4 ratio equal to 1 and a T_3/T_4 flow ratio also equal to 1, and knowing the K values, the distribution spaces for T_3 and T_4 and the T_4 blood concentration, only the T_3 concentration remains unknown. This may be calculated from the following formula:

TABLE III

$$\frac{SC\ T_4 \times K\ T_4 \times T_4\ DS}{SC\ T_3 \times K\ T_3 \times T_3\ DS} = \frac{TC\ T_4}{TC\ T_3} = 1$$

	DS (% day/70 kg)	K (% day)	SC (μg %)
T_4	7.25 (10)*	9.0 (10)	8.3 (25)
T_3	25.90 (25)	46.8 (25)	X

X = 0.5 μg %
SC = serum concentration
K = fractional rate of turnover
DS = distribution space
* (N) = number of observations
TC = concentration in the thyroid gland
T_4 = l-thyroxine
T_3 = l-triiodothyronine

We can now say:

(1) The blood T_3/T_4 ratio in normal subjects is 2/98.

(2) The normal T_3 serum concentration is 0.2 μg % (Sterling *et al.*, 1969).

(3) Assuming a thyroid T_3/T_4 ratio of 1, the blood T_3/T_4 ratio of iodine deficient subjects of Peumo would be 5.5/94.5 and the T_3 serum concentration would be 0.5 μg %.

In order to test this hypothesis we are currently measuring T_3 concentration in the serum of people from Peumo. We are using the T_3 determination method of Sterling *et al.*, which consists in removal of thyronines from serum by cation exchange resin, the separation of T_3 from T_4 by descending chromatography and finally quantification of the eluted T_3 by displacement methodology. Our technique was checked by Dr. Bellabarba at the University of Sherbrooke, running 10 duplicates of our samples. Our values are on average 1.2 times higher than those obtained by him.

The average T_3 serum concentration in 7 normal subjects of Santiago, with a urinary iodide excretion averaging 39.8 $\pm$ 11.7 μg/24 hr, was 0.35 $\pm$ 0.07 μg %. In 37 patients from Peumo the T_3 serum concentration was 0.56 $\pm$ 0.18 μg % and they have an average urinary iodide excretion of 38.2 $\pm$ 5.2 μg/24 hr. There is no statistically significant difference between T_3 concentration in Santiago and Peumo. Also, there is no correlation between T_3 concentration and type of goiter or urinary iodide excretion in the Peumo subjects.

These results show that there is a similar iodine deficiency in Peumo as in our supposed 'normal' control subjects. In both groups the T_3 serum concentration was elevated. The value of 0.56 μg % found in the Peumo subjects supports our previous speculation about the

T_3 serum level one should find in people living there and also indicates that the thyroid T_3/T_4 ratio in them is probably close to 1.

The T_4 disposal rate, calculated in 6 subjects, whose T_3 peripheral metabolism, we have studied simultaneously, is 40.1 μg/day, which is half Robbins and Rall's figure of 80.5 μg of T_4 per day. In these same patients the T_3 degradation rate is 62.2 μg/day, which is slightly less than double the figure obtained by the calculations we made, based on Fischer and Oddie's data of 33 μg/day.

These figures support the theory that the iodine-deficient subjects have a reduced T_4 secretion, and an increased T_3 secretion which explains their euthyroidism.

TABLE IV

L-thyroxine and l-triiodothyronine disposal rates of 6 subjects from Peumo as compared with normal subjects

	DS (1)	K (% day)	SC (μg/100 ml)	M (μg/day)	
				Peumo	Robbins and Rall's normal
T_4	6.59 ±0.38*	8.3 ±0.8	7.65 ±0.96	40.1 ±3.9	80.5
					Sterling's normal
T_3	18.90 ±1.9	48.0 ±3	0.72 ±0.12	62.2 ±9.03	33

* = standard error
DS = distribution space
K = fractional rate of turnover
SC = serum concentration
M = hormonal disposal rate

Since our values are 1.2 times higher than Bellabarba's our figure of T_3 disposal rate could be 52, still much higher than Sterling's.

ROLE OF TSH IN T3 SECRETION IN ENDEMIC GOITER

As mentioned before, Taurog *et al.* demonstrated that the T_3 concentration in the thyroid vein is considerably increased after TSH administration in rats.

Buttfield *et al.* (1966), working in the endemic goiter area of Eastern New Guinea, found that the serum TSH level estimated using the McKenzie method (1958) revealed a significant increase in goitrous, but not in non-goitrous natives, and this finding was reversed in patients who had received iodized oil treatment 3 months before. He concluded that the lower serum PBI and elevated serum TSH level in the goitrous compared with non-goitrous natives indicated a failure to adapt to an iodine deficiency.

Recently Adams *et al.*, in a paper presented to the VI International Thyroid Congress in Vienna, showed that people on a normal iodine intake (urinary iodide excretion of 200 to 450 μg/day) have mean TSH levels of 0.35 in New Zealand and 0.65 μU/ml in the U.S.A., by bioassay, and 0.66 (range 0.3-0.9) μU/ml by immunoassay, in contrast to mean level of TSH in natives from Nepal of 5 μU/ml; the latter have urinary iodide values averaging 20 μg/day, and plasma thyroxine values from 0.5 to 11.3 μg% (normal = 4.5-12). The serum TSH level of 60 μU/ml was found in natives from New Guinea. These have a much more profound iodine deficiency, as reflected by their urinary iodide excretion of 5 μg/day and plasma thyroxine values ranging from 0.3 to 2.3 μg%. The authors have suggested a gradation in TSH levels required to maintain apparent euthyroidism in subjects with varying levels of iodide intake.

Dr. Gianetti from our group, working in Dr. Forsham's laboratory in San Francisco, has recently found elevated basal levels and secretion rates of TSH in iodine-deficient rats, and this increases with time. She also found a correlation between thyroid size and TSH secretion ($r = 0.6$), and finally she has made the observation that pituitary TSH in the rat diminished during the first 15 days of an iodine-deficient diet, but then increased about the 30th day.

These results confirm those of Greer and Rockie (1969) who also pointed out that the absence of TSH, provoked by hypophysectomy in the rat performed at the 30th day of an iodine-deficient diet, suppresses thyroidal T_3 (Studer and Greer, 1965). They concluded that thyroidal iodine depletion is more important than TSH in producing high T_3/T_4 ratios, but both are required. A moderate level of TSH stimulation seems to be a permissive prerequisite. In the iodine replete thyroid, a marked reduction in the quantity of entering iodide will not increase the T_3/T_4 of newly synthesized iodo-thyronines.

It is possible therefore to conclude from this evidence, that in subjects from an iodine-deficient area, there exists an increased secretion of TSH and consequently of T_3.

T3 THYROTOXICOSIS IN IODINE DEFICIENCY

If iodine deficiency induces a qualitative modification of thyroid hormone secretion in favor of T_3, it is conceivable that patients who developed thyrotoxicosis under these conditions did so because of this hormone, or that at least it was involved to a major extent.

Since we have observed that 11% of our thyrotoxic patients had a normal PBI (mean 5.9 μg% – range 4.4 to 7.9) and also that in our hospital practice there exists a high prevalence of iodine-deficient subjects, we presume that this could influence the quality of the thyroid secretion in these patients.

We studied (Pineda *et al.*, 1970) 27 subjects with an unequivocal toxic diffuse goiter, without previous treatment, in which 11 had a normal PBI (mean 6.1 μg%, range 4.4 to 7.8). In 8 of these the thyroid suppression test with 75 μg of T_3 daily for 10 days was carried out without demonstrating any significant inhibition (Almeida *et al.*, 1963) of the 24-hr I^{131} thyroid uptake. The urinary iodide excretion of these patients had a significant correlation with PBI ($r = 0.62$, $p < 0.001$).

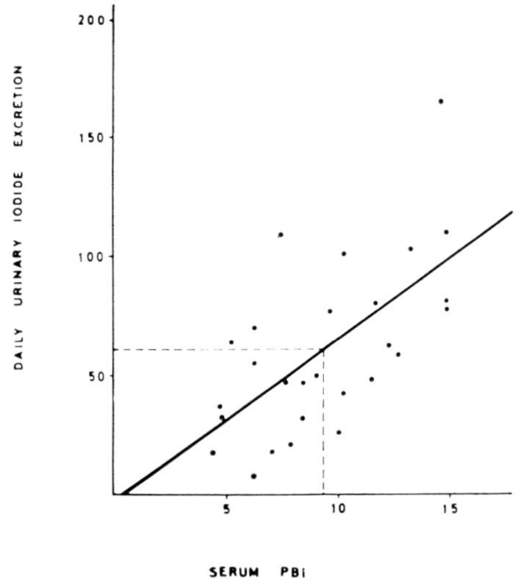

Fig. 1. Correlation between urinary iodide excretion and serum PBI.

This demonstrates the influence of iodine intake on the serum concentration of PBI, which seems to be independent of thyroid function (Barzelatto *et al.*, 1967; De Visscher *et al.*, 1961; Buttfield *et al.*, 1966).

Unfortunately, when we studied these patients, we did not have available T_3 determinations, so we had to rely on a chromatographic technique to evaluate the proportion of T_3 in the plasma. We found in these subjects, with normal PBI, that the percentage of endogenous labelled T_3, 2 hours after administering radioiodine, was 29.5% $\pm$ 8.1 of the hormonal I^{131}. On the other hand, in the patients with high PBI, this figure was only 7.0 $\pm$ 1.8%. This difference is statistically significant ($p = 0.005$). Furthermore, we found a correlation which was also significant ($p < 0.05$) between the percentage of T_3 and the urinary iodide excretion (r — 0.41).

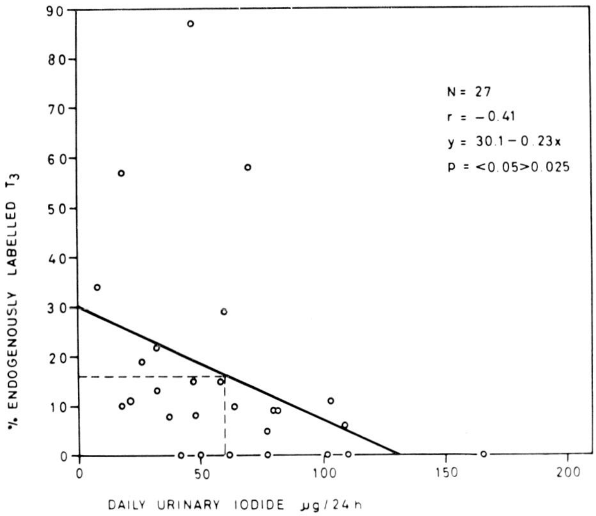

Fig. 2. Correlation between % endogenously labeled triiodothyronine and daily urinary iodide excretion.

Since PBI is essentially thyroxine, our results suggest that the lack of iodine, while limiting thyroxine production in hyperthyroidism, induces a greater participation of T_3 in the condition.

The predominating participation of T_3 in thyrotoxicosis has been occasionally reported in the literature (Rupp and Paschkis, 1962; Klein, 1960; Shimaoka, 1963). Recently Sterling *et al.* have reported 7 thyrotoxic patients with elevated T_3 and normal T_4 plasma levels, pointing this out as a clinical rarity. On the other hand, 3 of their patients were cases of recurrent thyrotoxicosis, after being treated by surgery or with radioactive iodine. We have intentionally excluded from our series patients of this type.

The possibility that T_3 thyrotoxicosis occurs more frequently in iodine-deficient areas might thus be due to the altered pattern of thyroid secretion induced by the lack of iodine.

REFERENCES

Adams, D. D., Kennedy, T. H., Utiger, R. D. (1970): Serum TSH concentrations by bioassay and immunoassay in iodine deficiency and other states. In: *Proceedings of VI Thyroid Congress*, Vienna.

ALMEIDA, F. A., MEDINA, M., BARZELATTO, J. and ATRIA, A. (1963): *La Prueba de Supresión con Triyodotironina, su Valor en Zonas de Endemia Bociosa.* IV Reunión Annual Sociedad Mexicana de Nutrición y Endocrinologia, Ixtapan de la Sal, Mexico.

BARZELATTO, J., BECKERS, C., STEVENSON, C., COVARRUBIAS, E., GIANETTI, A., BOBADILLA, E., PARDO, A., DONOSO, H. and ATRIA, A. (1967): Endemic goiter in Pedregoso (Chile). I. Description and function studies. *Acta endocr. (Kbh.)*, *54*, 577.

BECKERS, C., BARZELATTO, J., STEVENSON, C., GIANETTI, A., PARDO, A., BOBADILLA, E. and DE VISSCHER, M. (1965): Endemic goiter in Pedregoso (Chile). II. Dynamic studies on iodine metabolism. *Acta endocr. (Kbh.)*, *54*, 591.

BRAASCH, J. W., ALBERT, A., KEATING, F. R. and BLACK, B. M. (1955): A note on the iodinated constituents of normal thyroids and of exophthalmic goiters. *J. clin. Endocr.*, *15*, 732.

BUTTFIELD, I. H., BLACK, M. L., HOFFMAN, M. J., MASON, E. K., WALLBY, M. L., GOOD, B. F. and HETZEL, B. I. (1966): Studies of the control of thyroid function in endemic goiter in eastern New Guinea. *J. clin. Endocr.*, *26*, 1201.

CHOUFOER, I. C., VAN RHIJN, M., KASSENAAR, A. A. H. and QUERIDO, A. (1963). Endemic goiter in Western New Guinea: Iodine metabolism in goitrous and non-goitrous subjects. *J. clin. Endocr.*, *23*, 1203.

DE VISSCHER, M., BECKERS, C., VAN DER SCHRIECK, H. G., DE SMET, M., ERMANS, A. M., GALPERIN, H. and BASTENIE, P. A. (1961): Endemic goiter in the Uele region (Republic of Congo). I. General aspects and functional studies. *J. clin. Endocr.*, *21*, 175.

ERMANS, A. M., DUMONT, J. E. and BASTENIE, P. A. (1963): Thyroid function in a goitrous endemia. II. Non-hormonal iodine escape from the goitrous gland. *J. clin. Endocr.*, *23*, 550.

ERMANS, A. M. and DECOSTRE, D. (1968): Relationship between the degree of iodination of thyroglobulin and the distribution of iodoaminoacids in nontoxic goiter. In: *Third International Congress of Endocrinology, Abstract No. 361*, p. 145. ICS No. 157. Excerpta Medica, Amsterdam.

FELDMAN, J. D. (1957): Effect of estrogen on the peripheral utilization of thyroid hormones. *Amer. J. Physiol.*, *188*, 30.

FISCHER, D. A. and ODDIE, T. H. (1964): Whole-body counting of I^{131} labelled triiodothyronine. *J. clin. Endocr.*, *24*, 733.

GIANETTI, A. Personal communication.

GREER, M. A., GRIM, Y. and STUDER, H. (1968): Qualitative changes in the secretion of thyroid hormones induced by iodine deficiency. *Endocrinology*, *83*, 1193.

GREER, M. A. and ROCKIE, E. (1969): Effect of thyrotropin and the iodine content of the thyroid on the triiodothyronine/thyroxine ratio of newly synthesized iodothyronines. *Endocrinology*, *85*, 244.

GROSS, J. and PITT-RIVERS, R. (1952): The identification of 3-5-3′-triiodothyronine in human plasma. *Lancet*, I, 439.

HENINGER, R. W. and ALBRIGHT, E. C. (1966): Effect of iodine deficiency on iodine-containing compounds of rat tissues. *Endocrinology*, *79*, 309

INOUE, K. and TAUROG, A. (1968): Acute and chronic effects of iodide on thyroid radioiodine metabolism in iodine-deficiency rats. *Endocrinology* *83*, 279.

KLEIN, E. (1960): Über die Beziehungen zwischen dem thyreoidalen und peripheren Jodstoffwechsel bei Schilddrüsengesunden und Hyperthyreosen. *Acta endocr. (Kbh.)*, *34*, 137.

LARSON, F. C., TOMITA, K. and ALBRIGHT, E. C. (1955): The deiodination of thyroxine to triiodothyronine by kidney slices of rats with varying thyroid function. *Endocrinology*, *57*, 338.

MACKENZIE, J. M. (1958): Delayed thyroid response to serum from thyrotoxic patients. *Endocrinology*, *62*, 865.

MATSUDA, K. and GREER, M. A. (1965): Nature of thyroid secretion in the rat and the manner in which it is altered by thyrotropin. *Endocrinology*, *76*, 1012.

NOBEL, S. and BARNHART, F. (1969): Specific binding radioassay of serum thyroxine. *Clin. Chem.*, *15*, 509.

PARRA-JIMENEZ, N., RODRIGUEZ GARCIA, P., ROCHE, M. and GAEDE, K. (1962): Circulating iodothyronines in subjects from an endemic goiter area. *J. clin. Endocr.*, *22*, 757.

PINEDA, G., SILVA, E., GIANETTI, A., STEVENSON, C. and BARZELATTO, J. (1970): Influence of iodine deficiency upon PBI in hyperthyroidism. *J. clin. Endocr.*, *30*, 120.

PITT-RIVERS, R. and RALL, J. E. (1961): Radioiodine equilibrium studies of thyroid and blood. *Endocrinology*, *68*, 309.

PITT-RIVERS, R., STANBURY, J. B. and RAPP, B. (1955): Conversion of thyroxine to 3-5-3′-triiodothyronine *in vivo*. *J. clin. Endocr.*, *15*, 616.

Querido, A., Schret, K. and Tepstra, J. (1957): Hormone synthesis in the iodine-deficient thyroid gland. In: *Regulation and Mode of Action of Thyroid Hormones.* Ciba Foundation Colloquia on Endocrinology, Vol. X, pp. 124–132. Editors: G. E. W. Wolstenholme and E. C. P. Millar. Churchill, London.

Rall, J. E., Robbins, J. and Lewallen, G. J. (1964): cited in Robbins and Rall (1967).

Ramalingaswami, V., Subramanian, T. A. B. and Deo, M. G. (1961): The aetiology of Himalayan endemic goitre. *Lancet, 1,* 791.

Robbins, J. and Rall, J. E. (1967): The iodine-containing hormones. In: *Hormones in Blood,* 2nd Edition, Vol. 1, pp. 383–470. Editors: C. H. Gray and A. L. Bacharach. Academic Press, London.

Roche, J., Michel, R., Wolf, W. and Nuñez, J. (1956): Sur deux nouveaux constituants hormonaux du corps thyroide, la 3-3′-diiodothyronine et la 3-3′-5′-triiodothyronine. *Biochim. biophys. Acta (Amst.), 19,* 308.

Row, V. V., Kim, R. H., Ezrin, C. and Volpé, R. (1967): Nature of organic iodinated compounds in the circulation of euthyroid and hyperthyroid subjects stimulated with porcine thyrotropin. *J. clin. Endocr., 27,* 1674.

Rupp, J. J., and Paschkis K. E. (1962): The changing pattern of circulating iodinated aminoacids in a case of thyrotoxicosis. *Amer. J. Med., 30,* 472.

Shimaoka, K. (1963): Toxic adenoma of the thyroid with triiodothyronine as the principal circulating hormone. *Acta endocr. (Kbh.), 43,* 285.

Silva, E., and Stevenson, C. (1970): Efecto del trio y de la cavencia de yodo en la distribución de amino-acidos yodados en él tiroides de la rata. *Rev. med. Chile, 98,* 776.

Sterling, K., Bellabarba, D., Newman, E. S. and Brenner, M. A. (1969): Determination of triiodothyronine concentration in human serum. *J. clin. Invest., 48,* 1150.

Studer, H. and Greer, M. A. (1965): A study of the mechanisms involved in the production of iodine deficiency goiter. *Acta endocr. (Kbh.), 49,* 610.

Tata, J. R., Rall, J. E. and Rawson, R. W. (1957): Metabolism of l-thyroxine an 1-3-5-3′-triiodothyronine by brain tissue preparations. *Endocrinology, 60,* 83.

Taurog, A., Porter, J. and Thio, D. T. (1964): Nature of the I^{131} compounds released into the thyroid veins of rabbits, dogs and cats, before and after TSH administration. *Endocrinology, 74,* 902.

Weinert, H., Masui, H., Radichevich, I. and Werner, S. C. (1967): Materials indistinguishable from iodotyrosines in normal human serum and human serum albumin. *J. clin. Invest., 46,* 1264.

Werner, S. C. and Nauman, J. A. (1968): The thyroid. *Ann. Rev. Physiol., 30,* 213.

Zaninovich, A. A., Farah, H., Ezrin, C. and Volpé, R. (1966): Lack of significant binding of l-triiodothyronine by tyroxine-binding-globulin *in vivo* as demonstrated by acute disappearance of I^{131} labeled triiodothyronine. *J. clin. Invest., 45,* 1290.

STEROIDS – GONADOTROPINS

CONTENTS

SYNTHESIS OF STEROID HORMONES IN SYNCHRONIZED CELLS

PEDRO GARZON* and DAVID L. BERLINER**

Department of Anatomy, University of Utah Medical Center, Salt Lake City, Utah; Biochemistry Department, School of Medicine, Universidad de Guadalajara, Guadalajara, Jalisco, México; and Alza Corporation, Palo Alto, Calif.

INTRODUCTION

It is well known that the liver was thought for several years to be the most important organ regarding the metabolism of steroid hormones. However, experiments first developed in eviscerated rats demonstrated that extrahepatic tissues are capable of biotransforming progesterone and cortisol to a variety of metabolites (Berliner and Wiest, 1956; Berliner *et al.*, 1958). Goldman *et al.* (1957) initiated studies of the steroid metabolic capacity of human skin. Malkinson *et al.* (1959) showed that hydrocortisone was metabolized by human skin *in vitro* into a compound with a relative mobility (Rf) in paper chromatography similar to cortisone.

More recently, in 1964, Hsia *et al.* showed that skin from several different anatomic sites had different capacities to metabolize hydrocortisone. Their later studies (Hsia and Hao, 1966; 1967) demonstrated the interconversion of cortisol and cortisone by human skin. Other recent studies have shown the skin to possess a large capacity for biotransformation of steroid hormones. Some examples of this capacity are the interconversions of estrone and estradiol (Frost *et al.*, 1967; Weinstein *et al.*, 1968), interconversions of testosterone and androstenedione (Gomez and Hsia, 1968), the conversions of dehydroepiandrosterone (DHA) into testosterone, androstenedione and DHA-sulfate (Gallegos and Berliner, 1967; Faredin *et al.*, 1968), and the conversion of DHA into 7-oxygenated derivatives (Faredin *et al.*, 1969). More recently Frost *et al.* (1969) reported the saturation of the 4-5 double bond to form 5α-pregnanes, reduction of the 3-one to 3β-ol and reduction of the 20-one to 20α-ol as major metabolic pathways for progesterone in human skin and vaginal mucosa.

Fibroblasts, which make up a major portion of the cells in connective tissue of the skin, have shown to possess 5α, 5β, 20α, and 20β-steroid-dehydrogenase activity, and 6β and 21-hydroxylase activity *in vitro* (Sweat *et al.*, 1958; 1960; Garzon and Berliner, 1968; 1969; Berliner and Garzon, 1969). Therefore, this study is an attempt to link these metabolic capacities of fibroblasts with the ability of human skin to metabolize progesterone.

MATERIALS AND METHODS

Abdominal skin was obtained from a 46-year-old woman during an oophorectomy secondary to a cystic tumor. Abdominal skin was also obtained from a 60-year-old woman during nephrectomy secondary to necrotizing pyelonephritis.

---

* Present address: Depto. Bioquímica, Facultad de Medicina, Universidad de Guadalajara, Guadalajara, Jalisco, Mexico.

** Present address: Alza Corp., 950 Page Mill Road, Palo Alto, Calif.

All samples of abdominal skin were immediately immersed in warm Eagle's culture media supplemented with penicillin 100 U/ml and streptomycin sulfate 100 μg/ml (Eagle, 1959). A sample of skin obtained from the 46-year-old woman at the time of surgery was processed to separate dermis from the epidermal layer within one hour after it was obtained from the donor.

Progesterone-4-^{14}C (S.A. 46.7 mCi/mM) was purified by paper chromatography (Zaffaroni, 1950). Propylene glycol was used to solubilize progesterone-4-^{14}C in the culture media. Steroids used as carriers were purified by paper chromatography (Zaffaroni, 1950) and recrystallized. Solvents were distilled immediately before use. Radioactivity of the extracts and fractions were recorded using a gas-flow strip-scanner and a tricarb scintillator spectrometer. A Nuclear Chicago gas-flow counter was used to determine the specific activities of the recrystallized compounds.

Incubation of Skin Minces

Following an aseptic procedure, skin samples were separated into 1 g portions, minced and resuspended in Eagle's minimum essential media. Three samples were incubated with 2μCi of progesterone-4-^{14}C in each bottle.

Acetone was added to the first sample immediately after placing the radioactive steroid and served as a control. The other two samples were incubated for a period of five days. On the fifth day the media was tested for bacterial growth and the metabolic process was stopped by the addition of three volumes of warm acetone (50°C). Further extractions with acetone and chloroform were performed. Radioactivity of the final extracts was counted with a tricarb scintillator spectrometer before chromatography.

The extracts were chromatographed in the hexane-formamide system (Zaffaroni, 1950). Aliquots from the eluted radioactive peaks were counted to obtain the respective percentages of conversion and were identified as was described elsewhere (Garzon and Berliner, 1970; Sweat *et al.*, 1958). The more polar areas of the chromatograms were rechromatographed in a hexane-benzene system using known 6β-hydroxy-4-pregnene-3,20-dione as a carrier. A U.V. scanner (wavelength 240 mμ) was used to determine the location of the carrier in the paper chromatogram and the radioactive peak containing the carrier was divided into three aliquots. One aliquot was recrystallized three times in 70% methanol with known amounts of crystalline 6β-hydroxy-4-pregnene-3,20-dione added; another aliquot was oxidized with CrO_3 to 6-keto-4-pregnene-3,20-dione and rechromatographed in benzene-formamide, and the remaining portion was acetylated (Fieser, 1941) with acetic anhydride and pyridine (3 : 1) and rechromatographed in the heptane-formamide system (Zaffaroni, 1950).

Isolation and Incubation of Fibroblasts

Skin slices were washed thoroughly with sterile phosphate buffer solution (PBS), pH 7.4 to eliminate excess of media. Slices were transferred into a sterile 8-ounce bottle containing 0.25% trypsin-PBS (pH 7.4) and left at 37°C for 15 minutes; thereafter they were removed, placed keratin-side down on sterile gauze, and the dermis was lifted off with fine forceps (Gruckshank *et al.*, 1960; Medawar, 1948). The dermis was transferred into a sterile Erlenmeyer flask containing 0.25% trypsin PBS. This time trypsination was accompanied by stirring, using a magnetic stirrer at 37°C for 15 minutes. The effect of trypsin in the cell suspension was neutralized with calf serum, filtered into sterile test-tubes and centrifuged at 1200 rpm for 5 minutes. The remaining tissue was recovered from the gauze and trypsination was repeated.

RESULTS

Five fractions were separated by the hexane-formamide system. The following percentages of conversion were obtained by quantification of the recovered radioactivity after elution of the fractions: unknown (most polar fraction) – 5.6%; 20α-hydroxy-4-pregnene-3-one – 1.0%; 20β-hydroxy-4-pregnene-3-one – 0.5%; 4-pregnane-3,20-dione – 3.9%.

These metabolites were characterized as having been identified following the procedures as described elsewhere (Garzon and Berliner, 1970; Sweat *et al.*, 1958). In a hexane-benzene system the most polar fraction revealed the presence of 6β-hydroxy-4-pregnene-3,20-dione which constituted 1% of the total recovered radioactivity. This steroid had an Rf value of 0.34 in this system. Upon oxidation to 4-pregnene-3,6,20-trione, it revealed an Rf value of 0.68. The acetylated derivative in heptane-formamide system had an Rf of 0.20. Both, radioactive steroid and carrier, ran at the same rate.

Various crystallizations performed of the original metabolite with authentic 6β-hydroxy-4-pregnene-3,20-dione showed constant specific activities (Table I).

TABLE I

Crystallizations of 6β-hydroxy-4-pregnene-3,20-dione isolated from human skin.

Before crystallizations	First	Second	Third
339[b]	342[b]	347[b]	343[b]
(320–373)[a]	(340–344)	(329–344)	(335–354)

[a] Values in parentheses represent the minimum and maximum counts per minute per mg.
[b] Crystallizations from 70% methanol.

Primary explants showed a rapid fibroblast proliferation. Subcultures of the confluent fibroblast layer were performed twice within a one-week period. Cells grown on the cover-slips in Leighton tubes demonstrated a consistent fibroblast morphology (Fig. 1). No critical contamination was found.

Quantitation of the radioactive areas after selection of them with the proper carriers and subsequent procedures for their specific identification revealed the following percentages of conversion: unknown area (most polar fraction) – 8.1%; 20α-hydroxy-4-pregnene-3-one – 0.8%; 20β-hydroxy-4-pregnene-3-one – 0.3%; 4-pregnane-3,20-dione – 89.6%; 5α-pregnane-3,20-dione – 1.2%.

From the unknown area 6β-hydroxy-4-pregnene-3,20-dione constituted 0.5% of the total progesterone-4-^{14}C biotransformed; 6β-hydroxy-4-pregnane-3,20-dione, isolated from tissue-cultured fibroblasts was identified following similar procedures as those utilized for the 6β-hydroxy-4-pregnane-3,20-dione obtained from skin minces. After crystallization, this steroid exhibited constant specific activities (Table II).

TABLE II

Crystallizations of 6β-hydroxy-4-pregnene-3,20-dione isolated from human skin fibroblasts.

Before crystallizations	First	Second	Third
148[b]	152[b]	150[b]	149[b]
(143–151)[a]	(143–157)	(145–157)	(146–151)

[a] Values in parentheses represent the minimum and maximum counts per minute per mg.
[b] Crystallizations from 70% methanol.

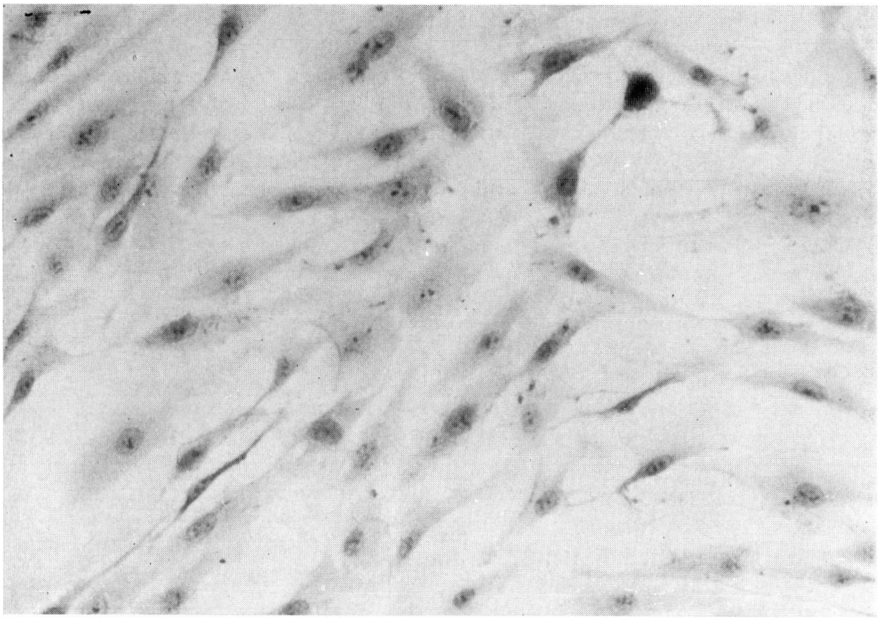

Fig. 1. Steroid 6β-hydroxylase activity by human skin and by human skin fibroblasts.

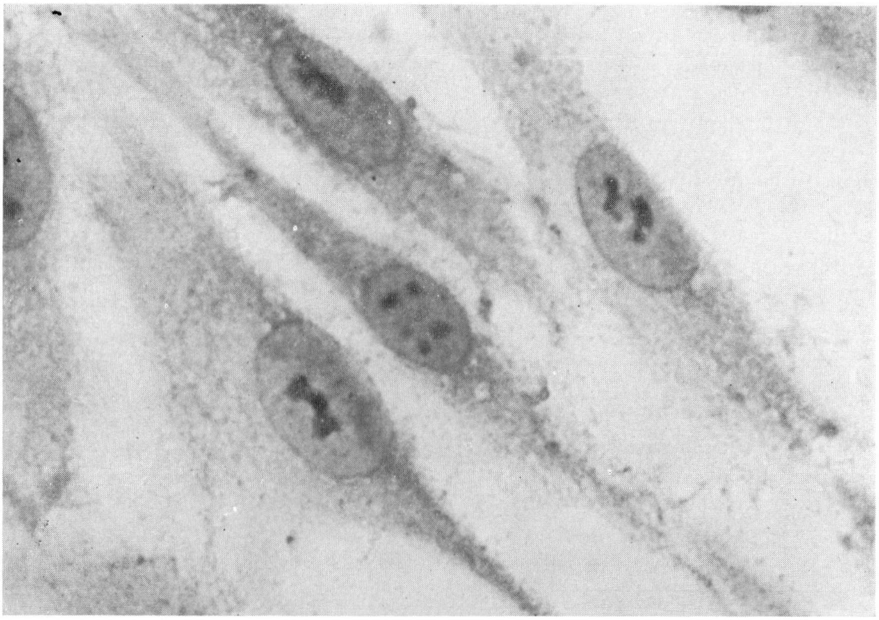

Fig. 2. Steroid 6β-hydroxylase in skin.

DISCUSSION

A summary of the literature pertaining to the production of 6-hydroxylated corticosteroids and 17-ketosteroids was performed by Dorfman (1957). Later researchers have reported the identification and isolation of 6β-hydroxysteroid derivatives from placenta (Berliner and Salhanik, 1956; Hogopian *et al.*, 1956), adrenal slices (Touchstone *et al.*, 1959), neoplastic testicular tissue (Dominguez 1961,), liver (Cohn *et al.*, 1961; Lipman *et al.*, 1962), human urine (Burstein *et al.*, 1954; Nadel *et al.*, 1956; Ulstrom *et al.*, 1960; Frantz *et al.*, 1961; Katz *et al.*, 1962), kidney and skeletal muscle (Lipman *et al.*, 1962). However, their physiological role is still obscure.

Experiments performed *in vivo* and *in vitro* (Ulstrom *et al.*, 1960; Frantz *et al.*, 1961; Katz *et al.*, 1962; Lipman *et al.*, 1962) using cortisol as a precursor indicates that 6β-hydroxylation may represent a truly compensatory route of metabolism for cortisol.

In recent studies we have shown that fibroblasts have the capacity to hydroxylate progesterone-4-^{14}C at the C-6 and C-21 position to form 6β-hydroxy-4-pregnene-3,20-dione and 21-hydroxy-4-pregnene-3,20-dione respectively (Garzon and Berliner, 1969; Berliner and Garzon, 1969). Therefore, hydroxylation at the C-6 position collaterally to the above-mentioned steroid hormone transformations by the skin, strengthens the idea that this organ plays an important role in the regulation and biotransformation of steroid hormones (Berliner and Dougherty, 1961). Cultivation of epidermal cells has been done in the past (Vernon *et al.*, 1957; Karasek, 1966; Klaus and Snell, 1967), but fibroblast overgrowth has constituted a serious problem. Gruckshank *et al.* (1960), using a modification of Medawar's technique, became successful in obtaining pure cultures of epidermal cells, except in one of his many cultures. Epidermal layers can easily be lifted off leaving a clean dermal surface due to the loosening effect of trypsin at the dermo-epidermal junction (Gruckshank *et al.*, 1960; Medawar, 1948). Then epidermal explants as well as dermal explants can be obtained with a certain degree of purity. This method, of course, does not exclude epidermal cell contamination, but it reduces the possibility of its occurring.

Knowing that the dermal layer contains an abundance of fibroblasts, the observed biotransformation of progesterone-4-^{14}C by primary explants established a closer linkage between metabolism of progesterone-4-^{14}C by minced human skin and fibroblasts grown *in vitro* obtained from skin slices from the same source. Thus, the presence of these enzymatic activities in both human skin and human skin fibroblasts supports its role as an organ of endocrinological importance.

Despite the above-mentioned results, it is difficult at this time to ascribe fibroblasts as the only cell in the skin capable of producing these metabolic changes. Nevertheless, there is no doubt that they contribute extensively to the general steroid metabolic pathways due to their ubiquitous distribution.

Pellets obtained after centrifugation were resuspended in Eagle's culture media and distributed in 8-ounce bottles and in Leighton tubes. Cells were allowed to grow at 37°C in an environment of 95% air and 5% CO_2. Confluent cultures obtained 96 hours after the second subculture were incubated with 1 μCi of progesterone-4-^{14}C (S.A. 46.7 mCi/mM for a five-day period. On the fifth day of incubation, bottles were observed for bacterial contamination. The above-mentioned procedures for the extraction and chromatography of the extracts were followed.

To determine the predominant cell type obtained from the skin slices, cells were grown on cover slips and fixed and stained daily with cresyl violet.

SUMMARY

Human skin randomly obtained has proven effective in metabolizing progesterone-4-^{14}C *in vitro* into 6-hydroxy-4-pregnene-3,20-dione among other previously identified metabolites. It has been demonstrated that human skin and human skin fibroblasts possess similar enzymatic capacities for the biotransformation of steroid hormones. The extensive metabolism of progesterone by the skin suggests that this organ plays a major role in the homeostatic mechanism which regulates steroid biotransformation.

REFERENCES

BERLINER, D. L. and DOUGHERTY, T. F. (1961): Hepatic and extrahepatic regulation of corticosteroids. *Pharmacol. Rev.*, *13*, 329.

BERLINER, D. L. and GARZON, P. (1969): Steroid-21-hydroxylase activity by fibroblasts during the cell cycle. *Steroids (Shrewsbury, Mass.)*, *14*, 409.

BERLINER, D. L., GROSSER, B. I. and DOUGHERTY, T. F. (1958): The metabolism of cortisol in eviscerated rats. *Arch. Biochem.*, *77*, 81.

BERLINER, D. L. and SALHANIK, H. A. (1956): The presence of 6β-hydroxylase in human placenta. *J. clin. Endocr.*, *16*, 903.

BERLINER, D. L. and WIEST, W. G. (1956): Extrahepatic metabolism of progesterone. *J. biol. Chem.*, *221*, 449.

BURSTEIN, S., DORFMAN, R. I. and NADEL, E. M. (1954): 6β-Hydroxycortisol, a new steroid in human urine. *Arch. Biochem.*, *53*, 307.

COHN, G. L., UPTON, U. and BONDY, P. K. (1961): The *in vivo* conversion of cortisol-4-^{14}C to 6β-hydroxycortisol-4-^{14}C by the human cirrhotic liver. *J. clin. Endocr.*, *21*, 1328.

DOMINGUEZ, O. V. (1961): Biosynthesis of steroid by testicular tumors complicating congenital adrenocortical hyperplasia. *J. clin. Endocr.*, *21*, 663.

DORFMAN, R. I. (1957): Biochemistry of steroid hormones. *Ann. Rev. Biochem.*, *27*, 523.

EAGLE, H. (1959): Amino acid metabolism in mammalian cell culture. *Science*, *130*, 432.

FAREDIN, I., FAZEKAS, A. G., TOTH, I., KOKAI, K. and JULESZ, M. (1969): Transformation *in vitro* of DHE-4-^{14}C into 7-oxygenated derivatives by normal human male and female skin tissue. *J. invest. Derm.*, *52*, 357.

FAREDIN, I., TOTH, I., FAZEKAS, A. G., KOKAI, K. and JULESZ, M. (1968): Conjugation *in vitro* of DHE-4-^{14}C sulfate by normal human female skin slices. *J. Endocr.*, *41*, 295.

FIESER, L. F. (1941): Solvents. In: *Experiments in Organic Chemistry, Part II*, p. 358. Editor: D. C. Heath. Boston, Mass.

FRANTZ, A. G., KATZ, F. H. and JAILER, J. W. (1961): 6β-Hydroxycortisol and other polar corticosteroids. Measurement and significance in human urine. *J. clin. Endocr.*, *21*, 1290.

FROST, P., GOMEZ, E. C., WEINSTEIN, G. D., LAMAS, J. and HSIA, S. L. (1969): Metabolism of progesterone-4-^{14}C *in vitro* in human skin and vaginal mucosa. *Biochemistry (Wash.)*, *8*, 948.

FROST, P., WEINSTEIN, G. D. and HSIA, S. L. (1967): Metabolism of estradiol 17β and estrone in human skin. *J. invest. Derm.*, *46*, 584.

GALLEGOS, A. J. and BERLINER, D. L. (1967): Transformation and conjugation of dehydroepiandrosterone by human skin. *J. clin. Endocr.*, *27*, 1214.

GARZON, P. and BERLINER, D. L. (1968): Enzymatic changes in the metabolism of progesterone during the 'S' stage of cell cycle. In: *Proceedings, 5th Annual National Meeting of the Reticuloendothelial Society, Vol. 5/6.*

GARZON, P. and BERLINER, D. L. (1969): Steroid 21-hydroxylase activity by fibroblasts during the life cell cycle. In: *51st Meeting of the Endocrine Society*, p. 78.

GARZON, P. and BERLINER, D. L. (1970): Enzymatic changes in the metabolism of progesterone during the 'S' phase of the cell cycle. *J. reticuloendoth. Soc.*, 7397.

GOLDMAN, L., FLATT, R., MIHINOY, J. S., MIER, J. and DASKALAKIS, E. C. (1957): Studies in local action of corticosteroids at cellular level in the skin of man. VIII. Partition paper chromatography of skin extracts. *J. invest. Derm.*, *29*, 1.

GOMEZ, E. C. and HSIA, S. L. (1968): *In vitro* metabolism of testosterone-4-^{14}C and 4-androstene-3,17-dione-4-^{14}C in human skin. *Biochemistry (Wash.)*, *7*, 24.

GRUCKSHANK, C. N. D., COOPER, J. R. and HOOPER, C. (1960): The cultivation of cells from adult epidermis. *J. invest. Derm.*, *34*, 338.

HAGOPIAN, M., PINCUS, G., CARLO, J. and ROMANOFF, E. B. (1956): Notes and comments. Isolation of an unknown substance and 6-ketoprogesterone from perfusates of human placentae. *Endocrinology, 58*, 387.

HSIA, S. L. and HAO, Y. L. (1966): Metabolic transformation of cortisol-4-^{14}C by human skin. *Biochemistry (Wash.), 5*, 1469.

HSIA, S. L. and HAO, Y. L. (1967): Transformation of cortisone to cortisol in human skin. *Steroids (Shrewsbury, Mass.), 10*, 489.

HSIA, S. L., WITTEN, V. H. and HAO, Y. L. (1964): *In vitro* metabolic studies of hydrocortisone-4-^{14}C in human skin. *J. invest. Derm., 43*, 407.

KARASEK, M. A. (1966): *In vitro* culture of human skin epithelial cells. *J. invest. Derm., 47*, 533.

KATZ, F. H., LIPMAN, M. M., FRANTZ, A. G. and JAILER, J. W. (1962): The physiologic significance of 6β-hydroxycortisol in human corticoid metabolism. *J. clin. Endocr., 22*, 71.

KLAUS, S. N. and SNELL, R. S. (1967): The response of mammalian epidermal melanocytes in culture to hormones. *J. invest. Derm., 48*, 356.

LIPMAN, M. M., KATZ, F. H. and JAILER, J. W. (1962): An alternate pathway for cortisol metabolism, 6β-hydroxycortisol production by human tissue slices. *J. clin. Endocr., 22*, 268.

MALKINSON, D. F., LEE, M. W. and CUTUKOVIC, I. (1959): *In vitro* studies of adrenal steroid metabolism in the skin. *J. invest. Derm., 32*, 101.

MEDAWAR, P. B. (1948): The cultivation of adult mammalian skin epithelium *in vitro*. *Quart. J. micr. Sci., 89*, 187.

NADEL, E. M., BURSTEIN, S. and DORFMAN, R. I. (1956): Isolation of polar reducing corticosteroids from human urine. *Arch. Biochem., 61*, 144.

SWEAT, M. L., BERLINER, D. L., BRYSON, M. J., NABORS, C. J., HASKELL, J. and HOLMSTROM, E. (1960): The synthesis and metabolism of progesterone in human and bovine ovary. *Biochim. biophys. Acta (Amst.), 40*, 289.

SWEAT, M. L., GROSSER, B. K., BERLINER, D. L., SWIM, H. E., NABORS JR., C. J. and DOUGHERTY, T. F. (1958): Metabolism of cortisol and progesterone by cultured uterine fibroblasts, stain U-12-705. *Biochim. biophys. Acta (Amst.), 28*, 591.

TOUCHSTONE, J. C., KASPAROW, M. and ROSENTHAL, O. (1959): Most polar steroids of human adrenal incubates. *Fed. Proc., 18*, 340.

ULSTROM, R. A., COLLE, E., BURLEY, J. and GUNVILLE, R. (1960): Adrenocortical steroid metabolism in newborn infants. II. Urinary excretion of 6β-hydroxycortisol and other popular metabolites. *J. clin. Endocr., 20*, 1080.

VERNON, P. P., SANFORD, K. K., EVANS, V. J., HYATT, G. W. and EARLE, W. R. (1957): Establishment of clones of epithelial cells from human skin. *J. nat. Cancer Inst., 18*, 709.

WEINSTEIN, G. D., FROST, P. and HSIA, S. L. (1968): *In vitro* interconversion of estrone and 17β-estradiol in human skin and vaginal mucosa. *J. invest. Derm., 51*, 4.

ZAFFARONI, A. (1950): Micromethods for the analysis of adrenocortical steroids. *Recent Progr. Hormone Res., 8*, 51.

STEROID AND GONADOTROPIN SECRETION IN THE POLYCYSTIC OVARY SYNDROME*

V. B. MAHESH, R. B. GREENBLATT, H. F. L. SCHOLER and J. O. ELLEGOOD

Department of Endocrinology, Medical College of Georgia, Augusta, Ga., U.S.A.

The various clinical signs and symptoms of the polycystic ovary (Stein-Leventhal) syndrome occur individually or in different combinations, in some non-endocrine and a variety of endocrine disorders. It is not surprising, therefore, that the criteria as to what constitute the polycystic ovary syndrome are rather vague and that this 'syndrome complex' may comprise a number of disorders of hormone secretion resulting from different etiologies.

Source of excessive androgens in the polycystic ovary syndrome

Most cases of the polycystic ovary syndrome, particularly those with hirsutism, have the association of elevated androgen secretion with secondary amenorrhea or oligomenorrhea and large pale polycystic ovaries. Considerable data on the secretion of androgens and the finding of polycystic ovaries had accumulated in virilizing adrenal tumors and congenital adrenal hyperplasia before much attention was diverted to the physiopathology of the polycystic ovary syndrome. Consequently, early reports of elevated urinary 17-ketosteroids in the polycystic ovary syndrome invariably implicated the adrenal as the main source of excessive androgens (Buxton and Vande Wiele, 1954; Perloff *et al.*, 1957; Gallagher *et al.*, 1958; Perloff *et al.*, 1958; Gemzell *et al.*, 1959; Brooks and Prunty, 1960; Herrmann *et al.*, 1960; Lipsett and Riter, 1960). However, the possibility of the secretion of androgens by the polycystic ovary was also mentioned repeatedly because of numerous reports that the level of urinary 17-ketosteroids showed a decrease after wedge-resection (Greenblatt, 1953; Gemzell *et al.*, 1959; Pesonen *et al.*, 1959; Greenblatt and Baldwin, 1960; Herrmann *et al.*, 1960; Lanthier, 1960; Goldzieher and Axelrod, 1962; Baulieu *et al.*, 1963; Gold and Goldberg, 1963).

Extensive studies were undertaken in our laboratory to establish the source of excessive androgens in the polycystic ovary syndrome (Mahesh and Greenblatt, 1961; 1962; 1963; 1964*a*; 1964*b*; 1968; Mahesh *et al.*, 1962; 1964; Mahesh, 1964). Fractionation and individual estimation of various urinary steroids showed that the majority of patients with this syndrome had elevated urinary 17-ketosteroids. The elevation was found in the 11-oxygenated-17-ketosteroid or the 11-deoxy-17-ketosteroid fraction or both. As 11-oxygenated-17-ketosteroids, with rare exceptions, arise from adrenal precursors, an elevation in that fraction indicated that the adrenal was a source of excessive androgens. The 11-deoxy-17-ketosteroids may arise from adrenal as well as ovarian precursors. Patients with elevation of this fraction could be divided into two groups based on the response to adrenal suppression with dexa-

* This investigation was supported by research grant #HD–04626–11 from the National Institute of Child Health and Human Development, National Institutes of Health, Bethesda, Maryland. Reagents for the radioimmunoassay of pituitary FSH and LH were kindly supplied by the National Pituitary Agency and the National Institute of Arthritis and Metabolic Diseases.

methasone. A number of patients showed adequate depression of the urinary 11-deoxy-17-ketosteroids, as compared to the normal with adrenal suppression, and therefore the source of excessive androgens was considered to be the adrenals. Others showed only a poor reduction of the elevated 11-deoxy-17-ketosteroids on adrenal suppression but showed a marked lowering only after the ovaries were further suppressed with large doses of stilbestrol. The source of excessive androgens was therefore considered to be the ovaries. In several patients it appeared that excessive androgen secretion was of adrenal as well as ovarian origin. Therefore patients with the polycystic ovary syndrome complex with excessive androgens could represent an adrenal disorder or an ovarian disorder, or a disorder involving both.

The secretion of excessive androgens by the polycystic ovary was a new concept that needed adequate confirmation. Patients having excessive androgens of ovarian origin showed a dramatic decrease in blood and urinary levels after wedge-resection of the ovary and a remarkable rise after stimulation of ovarian function with human pituitary gonadotropins. Furthermore, large quantities of Δ^4-androstenedione and/or dehydroepiandrosterone were isolated from ovarian tissue and ovarian vein blood in these cases. These data, along with urinary steroid excretion studies before and after adrenal suppression and ovarian stimulation, confirm that the ovary indeed may be a source of excessive androgens in the polycystic ovary syndrome. Our findings have been confirmed by other investigators using a variety of methods (Axelrod and Goldzieher, 1962; Short, 1962; Starka *et al.*, 1962; Baulieu *et al.*, 1963; Mac Donald *et al.*, 1963; Simmer, 1963; Jeffcoate *et al.*, 1968*a*; Jeffcoate *et al.*, 1968*b*). Studies using blood production rates and metabolic clearance rates of testosterone and Δ^4-androstenedione in the polycystic ovary syndrome have also appeared in literature (Bardin *et al.*, 1968; Horton and Neisler, 1968) and implied that there may be adrenal androgens that are not acutely dependent on ACTH and may not suppress with short courses of high-dose dexamethasone treatment, unlike the adrenal corticoids and 11-oxygenated-17-ketosteroids. The role of adrenal precursors in ovarian androgen production is not clear. Furthermore, studies with ovarian vein blood are conclusive as far as the role of the ovary is concerned. An adrenal involvement in addition to that, however, cannot be ruled out.

Factors contributing to ovulatory failure in the polycystic ovary syndrome

Patients with the polycystic ovary syndrome have disturbances in menstrual function, such as oligomenorrhea or secondary amenorrhea. Restoration of cyclic ovulatory menses may be achieved in most instances by the wedge-resection of the polycystic ovary and in others by the suppression of excessive adrenal androgens with glucocorticoids. Some cases require both wedge-resection and treatment with glucocorticoids. It has been postulated by several investigators that the problems with the polycystic ovary syndrome are hypothalamic. It is difficult to entertain the concept of a hypothalamic disorder because cyclic ovulatory menses result following the lowering of the level of circulating androgens in blood to normal levels. The action of these androgens may be direct or may be mediated through the peripheral conversion of these androgens to estrogens. The concept of a thick ovarian capsule has also not been borne out because removal of one ovary, without interfering with the contralateral ovary, has invariably resulted in the restoration of cyclic ovulatory menses. Therefore in all probability the primary factor responsible for anovulation in the polycystic ovary syndrome appears to be the abnormal steroid production by the ovary and/or the adrenal, which in turn modifies the pattern of gonadotropin secretion.

Gonadotropin secretion

The initial work on the secretion of gonadotropins in the polycystic ovary syndrome was done by urinary assays. The findings of several investigators showed normal levels for FSH and normal to elevated levels for LH (Ingersoll and McDermott, 1950; McArthur *et al.*, 1950; Keettel *et al.*, 1959; Taymor and Barnard, 1962; Butt *et al.*, 1963; Charles *et al.*, 1963). The relative insensitivity of the urinary methods, the need for large quantities of urine, and the presence of interfering material prevented precise evaluation of the alterations in gonadotropin secretion. The development of radioimmunoassays for serum FSH and LH has now made it possible to study the patterns in normal cyclic menses and in ovulatory failure (Faiman and Ryan, 1967; Odell *et al.*, 1967; Midgley and Jaffe, 1968; Odell *et al.*, 1968; Saxena *et al.*, 1968; Yen *et al.*, 1970). The observations made by various investigators indicated that near the time of ovulation there was a surge of both FSH and LH in the normal human menstrual cycle.

The surge of LH was expected at the time of ovulation on the basis of classical concepts in reproductive physiology. However the finding of a peak of FSH at this time was unexpected. In order to investigate the role of FSH in the rupture of the mature follicle, studies were carried out in our laboratory using experimental animals (Goldman and Mahesh, 1968; 1969). Pubertal female rats and adult cycling rats were found to show a sharp depletion of pituitary FSH and LH between 12 noon and 5 p.m. on the day of proestrus. Everett *et al.* (1949; Everett and Sawyer, 1950) established that in the rat the gonadotropins required for ovulation are released during this period. Radioimmunoassays of serum FSH and LH in the rat on the day of proestrus has confirmed the secretion of both FSH and LH during this critical ovulatory period (Eldridge *et al.*, 1970). Therefore, the pattern of gonadotropin secretion in the rat at the time of ovulation was similar to that found in the human. Rats with mature follicles

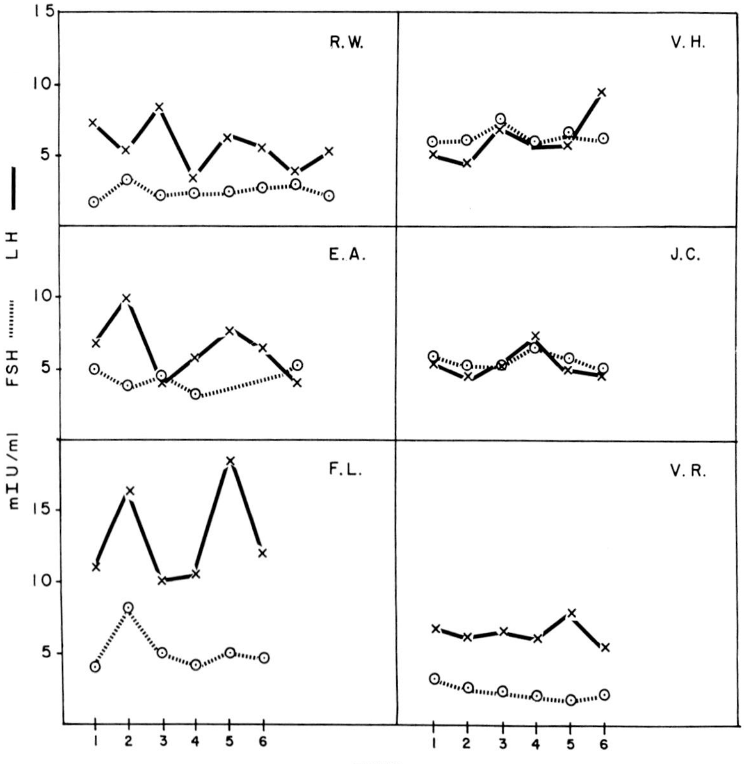

Fig. 1. Serum FSH and LH levels in 6 patients with the polycystic ovary syndrome. Patients did not receive any treatment for 3 months prior to and during the study.

were prepared by injecting pregnant mare serum gonadotropins on day 30 of age and blocking the ovulatory surge of gonadotropins by phenobarbital. Animals thus prepared ovulated when injected with either FSH or LH (Goldman and Mahesh, 1968). A role of FSH in the ovulatory process was further confirmed in the hamster by demonstrating that injection of a liberal excess of anti-LH during the 'critical ovulatory surge of gonadotropins' did not block ovulation, whereas a mixture of anti-FSH and anti-LH did. Furthermore, hamsters ovulated with exogenous FSH in the presence of a liberal excess of anti-LH (Goldman and Mahesh, 1969). Although FSH could bring about the rupture of the follicle to cause ovulation, preliminary evidence indicated that LH was required for progesterone secretion and therefore a synergistic role of FSH and LH was indicated at the time of ovulation. Because of species difference, confirmation of these concepts derived in experimental animals is necessary in the human.

Studies of serum gonadotropin levels in patients with the polycystic ovary syndrome in our laboratory showed that LH may be low, normal or elevated with sporadic peaks (Fig. 1). Serum FSH levels were in general lower than those found in the follicular phase of the normal menstrual cycle. The ovulatory surge in both FSH and LH was absent. Extensive work has been done by our group in the induction of ovulation with clomiphene citrate in patients

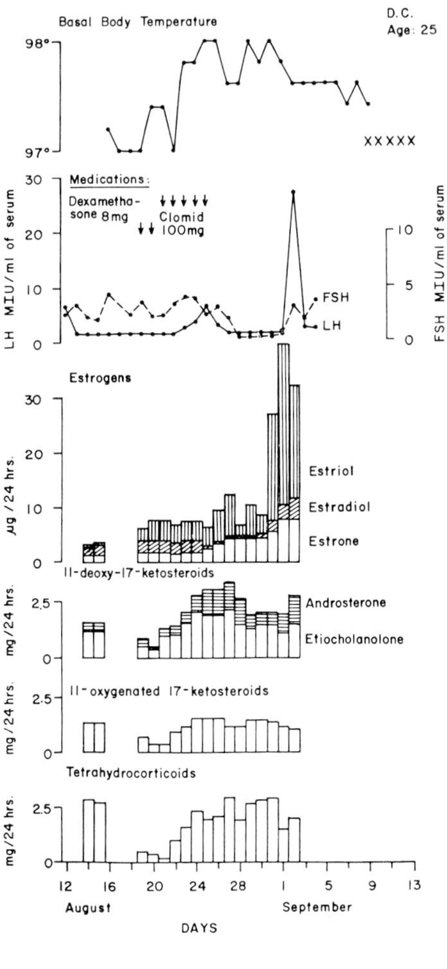

Fig. 2. Serum FSH and LH in a patient with the polycystic ovary syndrome treated with 100 mg clomiphene citrate for 5 days. Note a slight increase in serum LH while the patient was on clomiphene, followed by a peak in estrogens and LH on the 12th day of the start of clomiphene treatment. FSH levels did not show any significant change during the cycle and the patient did not ovulate on the basis of pregnanediol and other classical criteria of ovulation.

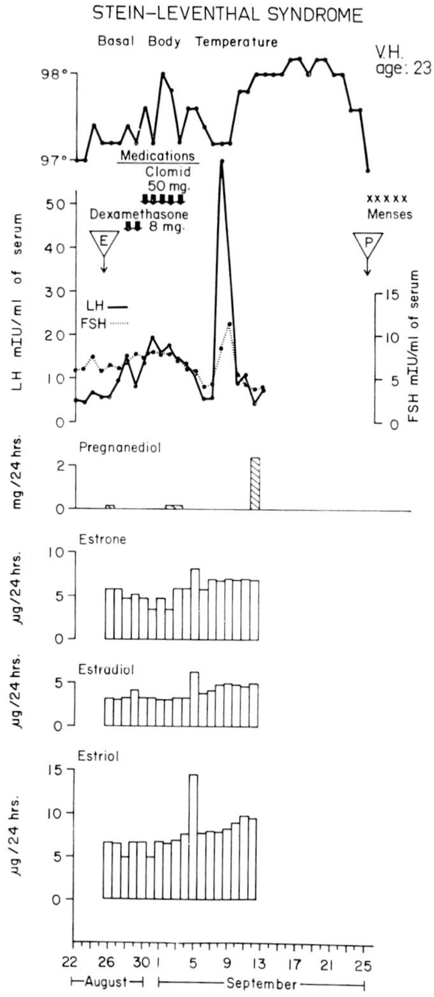

Fig. 3. Serum FSH and LH levels in a patient with the polycystic ovary syndrome treated with clomiphene for 5 days. Small increases occurred in serum FSH and LH during clomiphene treatment. The levels returned to low values after discontinuation of treatment. A peak in urinary estrogens was observed 8 days after the start of clomiphene followed by a surge of FSH and LH on the 10th day resulting in ovulation.

with the polycystic ovary syndrome (Greenblatt *et al.*, 1961; Greenblatt *et al.*, 1962; Roy *et al.*, 1963). It has been adequately demonstrated that clomiphene brings about the release of gonadotropins, resulting in ovulation. Patients with the polycystic ovary syndrome varied in their response to clomiphene, some showing very little change in the gonadotropin secretion pattern and lack of ovulation. Others showed a dramatic surge of LH similar to that observed in the normal menstrual cycle, but with very little or no change in FSH, and these patients also did not ovulate (Fig. 2). The patients that ovulated as a result of clomiphene treatment showed a peak in urinary estrogens, followed by a surge of both FSH and LH (Fig. 3). These results indicate that even in the human, FSH may have significance in the rupture of the follicle and ovulation. It may be of interest to note in this regard that Strott *et al.* (1970) observed that, in patients with the short luteal phase, the only consistent deviation from the normal was a dulled or misplaced FSH peak near the time of ovulation. The classical concept of the role of FSH in human ovulation therefore merits further re-evaluation and the possibility of a synergistic effect of both FSH and LH at the time of ovulation should be considered.

REFERENCES

AXELROD, L. R. and GOLDZIEHER, J. W. (1962): The polycystic ovary. III. Steroid biosynthesis in normal and polycystic ovarian tissue. *J. clin. Endocr.*, *22*, 431.

BARDIN, C. W., HEMBREE, W. C. and LIPSETT, M. B. (1968): Suppression of testosterone and androstenedione production rates with dexamethasone in women with idiopathic hirsutism and polycystic ovaries. *J. clin. Endocr.*, *28*, 1300.

BAULIEU, E. E., MAUVAIS-JARVIS, P. and COPPECHOT, C. (1963): Steroid studies in a case of Stein-Leventhal syndrome with hirsutism. *J. clin. Endocr.*, *23*, 374.

BROOKS, R. V. and PRUNTY, F. T. G. (1960): Patterns of steroid excretion in three types of hirsutism. *J. Endocr.*, *21*, 263.

BUTT, W. R., CROOKE, A. C., CUNNINGHAM, F. J. and PALMER, R. (1963): The effect of dexamethasone on the excretion of oestriol and follicle-stimulating hormone in patients with Stein-Leventhal syndrome. *J. Endocr.*, *26*, 303.

BUXTON, C. L. and VANDE WIELE, R. L. (1954): Wedge resection of polycystic ovaries; critical analysis of 40 operations. *New Engl. J. Med.*, *251*, 293.

CHARLES, D., BARR, W., BELL, E. T., BROWN, J. B., FOTHERBY, K. and LORAINE, A. J. (1963): Clomiphene in the treatment of oligomenorrhea and amenorrhea. *Amer. J. Obstet. Gynec.*, *86*, 913.

ELDRIDGE, J. C., SCHOLER, H. F. L. and MAHESH, V. B. (1970): Serum FSH and LH patterns in pubertal rats, in rats primed with PMS on day 30 and after castration. *Proceedings of the 52nd Meeting of the Endocrine Society*, St. Louis, Missouri, June 10–12, p. 157.

EVERETT, J. W. and SAWYER, C. H. (1950): A 24-hour periodicity in the LH-release apparatus of female rats, disclosed by barbiturate sedation. *Endocrinology*, *47*, 198.

EVERETT, J. W., SAWYER, C. H. and MARKEE, J. E. (1949): A neurogenic timing factor in control of the ovulatory discharge of luteinizing hormone in the cyclic rat. *Endocrinology*, *44*, 234.

FAIMAN, C. and RYAN, R. J. (1967): Serum follicle-stimulating hormone and luteinizing hormone concentrations during the menstrual cycle as determined by radioimmunoassays. *J. clin. Endocr.*, *27*, 1711.

GALLAGHER, T. F., KAPPAS, A., HELLMAN, L., LIPSETT, M. B., PEARSON, O. H. and WEST, C. D. (1958): Adrenal hyperfunction in idiopathic hirsutism and the Stein-Leventhal syndrome. *J. clin. Invest.*, *37*, 794.

GEMZELL, C. A., TILLINGER, K. G. and WESTMAN, A. (1959): A clinical study of ovarian pathology in the urinary excretion of 17-ketosteroids. *Acta endocr. (Kbh.)*, *30*, 387.

GOLD, J. J. and GOLDBERG, S. (1963): The excretion of free 17-ketosteroids in hirsutism. *Fertil. and Steril.*, *14*, 73.

GOLDMAN, B. D. and MAHESH, V. B. (1968): Fluctuations in pituitary FSH during the ovulatory cycle in the rat and a possible role of FSH in the induction of ovulation. *Endocrinology*, *83*, 97.

GOLDMAN, B. D. and MAHESH, V. B. (1969): A possible role of acute FSH-release in ovulation in the hamster, as demonstrated by utilization of antibodies to LH and FSH. *Endocrinology*, *84*, 236.

GOLDZIEHER, J. W. and AXELROD, L. R. (1962): Polycystic ovary. II. Urinary steroid excretion. *J. clin. Endocr.*, *22*, 425.

GREENBLATT, R. B. (1953): Cortisone in treatment of the hirsute woman. *Amer. J. Obstet. Gynec.*, *66*, 700.

GREENBLATT, R. B. and BALDWIN, K. R. (1960): The polycystic ovary syndrome (Stein-Leventhal syndrome). In: *Clinical Endocrinology, Vol. 1*, p. 498. Editor: E. B. Astwood. Grune and Stratton, New York.

GREENBLATT, R. B., BARFIELD, W. E., JUNGCK, E. C. and RAY, A. W. (1961): Induction of ovulation with MRL/41. *J. Amer. med. Ass.*, *178*, 101.

GREENBLATT, R. B., ROY, S., MAHESH, V. B., BARFIELD, W. E. and JUNGCK, E. C. (1962): Induction of ovulation. *Amer. J. Obstet. Gynec.*, *84*, 900.

HERRMANN, W., BUCKNER, F. and MORRIS, J. (1960): The problem of mild adrenal hyperplasia. *Fertil. and Steril.*, *11*, 74.

HORTON, R. and NEISLER, J. (1968): Plasma androgens in patients with the polycystic ovary syndrome. *J. clin. Endocr.*, *28*, 479.

INGERSOLL, R. M. and MCDERMOTT, W. B. (1950): Bilateral polycystic ovaries, Stein-Leventhal syndrome. *Amer. J. Obstet. Gynec.*, *60*, 117.

JEFFCOATE, S. L., BROOKS, R. V., LONDON, D. R., SMITH, P. M., SPATHIS, G. S. and PRUNTY, F. T. G.

(1968*a*): Secretion of C_{19}-steroids and oestrogens in the polycystic ovary syndrome; production and secretion rates. *J. Endocr.*, *42*, 213.

JEFFCOATE, S. L., BROOKS, R. V., LONDON, D. R., PRUNTY, F. T. G. and RHODES, P. (1968*b*): Secretion of C_{19}-steroids and oestrogens in the polycystic ovary syndrome. Ovarian studies *in vivo* and *in vitro* (including studies *in vitro* on a coincidental granulosa cell tumour). *J. Endocr.*, *42*, 245.

KEETTEL, W. C., BRADBURY, J. T. and STODDARD, F. J. (1959): Urinary 17-ketosteroids in the syndrome of polycystic ovaries and hyperthecosis. *Amer. J. Obstet. Gynec.*, *73*, 945.

LANTHIER, A. (1960): Observations on the polycystic ovary syndrome. *J. clin. Endocr.*, *20*, 1587.

LIPSETT, M. D. and RITER, B. (1960): Urinary ketosteroids and pregnanetriol in hirsutism. *J. clin. Endocr.*, *20*, 180.

MACDONALD, P., VANDE WIELE, R. and LIEBERMAN, S. (1963): Precursors of urinary 11-desoxy-17-ketosteroids of ovarian origin. *Amer. J. Obstet. Gynec.*, *86*, 1.

MAHESH, V. B. (1964): Steroid secretions of polycystic (Stein-Leventhal) ovaries. In: *Proceedings of the Second International Congress of Endocrinology, London*, p. 944. Editor: S. Taylor. ICS 83. Excerpta Medica, Amsterdam.

MAHESH, V. B. and GREENBLATT, R. B. (1961): Physiology and pathogenesis of the Stein-Leventhal syndrome. *Nature (Lond.,)* , *191*, 888.

MAHESH, V. B. and GREENBLATT, R. B. (1962): Isolation of dehydroepiandrosterone and 17-hydroxy-^{5}-pregnenolone from the polycystic ovaries of Stein-Leventhal syndrome. *J. clin. Endocr.*, *22*, 441.

MAHESH, V. B. and GREENBLATT, R. B. (1963): The *in vivo* conversion of dehydroepiandrosterone and androstenedione to testosterone in the human. *Acta endocr. (Kbh.)*, *41*, 400.

MAHESH, V. B. and GREENBLATT, R. B. (1964*a*): Steroid secretions of the normal and polycystic ovary. *Rec. Progr. Hormone Res.*, *20*, 341.

MAHESH, V. B. and GREENBLATT, R. B. (1964*b*): Urinary steroid excretion patterns in hirsutism. II. Effect of ovarian stimulation with human pituitary FSH on urinary 17-ketosteroids. *J. clin. Endocr.*, *24*, 1293.

MAHESH, V. B. and GREENBLATT, R. B. (1968): Hormonal studies in females with virilizing adrenal tumors. *Res. Steroids*, *3*, 221.

MAHESH, V. B., GREENBLATT, R. B., AYDAR, C. K. and ROY, S. (1962): Secretion of androgens by the polycystic ovary and its significance. *Fertil. and Steril.*, *13*, 413.

MAHESH, V. B., GREENBLATT, R. B., AYDAR, C. K., ROY, S., PUEBLA, R. A. and ELLEGOOD, J. O. (1964): Urinary steroid excretion patterns in hirsutism. I. Use of adrenal and ovarian suppression in the study of hirsutism. *J. clin. Endocr.*, *24*, 1283.

MCARTHUR, J. W., INGERSOLL, F. M. and WORCESTER, J. (1958): The urinary excretion of ICSH and FSH by women with diseases of the reproductive system. *J. clin. Endocr.*, *18*, 1202.

MIDGLEY, A. R. and JAFFEE, R. B. (1968): Correlation of serum concentrations of follicle-stimulating and luteinizing hormones during the menstrual cycle. *J. clin. Endocr.*, *28*, 1699.

ODELL, W. D., ROSS, G. T. and RAYFORD, P. L. (1967): Radioimmunoassay for luteinizing hormone in human plasma or serum. *J. clin. Invest.*, *46*, 248.

ODELL, W. D., PARLOW, A. F., CARGILLE, C. M. and ROSS, G. T. (1968): Radioimmunoassay for human follicle stimulating hormone. *J. clin. Invest.*, *47*, 2551.

PERLOFF, W. H., CHANNICK, B. J., SUPLICK, B. and CARRINGTON, E. R. (1958): Clinical management of idiopathic hirsutism. *J. Amer. med. Ass.*, *167*, 2041.

PERLOFF, W. H., HADD, H. E., CHANNICK, B. J. and NODINE, J. H. (1957): Hirsutism. *Arch. intern. Med.*, *100*, 981.

PESONEN, S., TIMONEN, S. and MIKKONEN, R. (1959): Symptoms and etiology of the Stein-Leventhal syndrome. *Acta endocr. (Kbh.)*, *30*, 405.

ROY, S., GREENBLATT, R. B., MAHESH, V. B. and JUNGCK, E. C. (1963): Clomiphene citrate: further observations on its use in induction of ovulation in the human and its mode of action. *Fertil. and Steril.*, *14*, 575.

SAXENA, B. B., DEUMURA, H., GANDY, H. M. and PETERSON, R. E. (1968): Radioimmunoassay of human follicle stimulating and luteinizing hormones in plasma. *J. clin. Endocr.*, *28*, 519.

SHORT, R. V. (1962): Further observations on the defective synthesis of ovarian steroids in the Stein-Leventhal syndrome. *J. Endocr.*, *24*, 359.

SIMMER, H. H. (1963): Androgen polyzystische Ovarien und Hirsutism. *Dtsch. med. Wschr.*, *88*, 1661.

STARKA, L., MATYS, Z. and JANATA, J. (1962): Der Nachweis von Dehydroepiandrosterone in menschlichen sklerocystischen Ovarien. *Clin. chim. Acta*, *7*, 776.

STROTT, C. A., CARGILLE, C. M., ROSS, G. T. and LIPSETT, M. B. (1970): The short luteal phase *J. clin. Endocr.*, *30*, 246.

TAYMOR, M. L. and BERNARD, R. (1962): Luteinizing hormone excretion in the polycystic ovary syndrome. *Fertil. and Steril.*, *12*, 501.

YEN, S. S. C., VELA, P. and RANKIN, J. (1970): Inappropriate secretion of follicle-stimulating hormone and luteinizing hormone in polycystic ovarian disease. *J. clin. Endocr.*, *30*, 435.

MECHANISM OF ACTION OF ESTROGENS – PHYSIOLOGICAL APPROACH THROUGH BINDING*

J. M. ROSNER,** J. C. MACOME, A. CASTRO VÁZQUEZ, ANA M. BRUNENGO, D. N. DE CARLI, BERTA IMAS, J. H. DENARI, ISABEL MARTÍNEZ, E. PEDROZA and D. P. CARDINALI

Instituto Latinamericano de Fisiología de la Reproduccion (ILAFIR), Universidad del Salvador, Casilla de Correo 10, San Miguel (P.B.A.), Republica Argentina

Recent research in the estrogen field has produced a revolution in knowledge, leading to a modification of current concepts. This is well illustrated by considering the classical definition of a hormone: a substance produced by specific tissues that enters the general circulation and exerts its effects at a distance from its source of origin (Russell, 1965). It is now established that several tissues, like the mammary gland, are able to produce estrogens (Adams and Wong, 1968); that the estrogens produced by the ovary can accumulate in the follicular fluid and exert their action by contiguity with the oviduct without entering the general circulation (Giorgi *et al.*, 1969); and finally estrogens, like other hormones, may act *in situ* (Schuetz, 1969). A new definition is required and that given by Mueller (1968), 'When the product of one cell type selectively modifies the function of another, we refer to the communicating molecule as a hormone', is perfectly compatible with the new facts.

By considering this definition at the molecular level it is unnecessary to become involved with different types of cells, circulation or distances. The work of Jensen *et al.* (1966), showing that estradiol is first distributed evenly through the body and two hours later is concentrated in the vagina, uterus, anterior hypophysis and anterior hypothalamus, makes it necessary indeed to review the concept of a 'target organ', introducing the time factor as an indispensable requirement. Lately, the oviduct has been added to the group of primary organs where estradiol will act (Rosner *et al.*, 1969) and the sympathetic ganglia of the posterior abdomen of the mouse have the highest uptake of radioactive estradiol (Carr and Williams, 1969).

By studying the early distribution of radioactive estradiol, it can be observed that there is a much higher uptake by the neocortex, hypothalamus and anterior hypophysis during the first few minutes than by the uterus and vagina (Pedroza García and Rosner, 1970) (Fig. 1). One hour after the injection of estradiol the uptake is reversed for every organ except the anterior hypophysis. Considering that the liver estradiol retention time is short but that this hormone increases the synthesis of several proteins (*e.g.*, corticosteroid binding globulin, thyroxine binding globulin) it is necessary to review the concept that a long retention time is always required for hormonal biological actions to take place.

Even a target organ cannot be considered as a whole in respect of the estradiol uptake.

---

* Research supported by grants from the Ford Foundation and Consejo Nacional de Investigaciones Científicas y Técnicas, R. Argentina.

**Member of the Carrera del Investigador, Consejo Nacional de Investigaciones Científicas y Técnicas, R. Argentina.

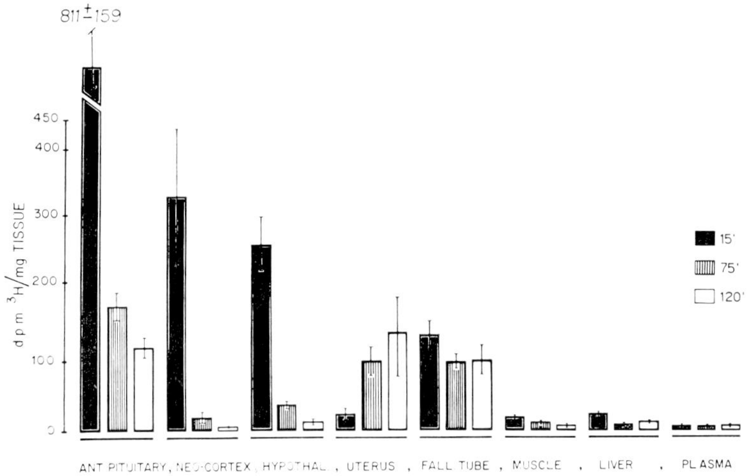

Fig. 1. Distribution of 6 μCi (SA 40 Ci/mmol.) of 17β-estradiol-6,7-³H in the female guinea pig.

When human females were injected with a tracer dose of tritiated estradiol the endometrium was the only one showing a significant difference between the estrogenic and progestational phase as compared to the myometrium and cervix ($p < 0.05$) (Martínez *et al.*, 1970). When the *in vitro* estradiol uptake by the human uterine cervix was studied in non-pregnant and full-term pregnant patients a significantly higher uptake was observed in the latter group ($p < 0.001$) (Martínez *et al.*, 1970) (Figs. 2, 3).

These *in vivo* and *in vitro* results suggest different levels of estrogen uptake which could mean different tissue thresholds. In a similar way the human fallopian tube shows a significant

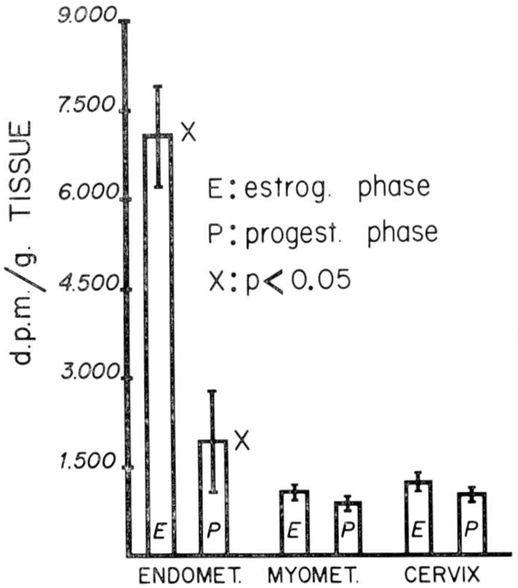

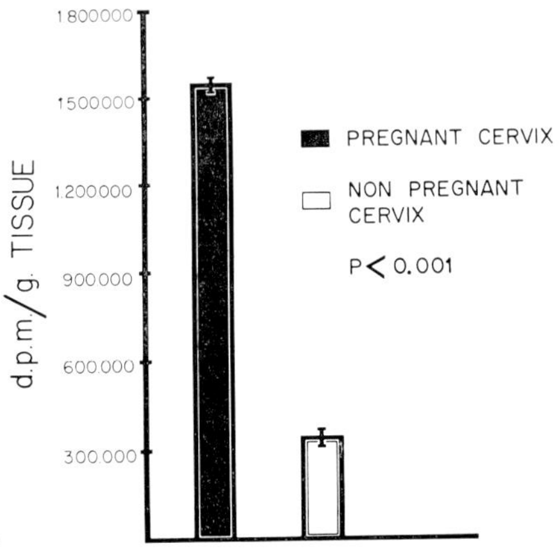

Fig. 2. In vivo uptake of tritiated estradiol by human endometrium, myometrium and cervix during the estrogenic (E) and progestational (P) phases.

Fig. 3. In vitro uptake of tritiated estradiol by human pregnant and non-pregnant cervix.

difference ($p < 0.02$) in the estradiol uptake between the ampulla and the isthmical portion in favor of the latter (Mendizábal *et al.*, 1970).

In rats' uteri, estradiol is not further metabolized (Jensen *et al.*, 1966) and influences directly the transcription and translation processes that take place in the nucleic acids (Hamilton, 1968). In the human uterus, Sweat *et al.* (1967) demonstrated that estradiol is partially metabolized to estrone. Macome *et al.* (1969) showed the same using uteri from pregnant rats. But even considering the two last situations, estradiol is the physiological estrogen in mammals. With the androgens the opposite is true. Testosterone needs to be metabolized to 5α-dihydrotestosterone by a 5α-reductase in order to act at the cellular level (Mauvais-Jarvis *et al.*, 1969) and the same occurs with progesterone which is metabolized to 5α-pregnane-3-20-dione by the uterine nucleus, as shown by Armstrong and King (1970).

After entering the uterine cell the estradiol is taken up by a cytosol protein with an M.W. of 200,000 (Gorski *et al.*, 1968), the complex being temperature- and pH-dependent. This protein has a sedimentation coefficient of 8 S (Giannopoulos and Gorski, 1970) or 9 S (Vonderhaar *et al.*, 1970) and it is formed by two subunits, only one being active in estrogen binding (Vonderhaar *et al.*, 1970). The active protein fraction is the carrier of estradiol from cytoplasm to the nucleus (Shyamala and Gorski, 1969). In the nucleus the carrier protein is transformed to a 5 S protein (Brecher *et al.*, 1970).

The supernatant protein has three functional characteristics: (1) specificity; (2) limited capacity; (3) carrier function.

(1) *Specificity:* It will only bind estradiol and no other hormones, such as testosterone, cortisol, etc. (Gorski *et al.*, 1968). Nevertheless, it has a weaker binding capacity for other natural and synthetic estrogens (Gorski *et al.*, 1968), and the simultaneous *in vivo* injection of chlormadinone and ^{3}H-estradiol depresses estradiol uptake (Macome *et al.*, 1970). When different doses of chlormadinone were used an inhibition of the anterior hypophysis uptake ($p < 0.01$) was obtained with an equimolecular amount (58 ng) of the progestagen; 1 μg was necessary to produce a significative diminution of the uterine uptake ($p < 0.01$). The anterior hypothalamus estradiol uptake was not modified by even 100 μg of intravenous chlormadinone. Kato *et al.* (1968) have observed that clomiphene markedly depresses the estradiol

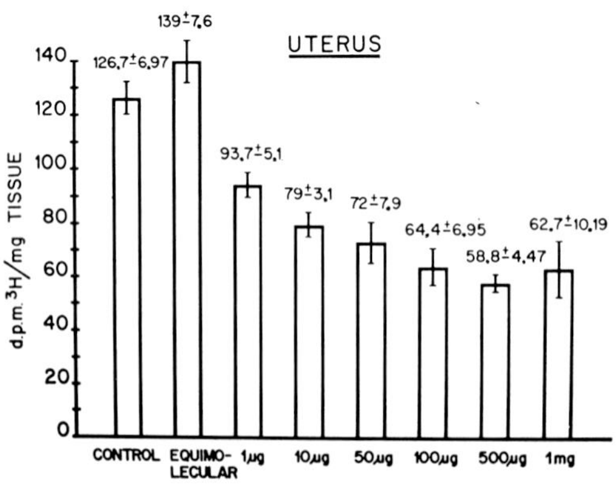

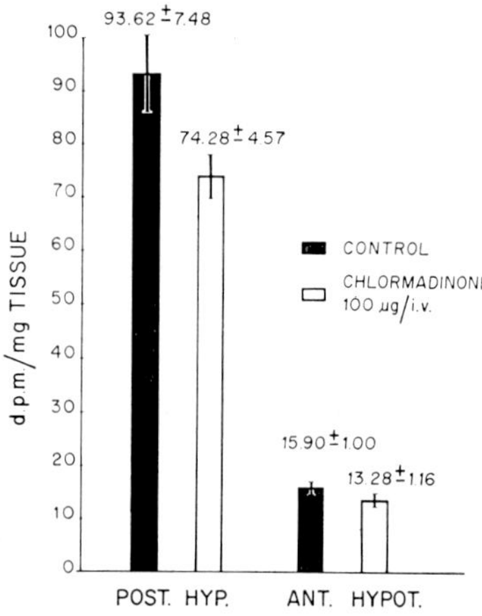

Fig. 4. Effect of different doses of chlormadinone acetate on the *in vivo* uptake of tritiated estradiol by the rat uterus.

Fig. 5. Effect of 100 μg of chlormadinone acetate on the *in vivo* uptake of tritiated estradiol by the rat anterior hypothalamus and posterior hypophysis.

TABLE I

Effect of 100 μg of chlormadinone acetate on the in vivo *subcellular distribution of 2.7 μCi (SA 40 Ci/mmol) of 6,7-³H estradiol-17β in the rat uterus.*

	Nucleus	Mitochondria	Microsomes	Supernatant
Estradiol	9.275 ± 400	517 ± 65	343 ± 43	2.668 ± 182
Estradiol + chlormadinone	3.981 ± 663	440 ± 99	335 ± 48	2.121 ± 316

Expressed as dpm/mg, mean ± S.E. p < 0.005, Student's test.

uptake by the anterior hypophysis and a smaller depression was observed in the anterior hypothalamus. By ultracentrifugation studies it was demonstrated that chlormadinone modifies the intracellular distribution of ^{3}H-17β-estradiol, by significantly depressing the amount of estradiol bound to the nucleus (Denari and Rosner, 1970) (Figs. 4, 5) (Table I).

Zimmering *et al.* (1970) describe two binding modes of 17β-estradiol to the 8 S receptor when studied by equilibrium dialysis at 5°C. The first is observed at low concentration of free estradiol and is consistent with homogeneous independent binding sites. Above a critical concentration of estradiol a second binding mode occurs which is characterized by dependent cooperative binding. Sulphydryl blocking reagents (Jensen *et al.*, 1967) and iodination (Puga and Bresciani, 1970) disrupt the estradiol receptor complex, which suggests that sulphydryl groups and aromatic amino acids are involved in the estradiol binding. The *in vitro* binding of estradiol to uterine proteins is enhanced by several cations, Zn having the maximal effect (Emanuel and Oakey, 1969).

(2) *Limited Capacity:* The 8 S supernatant uterine protein has a limited capacity to bind estradiol which is determined by the number of binding sites. The ability to bind estradiol could be enhanced by increasing the number of binding sites as is done by estrogen priming (Gorski *et al.*, 1968) or by making more estrogen available to the binding protein. It is known that estradiol releases histamine in the uterus of the spayed rat (Spaziani and Szego, 1958) and histamine can mimic several estrogenic effects (Hechter *et al.*, 1942; Holden, 1939; Spaziani, 1963; Astwood, 1938; Leonard, 1963; Szego and Lawson, 1964).

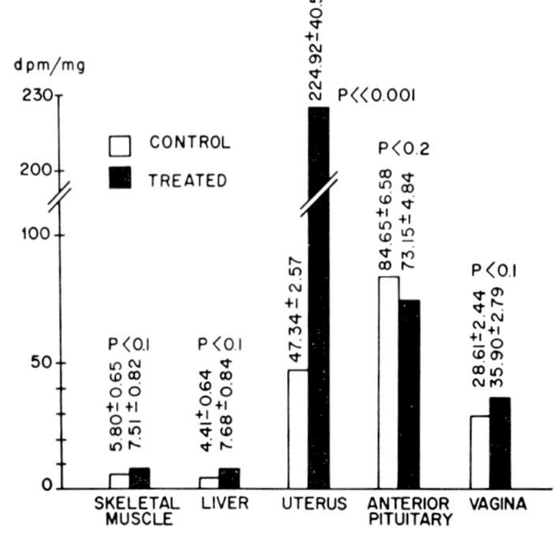

Fig. 6. Effect of simultaneously injected histamine dihydrochloride (50 mg s.c.) on the *in vivo* distribution of tritiated estradiol in the rat.

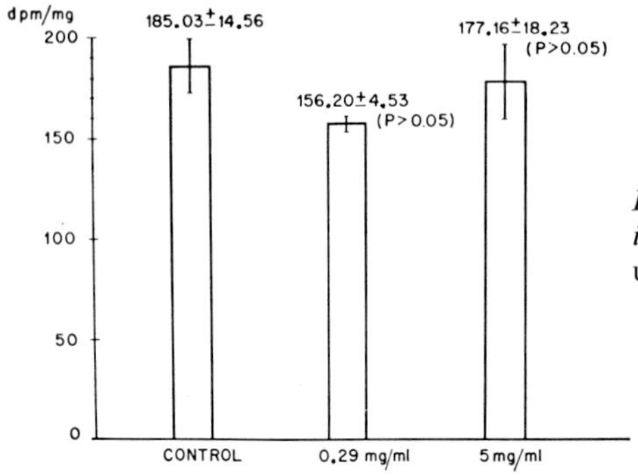

Fig. 7. Effect of histamine dihydrochloride on the *in vitro* uptake of tritiated estradiol by the rat uterus added simultaneously to the incubation flask.

Decidual formation, which requires estrogens (Yochim and De Feo, 1962) is preceded by uterine histamine release (Shlesnyak, 1959). The possible regulation by histamine of the estrogenic effects was studied in our laboratory by simultaneous *in vivo* injection of histamine dihydrochloride and tritiated 17β-estradiol in ovariectomized rats (Castro *et al.*, 1971). Histamine specifically increased the estradiol uptake by the uterus ($p < 0.001$) without modifying uptake by the other target organs (Fig. 6). Histological examination of the uterus showed marked dilatation of the vascular bed and endometrial edema.

Since histamine did not increase the *in vitro* uptake of estradiol (Fig. 7), the *in vivo* results suggest a possible vascular mechanism. The injection of histamine also enhances the nuclear incorporation of ^{3}H-17β-estradiol when studied by differential centrifugation (Castro *et al.*, 1970) (Table II).

TABLE II

Effect of 50 mg of histamine dihydrochloride on the in vivo *subcellular distribution of 5.76 × 10⁶ dpm (SA 40 Ci/mmol) of 6, 7-³H estradiol-17β in the rat uterus.*

	Control %	Histamine %
Nuclear fraction	49.6 ± 2.0	57.7 ± 1.3*
Cytoplasmic fraction	50.4 ± 2.0	42.3 ± 1.3

* Significance: $P < 0.01$.

(3) *Carrier Function:* The cytosol protein is specifically induced by a single injection of 17β-estradiol into immature rats or mature ovariectomized rats. The injection of estradiol increases the incorporation of labeled amino acids into a specific soluble protein (induced protein) (Barnea and Gorski, 1970). The induced protein was not detected when uterine proteins were labeled with radioactive amino acids prior to estrogens, which indicates *de novo* synthesis of this protein.

The stimulation of hormone-specific synthesis becomes detectable 30 minutes after estradiol administration and, reaching a maximum at 1 hour, rapidly declines to control level 4 hours later. There is no detectable increase in the rate of synthesis of other uterine proteins until after the synthesis of estrogen-specific proteins has begun (Mayol and Thayer, 1970).

With the aims of achieving a better understanding of the estrogen mechanism of action and controlling their effects, two approaches have been utilized. Ferin *et al.* (1969) have

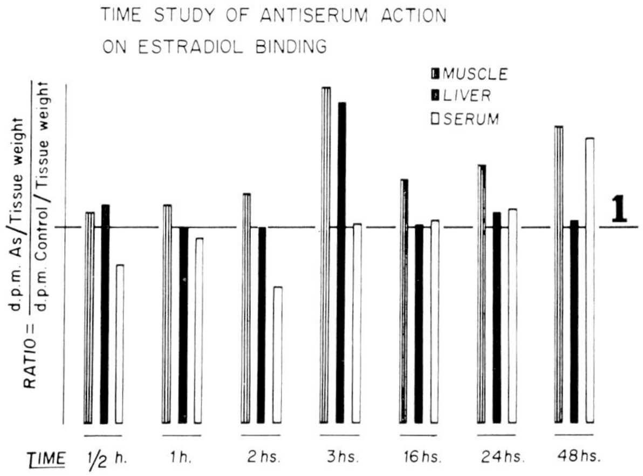

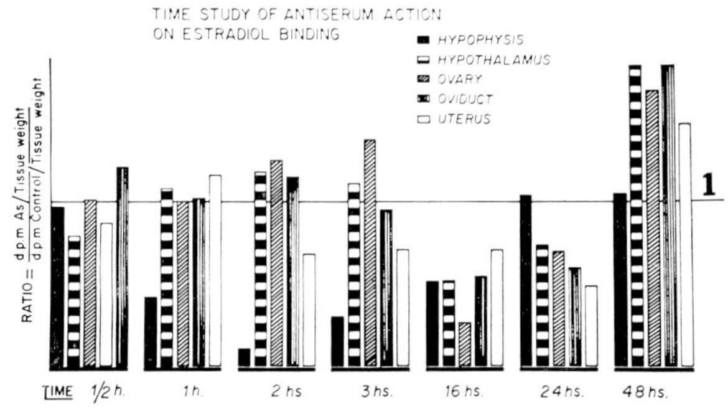

Figs. 8 and *9*. An optimal dose of rabbit antiserum against a total extract of rat uterus was injected intravenously to mature female rats at different time intervals prior to the tritiated estradiol injection. The bars represent the ratio of tritiated estradiol uptake inhibition by the antiserum compared with the controls injected with normal rabbit serum, normal rat serum or rabbit antiserum to normal rat serum.

developed a technique for obtaining antibodies against 17β-estradiol by using an albumin-estrogen complex. In our laboratory antibodies to the supernatant and nuclear fraction and total uterine rat homogenates have been prepared (Brunengo *et al.*, 1970). In this presentation we will discuss the preliminary results obtained after the injection of antibodies against the total uterine extract.

After performing a dose-response experiment and determining the optimal effective dose a time study of the inhibition of ^{3}H-17β-estradiol uptake was undertaken. In relation to the inhibition of estradiol uptake by the previously injected antiserum (30 minutes to 48 hours previous to estradiol injection), the organs studied can be divided into two groups. The liver, muscle and serum estradiol uptake was not modified by the antiserum. The first inhibitory effect is produced in the hypophysis, appearing 1 hour after the antiserum injection and is still observed 16 hours after the injection of antiserum. Hypothalamus, oviduct, ovary and uterus behaved similarly, inhibition starting 16 hours after the antiserum injection and being observed 24 hours after, but not 48 hours later (Figs 8, 9).

The experiments discussed in this paper offer encouraging results, opening new possibilities for a better comprehension of the mechanism of action of estrogen but will necessarily be superseded by new discoveries.

REFERENCES

ADAMS, J. B. and WONG, M. S. F. (1968): Paraendocrine behaviour of human breast carcinoma: *in vitro* transformation of steroids to physiologically active hormones. *J. Endocr.*, *41*, 41.

ARMSTRONG, O. T. and KING, E. R. (1970): Conversion of progesterone to 5α-pregnan-3,20 dione (5α-P) by uterine nuclei and its possible significance. *Fed. Proc.*, *29*, 250.

ASTWOOD, E. B. (1938): A six-hour assay for the quantitative determination of estrogen. *Endocrinology*, *23*, 25.

BARNEA, A. and GORSKI, J. (1970): Estrogen-induced protein. Time course synthesis. *Biochemistry*, *9*, 1899.

BRECHER, P. I., NUMATA, M., DE SOMBRE, E. R. and JENSEN, E. V. (1970): Conversion of uterine 4 S estradiol-receptor complex to 5 S complex in a soluble system. *Fed. Proc.*, *29*, 249.

BRUNENGO, A. M., IMAS, B., SALMORAL, E. and ROSNER, J. M. (1970): Unpublished results.

CARR, I. and WILLIAMS, M. A. (1969): Binding of tritiated oestradiol by certain cells in autonomic ganglia in the mouse. *J. Endocr.*, *43*, 131.

CASTRO, A., DE CARLI, D. N., MACOME, J. C. and ROSNER, J. M. (1971): The effect of chlormadinone acetate on the *in vivo* uptake of 6, 7-^{3}H-estradiol 17β by the rat uterus and hypophysis. In: *Proceedings, III International Congress on Hormonal Steroids, Hamburg, 1970.* Editor: V. James, ICS 219. Excerpta Medica, Amsterdam.

DENARI, J. H. and ROSNER, J. M. (1970): Unpublished results.

EMANUEL, M. B. and OAKEY, R. E. (1969): Effect of Zn^{++} on the binding of oestradiol-17β to a uterine protein. *Nature*, *223*, 68.

FERIN, M., ZIMMERING, P. E. and VANDE WIELE, R. L. (1969): Effects of antibodies to estradiol-17β on PMS-induced ovulation in immature rats. *Endocrinology*, *84*, 893.

GIANNOPOULOS, G. and GORSKI, J. (1970): Search for the native state of the estrogen receptor in rat uterus: isolation of a new form of estrogen-specific binding protein. *Fed. Proc.*, *29*, 469.

GIORGI, E. P., ADDIS, M. and COLOMBO, G. (1969): The fate of free and conjugated oestrogens injected into the graafian follicle of equines. *J. Endocr.*, *45*, 37.

GORSKI, J., TAFT, D., SHYAMALA, G., SMITH, D. and NOTIDES, A. (1968): Hormone receptors: studies on the interaction of estrogen with the uterus. *Recent Progr. Hormone Res.*, *24*, 45.

HAMILTON, T. (1968): Control by estrogen of genetic transcription and translation. *Science*, *161*, 649.

HECHTER, O., KROHN, L. and HARRIS, J. (1942): The effect of estrogen on the permeability of the uterine capillaries. *Endocrinology*, *29*, 386.

HOLDEN, R. B. (1939): Vascular reactions of the uterus of the immature rat. *Endocrinology*, *25*, 593.

JENSEN, E. V., HURST, D. J., DE SOMBRE, E. R. and JUNGBLUT, P. W. (1967): Sulfhydryl groups and estradiol-receptor interaction. *Science*, *158*, 385.

JENSEN, E. V., JACOBSON, H. I., FLEISHER, J. W., SAHA, N. N., GUPTA, G. N., SMITH, S., COLUCCI, V., SHIPLACOFF, D., NEUMANN, H. G., DE SOMBRE, E. R. and JUNGBLUT, P. W. (1966): Estrogen receptors in target tissues. In: *Steroid Dynamics*, p. 133. Editors: G. Pincus, T. Nakao and J. F. Tait. Academic Press, New York.

KATO, J., KOBAYASHI, T. and VILLEE, C. A. (1968): Effect of clomiphene on the uptake of estradiol by the anterior hypothalamus and hypophysis. *Endocrinology*, *82*, 1250.

LEONARD, S. L. (1963): Effect of histamine and serotonin in stimulating phosphorylase activity in the rat uterus. *Endocrinology*, *72*, 865.

MACOME, J. C., CASTRO, A. J., DEL RIO, P. O., BECCUTI, J. and ROSNER, J. M. (1969): Estudio de la acción del 17α-etinil-Δ4-estren-17β-ol (Linestrenol) durante los primeros días de la preñez de la rata. In: *Proceedings, III Meeting, Asociación Latino Americana de Investigaciónes en Reproducción Humana (A. L. I. R. H.) Bahía, Brasil*, p. 31.

MACOME, J. C., DE CARLI, N. and ROSNER, J. M. (1970): The effect of chlormadinone acetate on the *in vivo* uptake of 6, 7-^{3}H-estradiol-17β by the rat uterus and hypophysis. In: *Proceedings of III International Congress on Hormonal Steroids, Hamburg, 1970.* Editor: V. James. ICS 219. Excerpta Medica, Amsterdam.

MARTINEZ, I., MENDIZABAL, A., ROSNER, J. M. and MACOME, J. C. (1970): Captación de 17β-estradiol-6, 7-^{3}H *in vivo* por distintos segmentos del útero humano. In: *Proceedings, IV Meeting, Asociación Latino Americana de investigaciones en Reproducción Humano (A.L.I.R.H.), México,* p. 34.

MAUVAIS-JARVIS, P., BERCOVICI, J. P. and GAUTHIER, F. (1969): *In vivo* studies on testosterone metabolism by skin of normal males and patients with the syndrome of testicular feminization. *J. clin. Endocr.*, *29*, 417.

MAYOL, R. F. and THAYER, S. A. (1970): Synthesis of estrogen specific proteins in the uterus of the immature rat. *Biochemistry, 9*, 2482.

MENDIZABAL, A., ROSNER, J. M., MARTINEZ, I. and SPALTRO, N. A. (1970): Captación de 17β-estradiol 6, 7-^{3}H por la trompa de falopio humana. In: *Proceedings, VI Latin-American Congress of Obstetrics and Gynecology, San José, Costa Rica.*

MUELLER, G. C. (1968): Estrogen action and genetic expression in the uterus. In: *Biogenesis and Action of Steroid Hormones*, p. 1. Editors: R. I. Dorfman, K. Yamasaki, M. Dorfman. Geron-X, Los Altos, Calif.

PEDROZA GARCIA, E. and ROSNER, J. M. (1970): Unpublished results.

PUGA, G. A. and BRESCIANI, F. (1970): Binding activity of oestrogen receptors destroyed by iodination. *Nature, 225*, 1251.

ROSNER, J. M., MACOME, J. C., CASTRO VAZQUEZ, A. and DE CARLI, D. N. (1969): Captación de estradiol-6, 7-^{3}H por el oviducto de rata. In: *Proceedings, 2das. Jornadas Rioplatenses de Endocrinología y Metabolismo, Salta, Argentina*, p. 34.

RUSSELL, J. A. (1965): The hormones. In: *Physiology and Biophysics*, p. 1085. Editors: T. C. Ruch and H. D. Patton. W. B. Saunders, Philadelphia.

SCHUETZ, A. W. (1969): Oogenesis: processes and their regulation. In: *Advances in Reproductive Physiology*, vol. 4, p. 99. Editor: A. Mc Laren. Logos Press, London.

SHLESNYAK, M. C. (1959): Fall in uterine histamine associated with ovum implantation in pregnant rat. *Proc. Soc. exp. Biol. (N.Y.) 100*, 380.

SHYAMALA, G. and GORSKI, J. (1969): Estrogen receptors in the rat uterus. *J. biol. Chem., 244*, 1097.

SPAZIANI, E. (1963): Relationship between early vascular responses and growth in the rat uterus: stimulation of cell division by estradiol and by vasodilating amines. *Endocrinology, 72*, 180.

SPAZIANI, E. and SZEGO, C. M. (1958): The influence of estradiol and cortisol on uterine histamine of the ovariectomized rat. *Endocrinology, 63*, 669.

SWEAT, M. L., BRYSON, M. J. and YOUNG, R. B. (1967): Metabolism of 17β-estradiol and estrone by human proliferative endometrium and myometrium. *Endocrinology, 81*, 167.

SZEGO, C. M. and LAWSON, D. A. (1964): Influence of histamine on uterine metabolism: stimulation of incorporation of radioactivity from amino acids into protein, lipid and purines. *Endocrinology, 74*, 372.

VONDERHAAR, B. K., KIM, U. H. and MUELLER, G. C. (1970): Estradiol induced modifications of the soluble estrogen receptors in rat uterus. *Fed. Proc., 29*, 249.

YOCHIM, J. M. and DE FEO, V. J. (1962): Control of decidual growth in the rat by steroid hormones of the ovary. *Endocrinology, 71*, 134.

ZIMMERING, P. E., KAHN, I. and LIEBERMAN, S. (1970): Estradiol and progesterone binding to a fraction of ovine endometrial cytoplasm. *Biochemistry, 9*, 2498.

LOCI OF ACTION OF PROLACTIN AND LUTEINIZING HORMONE IN THE HAMSTER OVARY DURING LACTATION. THE INTERSTITIAL TISSUE

A. B. FAJER

Department of Physiology, School of Medicine, University of Maryland, Baltimore, Md 21201, U.S.A.

It is well established that the hamster does not show a post-partum ovulation (Greenwald, 1965).

At parturition, vesicular follicles undergo atresia and corpora lutea are destroyed by luteolysis. The interstitial tissue becomes the dominant element in the histological picture (Fig. 1).

It is accepted that, in the adult hamster, the interstitial cells originate from theca interna cells of regressing follicles (Nakano, 1960; Guraya and Greenwald, 1965). However it was also proposed that interstitial cells may derive from the granulosa cells of preantral follicles (Knigge and Leatham, 1956).

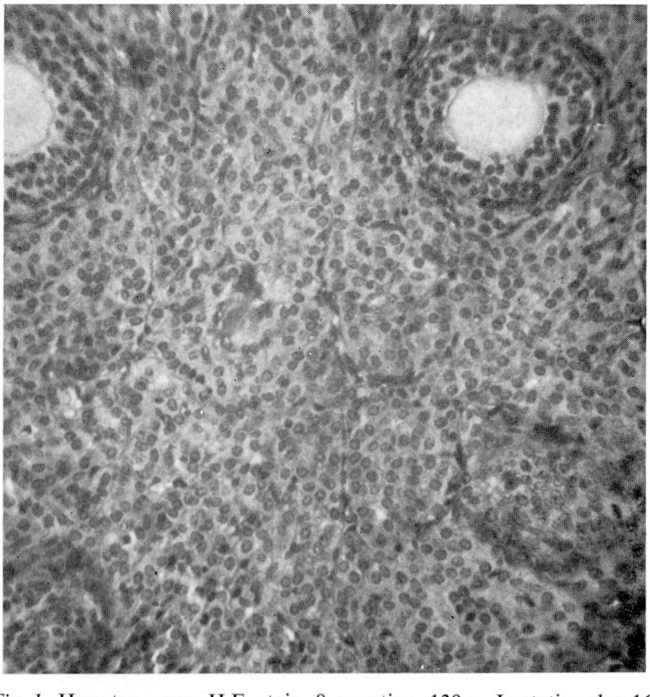

Fig. 1. Hamster ovary. H.E. stain, 8 μ section, 130×. Lactation day 16.

After removal of suckling young, follicular development begins in a fashion similar to that described in the cyclic hamster and ovulation occurs four days later.

Determination of pituitary FSH and LH (Greenwald *et al.*, 1967) would tend to confirm the idea that FSH secretion is diminished during lactation and LH and prolactin are the predominant hormones.

Biologically it is apparent that during lactation the ovary is not secreting large amounts of active hormones but there is no data on this point. Study of the lactational anestrus in the hamster required then the study of the ovarian secretion and consequently of the interstitial cells.

INTERSTITIAL TISSUE DURING THE ESTROUS CYCLE

It has been shown histochemically that the interstitial cells are active during the estrous cycle (Guraya and Greenwald, 1965). There are changes in the amount of demonstrable lipids during the periovulatory period.

Determinations of ovarian free and esterified cholesterol (Hoffman and Fajer, 1970) have shown that there is a significant drop in esterified cholesterol during the evening preceding ovulation. The cholesterol ester concentration drops from 5.8 mg% to 1.8 mg% from day 1 to day 2 of the cycle. At the same time no significant changes are seen in free cholesterol concentrations. Free cholesterol rises from 0.340 mg% on day 2 to 0.480 mg% on day 3 and 0.490 mg% on day 4, to drop again at the time when the corpus luteum regresses (Fig. 2).

In the hamster, there is a preovulatory rise in progesterone blood concentration (Norris, 1955; Lukaszewska and Greenwald, 1970). We have shown that an increased progesterone secretion can be detected at 8:00 p.m. on the night of ovulation. The concentration rises

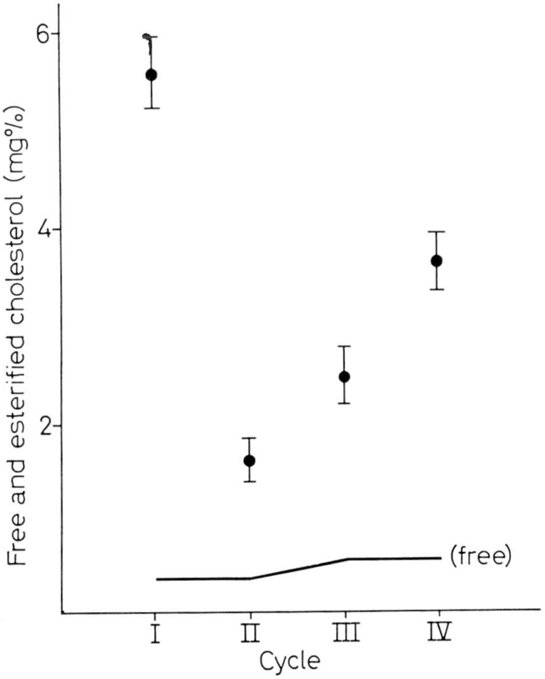

Fig. 2. Free and esterified cholesterol in the hamster ovary during the estrous cycle.

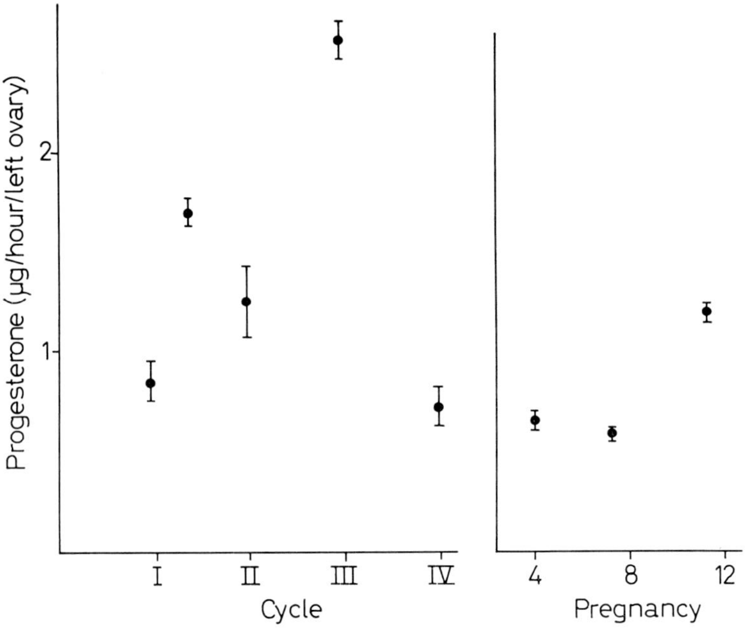

Fig. 3. Ovarian venous concentrations of progesterone during the estrous cycle and pregnancy.

from 0.87 $\pm$0.09 μg/hour/ovary on the morning of day 1 to 1.29 $\pm$0.17 μg/hour/ovary at 8:00 p.m. on the same day. In contrast with the peripheral levels, the concentration of progesterone in the ovarian blood on day 3 of the cycle is higher, 2.5 $\pm$0.08 μg/hour/ovary, than those of the night of day 1 (Fig. 3).

The preovulatory surge of progesterone is of non-luteal origin and the interstitium must be the major source.

It is important to note that in the hamster the ovarian secretion of progesterone shows no increase before the formation of the placenta. This indicates that maintenance of the luteal tissue is the main event in the transformation of the cyclic corpora into corpora of pregnancy.

STEROIDS IN THE OVARIAN VENOUS BLOOD DURING LACTATION

Ovarian venous blood was collected under Nembutal anesthesia. Ether extracts of large samples, equivalent to 120 minutes' blood flow obtained from 5 or 6 animals were analyzed using different thin-layer chromatographic systems and gas-liquid chromatography (SE-30 and QF-1 columns). Five steroids were found in concentrations that allowed chromatographic identification: pregnenolone (Δ^5-pregnen-3βol-20-one), progesterone, 5α-pregnane-3,20-dione, 5β-pregnane-3,20-dione and pregnanolone (3α-hydroxy-5β-pregnan-20-one).

Pregnenolone is quantitatively the most important steroid found (Table I). The concentrations rise from 2.4 $\pm$0.5 μg/hour/ovary to 6.5 $\pm$1.0 μg/hour/ovary during days 2 to 16 of lactation. These values give a daily secretion of 115 to 312 μg. Pregnenolone is biologically an inactive steroid but shows anti-estrogenic activity at the uterine level when tested simultaneously with estrogens. Pregnanolone is quantitatively the second most important compound found. Its concentration varied between 1.70 and 2.65 μg/hour/ovary between days 2 and 16.

TABLE I

Steroids in hamster ovarian venous blood during lactation

Steroids	Day 2 – Day 4 µg/animal/day	Day 7 – Day 8 µg/animal/day	Day 10 – Day 12 µg/animal/day	Day 15 – Day 16 µg/animal/day
Pregnenolone	115.68 ± 24.92*	115.04 ± 21.70	198.96 ± 33.32	312.96 ± 53.14
Progesterone	—	—	—	—
5α-Pregnanedione	23.52 ± 5.07	22.20 ± 3.70	27.48 ± 5.02	28.80 ± 4.37
5β-Pregnanedione	7.20 ± 1.83	2.78 ± 0.71	1.28 ± 0.42	1.71 ± 0.65
Pregnanolone	81.44 ± 17.95	78.72 ± 14.99	94.92 ± 16.22	128.08 ± 21.59

* Standard error of the mean.

Smaller concentrations of 5α pregnanedione and even smaller of 5β pregnanedione were also consistently found.

With the methods used no 20α or 20β hydroxy-progesterone could be detected.

Progesterone values are not given in Table I, but progesterone was always present in concentrations varying between 0.10 and 0.15 µg/hour/ovary. These concentrations are remarkably lower than those found during the estrous cycle. These findings open the possibility of studying the metabolism of the isolated interstitial cells and their response to gonadotropins.

TABLE II

Hamster ovarian blood during pregnancy

	Day 6		Day 9	
Steroids	µg/ovary/hr	µg/animal/day	µg/ovary/hr	µg/animal/day
Pregnenolone	0.03	1.44	0.50	24.00
Progesterone	0.09	4.32	1.75	84.00
5α-Pregnanedione	—	—	0.013	0.624
5β-Pregnanedione	—	—	0.013	0.624
Pregnanolone	—	—	0.05	2.40

These compounds are detectable during pregnancy but the concentrations are very different from those described above (Table II). During day 9 of pregnancy, progesterone concentration is 3.5 times higher than that of pregnenolone. The concentrations of the progesterone metabolites are very low.

INFLUENCE OF LUTEINIZING HORMONE AND PROLACTIN ON THE METABOLISM OF PROGESTERONE AND PREGNENOLONE IN VITRO

The demonstration of pregnenolone, progesterone and progesterone metabolites in the ovarian venous blood raises the following points:

(1) Since pregnenolone concentrations are higher than those of progesterone, there seems

to be a block in one of the two enzymatic steps between the two compounds. How is this block regulated?

(2) The concentrations of the metabolites are higher than those of progesterone. Are they produced by the ovary? In case of an affirmative answer, is 5α-pregnanedione correspondent to 20α hydroxy-progesterone in the rabbit? In this case is the conversion regulated by LH and prolactin?

We have data concerning the second question. It was possible to demonstrate that progesterone-H^3 is converted *in vitro* to pregnanedione-H^3. Using ovaries of lactating animals (days 10–12 of lactation), the conversion of progesterone to pregnanedione was 6.9% after 3 hours of incubation, under 95% O_2 – 5% CO_2 with 1 mg/ml glucose added to the medium (Table III).

TABLE III

Pregnanedione-H^3 formed from progesterone-H^3

	With LTH		With LH		Control	
	% conversion	$\sin^{-1}$ trans-formation	% conversion	$\sin^{-1}$ trans-formation	% conversion	$\sin^{-1}$ trans-formation
	0.49	4.01	13.2	21.30	7.6	16.00
	0.38	3.53	11.4	19.73	7.0	15.34
	0.34	3.34	15.9	23.50	6.4	14.65
	0.33	3.29			7.1	15.45
					6.8	15.12
					6.3	14.54
					7.2	15.56
ΣX		14.17		64.53		106.66
$\bar{X}$	0.38	3.54	13.4	21.51	6.9	15.24
ΣX^2		50.52		1395.21		1626.78
n		4		3		7
σ		0.28		1.55		0.78
$\sigma/\sqrt{n-1}$	0.00	0.16	0.04	1.09	0.00	0.19

Progesterone-H^3 23.0 $\pm$2.0 μg (2.5 nc)/5 ml of medium
LTH (NIH S_7) 6 μg/5 ml of medium
LH (NIH S_{11}) 13 μg/5 ml of medium

It was possible to show a definitive influence of LH and prolactin on this process. LH added to the medium (2.6 μg/ml; NIH-S_{11}) increased the formation of pregnanedione to 13.4% $\pm$0.04 and prolactin (1.2 μg/ml, NIH-S_7) reduced it to 0.38% (Fig. 4).

The activity of prolactin *in vitro* is an unexpected finding. However we were also able to show that prolactin increases conversion of labeled cholesterol to progesterone when added to incubated ovaries of *hypophysectomized* animals luteinized by the administration of exogenous FSH and LH (Fajer and Sharma, 1969). Pregnanedione-H^3 can also be detected when pregnenolone-H^3 is added to the medium. The conversion rate is only 2.8%. The addition of LH to the medium raises this rate to 11% but no effect can be shown with prolactin (Fig. 5).

The lower conversion of pregnenolone was foreseeable but no explanation can be offered for the lack of action by prolactin. Compounds similar to those described in this presentation were described previously in the rat. They resulted from incubations of labeled progesterone with different ovarian tissue preparations (Weist, 1963; Zmigrod and Lindner, 1969) or were

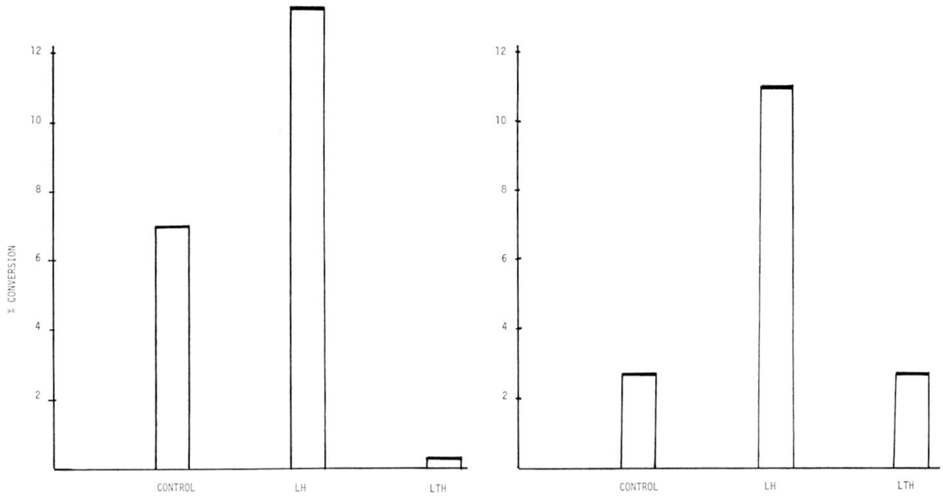

Fig. 4. Pregnanedione-H^3 formed from progesterone-H^3.

Fig. 5. Pregnanedione-H^3 formed from pregnenolone-H^3.

present in extracts of ovarian tissues (Fajer and Holzbauer, 1968; Holzbauer, 1969).

In summary it can be stated that the ovary of the lactating hamster with its hypertrophied interstitium is a very active organ with a peculiar steroid metabolism.

REFERENCES

FAJER, A. B. and HOLZBAUER, M. (1968): Pregnenolone, progesterone, and 20-dihydroprogesterone in rat ovarian blood and ovaries during the estrous cycle. *J. Physiol. (Lond.)*, *196*, 99.

FAJER, A. B. and SHARMA, D. (1969): On the loci of action of prolactin and LH in the corpus luteum (Abstract). In: *Program, 51st Meeting of the Endocrine Society*, *38*, 6.

GREENWALD, G. S. (1965): Histologic transformation of the ovary of the lactating hamster. *Endocrinology*, *77*, 64.

GREENWALD, G. S., KEAVER, J. E. and GRADY, K. L. (1967): Ovarian morphology and pituitary FSH and LH concentration in the pregnant and lactating hamster. *Endocrinology*, *80*, 851.

GURAYA, S. S. and GREENWALD, G. S. (1965): A histochemical study of the hamster ovary. *Amer. J. Anat.*, *116*, 257.

HOFFMAN, D. C. and FAJER, A. B. (1970): Progesterone concentration in ovarian venous blood of the hamster during the estrous cycle and pregnancy. *Fed. Proc.*, *29*, 250.

HOLZBAUER, M. (1969): Pregnenolone and metabolites of progesterone in the ovary. *J. Physiol. (Lond.)* *204*, 8.

KNIGGE, K. M. and LEATHAM, J. H. (1956): Growth and atresia of follicles in the ovary of the hamster. *Anat. Rec.*, *124*, 679.

LUKASZEWSKA, N. H. and GREENWALD, G. S. (1970): Progesterone levels in the cyclic and pregnant hamster. *Endocrinology*, *86*, 1.

NAKANO, A. (1960): Histological studies of the prenatal and postnatal development of the ovary in the golden hamster. *Okajimas Folia anat. jap.*, *35*, 183.

NORRIS, W. W. JR. (1955): Free progestin levels in the blood plasma of hamsters during the estrous cycle. *Biol. Abstr.*, 3, no. 17449.

WIEST, W. (1963): *In vitro* metabolism of progesterone and 20α-hydroxy-pregnen-4-en-3-one by tissues of the female rat. *Endocrinology*, *73*, 310.

ZMIGROD, A. and LINDNER, H. R. (1969): Metabolism of progesterone by the rat ovary: formation of 3β-hydroxy-5α pregnan-20-one by ovarian microsomes. *Acta endocr. (Kbh.)*, *61*, 618.

FSH AND LH IN THE SERUM AND URINE OF NORMAL CHILDREN AND ADULTS AND IN ENDOCRINE DISORDERS

ANN JOHANSON

Department of Pediatrics, University of Virginia, Charlottesville, Va., U.S.A.

In the last few years, we have been engaged in the development of specific radioimmunoassays for luteinizing hormone and follicle-stimulating hormone, and their application to measurement of levels in serum and urine of children. Prior to this time, information on gonadotropin levels in children had been very limited and was confined almost exclusively to measures of total urinary gonadotropins. We have determined serum LH and FSH in 249 normal children, aged 2–18 years, and urine LH and FSH in 91 and 83, respectively, norma

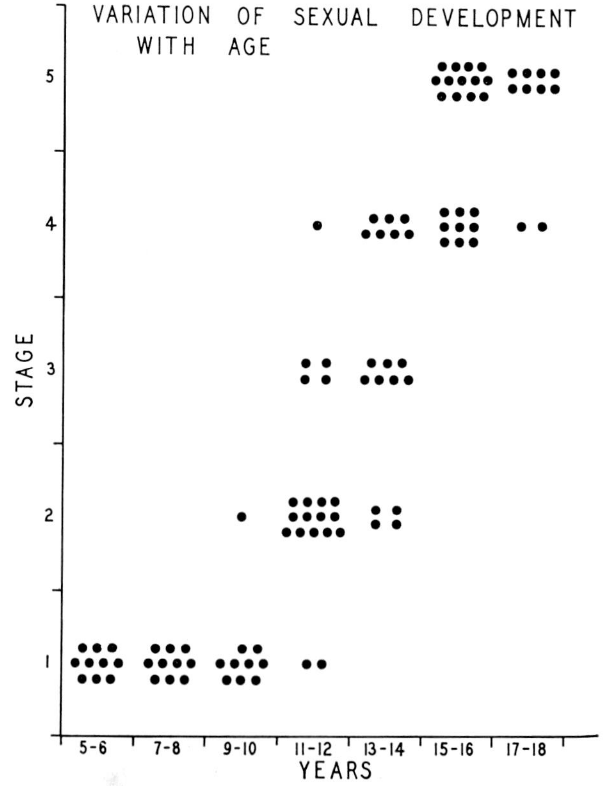

Fig. 1. Stages of sexual development versus chronological age in 100 normal males. (The shaded areas represent one S.D. from the mean. Fig. 1–11, 15, 17–19.)

boys 5–18 years old. In addition, over 100 patients with disorders of sexual development have had determinations of serum LH and FSH.

Double antibody radioimmunoassay techniques of Midgley (1967; 1969) have been used. Purified pituitary preparations of LH (822.2) and FSH (780,869), supplied by Dr. Leo Reichert and the National Pituitary Agency, were iodinated with I^{131} or I^{125}. Specific antisera against human FSH and chorionic gonadotropin prepared in rabbits by Dr. Rees Midgley and subsequently supplied by the National Pituitary Agency were used. A urine extract, the 2nd International Reference Preparation of Human Menopausal Gonadotropin, was used as the standard. A crude pituitary preparation was used as standard for some of the serum determinations, but since a constant factor for conversion to international units of the 2nd IRP was observed at all levels, within our range of determinations, all values are reported in milli-international units of 2nd IRP. Sheep antiserum against rabbit gamma globulin was used for the second antibody.

Early morning serum samples and 24-hour urine collections were obtained from 100 normal boys, 5–18 years of age, who were between the 20th and 80th percentile for height and weight. Their sexual development was assessed according to Tanner's classification (Tanner, 1962). Only one of ten 9–10-year-olds had early pubertal development, which for the most part occurred in the 11–12-year age group. Almost all 17–18-year-olds had adult male sexual development (Fig. 1).

Serum LH rises significantly from prepubertal levels (mean 3.4 mIU/ml) in the 9–10-year-old group (mean 4.8 mIU/ml) (Johanson *et al.*, 1969). This rise precedes clinical evidence of virilization. Levels not significantly different from adult levels are reached in the 13–14-year-old group, before any boys have attained adult sexual development clinically. The mean

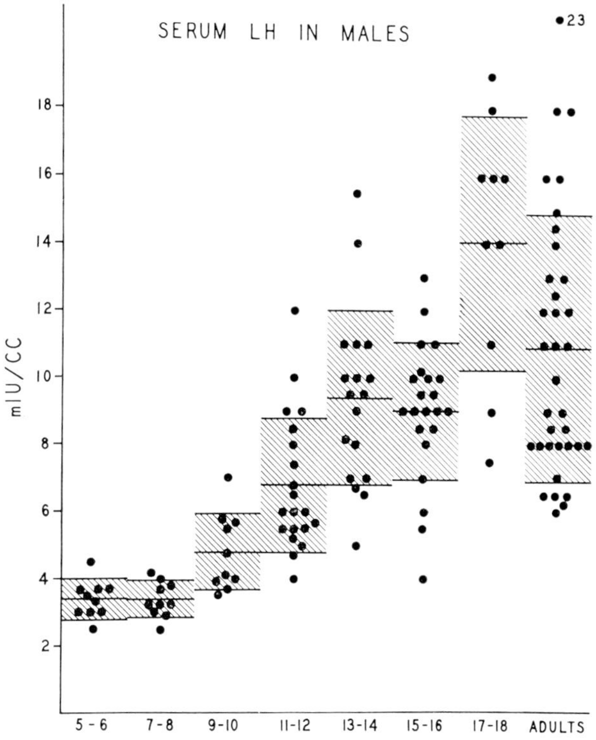

Fig. 2. Serum LH versus chronological age in normal males.

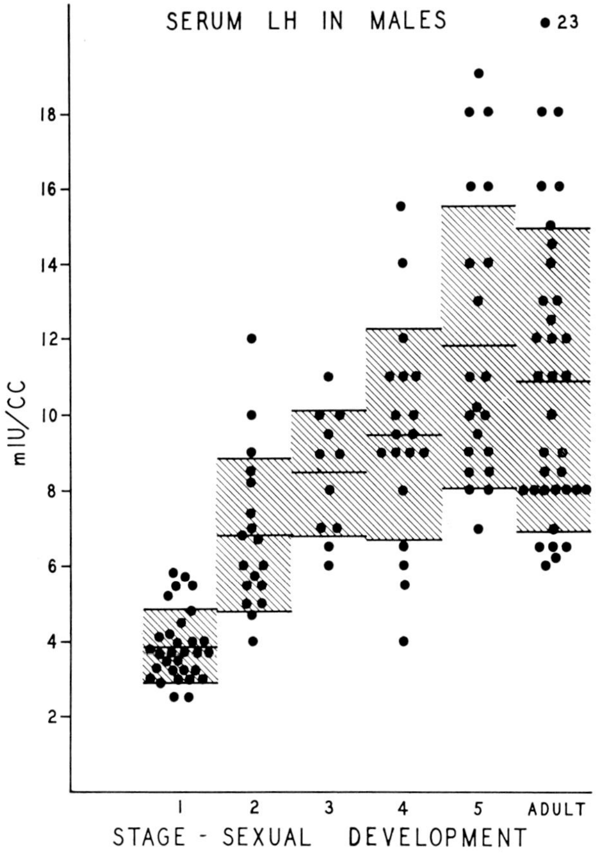

Fig. 3. Serum LH in normal males versus stage of sexual development.

level in the 17–18-year-old group is higher than that in adults, though not significantly so. There is a three–fold rise in mean LH from pre-adolescence to maturity (Fig. 2).

The expected rise in serum LH is observed with advancing stage of sexual development. Because of considerable range in most groups, values differ significantly only between stages 1 and 2, and stages 1, 3 and 5 (adult levels being essentially the same as those of stage 5) (Fig. 3).

Serum FSH levels in the same normal boys increase (Raiti *et al.*, 1969*a*), as do LH–levels, at the age of 9–10 years, before the boys mature to stage 2 sexual development. After 13 years of age no significant increment in mean levels is observed. Considerable overlap of values exists for all groups, even when prepubertal and adult values are compared, which is not true for serum LH. Mean serum FSH levels rise less than two times from prepuberty to adulthood (Fig. 4).

Serum FSH levels rise with progressive sexual development to the adult mean by stage 3 (Fig. 5).

Immunoassayable LH (in international units of 2nd IRP) extracted from 24-hour urines (Baghdassarian *et al.*, 1970) is seen to rise significantly only after 11 years of age, when clinical sexual maturation is also first occurring. This is in contrast to the earlier rise of serum LH that was observed in 9-10-year-olds. Mean values are significantly higher in each age group until adult levels are reached by 17- and 18-year-olds. There is very distinct separation of all prepubertal and most early pubertal levels from adult levels, which are not so clearly separate

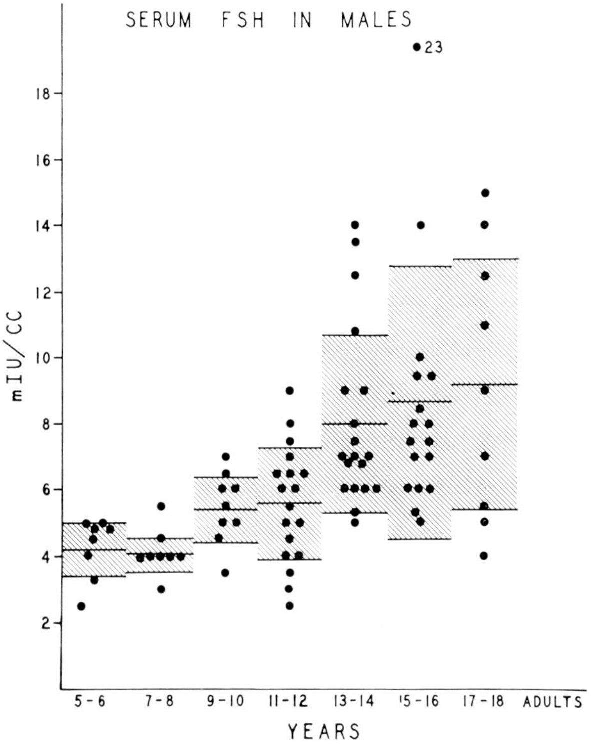

Fig. 4. Serum FSH versus chronological age in normal males.

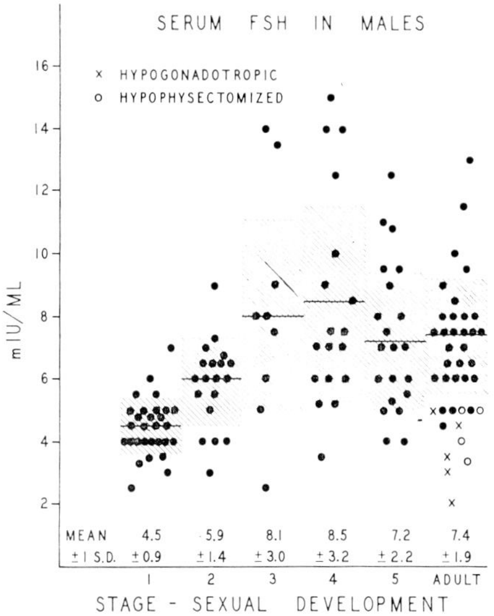

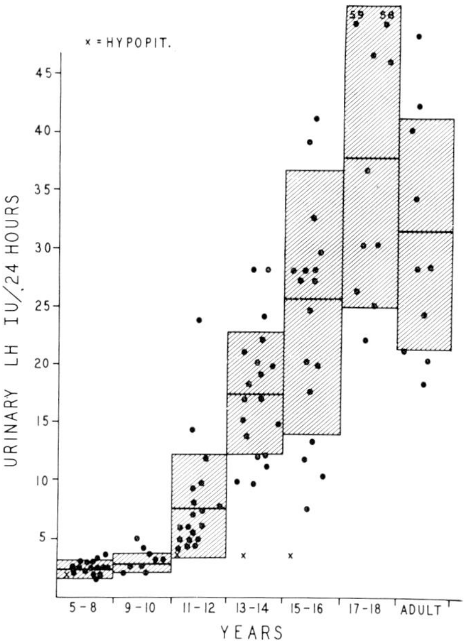

Fig. 5. Serum FSH in normal males versus stage of sexual development.

Fig. 6. Urinary LH excretion versus chronological age in normal males.

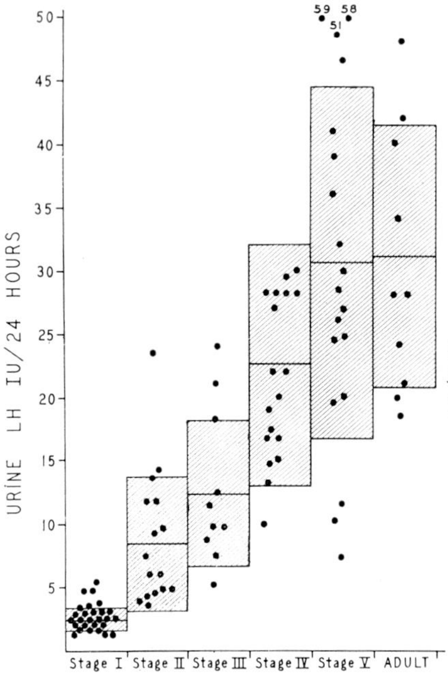

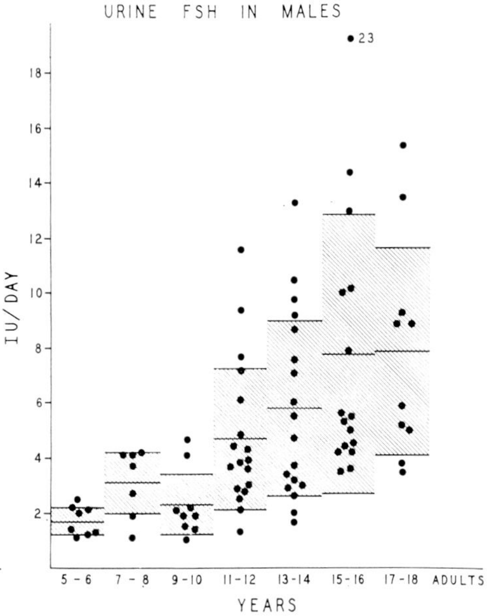

Fig. 7. Urinary LH excretion in normal males versus stage of sexual development.

Fig. 8. Urinary FSH excretion versus chronological age in normal males.

by serum LH determination and not at all distinct when serum FSH is measured. Mean urinary LH excretion in adults is 13 times that in prepubertal boys (Fig. 6).

The rise in urinary LH excretion with progressive stage of sexual development occurs in a step-wise manner (Fig. 7).

Urinary excretion of FSH, like urinary LH, first increases significantly after 11 years, concomitant with clinical sexual maturation (Raiti *et al.*, 1969*b*). Overlap of prepubertal and adult levels does occur. Mean levels increase four times from childhood to maturity. When urinary FSH excretion is plotted against stage of sexual development there is overlap of values at all stages (Fig. 8).

The data thus far presented have been summarized in Figure 9, which plots serum and urinary FSH and LH and 17KS excretion for stage of pubertal development. All parameters rise progressively to stage 4. Serum LH rises more than serum FSH. Urinary LH is seen to have the most striking and clearly separable levels between early and late stages of development (Fig. 9).

Serum LH level determinations were made in 149 endocrinologically normal girls aged 2–20 years. Prepubertal mean and range were comparable to those in boys. Throughout the prepubertal period of 2–9 years, levels are constant. As in the boys, a significant increase in levels is found after 9 years of age. This is coincident with incipient sexual development. Adult mean follicular phase level is significantly greater than mean luteal phase level and similar to adult male mean level. Adult luteal phase levels overlap prepubertal levels. The very high levels are midcycle peaks and were not used in computing means. Exemplary hypogonadotropic levels are seen to overlap prepubertal levels, but not adult levels (Fig. 10). Progressive rise of means is observed as sexual development proceeds (Fig. 11). Stage 1 is prepubertal; in stage 2 appearance of breast tissue has occurred; in stage 3 sexual hair has

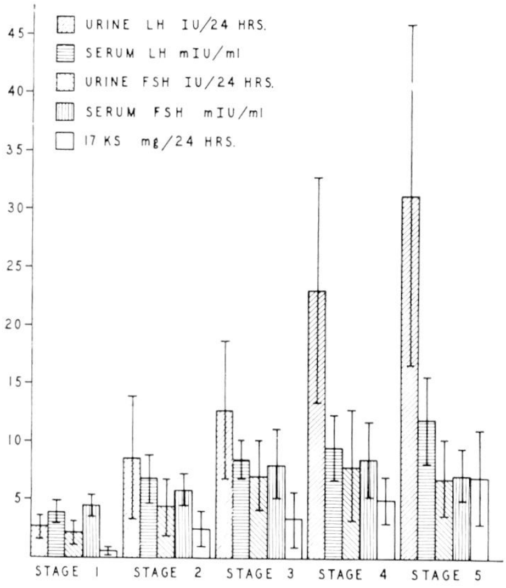

Fig. 9. Summary of interrelationship of urinary FSH, LH, and 17-KS excretion and serum FSH and LH concentrations in normal males versus stage of sexual development.

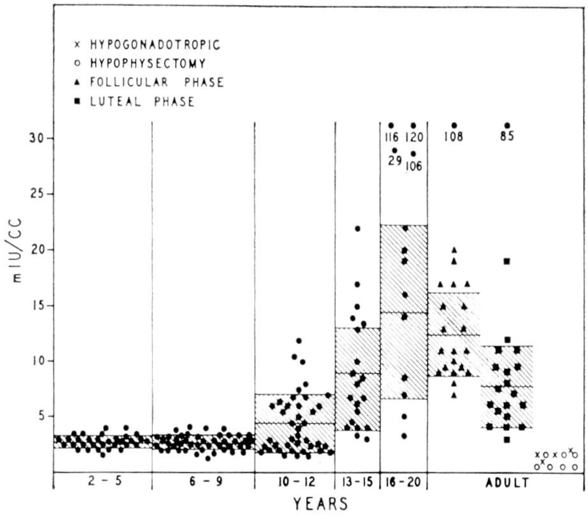

Fig. 10. Serum LH in normal females versus chronological age.

appeared; and stage 4 denotes menarche. Serum FSH levels in girls have been determined (Penny *et al.*, 1971) and at all ages, except 11–12 years, are the same as levels in boys. At this age, they are higher in girls, perhaps reflecting earlier puberty. The mean level in girls 2–4 years old is slightly but significantly *less* than that in 5–8-year-old girls. It therefore appears that there may be a progressive rise in FSH in girls throughout the preadolescent period and well preceding the more striking increment observed around the time of puberty. We do not have FSH data on boys younger than 5 years, and so are unable to speculate on a similar occurrence in males.

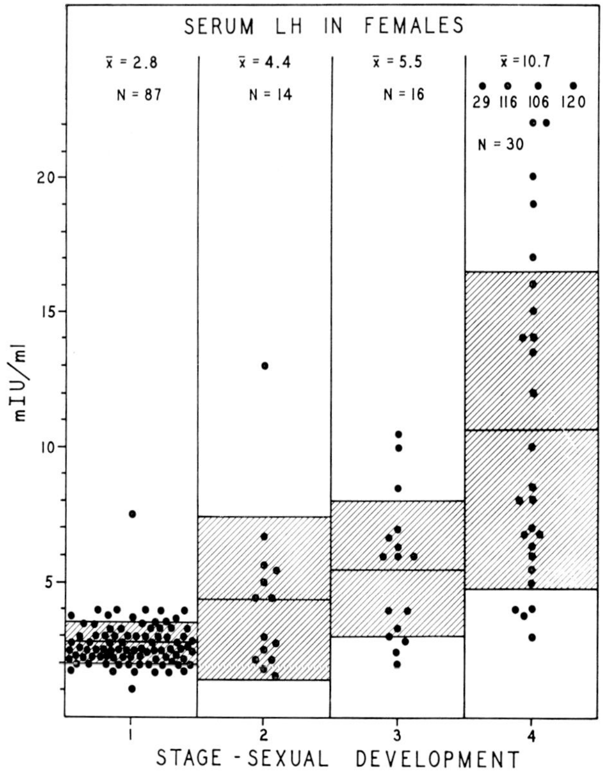

Fig. 11. Serum LH in normal female children versus stage of sexual development.

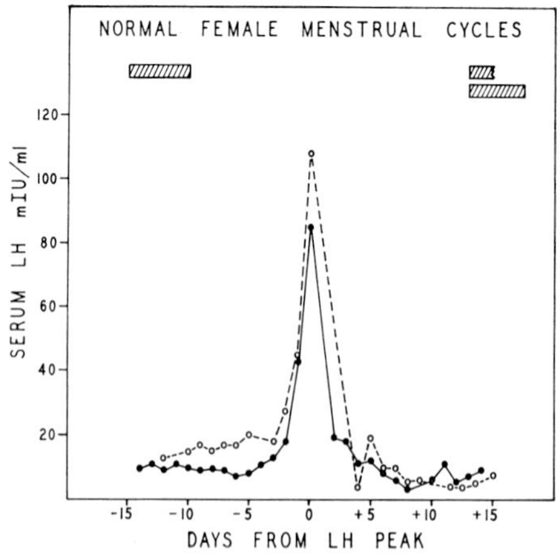

Fig. 12. Serum LH concentrations during normal menstrual cycle in 2 normal females.

Serum LH levels during normal menstrual cycles in 2 adult females show several characteristics typical of normal cycles: higher follicular than luteal phase levels, sharp midcycle peaks occurring over 2-day periods and irregular luteal phase levels. FSH levels from the same and other cycles have shown lower but simultaneous midcycle peaks, small follicular

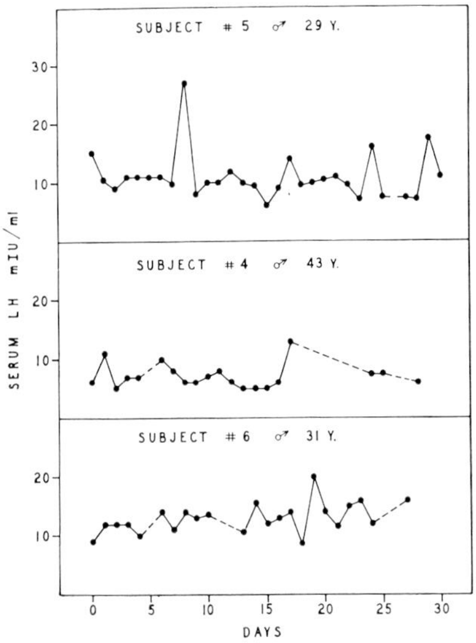

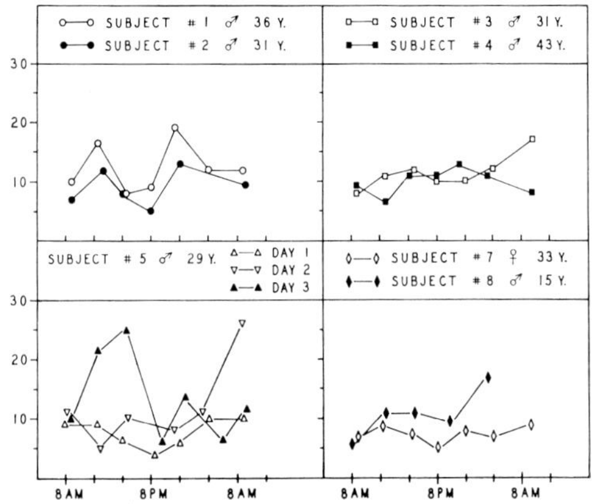

Fig. 13. Daily variability of serum LH concentration.

Fig. 14. Diurnal variability of serum LH concentration.

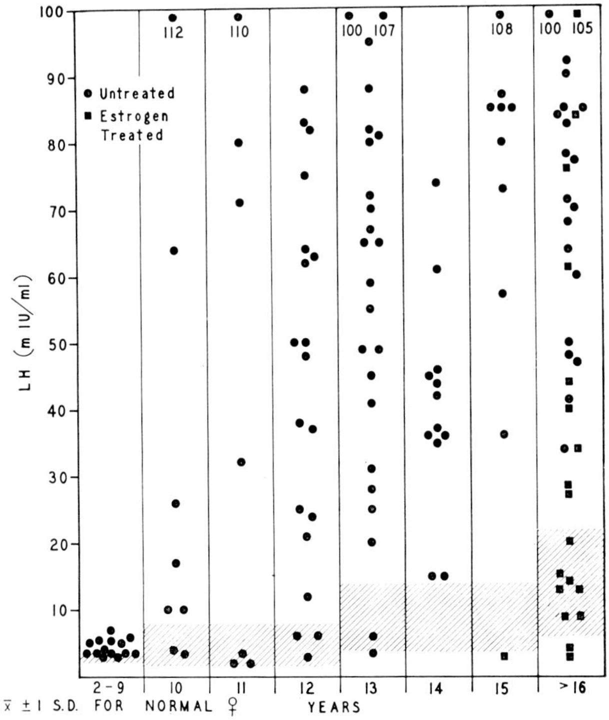

Fig. 15. Serum LH in patients with gonadal agenesis.

phase peaks and higher follicular than luteal phase levels. These features are even more apparent from urinary excretion levels. Urinary LH peaks are broader, persisting for 4 or 5 days and there usually is a 'shoulder' on the descent limb of the LH midcycle peak before falling to low luteal levels. A late luteal phase rise is observed in urinary FSH (Fig. 12).

Recent data from our laboratory on urinary FSH and LH in perimenarchal girls indicate that even in 1–12-month post-menarchal girls, regular midcycle, presumably ovulatory, peaks occur (in 9 of 9 cycles observed). Other characteristics of normal adult cycles also were observed, *i.e.* broad LH peaks extending over 4–5 days, higher follicular than luteal phase levels of both LH and FSH, and follicular phase peaks of FSH. One premenarchal girl (12½) who presumptively is within 1 year of menarche, over a 3-month period was observed to have on at least 2 days simultaneous peaks of LH and FSH. These levels were comparable to normal adult midcycle peak levels (Hayes and Johanson, in press).

Daily variation of serum LH in 3 adult males is shown to be considerable. Serum FSH varies minimally day-to-day and urinary LH very little (Fig. 13).

Diurnal variation of serum LH in six males (one on each of 3 different days) and one female is also considerable and inconstant in its pattern from one individual to another and in one individual from day to day. The wide fluctuations in serum LH as opposed to urine LH and serum FSH may be due to the much shorter half-life in blood of serum LH than FSH (Yen *et al.*, 1970) (Fig. 14).

Over 130 sera from 51 female patients with gonadal dysgenesis (Turner's syndrome) have been evaluated. Mean prepubertal LH levels in these girls is slightly higher than normal, but there is enough overlap so that there is little diagnostic significance in this test at that time. LH levels rise tremendously in many girls as early as 10 years. However even in 13- and

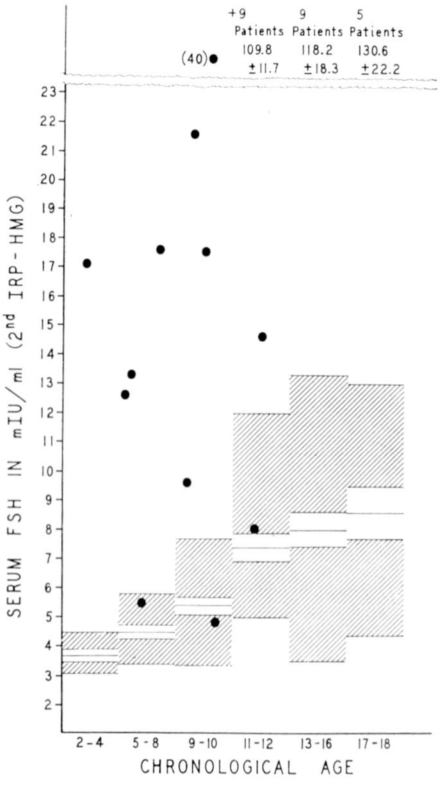

Fig. 16. Serum FSH in patients with gonadal agenesis. Cross-hatched is range of normal, ± SEM is white.

14-year-olds a number of untreated patients had levels within the normal range. Many of the patients receiving 1.25 mg of Premarin did not have suppressed levels of LH (Penny *et al.*; Guyda *et al.*, 1969) (Fig. 15).

In contrast, when 35 untreated girls were evaluated, 8 of 10, who were 5 to 11 years of age, had elevated serum FSH. After 11 years, only 1 of 25 had a normal FSH. Serum FSH levels therefore seem to be diagnostically much more significant than LH in agonadal states (Fig. 16).

Serum LH in sexually precocious girls is normal for *stage* of sexual development, but means for age groups are significantly higher in sexual precocity than normal. However, over 50% of untreated precocious girls had LH levels within the range of normal for age. Recent data indicate that 90% of precocious girls have serum FSH levels greater than normal for their age. Again FSH may be a more sensitive indicator of altered pituitary gonadal function. Medroxyprogesterone inconstantly suppressed LH to normal (Fig. 17).

Serum LH levels shown here and serum FSH levels in premature thelarche and premature

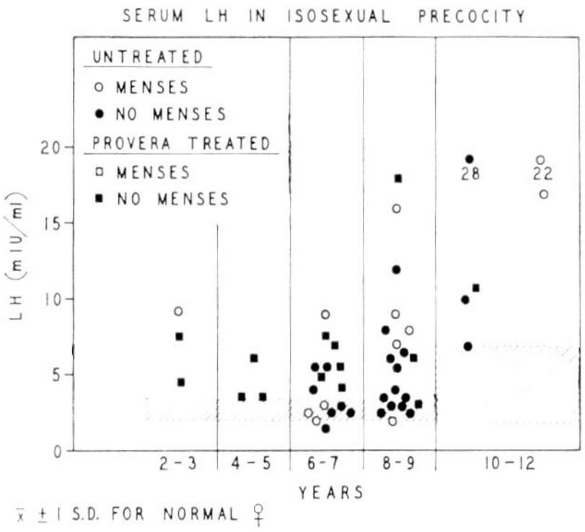

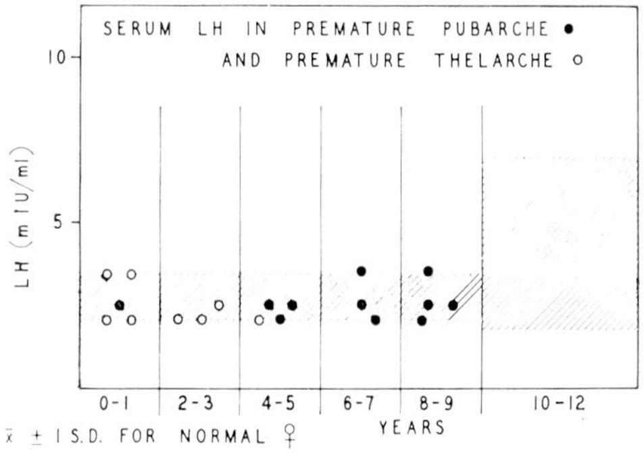

Fig. 17. Serum LH in patients with isosexual precocity versus chronological age.

Fig. 18. Serum LH in premature pubarche and premature thelarche versus chronological age.

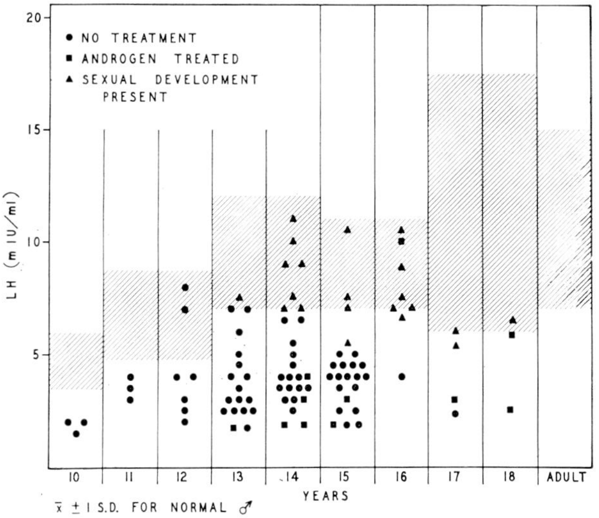

Fig. 19. Serum LH in patients with constitutional delay of growth and adolescence.

pubarche are within normal range for age. Levels of both hormones in boys with adolescent gynecomastia are also normal for age and sexual development (Fig. 18).

Most serum LH levels of boys constitutionally delayed in height and bone age by at least $1\frac{1}{2}$ years are below the normal range for age. Forty per cent of the boys had levels that were even less than expected for stage of development. All FSH levels were within expected range for sexual development (Fig. 19).

In conclusion, data has been presented on normal levels for LH and FSH in serum and urine. All subjects tested had measurable gonadotropin. Serum and urine LH increase significantly more than FSH from childhood to adulthood. Urinary LH is the parameter that most clearly distinguishes prepubertal and early pubertal individuals from mature adolescents and adults. A rise in serum FSH, but not LH, is observed between early and late prepubertal age groups of females. In sexual precocity and gonadal agenesis serum FSH is almost always elevated for age, while LH may be within the normal range. This apparent dichotomy between FSH and LH suggests independent feedback mechanisms and maturation processes and/or different thresholds for inhibiting agents. Premature thelarche and pubarche, and adolescent gynecomastia are associated with normal levels of gonadotropins and therefore probably are not associated with pituitary-gonadal disturbances.

REFERENCES

BAGHDASSARIAN, A., GUYDA, H., JOHANSON, A., MIGEON, C. J. and BLIZZARD, R. M. (1970): The urinary excretion of radioimmunoassayable luteinizing hormone (LH) in normal children and adults, according to age and stage of sexual development. *J. clin. Endocr., 31,* 428.

GUYDA, H. J., JOHANSON, A. J., MIGEON, C. J. and BLIZZARD, R. M. (1969): Serum luteinizing hormone by radioimmunoassay in disorders of adolescent development. *Pediat. Res., 3,* 538.

HAYES, A. and JOHANSON, A. (1971). *Pediat. Res.* In press.

JOHANSON, A. J., GUYDA, H., LIGHT, C., MIGEON, C. J. and BLIZZARD, R. M. (1969): Serum luteinizing hormone by radioimmunoassay in normal children. *J. Pediat., 74,* 416.

MIDGLEY, A. R., JR. (1967): Radioimmunoassay for human follicle stimulating hormone. *J. clin. Endocr., 27,* 295.

MIDGLEY, A. R., JR. (1969): A method for human chorionic gonadotropin and human luteinizing hormone. *Endocrinology, 79,* 10.

PENNY, R., GUYDA, H., BAGHDASSARIAN, A., JOHANSON, A. and BLIZZARD, R. (1970): Correlation of serum follicular stimulating hormone (FSH) and luteinizing hormone (LH) as measured by radioimmunossay in disorders of sexual development. *J. clin. Invest., 49,* 1847.

RAITI, S., JOHANSON, A., LIGHT, C., MIGEON, C. J. and BLIZZARD, R. M. (1969*a*): Measurement of immunologically reactive follicle stimulating hormone in serum of normal male children and adults. *Metabolism, 18,* 234.

RAITI, S., LIGHT, C. and BLIZZARD, R. M. (1969*b*): Urinary follicle stimulating hormone excretion in boys and adult males as measured by radioimmunoassay. *J. clin. Endocr., 29,* 884.

TANNER, J. M. (1962): *Growth at Adolescence.* Blackwell Scientific Publications, Oxford.

YEN, S. S. C., LLERENA, L. A., PEARSON, O. H., and Little A. S. (1970): Disappearance rates of endogenous follicle-stimulating hormone in serum following surgical hypophysectomy in man. *J. clin. Endocr., 30,* 325.

ACTION OF HMG, HCG AND PURIFIED FSH AND LH ON THE TESTIS OF HYPOPHYSECTOMIZED PATIENTS

ROBERTO E. MANCINI and OSCAR VILAR

Centro de Investigaciones sobre Reproducción, Facultad de Medicina,
Universidad de Buenos Aires, Argentina

INTRODUCTION

Our understanding of the mechanism of spermatogenesis, a rhythmical and synchronous process of cell proliferation and differentiation, has only begun to deepen in the course of the last few years. On the other hand, remarkable progress has been recorded in the study of the interstitial or Leydig cells, in which studies of steroidogenesis have offered proof of testosterone production.

Because the attention of research workers has been attracted mainly by the morphological changes, the microscopic and electron-microscopic basis of the development of human spermatogenesis (Mancini *et al.*, 1960; 1963; Vilar *et al.*, 1962) and its dynamics in adult testes have been better understood (Heller and Clermont, 1964). However, little is known of the metabolism of nucleoproteins, proteins, lipids and carbohydrates (Means and Hall, 1968; Leidermann and Mancini, 1969; Yokoe and Hall, 1970; Fabbrini *et al.* 1968) or of gonadotrophic factors, other pituitary trophins or locally-acting steroid hormones (Heller *et al.*, 1950; Dvoskin, 1947; Mancini *et al.*, 1966), which are assumed to participate in the well-balanced unwinding of the successive spermatogenenic phases, *i.e.*, spermatogonial, spermatocytic, spermiogenic.

As regards the effect of gonadotrophins and following the attention paid recently to the study of human pituitary (HPG) and urinary menopausal (HMG) gonadotrophins and their striking effects on ovulation, the problem of the mechanisms of the gonadotrophic regulation of human spermatogenesis has been re-examined. The classic preparations of chorionic gonadotrophin (HCG) or serum gonadotrophin (PMS) or both were often used in the past in cases of hypogonadism or in normo-endocrine sterile patients (Heller and Nelson, 1948; Maddock, 1949; Bartler *et al.*, 1952) in an attempt to stimulate or restore human spermatogenesis.

After it had been observed that HMG may induce complete spermatogenesis and the development of Leydig cells in hypophysectomized rats (Borth *et al.*, 1954), its administration to humans led to promising results, particularly in cases of hypogonadotrophic hypogonadism. Thus treatment with pituitary gonadotrophin (HPG) or menopausal gonadotrophin (HMG) combined with chorionic gonadotrophin, proved to be useful in the stimulation of spermatogenesis in patients partially (Gemzell and Kjessler, 1964) or totally (McLeod *et al.*, 1966) hypophysectomized and in cases of prepuberal hypogonadotrophic hypogonadism (Johnsen, 1966; Paulsen, 1968; Crooke *et al.*, 1968). Nevertheless, the necessity for a better assessment of the effect of single or combined doses and different periods of treatment with the gonadotrophin preparations HMG and HCG, either for induction, or on the whole spermatogenic process, and on each one of its three main phases (spermatogonial, spermatocytic, spermiogenic), has led us to study their effects on hypophysectomized adult patients (Mancini *et al.*, 1969), in cases of prepuberal hypogonadotrophic hypogonadism (Rosemberg, 1968) and in children aged six or eight (Bergada and Mancini, 1970).

Although it is now generally agreed that both FSH and LH contained in these gonadotrophin preparations are needed simultaneously for the development of a seminiferous epithelium, several points still remain to be clarified: (1) The separate actions of purified preparations of FSH and LH. (2) Effect of successive administration of FSH and LH and *vice versa*. (3) Effect of simultaneous treatment with FSH and LH at different ratios. (4) Cell stage reached by germinal and Sertoli cell population induced by these three hormonal schedules. (5) To what extent Leydig cell differentiation and function is necessary for development of germinal, Sertoli cell and tubular wall structures. (6) If development and regression of peritubular hyalinization are under FSH or LH control or both.

The availability of highly purified preparations of human urinary FSH and LH (Donini, 1969) recently prompted us to carry an investigation in eunuchs and in hypophysectomized patients (Mancini, 1970). Urinary gonadotrophins and steroids being completely absent or very low, these conditions were taken as basic models for the elucidations of the mechanism of regulation of human spermatogenesis.

In the following text a short review of our previous studies on the single or combined effect of HCG, HMG and purified FSH and LH on hypophysectomized patients will be made.

I – EFFECT OF HMG AND HCG ON THE RECOVERY OF SPERMATOGENESIS OF HYPOPHYSECTOMIZED PATIENTS

Six adult patients aged between 32 and 53 years operated on for hypophyseal chromophobe adenoma, followed by X-irradiation and with no previous gonadotrophic treatment, were selected for this study.

Unilateral testicular biopsies were obtained in each case at different periods of time from 6 months to 10 years after operation, before starting treatment, and repeated in the same gland at the end of the period of administration of hormones.

The diameter and thickness of the wall of the seminiferous tubules were measured, while a cell-counting technique (Mancini *et al.*, 1960; Mancini *et al.*, 1963) was used to detect the numerical variations in the cells of the germinal epithelium and the interstitial Leydig cells. Moreover histochemical methods, already described in papers mentioned above and electron-microscopic examination were carried out on the same material.

As examination of the biopsies showed that the regression of seminiferous epithelium, tubule wall and interstitial cells was of different degrees, the patients were categorized as follows: (*a*) Group I, showing seminiferous tubules containing Sertoli, spermatogonial cells and primary spermatocytes mostly up to the pachytene stage, moderate hyalinosis of tubule wall and low number of Leydig cells. (*b*) Group II having seminiferous tubules containing only spermatogonial and Sertoli cells, severe hyalinization of the tubule wall and few or more Leydig cells. It is noted that this histological picture was the predominant one in all sections of the biopsies.

Both groups mentioned above, comprising 3 patients, were treated after a control biopsy with only one of the following hormones: (1) human chorionic gonadotrophin (HCG), 2000 IU divided in 2 doses/week; (2) human menopausal gonadotrophin (HMG), (Pergonal-500, FSH 75 I.U., and LH, 75 I.U., 2nd IRP), 3 ampoules every other day/week; (3) HMG, 3 ampoules plus HCG 2000 I.U./week.

Concerning hypophysectomy, although complete removal was attempted in all cases, none proved to be complete. In the following paragraphs we will discuss the action of different gonadotrophins on the testes of adult hypophysectomized patients and will demonstrate the influence of two gonadotrophic preparations containing different FSH-LH ratios on the recovery of the three main phases of the spermatogenic process.

With regard to the regression of the gonad after hypophysectomy, some relationship between the time elapsed after operation and the progressive deterioration of the gland was noticed. This assumption, which seems to be supported by the fact that only arrest at the spermiogenic phase is present in another group of similar patients a few months after hypophysectomy (Mancini *et al.*, 1968), should, however, be evaluated by taking into consideration the condition of the gonad before operation, the amount of pituitary gland removed and the persistence of other pituitary functions (Luft *et al.*, 1958). However it was claimed that 14 weeks are necessary to obtain complete atrophy of the gonad based on a study of an adult hypophysectomized diabetic patient (McLeod *et al.*, 1966). Therefore, we would emphasize that the cases reported here represent postpuberal hypogonadotrophic conditions developed after hypophysectomy and that the results obtained by the treatment can be only ascribed to the amount and quality of the gonadotrophins used.

The different degrees in the apparent synchronous regression of the three structures of testis, germinal epithelium, tubule wall and Leydig cells constituted our main criteria to substantiate the proposed classification of the patients in Groups I and II. It is interesting to point out that disappearance of Leydig cell population was paralleled by a similar change in the spermiogenic and meiotic phases. This seems to confirm the assumption that, in the human, Sertoli and spermatogonial cells may persist in the absence of detectable gonadotrophins and of mature Leydig cells (Albert, 1961). The reduction in the germinal cell population was also accompanied by clear signs of cellular damage in the spermatogonial and Sertoli cells, seen more frequently in Group II than in Group I. In spite of reduction in tubular diameter, the decreased number of Sertoli cells paralleled by signs of involution suggests that disappearance of these cells may accompany the regression of germinal epithelium after hypophysectomy. The parallel regression of germinal and Leydig cells during the involution of the gonad makes it difficult to conclude from our cases whether or not gonadotrophic insufficiency in man may primarily induce the regression of Leydig cells or that of seminiferous epithelium.

Regarding the effect of the hormones administered, the classification of our patients into two groups according to the various cytological levels at which the regression of the germinal epithelium had stopped, enables us to evaluate on a uniform histological basis the action of gonadotrophins on the restoration of different phases of spermatogenesis. Based on rat experiments (Woods and Simpson, 1961), the term restoration, recovery or repair seems to be adequate in our cases, and differs from that of initiation of spermatogenesis, applicable to the action of gonadotrophins on prepuberal testis or on prepuberal hypogonadal patients.

By comparing the effects of gonadotrophins used, HCG, rich in LH activity, revealed a stimulating effect on the spermatogonial phase, and appears capable of promoting the development of spermatocytes not beyond the pachytene stage, together with the stimulation of Leydig cells, enlargement of seminiferous tubules and disappearance of hyalinization. This result, verified especially in Group II, would explain why in Group I there was only an increased number of pre-existent primary spermatocytes, but no further development to the next cellular phase. The effect of HMG containing both FSH and LH activity in an equal ratio was similar to that of HCG, as far as tubule diameter and decrease of hyalinization is concerned, but was higher on germinal cells and lower in its ability to develop mature Leydig cells. The above appears reflected in the stimulation of spermatogonial, spermatocyte and spermiogenic phase in Group I and in the development of spermatocytes and few spermatids in Group II. The addition of HCG to HMG not only reinforces considerably the effect of the latter hormone on Leydig cells, tubular hyalinosis and first phases of spermatogenesis, but is also apparent in the greater development of spermatids and spermatozoa in Group I and of spermatids in Group II. That, in this condition, Sertoli cells may recover their normal cytological aspect but not their normal number raises the question of the probable existence of a numerical relationship between both cell populations in the spermatogenesis of normal adult subjects, as was suggested in rat testis (Roosen-Runge, 1962).

The favorable action of HCG on the first phases of spermatogenesis might be explicable by its homologous origin and probably because the simultaneous stimulation of Sertoli and of Leydig cells, the latter being able to secrete steroid hormones, supposedly needed for seminiferous tubule maintenance. This appears to be supported by the use of HMG added with HCG, which results in the completion of the germinal cell line together with full development of Leydig cells and repair of Sertoli cells. The fact that this stimulating effect on all germinal cell phases does not reach the level of the whole germinal cell population seen in normal adult subjects (Mancini *et al.*, 1960; 1963) indicates that, with the doses of hormones used, with a ratio favorable to LH over FSH, only a qualitative progression of spermatogenesis was predominantly achieved. Whether or not results obtained in these cases would be a matter of duration of treatment with HMG or HCG rather than the FSH-LH will be considered in the next section. Similar results in the restoration of spermatogenesis which also favor the combined use of HMG and HCG, instead of HMG or HCG alone, were obtained by us in the group of hypophysectomized patients mentioned above, showing arrest at the spermiogenic phase (Mancini *et al.*, 1968). However, our findings on the progression of germinal cells from one phase to another under the action of gonadotrophins did not allow evaluation of the dynamics involved in this process. Our current studies applying the proposed histogram (Heller and Clermont, 1964) may help to determine if the frequency of the stages, ratio between germinal cells, and duration of the whole process are different from those of normal subjects.

In the hypophysectomized case, HMG alone could develop a few spermatozoa without Leydig cell stimulation in a testicle with only spermatogonial cells; however, addition of HCG to HMG produced Leydig cell development and a normal testicular biopsy (McLeod *et al.*, 1966). In a partially hypophysectomized patient showing the presence of the germinal cell phases up to the spermatids, treatment with a hypophyseal gonadotrophin rich in FSH restored the spermatogenesis in three weeks. This result was attributed to the effect of this hormone on the spermatid stage, but no information on LH content and on possible changes in the earlier germinal phases was reported (Gemzell and Kjessler, 1964). These discrepancies may be explained by the fact that the potency of both FSH and LH in the gonadotrophin preparations currently used was variable, or by the total doses administered, assuming that testicular response is dose dependent. Contrary to earlier reports (Bartler *et al.*, 1962), the necessity of both FSH and LH for the completion of spermatogenesis, and the assumption that LH present in the doses of HMG usually employed is insufficient, appears also to be supported by the inability of HMG alone, in contrast to HMG plus HCG, to stimulate the spermatogenic process in the immature testis in cases of prepuberal hypogonadism (Johnsen, 1966; Paulsen, 1968; Crooke *et al.*, 1968). In addition, it was recently reported that HMG alone may induce in prepuberal children after prolonged administration, only an enlargement of seminiferous tubules, slight Leydig and Sertoli cell maturation, and initiation of spermatogenesis up to leptotene or pachytene spermatocytes. Addition of HCG may give rise to a spermatid phase (Rosemberg *et al.*, 1968; Bergadá and Mancini, 1970). The lack of changes in secondary sexual signs and in the excretion of androgen metabolites in these cases, and in eunuchoidal patients as well, treated with HMG alone, suggests that Leydig cell stimulation was not sufficient to bring about full secretory activity. Whether or not some degree of Leydig cell function is necessary for full tubular development in the human being has not yet been definitely proved. However, contrary to some reported data (Johnsen, 1962), it has been demonstrated that in the human testis, during puberal maturation, spermatogenesis may start in the absence of Leydig cells and in the presence of their precursors such as fibroblast-like cells, but the full meiotic and subsequent spermiogenic process are accompanied by development of mature Sertoli and secretory Leydig cells (Mancini *et al.*, 1960; 1963).

That the Sertoli cell may be subjected to gonadotrophin control in parallel with Leydig cells is supported by our findings on the simultaneous stimulation exhibited by these cells when HCG or HMG affects the germinal cells. Whether Leydig cell activity is needed not only for germinal cell development but also for Sertoli cell function has not yet been clearly demonstrated.

II – EFFECT OF URINARY PURIFIED FSH AND LH

Four adult hypophysectomized patients similar to those described in the preceding section were used. Separate, successive and simultaneous effects of urinary purified FSH and LH were tried. To this purpose the first patient received a weekly amount of around 800 I.U. of FSH divided in 3 doses given during 16 weeks. After withdrawal of the hormone, the same dose of LH was administered during same period. To the second patient a similar dose of LH was first administered followed after withdrawal by a similar one of FSH during the same period. A combined dose of 400 I.U. of both FSH and LH was given to the third patient. Finally 800 I.U. of LH and 200 I.U. of FSH were administered to the fourth patient. Biopsies were taken before and at the end of each hormonal treatment and studied as already described. Histological examination showed severe peritubular hyalinization, only Sertoli and spermatogonial cells inside the tubules and no detectable Leydig cells. Thus, these cases belong to Group II, patients with the most advanced testicular damage, already described in the preceding section.

Results obtained in these patients confirmed those previously observed in eunuchs (Mancini *et al.*, 1970), as regards the impossibility of low or high doses of FSH or LH alone or administered successively to restore spermatogenesis. This also corroborates the predominant effect of FSH and LH in repairing the mature Sertoli cells without modifying their number and the more extended action of higher doses of LH. Changes in this cell appear to be reflected in the nuclear structures, mainly by the size and features of the nucleoli. The absence of apparent changes in spermatogonial cells suggest that FSH is incapable by itself of initiating or continuing spermatogenesis. This predominant effect on Sertoli cells appears to depend only on the FSH activity as the amount of LH contaminant is negligible. Moreover, the development of Sertoli cells has been induced in the lamb by injecting ovine pituitary FSH (Courot, 1962). Hypertrophy of these cells was also obtained after intra-testicular injection of the same hormone in the rat (Murphy, 1965). Using immunohistochemical techniques, a selective accumulation of Sertoli cells in the rat was reported at the optical and electron-microscopic level after intravenous injection of native or labeled FSH. Participation of pinocytosis of vesicles in the uptake of the hormone was evident (Mancini *et al.*, 1967; Castro *et al.*, 1970). Lack of effect on the remaining structures of the testis favor the idea of a direct action of FSH upon Sertoli cells. The earlier contention that this cell plays a role in the spermatogenic process appears to be supported not only by its participation in the intratubular diffusion of serum proteins (Mancini *et al.*, 1965), but also by the fact that during normal puberty, advanced meiosis and spermiogenesis are accompanied by the maturation of Sertoli cells (Mancini *et al.*, 1960; 1963). All these data strongly suggest that development and function of Sertoli cells may be under gonadotrophin control or that they may act as an intermediate site of FSH storage for ultimate action on the spermatogenic process or both.

As only LH induces an additional increment of spermatogonial cells and development of primary spermatocytes coinciding with differentiation of interstitial Leydig cells together with regression of hyalinosis, one may speculate that LH has a direct effect on Sertoli cells and an indirect one on spermatogonial cells which is mediated by Leydig cells. The probability of the dual action of LH is supported by a previous experience in the use of large doses of HCG alone as detailed in the preceding section, which induces spermatogenesis up to the pachytene stage, differentiation of Leydig cells, secretion of steroids, enlargement of tubular diameter and regression of hyaline material. However the possibility that the supposed direct effect of LH might also be mediated by some activated function of the intertubular fibroblast-like cells cannot be excluded.

The successive use of FSH and LH or *vice versa* points to the lack of an additive effect of both hormones, except for the maturation of Sertoli cells. The inefficiency of FSH to preserve the stimulating action of previously administered LH was evident. These findings, which may merely reflect the separate specific action of each hormone on the testis, not only verifies the more striking effect of LH but also substantiates the contention of the need of a simultaneous action of both hormones. The more relevant action of FSH and LH given at the same time (stimulation up to advanced meiotic phase) even at lower doses than those administered separately in patients of this group, or rather with a higher LH/FSH ratio (stimulation up to spermiogenic phase), points again to the importance of a simultaneous need for both gonadotrophins and an excess of LH. This appears to be corroborated by the patient already mentioned (see preceding section) treated with HMG added to HCG. These results also agree with those obtained in hypophysectomized patients in which administration of HMG precedes that of HCG (McLeod *et al.*, 1966).

Coincidentally it has been shown in hypophysectomized rats that FSH stimulates Sertoli cell development but only both hormones establish complete spermatogenesis (Lostroh, 1969). Also a ratio favorable to LH over FSH is required for the recovery of spermatogenesis; besides the 'gametogenic' action, LH unequivocally causes some stimulation of Leydig cells, which may not appear reflected by changes in the adnexal glands (Woods and Simpson, 1961). Current studies on hypophysectomized rats show that human urinary FSH and LH started 80 days post operation, produces recovery of spermatogenesis after 50 days, which is more evident if the ratio is in favor of LH (Vilar, 1970).

Whether or not the doses, ratio and period of time of the administration of both FSH and LH used in our cases for the stimulation of spermatogenesis, would be the same as that needed for the maintenance of this process, remain an open question.

III – EFFECT OF FSH AND LH ON PERITUBULAR HYALINIZATION

It was postulated that peritubular hyalinization is an unspecific process consequent to spermatogenic failure (Nelson and Heller, 1945), or that it damages secondarily the seminiferous epithelium (Johnsen, 1967) or that there is an apparent synchrony between hyalinization and regression of germinal epithelium and Leydig cells (Mancini *et al.*, 1969). Histochemical and ultrastructural studies in adult normal subjects showed that the seminiferous tubule wall is mainly composed of an acellular basal lamina adjacent to the germinal epithelium and an outer cellular layer in which fibrils arranged in compact bundles and flattened cells are present (Mancini *et al.*, 1964). Immunochemical analysis of this structure revealed the existence of two classes of glycoproteins, one corresponding to collagen and the other to reticulin substance (Denduchis *et al.*, 1969).

Similar studies have been made in our group of hypophysectomized patients (Seiguer *et al.*, 1970). Our findings at the optical level confirm previous observations of other authors who suggested that the connective tissue layer adjacent to the seminiferous epithelium is the place where hyalinization develops. When this process develops, the basal lamina appears disaggregated in some areas. The underlying cellular layer increases in thickness, the cell exhibits regressive changes, and deposition of an amorphous substance appears in between the fibrils, which show absence of characteristic electron density and cross striation. The incipient hyaline formation precedes immediately or appears simultaneously with several changes in the collagen fibril structure. These changes begin when the fibril cross-bandage becomes less well defined and end with the complete disappearance of the fibril. A process affecting the structure of collagen may take place in the first steps of hyalinization, although there are no data proving the existence of collagenolytic substances in the testis during hyalinization. Our results at the optical level showing absence of demonstrable collagen or reticulin fibrils within the hyaline, fragmented elastic fibers in the outer layers and weak or negative results obtained with labeled antibodies against testicular collagen or glycoprotein substances, also support the interpretation as a collagen breakdown. In addition it was recently reported by us that soluble and insoluble collagen as measured by hydroxyproline, show significantly lower values in testicular biopsies of hypophysectomized patients with advanced hyalinosis, than in normal subjects (Setchell *et al.*, 1969).

It is difficult to trace the origin of the dense and amorphous material which constitutes the principal hyaline component, mainly because a sequential study at different periods of time after hypophysectomy was not performed. The density of the interfibrillar substance increases while the collagen fibril undergoes dissolution, giving rise to the possibility that the former could represent material arising from collagen degradation. Nevertheless, the amorphous substance present in the first steps of hyalinization has the low density and homogeneous texture of fixed blood plasma. Since serum proteins normally accumulate in the peritubular tissue (Johnsen, 1966) their absence in the hyaline tissue as shown by immunofluorescent technics may be explicable as a consequence of an altered function of the structures of the tubule wall, claimed to operate as a diffusion-barrier (Ross, 1967). Instead the presence of some acid mucopolysaccharides and the lytic action of collagenase tend to suggest the presence of a complex amorphous collagenous substance linked with polysaccharide. The peritubular cells exhibited cytologic damage at the same time as the early signs of connective tissue changes appeared. These observations suggest a close relationship between peritubular cell function and the surrounding connective tissue structures. This assumption is also backed by the presence of ribosomes in the peritubular cell cytoplasm in the normal seminiferous tubule suggesting active protein synthesis. It has been proposed that these cells not only may act as contractile ones (Ross, 1967) but also may be engaged in the maintenance of the connective tissue of the tubular wall as was deduced from a histochemical study during development of the human puberal testis (Mancini *et al.*, 1964).

Concerning the effect of gonadotrophins on the peritubular hyalinization in our group of hypophysectomized patients, it is interesting to note, as was described in preceding sections, that only high doses of HCG or purified LH may induce regression of the lesion with parallel replacement of the hyaline tissue by normal connective tissue fibrils and morphological repair of peritubular cells. This observation, which confirms earlier findings on hypogonadal hypogonadotrophic subjects treated with HCG (Nelson, 1953), makes it likely that Leydig cells might be implicated through the local action of secreted steroids on peritubular collagen metabolism. The fact that FSH does not modify the hyaline, but HMG does but slightly and is accompanied by poor development of Leydig cells, strongly supports the participation of these cells in the recovery of the normal structure of the tubule wall in this pathological condition. However as it was reported that intravenously injected labeled LH localized in the cytoplasm of some peritubular cells of the seminiferous tubule of the rat testis (Mancini *et al.*, 1967), the possible existence of a direct trophic action of LH on these cells could not be categorically discarded in normal conditions.

REFERENCES

Albert, A. (1961): In: *Sex and Internal Secretion, Vol. 1*, p. 305. Editor: W. C. Young. Williams and Wilkins, Baltimore, Md.

Bartler, F. C., Sniffen, R. C., Simmons, F. A., Albright, A. and Howard, R. P. (1952): Effects of chorionic gonadotropin in male eunuchoidism with low follicle stimulating hormone; aqueous solution versus oil and beeswax suspension. *J. clin. Endocr.*, *12*, 1532.

Bergadá, C. and Mancini, R. E. (1969): Effect of human gonadotropins (HMG and HCG) on prepuberal testes. *Acta europ. fertil.* (in press).

Borth, R., Lunenfeld, B. and de Wattewille, H. (1954): Activité gonadotrope d'un extrait d'urine des femmes à ménopause. *Experientia (Basel)*, *10*, 266.

Castro, A. E., Seiguer, A. C. and Mancini, R. E. (1970): Electron-microscopic study on the localization of labeled gonadotropins in the Sertoli and Leydig cells of the rat testis. *Proc. Soc. exp. Biol. (N.Y.)*, *133*, 582.

COUROT, M. (1962): Actions des hormones gonadotropes sur le testicule de l'agneau impubère; réponse particulière de la lignée sertolienne. *Ann. Biol. anim.*, *2*, 157.

CROOKE, A. C., DAVIES, A. G. and MORRIS, R. (1968): Treatment of eunuchoidal men with human chorionic gonadotropin and follicle stimulating hormone. *J. Endocr.*, *42*, 441.

DENDUCHIS, B., GONZALEZ, N. and MANCINI, R. E. (1970): Collagen content of testis from hypophysectomized patients before and after treatment with gonadotropins. *Acta europ. fertil.* (in press).

DENDUCHIS, B., LUSTIG, L., GONZALEZ N. and MANCINI, R. E. (1969): Physicochemical and immunological study of connective tissue structures of the human testis. *Acta europ. fertil.*, *1*, 595.

DONINI, S. and DONINI, P. (1969): Radioimmunoassay employing polymerized antisera. In: *Karolinska Symposia on Research Methods in Reproductive Endocrinology. 1st Symposium: Immunoassay of Gonadotropins*, p. 257. Editor: E. Diczfalusy. Stockholm.

DVOSKIN, S. (1947): Reinitiation of spermatogenesis by pellets of testosterone and its esters in hypophysectomized rats. *Anat. Rec.*, *99*, 329.

FABBRINI, A., RE, M. and SPERA, G. (1968): Histochemical demonstration of 14-amylophosphorylase in the human testis under normal and pathological conditions. *Experientia (Basel)*, *24*, 789.

GEMZELL, C. A. and KJESSLER, B. (1964): Treatment of infertility after partial hypophysectomy with human pituitary gonadotropins. *Lancet*, *1*, 644.

HELLER, C. G. and CLERMONT, Y. (1964): Kinetics of the germinal epithelium in man. *Recent Progr. Hormone Res.*, *20*, 545.

HELLER, C. G. and NELSON, W. O. (1948): Classification of male hypogonadism and a discussion of the pathologic physiology and treatment. *J. clin. Endocr.*, *8*, 345.

HELLER, C. G., NELSON, W. O., HILL, I. B., HENDERSON, E., MADDOCK, W. O., JUNCK, E. C., PAULSEN, A. C. and MORTIMORE, G. E. (1950): Improvement in spermatogenesis following depression of the human testis with testosterone. *Fertil. and Steril.*, *1*, 415.

JOHNSEN, S. G. (1962): Management of male hypogonadism. A clinical endocrinological synopsis. *Acta endocr. (Kbh.)*, *66*, 1.

JOHNSEN, S. G. (1966): A study of human testicular function by the use of human menopausal gonadotropin and of human chorionic gonadotropin in male hypogonadotropic eunuchoidism and infantilism. *Acta endocr. (Kbh.)*, *53*, 315.

JOHNSEN, S. G. (1967): The mechanism involved in testicular degeneration in man. *Acta endocr. (Kbh.)*, *124*, 17.

LEIDERMAN, B. and MANCINI, R. E. (1969): Glycogen content in the rat testis from postnatal to adult ages. *Endocrinology*, *85*, 607.

LOSTROH, A. J. (1969): Regulation by FSH and ICSH (LH) of reproductive function in the immature male rat. *Endocrinology*, *85*, 438.

LUFT, R. H., OLIVECRONA, D., IKKOS, L. B., NILSSON, H. and MOSSBERG, H. (1958): In: *Endocrine Aspects of Breast Cancer*, p. 27. Editor: R. A. Currie. Livingstone, Edinburgh.

MADDOCK, O. W. (1949): Antihormone formation complicating pituitary gonadotropin therapy in infertile men. *J. clin. Endocr.*, *9*, 213.

MANCINI, R. E., CASTRO, A. and SEIGUER, A. C. (1967): Histologic localization of follicle-stimulating and luteinizing hormones in the rat testis. *J. Histochem. Cytochem.*, *15*, 516.

MANCINI, R. E., DONINI, P., VILAR, O. and PÉREZ LLORET, A. (1970): Effect of human urinary FSH and LH on the recovery of spermatogenesis in hypophysectomized patients (unpublished).

MANCINI, R. E., LAVIERI, J. C., MÜLLER, F., ANDRADA, J. A. and SARACENI, D. J. (1966): Effect of prednisolone upon normal and pathologic human spermatogenesis. *Fertil. and Steril.*, *17*, 500.

MANCINI, R. E., NARBAITZ, R. and LAVIERI, J. C. (1960): Origin and development of germinative epithelium and Sertoli cells in the human testis. Cytological, cytochemical and quantitative study. *Anat. Rec.*, *136*, 477.

MANCINI, R. E., SEIGUER, A. C. and PÉREZ LLORET, A. (1968): Effect of different gonadotropins preparations on the testis of hypophysectomized patients. In: *Gonadotropins*, p. 503. Editor: E. Rosemberg. Geron-X Publishing Co., Los Altos, Calif.

MANCINI, R. E., SEIGUER, A. C. and PÉREZ LLORET, A. (1969): Effect of gonadotropins on the recovery of spermatogenesis in hypophysectomized patients. *J. clin. Endocr.*, *29*, 467.

MANCINI, R. E., VILAR, O., DELLACHA, J. M., DAVIDSON, O. W. and CASTRO, A. (1965): Extravascular and intratubular diffusion of labeled serum proteins in the rat testis. *J. Histochem. Cytochem.*, *13*, 376.

MANCINI, R. E., VILAR, O., LAVIERI, J. C. and HEINRICH, H. (1963): Development of Leydig cells in the normal human testis. A cytological, cytochemical and quantitative study. *Amer. J. Anat.*, *112*, 113.

MANCINI, R. E., VILAR, O., PÉREZ DEL CERRO, M. and LAVIERI, J. C. (1964): Changes in the stromal connective tissue of the human testes. A histological, histochemical and electron microscopy study. *Acta physiol. lat.-amer.*, *14*, 382.

MCLEOD, J., PAZIANOS, A. and BRONSON, S. R. (1966): Restoration of human spermatogenesis and of reproductive tract with urinary gonadotropins following hypophysectomy. *Fertil. and Steril.*, *17*, 7.

MEANS, A. R. and HALL, P. F. (1968): Protein biosynthesis in the testis. I. Comparison between stimulation by FSH and glucose. *Endocrinology*, *82*, 597.

MURPHY, H. (1965): Intratesticular assays of FSH in hypophysectomized rats. *Proc. Soc. exp. Biol. (N.Y.)*, *118*, 1202.

NELSON, W. O. (1953): Some problems of testicular function. *J. Urol. (Baltimore)*, *69*, 325.

NELSON, W. O. and HELLER, C. G. (1945): Hyalinisation of the seminiferous tubules associated with normal or failing Leydig cell function. *J. clin. Endocr.*, *5*, 13.

PAULSEN, C. A. (1968): Effect of human chorionic gonadotropin and of human menopausal gonadotropin therapy on testicular function. In: *Gonadotropins*, p. 491. Editor: E. Rosemberg. Geron-X Publishing Co., Los Altos, Calif.

ROOSEN-RUNGE, E. C. (1962): The process of spermatogenesis in mammals. *Biol. Rev.*, *37*, 343.

ROSEMBERG, E., MANCINI, R. E., CRIGLER, J. F. and BERGADÁ, C. (1968): Effect of human menopausal gonadotropin on prepuberal testes. In: *Gonadotropins*, p. 527. Editor: E. Rosemberg. Geron-X Publishing Co., Los Altos, Calif.

ROSS, M. H. and LONG, I. R. (1966): Contractile cells in human seminiferous tubules. *Science*, *153*, 1271.

SEIGUER, A. C., PÉREZ LLORET, A. and MANCINI, R. E. (1970): Histogenesis of the hyalinization of human seminiferous tubules. Electronmicroscopical and histochemical study. *Lab. Invest.* (in press).

SETCHELL, B. P., VOGLMAYR, J. K. and WAITES, G. M. H. (1969): A blood testis barrier restricting passage from blood into rete testis fluid but not into the lymph. *J. Physiol. (Lond.)*, *200*, 73.

VILAR, O. (1971): Effect of human menopausal gonadotropins on the testes of the adult hypophysectomized rat. *Acta physiol. lat.-amer.* (in press).

VILAR, O., PÉREZ DEL CERRO, M. and MANCINI, R. E. (1962): Sertoli cell as a 'bridge cell' between the basal membrane and the germinal cells. *Exp. Cell Res.*, *27*, 158.

WOODS, M. C. and SIMPSON, M. E. (1961): Pituitary control of the testis of the hypophysectomized rat. *Endocrinology*, *69*, 91.

YOKOE, Y. and HALL, P. F. (1970): Testicular phospholipids. I Action of follicle stimulating hormone (FSH) upon biosynthesis of phospholipids in rat testis. *Endocrinology*, *86*, 18.

ANDROGENS

CONTENTS

BIOSYNTHESIS OF ANDROGENS IN MAN

RALPH I. DORFMAN

Professor of Pharmacology, Stanford University School of Medicine, Palo Alto, California, U.S.A.

The term androgen biosynthesis has usually been used to specify a process by which androgens arise from a sequence of inactive precursors within a given endocrine gland. It is now recognized that such a view is much too limited. Within the broader definition, a biosynthetic change may be defined as a conversion of an inactive compound to an androgen or a modification of a weakly active androgen to one having a significantly increased androgen potency. A special case of a biosynthetic reaction to androgen could also involve a change in the type of biological activity. The conversion of progesterone to androst-4-ene-3,17-dione could be such an example. On the basis of progestational activity, the reaction is strictly one of inactivation, while on the basis of the property of androgenicity the overall reaction is biosynthetic.

The biosynthetic changes need not be confined to a single gland nor does the gland need to be an endocrine gland. It is recognized that non-endocrine glands and target tissues may be the site of androgen biosynthesis. Two such examples will be discussed in this communication.

GENERAL STATEMENT

Androgens are formed by the testis, the ovary, the adrenal, and the placenta of pregnancy, and the routes overlap from tissue to tissue. The general plan involves the conversion of C_{27} sterols to C_{21} steroids and thence to C_{19} androgens. Androgen biosynthetic stimulatory mechanisms involved in androgen biosynthesis seem to influence primarily conversions from the C_{27} sterols to the C_{19} androgens. The principal regulators have been identified as anterior pituitary luteinizing hormone (LH), also known as interstitial cell stimulating hormone.

Brady and Gurin (1951) demonstrated the conversion of acetate to testosterone in the human testis. Since acetate was known to be convertible to cholesterol, Ungar and Dorfman (1953) tested the hypothesis that acetate and cholesterol were in fact precursors of androgens. In this study, acetate labeled with ^{14}C in the carboxyl position was administered to a patient bearing a virilizing adrenal tumor, and ^{14}C-containing androsterone, dehydroepiandrosterone and androst-5-ene-3β, 17β-diol were isolated from the urine. 3-^{14}C-Cholesterol was converted to both androsterone and etiocholanolone. In a later study, Savard *et al.* (1952) perfused ^{14}C-labeled acetic acid through a human testis and isolated labeled testosterone and androst-4-ene-3,17-dione from the perfusate.

Slaunwhite and Samuels (1956) in the rat testis and Savard *et al.* (1956) indicated that progesterone and 17α-hydroxyprogesterone were important intermediates in the formation of androgens. This route involves the sequence of progesterone $\rightarrow$ 17α-hydroxyprogesterone $\rightarrow$ androst-4-ene-3,17-dione $\rightarrow$ testosterone. This biosynthetic pathway from progesterone to testosterone presupposes the formation of C_{21} steroids. A route from cholesterol to pregnenolone and progesterone has been established with considerable certainty.

CHOLESTEROL TO PREGNENOLONE

The biosynthetic studies of cholesterol to pregnenolone were initiated in our laboratory and reported in 1960 by Shimizu *et al.* This paper proved the conversion of cholesterol to pregnenolone through the intermediate, 20α-hydroxycholesterol. In this study, labeled 20α-hydroxycholesterol was cleaved to isocaproic acid and pregnenolone. The initial studies were done in adrenal homogenates but it was soon shown that the human placenta and the rat testes performed these transformations as well, as was demonstrated by Shimizu *et al.* (1961). Rat liver homogenates did not perform these transformations.

20α, 22R-Dihydroxycholesterol, when incubated with adrenal homogenate, was also converted into pregnenolone. In another study, Chaudhuri *et al.* (1962) showed that 22-hydroxycholesterol could also serve as a precursor of pregnenolone. Thus, the pathway from cholesterol to pregnenolone involves the hydroxylation, either at position 20α or position 22R, which in turn leads to a dihydroxycholesterol compound. This 20,22-dihydroxy derivative under the action of a desmolase yields pregnenolone and isocaproic aldehyde. However, in most of the experimental studies the *in vitro* systems contained a dehydrogenase which oxidized the aldehyde to isocaproic acid.

Burstein *et al.* (1970) have recently demonstrated that the human adrenal does in fact convert cholesterol to pregnenolone.

Tables I and II summarize the many *in vitro* and *in vivo* perfusion studies, respectively, that have been reported and have contributed to a definition of the biosynthetic pathways to androgens. The information contained in these tables has been in effect the basis for the pathways of biosynthesis in the figures.

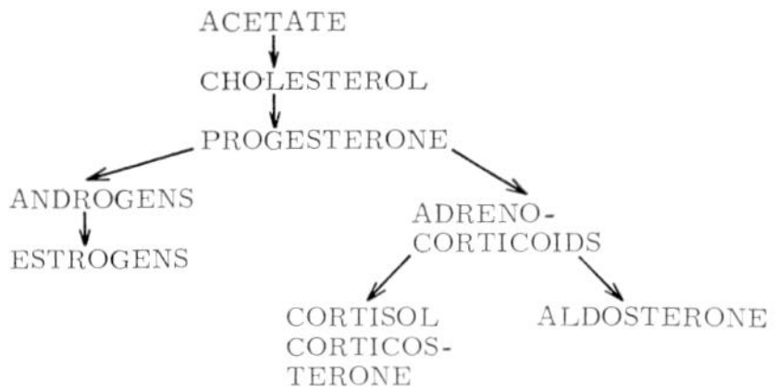

Fig. 1. Biosynthesis of steroid hormones.

Figure 1 presents the overview of steroid hormone biosynthesis which has general application in both sexes and in all the species studied. The general pattern of steroid biosynthesis is also repetitive in the steroid hormone-producing glands. Recently biosynthetic reactions in tissues other than the classical endocrine glands have assumed major importance and will be dealt with in another section of this communication.

Acetate is transformed into cholesterol, which is a basic precursor for steroid hormones including androgens. Cholesterol is probably the principal sterol precursor but most likely not the exclusive precursor, since cholestenone does seem to undergo cleavage in certain steroid-producing tissues to pregnenolone (unpublished observations).

The biosynthesis of androgens from cholesterol proceeds by way of a well-defined series of reactions through C_{21}. At least in the rat, a pathway from cholesterol to androgens not involving C_{21} steroids has been reported. This reaction involves the complete removal of the C_8 sidechain, leaving the androgen dehydroepiandrosterone.

Figure 1 also includes the biosynthetic pathways to corticoids and estrogens, which will not be discussed further in this communication.

Figure 2 defines the outline of androgen biosynthesis in human testes from acetate and cholesterol. The androgens in this figure are androst-4-ene-3,17-dione and dehydroepiandrosterone, which are relatively weak androgens. This figure also indicates three subsections labeled A, B, and C, which are expanded in detail in Figures 3, 4, and 5.

TABLE I

Biosynthesis of androgens in vitro
Human

Substrate	Product	Test system	Reference
Acetate	Dehydroepiandrosterone	Ovary	Noall *et al.* (1962)
	Dehydroepiandrosterone	Ovarian slices	Noall *et al.* (1962)
	17α-Hydroxyprogesterone 17α-Hydroxypregnenolone	Ovary (follicular cyst linings) minced	Ryan and Smith (1961)
	17α-Hydroxyprogesterone	Slice corpus luteum	Hammerstein *et al.* (1964)
	17α-Hydroxyprogesterone	Slices malignant testicular tumor	Engel, F. L. *et al.* (1964)
	17α-Hydroxypregnenolone 17α-Hydroxyprogesterone	Testis slices	Engel, F.L. *et al.* (1964)
	Dehydroepiandrosterone Androst-4-ene-3, 17-dione 11β-Hydroxyandrost-4-ene-3, 17-dione	Fetal (12–23 weeks) adrenal slices	Bloch and Benirschke (1962)
	Dehydroepiandrosterone Androst-4-ene-3, 17-dione 11β-Hydroxyandrost-4-ene-3, 17-dione	Adrenal slices (fetal)	Bloch and Benirschke (1959)
	Androst-4-ene-3, 17-dione Testosterone Dehydroepiandrosterone	Ovarian stromal tissues	Savard and Rice (1965)
	17α-Hydroxyprogesterone	Stromal ovarian tissue	Savard and Rice (1965)
	Androst-4-ene-3, 17-dione	Corpus luteum slices	Rice *et al.* (1964*a*)
	Dehydroepiandrosterone Testosterone Androst-4-ene-3, 17-dione	Ovarian stroma (luteal phase)	
	Dehydroepiandrosterone Androst-4-ene-3, 17-dione Testosterone	Male pseudo-hermaphrodite testis slice	Cleveland *et al.* (1965)
	Pregnenolone Progesterone 17α-Hydroxyprogesterone Dehydroepiandrosterone Androst-4-ene-3, 17-dione 11β-Hydroxyandrost-4-ene-3, 17-dione	Adrenal slice	Bloch *et al.* (1956)
	Testosterone	Testis tumor slices (grown in hamster)	Wotiz *et al.* (1960)
	5α-Androst-16-en-3α-ol	Testicular slices	Gower and Haslewood (1961)

(continued next page)

Substrate	Product	Test system	Reference
	Dehydroepiandrosterone Androst-4-ene-3, 17-dione	Fetal adrenal slice	Bloch and Benirschke (1962)
	Testosterone	Ovarian slices (Stein-Leventhal)	Leon *et al.* (1962)
	Dehydroepiandrosterone Androst-4-ene-3, 17-dione 11β-Hydroxyandrost-4-ene-3, 17-dione	Malignant testis tumor	Engel, F. L. *et al.* (1964)
	17α-Hydroxyprogesterone	Ovarian stroma and corpus luteum	Rice *et al.* (1964*a*)
	(Preliminary) Testosterone Androst-4-ene-3, 17-dione (Also 17α-Hydroxy-progesterone)	Stein-Leventhal ovary	O'Donnell and McCaig (1959)
	Testosterone	Testis homogenate	Rabinowitz and Oleksyshyn (1956)
	Androst-4-ene-3, 17-dione Dehydroepiandrosterone	Ovary (follicular cyst linings) minced	Ryan and Smith (1961)
	Androst-4-ene-3, 17-dione 11β-Hydroxyandrost-4-ene-3, 17-dione Adrenosterone	Slices interstitial cell tumor 3–10/12-year-old boy	Engel, L. L. *et al.* (1966)
	Testosterone	Ovarian stromal slice	Rice *et al.* (1964*b*)
	Androst-4-ene-3, 17-dione	Slice corpora lutea	Hammerstein *et al.* (1964)
	Androst-4-ene-3, 17-dione Dehydroepiandrosterone 11β-Hydroxyandrost-4-ene-3, 17-dione	Slices malignant testicular tumor	Engel, F. L. *et al.* (1964)
	17α-Hydroxyprogesterone	Interstitial cell tumor 3–10/12-years old	Engel, L. L. *et al.* (1966)
ACTH stimulation	Dehydroepiandrosterone Androst-4-ene-3, 17-dione 11β-Hydroxyandrost-4-ene-3, 17-dione	Adrenal (normal and abnormal) slices	Cohn and Mulrow (1963)
None	Androst-4-ene-3, 17-dione Dehydroepiandrosterone	Polycystic ovary	Kokhanenko (1965)
None	11β-Hydroxyandrost-4-ene 3, 17-dione	Adrenal adenoma	Nowaczynski and Koiw (1963)
Androst-4-ene-3, 17-dione 17α-Hydroxy-pregnenolone	Testosterone Dehydroepiandrosterone	Testis from patient with testicular feminization *in vitro*	Neher *et al.* (1965)

(continued next page)

Substrate	Product	Test system	Reference
Androst-4-ene-3,-17-dione	19-Hydroxyandrost-4-ene-3, 17-dione	Placental microsome	Longchampt *et al.* (1960)
	Testosterone	Placental homogenate supernatant	McKerns and Nordstrand (1964)
	Testosterone 6β-Hydroxyandrost-4-ene-3, 17-dione	Surviving slices corpus luteum	Huang (1967)
	Testosterone	Ovarian slices	Sandor and Lanthier (1960)
	Testosterone 6β-Hydroxyandrost-4-ene-3, 17-dione	Corpus luteum slices (26th day)	Huang (1966)
Pregnenolone	17α-Hydroxypregnenolone 17α-Hydroxyprogesterone	Granulosa cell multilocular cystadenoma	Griffiths *et al.* (1966*a*)
	17α-Hydroxypregnenolone 17α-Hydroxyprogesterone	Ovarian cystadeno-carcinoma	Plotz *et al.* (1966)
Progesterone	17α-Hydroxyprogesterone		
Pregnenolone	17α-Hydroxypregnenolone 17α-Hydroxyprogesterone	Homogenate testicular feminization	Neher *et al.* (1965)
17α-Hydroxy-pregnenolone	17α-Hydroxyprogesterone		
Progesterone	17α-Hydroxyprogesterone		
Pregnenolone	Dehydroepiandrosterone sulfate 17α-Hydroxypregnenolone sulfate	Adrenal homogenate fetus	Villee, C. A. *et al.* (1965)
17α-Hydroxy-pregnenolone	Dehydroepiandrosterone sulfate 17α-Hydroxypregnenolone		
Dehydroepi-androsterone	Dehydroepiandrosterone sulfate 16α-Hydroxydehydroepi-androsterone Androst-4-ene-3, 17-dione 11β-Hydroxyandrost-4-ene-3, 17-dione		
Pregnenolone Progesterone	17α-Hydroxyprogesterone	Gonad (testicular feminization)	Gwinup *et al.* (1966)
Pregnenolone and 17α-Hydroxy-progesterone	Androst-4-ene-3, 17-dione (presumptive)	Ovary (normal and Stein-Leventhal)	Lanthier and Sandor (1960*a*)
Pregnenolone	Testosterone Androst-4-ene-3, 17-dione	Fetal testis	Acevedo *et al.* (1961*a*)

(continued next page)

Substrate	Product	Test system	Reference
	Dehydroepiandrosterone	Adrenal homogenate	Goldstein *et al.* (1960)
	Androst-4-ene-3, 17-dione Testosterone 16α-Hydroxyprogesterone 17α-Hydroxyprogesterone	Testis 15–1/2 years Delayed sexual maturation	Villee, D. B. *et al.* (1965)
	Testosterone Androst-4-ene-3, 17-dione Dehydroepiandrosterone Androst-5-ene-3β, 16α, 17β-triol	Minced fetal testis	Acevedo *et al.* (1963)
	Dehydroepiandrosterone	Krukenberg tumor of ovary plus HCG	Ganis *et al.* (1965)
	17α-Hydroxypregnenolone 17α-Hydroxyprogesterone	Tumor adrenal	Weliky and Engel (1963)
Pregnenolone sulfate	17α-Hydroxypregnenolone sulfate	Hyperplastic adrenal homogenate	Calvin and Lieberman (1964)
Pregnenolone	Dehydroepiandrosterone (0.4%)	Microsomes and soluble portion of cystadenocarcinoma	Plotz *et al.* (1966)
17α-Hydroxy-pregnenolone	Dehydroepiandrosterone (0.7%) Androst-4-ene-3, 17-dione (0.05%)		
Progesterone	Androst-4-ene-3, 17-dione (0.5%) Testosterone (0.4%)		
Androst-4-ene-3, 17-dione	Testosterone (1.7%)		
Testosterone	Androst-4-ene-3, 17-dione (4.9%)		
Pregnenolone	Testosterone 17α-Hydroxyprogesterone 17α, 20α-Dihydroxy-4-pregnen-3-one 17α, 20β-Dihydroxy-4-pregnen-3-one 17α-Hydroxy-5-pregnenolone Dehydroepiandrosterone 6β-Hydroxy-4-androstene-3, 17-dione 16α-Hydroxy-4-androstene-3, 17-dione 3β, 20β-Dihydroxy-5-pregnene 6α-Hydroxyestradiol-17β 6-Ketoestradiol-17β 5-Pregnenolone	Testis mince 16-year-old	Axelrod (1965)

(continued next page)

Substrate	Product	Test system	Reference
	Testosterone 17α-Hydroxyprogesterone 17α, 20α-Dihydroxy-4-pregnen-3-one 17α, 20β-Dihydroxy-4-pregnen-3-one 6β-Hydroxy-4-androstene-3, 17-dione 3β, 20β-Dihydroxy-5-pregnene Estrone 5-Pregnenolone	Testis mince 61-year-old male prostatic cancer	
17α-Hydroxy-progesterone	Testosterone 17α, 20α-Dihydroxy-4-pregnen-3-one 17α, 20β-Dihydroxy-4-pregnen-3-one 4-Androstene-3, 17-dione 17α-Hydroxyprogesterone		
17α-Hydroxy-pregnenolone	Dehydroepiandrosterone	Adrenal adenoma	Cohn *et al.* (1963)
	11β-Hydroxyandrosta-4-diene-3, 17-dione	Adrenal tumor	Weliky and Engel (1961)
	Testosterone	Testis mince	Carstensen (1961)
	Dehydroepiandrosterone	Adrenal tumor slices	Lebeau *et al.* (1964)
Dehydroepi-androsterone sulfate	Dehydroepiandrosterone	Arrhenoblastoma ovary	Sandberg and Jenkins (1965*a*)
Dehydroepi-androsterone Testosterone Dehydroepi-androsterone ammonium sulfate	Testosterone Androst-4-ene-3, 17-dione 16α-Hydroxytestosterone	Normal adult testis homogenate	Dixon *et al.* (1965)
Dehydroepi-androsterone	Androst-4-ene-3, 17-dione Testosterone	Granulosa cell multilocular cystadenoma	Griffiths *et al.* (1966a)
	Testosterone	Skin brei	Cameron *et al.* (1966)
	Androst-4-ene-3, 17-dione 3β-Hydroxyandrost-5-ene-7, 17-dione	Homogenate adrenal in vitro	Neville and Webb (1965)
	Androst-4-ene-3, 17-dione	Fetal adrenals	Sakhatskaya and Burova (1966)

(continued next page)

Substrate	Product	Test system	Reference
Dehydroepiandrosterone sulfate	Dehydroepiandrosterone	Homogenate of fetal tissues 13 weeks-placenta+ 17 weeks-placenta+ kidney+ lung+ liver+ (Placenta most active)	French and Warren (1965)
Dehydroepiandrosterone	19-Hydroxydehydroepiandrosterone	Polycystic ovaries microsomal plus cytoplasmic fraction	Starka *et al.* (1966)
	Dehydroepiandrosterone sulfate	Adrenal	Wallace and Lieberman (1963)
Dehydroepiandrosterone	Testosterone	Ovarian arrhenoblastoma	Sandberg *et al.* (1966)
Progesterone	Testosterone Androst-4-ene-3, 17-dione		
		Adenoma and normal adrenal	Ichii *et al.* (1962)
	17α-Hydroxyprogesterone Testosterone	Testis tissue Feminization syndrome	Colla *et al.* (1966)
	Androst-4-ene-3, 17-dione	Placenta	Warren and Cheatum (1964)
	17α-Hydroxyprogesterone	Testis 15-week-old fetus	Bloch *et al.* (1962)
		Fetal adrenal (7 weeks)	Sakhatskaya and Burova (1965)
	Testosterone Androst-4-ene-3, 17-dione 17β-Estradiol 16α-Hydroxyprogesterone 17α-Hydroxyprogesterone	Dysgenetic gonad 18-year-old girl	Griffiths *et al.* (1966*b*)
	Androst-4-ene-3, 17-dione	Granulosa cell tumor slices	Loutfi and Hagerman (1965)
	Androst-4-ene-3, 17-dione Testosterone Also 17α-Hydroxyprogesterone 20α-Hydroxypregn-4-en-3-one 20β-Hydroxypregn-4-en-3-one	Ovarian arrhenoblastoma	Savard *et al.* (1961)
	20α-Hydroxypregn-4-en-3-one 17α-Hydroxyprogesterone Testosterone Androst-4-ene-3, 17-dione	Testis homogenate (prostatic cancer) In microsomes 17α-Hydroxylase C_{17}-C_{20} Lyase 17β-Dehydrogenase	Murota *et al.* (1966)

(continued next page)

Substrate	Product	Test system	Reference
	Testosterone Androst-4-ene-3, 17-dione	Testicular tumor homogenate	Dominguez (1961)
	Testosterone	Brenner tumor of ovary stimulated with CG	Hamwi *et al.* (1963)
	Testosterone Androst-4-ene-3, 17-dione	Brenner cell tumor ovary	Besch *et al.* (1963)
Androst-4-ene-3, 17-dione	Testosterone		
Progesterone	17α-Hydroxyprogesterone (16%) Androst-4-ene-3, 17-dione (0.6%) Testosterone (24%) 17β-Estradiol (0.05%)	Testicular feminization gonad	French *et al.* (1965)
Testosterone	17β-Estradiol (0.23%)		
Progesterone	Androst-4-ene-3, 17-dione	Homogenate adrenal adenoma	Roversi *et al.* (1963)
	Androst-4-ene-3, 17-dione 11β-Hydroxyandrost-4-ene-3, 17-dione	Adrenal tumor	Adadevoh and Engel (1964)
Pregnenolone	Progesterone 17α-Hydroxyprogesterone Androst-4-ene-3, 17-dione 17β-Estradiol	Theca cells ovary	Ryan and Petro (1966)
Progesterone	17α-Hydroxyprogesterone Androst-4-ene-3, 17-dione 17β-Estradiol		
Progesterone Androst-4-ene-3, 17-dione 17α-Hydroxyprogesterone	Testosterone Androst-4-ene-3, 17-dione	Lipoid cell tumor (ovarian homogenate)	Sandberg *et al.* (1962)
	17α-Hydroxyprogesterone		
Progesterone 17α-Hydroxyprogesterone	Androst-4-ene-3, 17-dione Testosterone	Testis homogenate (Klinefelter syndrome 47 chromosomes XXY)	Slaunwhite *et al.* (1962)
		Testis (Klinefelter type)	Slaunwhite *et al.* (1962)
Progesterone	Testosterone Androst-4-ene-3, 17-dione	Normal adrenal and virilizing adenoma	Ichii *et al.* (1962)

(continued next page)

Substrate	Product	Test system	Reference
	17α-Hydroxyprogesterone 11β-Hydroxyandrost-4-ene-3, 17-dione	Cushing's adrenal homogenate	Villee, D. B. *et al.* (1962)
	17α-Hydroxyprogesterone	Fetal testis	Acevedo *et al.* (1961*b*)
	17α-Hydroxyprogesterone	Placenta	Little and Shaw (1961)
		Slices ovary	Ota (1963)
		Slice corpus luteum	Rice *et al.* (1964*c*)
	Testosterone	Adrenal homogenate	Kase and Kowal (1962)
	17α-Hydroxyprogesterone	Fetal testis mince	Bloch *et al.* (1962)
		Feminizing testis	Griffiths *et al.* (1963)
	Androst-4-ene-3, 17-dione	Homogenate of new born adrenal	Villee, C. A. and Loring (1965)
Pregnenolone	Androst-4-ene-3, 17-dione Dehydroepiandrosterone		
Progesterone	Corticosterone Cortisol	Adrenal (neonatal)	Lanman and Silverman (1957)
	17α-Hydroxyprogesterone Testosterone Androst-4-ene-3, 17-dione	Ovary (idiopathic hirsutism)	Goldzieher and Axelrod (1960)
	Testosterone 17α-Hydroxyprogesterone 16α-Hydroxyprogesterone	Fetal testis homogenate	Bloch (1964)
	17α-Hydroxyprogesterone	Testis mince	Acevedo *et al.* (1963)
	Androst-4-ene-3, 17-dione	Minced ovary	Warren and Salhanick (1961)
Progesterone 17α-Hydroxy-progesterone	Testosterone Androst-4-ene-3, 17-dione	Ovarian homogenate	Kase *et al.* (1961)
Progesterone	Androst-4-ene-3, 17-dione (Also 17α-Hydroxy-progesterone)	Adrenal fetal zone	Solomon *et al.* (1958)
Pregnenolone	19-Hydroxyandrost-4-ene-3, 17-dione (2.6%) Testosterone (6.1%) Dehydroepiandrosterone (14.2%) Androst-4-ene-3, 17-dione (17.1%)	Testis from testicular feminization patient	Gwinup *et al.* (1966)
Progesterone	19-Hydroxyandrost-4-ene-3, 17-dione (2.1%) Testosterone (6.8%) Androst-4-ene-3, 17-dione (9.2%)		

(continued next page)

Substrate	Product	Test system	Reference
	17α-Hydroxyprogesterone (I) Testosterone (II) Androst-4-ene-3, 17-dione (III)	Comparative formation from testis % Normal Infertile I 20 26 II 26 1.5 III 1 5	Danezis (1966)
	Androst-4-ene-3, 17-dione 11β-hydroxyandrost-4-ene-3, 17-dione	Fetal adrenal homogenate	Villee, D. B. and Villee, C. A. (1964)
Pregnenolone	Dehydroepiandrosterone 16α-Hydroxyepiandrosterone		
Progesterone	Testosterone	Testicular homogenate Testicular feminization	Neher *et al.* (1965)
Androst-4-ene-3, 17-dione	Testosterone	Homogenate testis and adenoma in testicular feminization	
Pregnenolone 17α-Hydroxy-pregnenolone	Dehydroepiandrosterone Testosterone		
Progesterone	Androst-4-ene-3, 17-dione Testosterone	Minced fetal testis	Bloch *et al.* (1962)
	Testosterone Androst-4-ene-3, 17-dione	Ovarian lipoid cell homogenate	Rosner *et al.* (1964)
Progesterone 17α-Hydroxy-progesterone	5α-Androstane-3, 17-dione	Minced granulosa cell tumor ovary	Bryson *et al.* (1963)
Progesterone	Androst-4-ene-3, 17-dione	Normal placenta soluble homogenate supernatant	Little *et al.* (1963)
	Testosterone Androst-4-ene-3, 17-dione	Masculinovo-blastoma ovary homogenate	Bryson *et al.* (1962)
	Androst-4-ene-3, 17-dione	Homogenate of a virilizing adrenal adenoma	Roversi *et al.* (1963)
	Testosterone Androst-4-ene-3, 17-dione	Fetal (15 weeks) testis mince	Bloch, E. *et al.* (1962)
Progesterone 17α-Hydroxy-progesterone	Testosterone Androst-4-ene-3, 17-dione	Normal adrenal homogenate	Kase and Kowal (1962)
Progesterone	Androst-4-ene-3, 17-dione	Arrhenoblastoma	Wiest *et al.* (1959)

(continued next page)

Substrate	Product	Test system	Reference
	Androst-4-ene-3, 17-dione Testosterone	Fetal testis mince	Acevedo *et al.* (1961*a*)
	17α-Hydroxyprogesterone	Masculinovo-blastoma homogenate	Bryson *et al.* (1962)
	19-Hydroxyandrost-4-ene-3, 17-dione Testosterone	Polycystic ovaries (preparation not specified)	Axelrod and Goldzieher (1962)
Pregnenolone	19-Hydroxyandrost-4-ene-3, 17-dione Dehydroepiandrosterone		
Testosterone	19-Hydroxyandrost-4-ene-3, 17-dione		
Progesterone	Testosterone (not through 17α-hydroxyprogesterone)	Rat testis homogenate	Forchielli *et al.* (1961)
	Testosterone	Feminizing testis	Gwinup *et al.* (1965)
17α-Hydroxy-progesterone	Androst-4-ene-3, 17-dione	Testicular tumor homogenate	Dominguez (1961)
		Ovarian slices	Lanthier and Sandor (1960*b*)
Testosterone	Androst-4-ene-3, 17-dione Adrenosterone 11β-Hydroxyandrost-4-ene-3, 17-dione 11β-Hydroxytestosterone	Adrenal homogenate	Chang *et al.* (1963)
	11β-Hydroxyandrost-4-ene-3, 17-dione	Adrenal	Engel, L. and Dimoline (1963)
	5α-Androstane-3, 17-dione 5β-Androstane-3, 17-dione 16α-Hydroxyandrost-4-ene-3, 17-dione	Supernatant homogenate placenta	Löke (1964)
Testosterone Pregnenolone	Androst-4-ene-3, 17-dione Dehydroepiandrosterone Androst-4-ene-3, 17-dione Testosterone	Interstitial cell tumor of testis homogenate	Gual *et al.* (1962*b*)
Testosterone	Androst-4-ene-3, 17-dione 11β-Hydroxyandrost-4-ene-3, 17-dione 11β-Hydroxytestosterone	Normal adrenal	Chang *et al.* (1963)
Cholesterol Pregnenolone	Dehydroepiandrosterone 11β-Hydroxyandrost-4-ene-3, 17-dione	Adrenal adenoma homogenate	Goldstein *et al.* (1963)
Pregnenolone Progesterone	11β-Hydroxyandrost-4-ene-3 17-dione	Minced fetal adrenals	Villee, D. B. and Driscoll (1965)

(continued next page)

Substrate	Product	Test system	Reference
Progesterone 17α-Hydroxy-progesterone	Testosterone Androst-4-ene-3, 17-dione	Feminizing adrenal tumor	West *et al.* (1964)
Androst-4-ene-3, 17-dione	Testosterone 6β-Hydroxyandrost-4-ene-3, 17-dione		
Testosterone	Androst-4-ene-3, 17-dione 6β-Hydroxyandrost-4-ene-3, 17-dione		
Pregnenolone	Androst-4-ene-3, 17-dione Testosterone Dehydroepiandrosterone	Homogenate testis 'Testicular feminization'	Kase and Morris (1965)
Progesterone	Androst-4-ene-3, 17-dione Testosterone		
3β, 16α-Dihydroxy-androst-5-en-17-one	16α-Hydroxyandrost-4-ene-3, 17-dione	Placenta	Colás *et al.* (1964)
20α-Hydroxy-cholesterol	Dehydroepiandrosterone sulfate	Adrenal slice	Shimizu (1966)
Progesterone 17α-Hydroxy-progesterone	Androst-4-ene-3, 17-dione Testosterone	'Klinefelter' testes	Slaunwhite *et al.* (1962)
Dehydroepi-androsterone Progesterone	Androst-4-ene-3, 17-dione Testosterone	Arrhenoblastoma homogenate	Sandberg and Jenkins (1965*b*)
Pregnenolone Dehydroepi-androsterone	Androst-4-ene-3, 17-dione	Adrenal	Villee, C. A. and Loring (1964)
Pregnenolone Progesterone	Testosterone Androst-4-ene-3, 17-dione	Hyperplastic adrenals	Huseby and Dominguez (1964)
Progesterone	Testosterone Androst-4-ene-3, 17-dione 17α-Hydroxyprogesterone	Normal ovary minced	Kumari and Goldzieher (1966)
Pregnenolone	Testosterone Androst-4-ene-3, 17-dione Dehydroepiandrosterone Progesterone		
Androst-4-ene-3β, 17β-diol	Testosterone Androst-4-ene-3, 17-dione	Hyperplastic adrenal (female)	Colla *et al.* (1964)
Cortisone	Adrenosterone	Placental homogenate	Roversi and Polvani (1963)
Androst-5-ene-3β, 17β-diol-17α-H^3	Testosterone-17α-H^3 (without androst-4-ene-3, 17-dione as intermediate)	Placenta and adrenal tumor homogenate	Baulieu *et al.* (1963)
Cholesterol Pregnenolone	Dehydroepiandrosterone	Adrenal homogenate (adenoma)	Gual *et al.* (1962*a*)

(continued next page)

Substrate	Product	Test system	Reference
Androst-5-ene-3β, 7β, 17β-triol	Androst-5-ene-3β, 7β-diol-17-one	Placental brei	Cédard *et al.* (1964)
17α, 20α-Dihydroxy-cholesterol	Dehydroepiandrosterone	Normal adrenal slices	Shimizu (1965)
20α-Hydroxy-cholesterol	Dehydroepiandrosterone Androst-4-ene-3, 17-dione 11β-Hydroxyandrost-4-ene-3, 17-dione		
Androst-5-ene-3β, 17β-diol	Testosterone	Adrenal tumor placenta	Baulieu *et al.* (1963)
Cholesterol	Dehydroepiandrosterone	Fetal adrenal homogenate	Villee, D. B. *et. al* (1959)
Cholesterol	17α-Hydroxyprogesterone	Testis homogenate	Menon *et al.* (1965)
Progesterone	17α-Hydroxyprogesterone 20α-Hydroxypregn-4-ene-3-one 16α-Hydroxyprogesterone Androst-4-ene-3, 17-dione 19-Hydroxyandrost-4-ene-3, 17-dione	Polycystic ovary medulla	Axelrod and Goldzieher (1967*a*)
Dehydroepi-androsterone sulfate	Dehydroepiandrosterone Testosterone	Sliced polycystic ovarian tissue (Stein-Leventhal syndrome)	Loriaux *et al.* (1967)
Pregnenolone	Testosterone Androst-4-ene-3, 17-dione	Human hilus-cell tumor Ovary 58-year-old woman	Fahmy *et al.* (1967)
Dehydroepi-androsterone sulfate	Testosterone Dehydroepiandrosterone Androst-4-ene-3, 17-dione		
Pregnenolone	17α-Hydroxypregnenolone 16α-Hydroxytestosterone 19-Hydroxytestosterone Androst-4-ene-3, 17-dione 19-Hydroxyandrost-4-ene-3, 17-diol 16α-Hydroxyprogesterone Progesterone 17α-Hydroxyprogesterone 17α, 20α-Dihydroxypregn-4-en-3-one 17α, 20β-Dihydroxypregn-4-en-3-one 20α-Hydroxypregn-4-en-3-one Dehydroepiandrosterone Androst-5-ene-3β, 17β-diol Testosterone Pregn-5-ene-3β, 20β-diol Pregn-5-ene-3β, 20α-diol	Polycystic ovarian tissue	Axelrod and Goldzieher (1967*a*)

(continued next page)

Substrate	Product	Test system	Reference
Pregnenolone	Pregn-5-ene-3β, 20β-diol 17α-Hydroxyprogesterone 17α, 20α-Dihydroxypregn-4-en-3-one Dehydroepiandrosterone Testosterone Androst-4-ene-3, 17-dione	Normal human ovary	Axelrod and Goldzieher (1967*a*)
Progesterone	17α-Hydroxyprogesterone 16α-Hydroxyprogesterone	Polycystic ovarian tissue	
Pregnenolone	17α-Hydroxyprogesterone Dehydroepiandrosterone Androstene-4-ene-3, 17-dione Testosterone	Stroma homogenate	Leymarie and Savard (1968)
Progesterone	Androst-4-ene-3, 17-dione Testosterone 17α-Hydroxyprogesterone		
Pregnenolone	Dehydroepiandrosterone	Pregnancy medullary portion of ovary homogenate	Leymarie and Savard (1968)
Progesterone	17α-Hydroxyprogesterone Androst-4-ene-3, 17-dione Testosterone Estrone and Estradiol-17β (not detected)		
Pregnenolone	Dehydroepiandrosterone	Pregnancy cortical portion of ovary homogenate	
Progesterone	17α-Hydroxyprogesterone Androst-4-ene-3, 17-dione Testosterone Estrone Estradiol-17β		
Progesterone	Testosterone	Minced adrenal congenital hyperplasia 5-year-old boy	Axelrod and Goldzieher (1967*b*)
Pregnenolone	Dehydroepiandrosterone Testosterone	Minced ovary congenital hyperplasia 20-year-old female	
Androst-4-ene-3, 17-dione	Testosterone		
Dehydroepi-androsterone sulfate	Dehydroepiandrosterone 19-Hydroxydehydroepi-androsterone 19-Hydroxydehydroepi-androsterone sulfate	Full-term placenta mitochondria-free supernatant	O'Kelly and Grant (1967)
Pregnenolone	Androst-4-ene-3, 17-dione	Fetal adrenals in culture then homogenized	Villee, D. B. (1968)
Progesterone			

(continued next page)

Substrate	Product	Test system	Reference
Dehydroepi-androsterone sulfate	Dehydroepiandrosterone Testosterone	Polycystic ovarian tissue	Loriaux, D. L. *et al.* (1967)
	Dehydroepiandrosterone Androst-4-ene-3, 17-dione Testosterone	Corpus luteum of early pregnancy	Fahmy *et al.* (1968)
Pregnenolone	Androst-4-ene-3, 17-dione	Male adrenal brei	Axelrod and Goldzieher (1968)
Dehydroepi-androsterone	Androst-5-ene-3β, 17β-diol Androst-4-ene-3, 17-dione Testosterone	Cortical stroma and corpus luteum of pregnancy	Flickinger *et al.* (1968)
Pregnenolone sulfate	Dehydroepiandrosterone sulfate 16α-Hydroxydehydroepi-androsterone sulfate	Fetal adrenal homogenate (12, 15, 19 weeks)	Pérez-Palacios *et al.* (1968)
Progesterone	Testosterone and androst-4-ene-3, 17-dione	Homogenate of testis tissue and interstitial cell tumor	Sharma *et al.* (1967)
17α-Hydroxy-progesterone			
Pregnenolone	Pregnenolone sulfate 17α-Hydroxypregnenolone sulfate	Homogenized feminizing Leydig cell tumor of testis	Pierrepoint *et al.* (1966)
	Pregnenolone sulfate 17α-Hydroxypregnenolone sulfate Dehydroepiandrosterone sulfate	Minced of above	
Acetate	Cholesterol sulfate Dehydroepiandrosterone sulfate Pregnenolone sulfate 17α-Hydroxypregnenolone sulfate	Testicular feminization Gonad slices and fetal adrenal (20 weeks)	Jaffe *et al.* (1968)
Progesterone 17α-Hydroxy-progesterone	Androst-4-ene-3, 17-dione Testosterone 19-Hydroxyandrost-4-ene-3, 17-dione	Metastatic luteinized granulosa cell tumor homogenate	Besch *et al.* (1966)
17α-Hydroxy-progesterone	Testosterone Androst-4-ene-3, 17-dione	Testicular feminization syndrome gonad slices	French *et al.* (1967)
Testosterone	17β-Hydroxy-5α-androstan-3-one 5α-Androstane-3α, 17β-diol	Slices of skin from various regions	Wilson and Walker (1969)

(continued next page)

Substrate	Product	Test system	Reference
	5α-Androstane-3, 17-dione Androst-4-ene-3, 17-dione 5α-Androstane-3α, 17β-diol 17β-Hydroxy-5α-androstan-3-one	Newborn infant prepuce	
Androst-5-ene-3β, 17β-diol	Testosterone	Post-menopausal ovarian tissue	Pesonen *et al.* (1968)
Progesterone	Testosterone Androst-4-ene-3, 17-dione	Slices of normal ovary	Jeffcoate and Prunty (1968)
Progesterone	Testosterone Androst-4-ene-3, 17-dione 11β-Hydroxyandrost-4-ene-3, 17-dione	Hilar cell tumor of ovary	Jeffcoate and Prunty (1968)
Pregnenolone	Testosterone Epitestosterone Dehydroepiandrosterone Androst-4-ene-3, 17-dione		
Dehydroepi-androsterone	Androst-4-ene-3, 17-dione 11β-Hydroxyandrost-4-ene-3, 17-dione Testosterone	Homogenate normal adrenal	Neville *et al.* (1969*a*)
Dehydroepi-androsterone	Androst-5-ene-3β, 17β-diol Testosterone Androst-4-ene-3, 17-dione	Normal homogenized testis (57–72 years)	Rosner and Macome (1970)
Androst-5-ene-3β, 17β-diol	Testosterone		
Pregnenolone	16α-Hydroxydehydroepi-androsterone Dehydroepiandrosterone Androst-4-ene-3, 17-dione Testosterone	Adrenal anencephalic infant	Shahwan *et al.* (1969)
Dehydroepi-androsterone	Androst-4-ene-3, 17-dione 7-Ketodehydro-epiandrosterone	Adenoma homogenate Cushing's syndrome with virilism	Neville *et al.* (1969*b*)
Dehydroepi-androsterone 17α-Hydroxy-pregnenolone	Dehydroepiandrosterone Androst-4-ene-3, 17-dione 11β-Hydroxyandrost-4-ene-3, 17-dione Dehydroepiandrosterone	Adrenal tumor Cushing's syndrome	Cameron *et al.* (1969)
Dehydroepi-androsterone	Androst-5-ene-3β, 17β-diol sulfate		
Dehydroepi-androsterone	Androst-4-ene-3, 17-dione Testosterone 5α-Androstane-3, 17-dione 5α-Androstane-3β, 17β-diol Androst-5-ene-3β, 17β-diol Epiandrosterone	Placental brei (4 to 24 weeks)	Smith and Axelrod (1969)

TABLE II

Biosynthesis of androgen by perfusion
Human

Substrate	Product	Gland	Reference
Acetate	Testosterone Androst-4-ene-3, 17-dione	Testis	Savard *et al.* (1952)
None	11β-Hydroxyandrost-4-ene-3, 17-dione	Adrenals (Cushing's and Conn syndromes)	Shriefers *et al.* (1963)
Testosterone	Androst-4-ene-3, 17-dione	Placenta	Bolté *et al.* (1964)
Androst-5-ene-3β, 7β, 17β-triol	Androst-5-ene-3β, 17β-diol-7-one Androst-5-ene-3β-ol-7, 17-dione	Placenta	Cédard *et al.* (1964)
Dehydroepi-androsterone	Androst-5-ene-3β, 17β-diol	Placenta	Varangot *et al.* (1965)
Cholesterol sulfate	Dehydroepiandrosterone sulfate Androst-5-ene-3β, 17β-diol-3-monosulfate	Human (adrenocortical carcinoma) infused in splenic artery	Roberts *et al.* (1964)
Acetate Cholesterol	Testosterone Dehydroepiandrosterone	Testis 58-year-old man	Knapstein *et al.* (1968)
Pregnenolone Progesterone	Androst-4-ene-3, 17-dione	Ovarian slices	Aakvaag (1969)
Dehydroepi-androsterone sulfate	Dehydroepiandrosterone Androst-5-ene-3β, 17β-diol Testosterone	Normal and polycystic ovaries	Loriaux and Noall (1967)
Androst-4-ene-3, 17-dione	Testosterone		
Androst-4-ene-3, 17-dione	Testosterone	Testis from patient with testicular feminization	Wade *et al.* (1968)
17α-Hydroxy-pregnenolone	Dehydroepiandrosterone sulfate	Mid-term fetus	Pion *et al.* (1967)
Dehydroepi-androsterone Dehydroepi-androsterone sulfate	Testosterone Androst-4-ene-3, 17-dione	Testis *In vivo* perfusion	Knapstein *et al.* (1967*a*)
Progesterone	Testosterone Androst-4-ene-3, 17-dione	Testis *In vivo* perfusion	Knapstein *et al.* (1967*b*)
Dehydroepi-androsterone	Androst-5-ene-3β, 17β-diol Testosterone	*In situ* and *in vivo* testis perfusion	Yamaji *et al.* (1968)
Pregnenolone	Progesterone Dehydroepiandrosterone	Breast cancer *In vivo* perfusion (undergoing adrenalectomy)	Deshpande *et al.* (1969)
17α-Hydroxy-pregnenolone	Dehydroepiandrosterone		
Dehydroepi-androsterone	Androst-4-ene-3, 17-dione		
17α-Hydroxy-progesterone	Androst-4-ene-3, 17-dione		

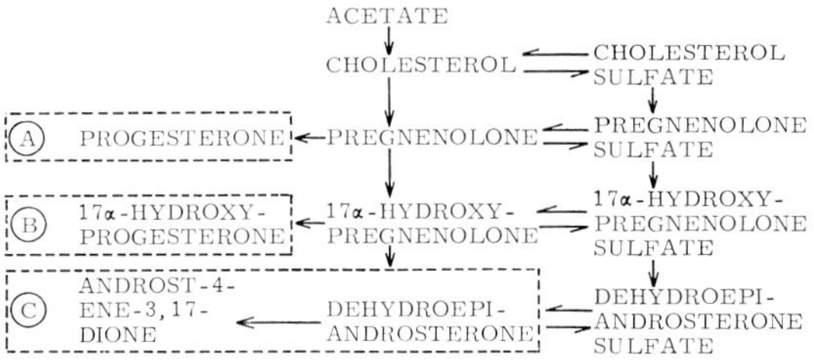

Fig. 2

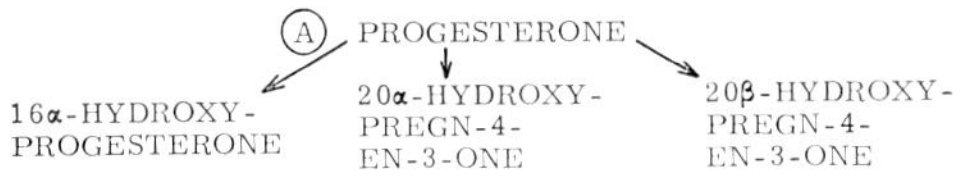

Fig. 3

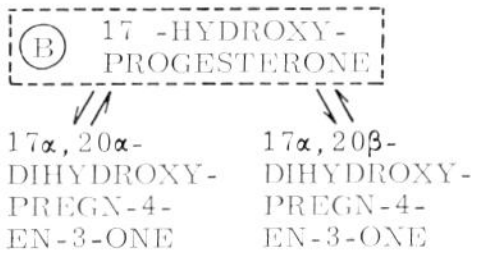

Fig. 4

Figs. 2–5. Biosynthesis of androgens – human testis.

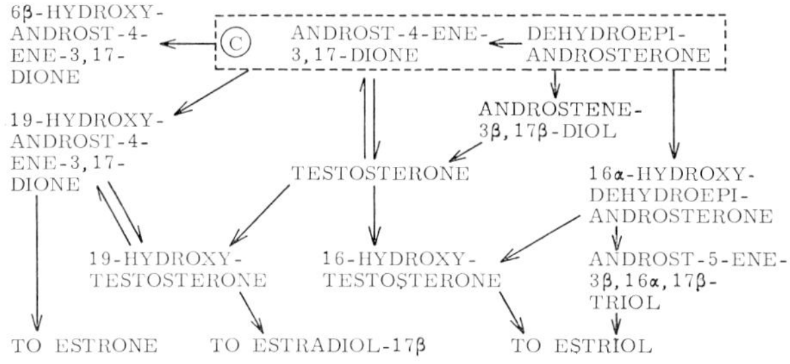

Fig. 5

Figures 3 and 4 list the steroid metabolism changes in progesterone and 17α-hydroxy-progesterone, respectively, which are not directly related to androgen biosynthesis.

Figure 5 is directly related to androgen biosynthesis. As indicated in this figure, the 16α- and 19-hydroxylated derivatives are neutral precursors of importance to estrogen biosynthesis. The function and/or relationship for the addition of the 6β-hydroxy group is not known. Two independent pathways to testosterone biosynthesis are indicated, one directly from androst-4-ene-3,17-dione and the second from dehydroepiandrosterone through androst-5-ene-3β,17β-diol.

Interstitial cell tumors of the testis have an unique capability in that 11β-hydroxylase is present, forming significant quantities of 11β-hydroxyandrost-4-ene-3,17-dione.

The basic biosynthetic sequence of reactions leading to the androgens androst-4-ene-3, 17-dione and dehydroepiandrosterone and the sulfate of the latter compound in the human ovary is precisely the same as the reactions already described for the biosynthetic reactions leading to androgens in the human testis (Fig. 6). The expanded metabolic changes for sections D and E of Figure 6 are presented in Figures 7 and 8 and require no further comments, since these are not biosynthetic routes to androgens.

The biosynthesis of androgens in the ovary is detailed in Figure 9 and, as in the testis, two routes to testosterone are indicated. An added androgen, epitestosterone, is described and its probable close relationship to androst-4-ene-3,17-dione indicated.

The human adrenal produces androgens; Figure 10, outlining the principal biosynthetic

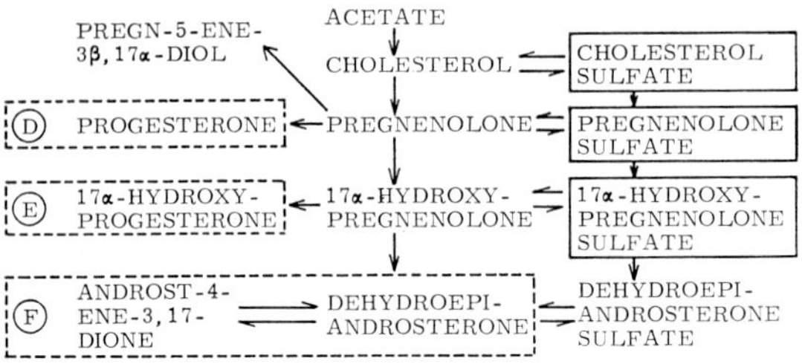

Fig. 6

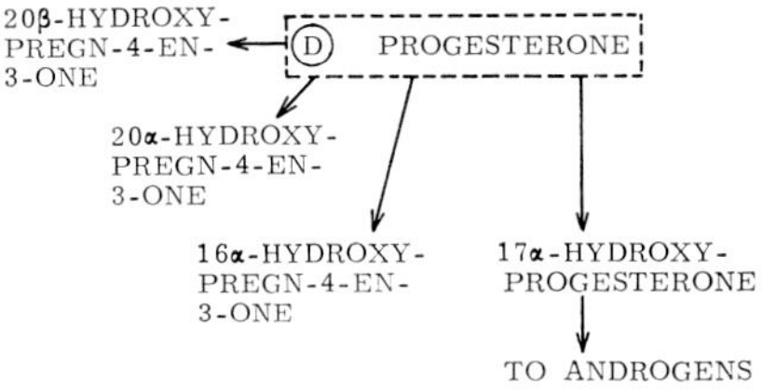

Fig. 7

Figs. 6–9. Biosynthesis of androgens – human ovary.

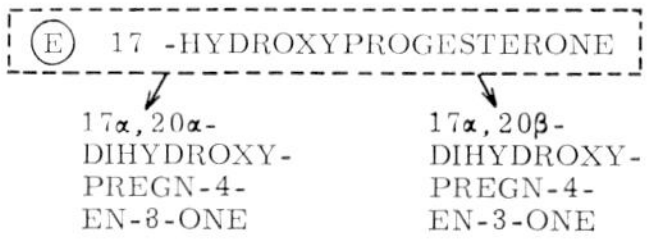

Fig. 8

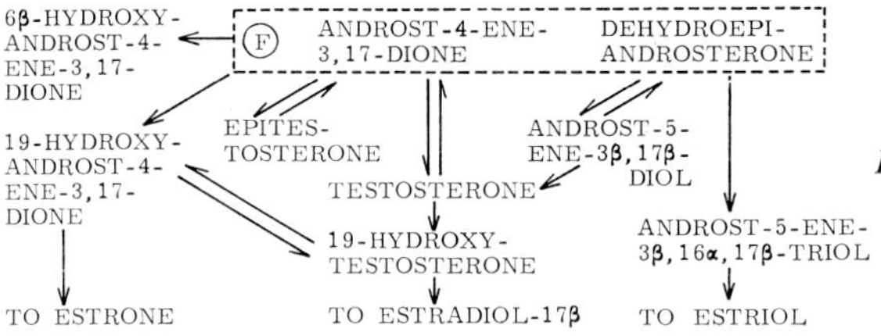

Fig. 9

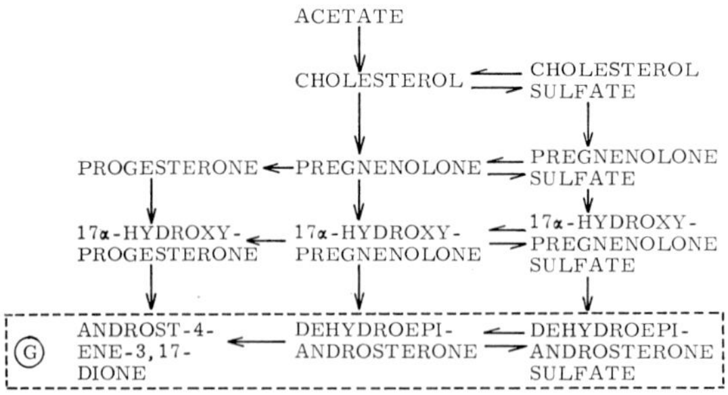

Fig. 10

Figs. 10–11. Biosynthesis of androgens – human adrenal.

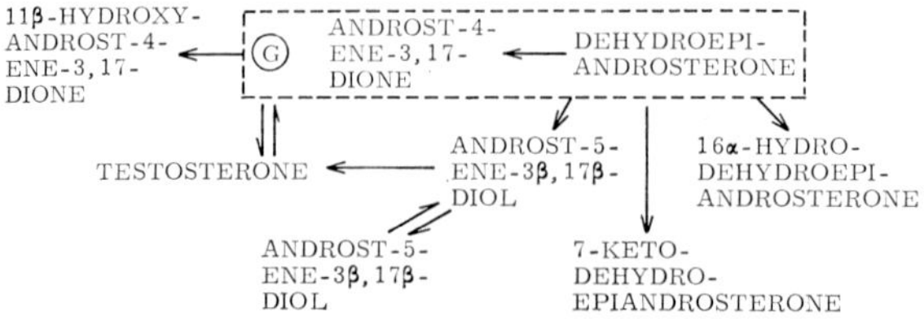

Fig. 11

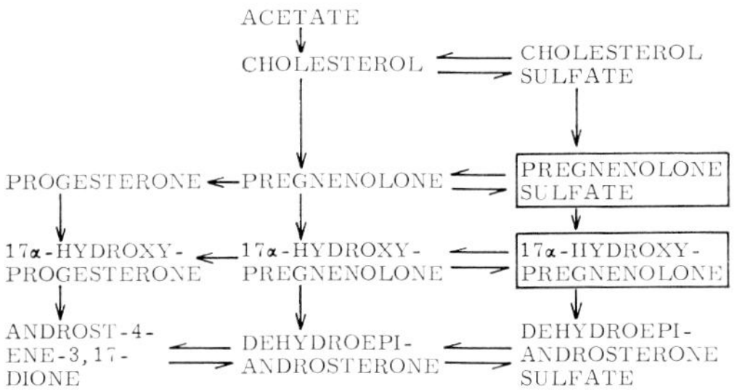

Fig. 12

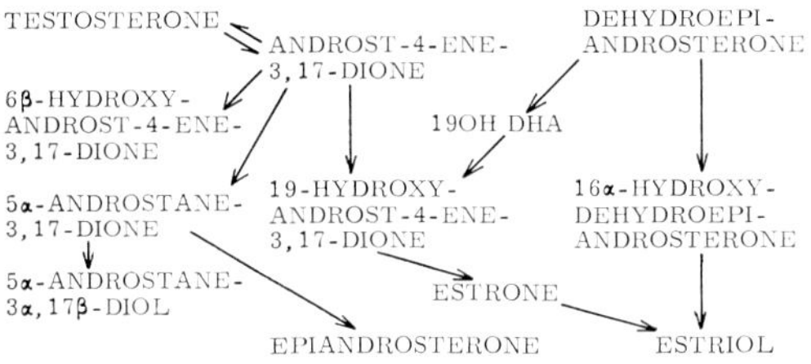

Figs. 12–14. Biosynthesis of androgens – human placenta.

Fig. 13

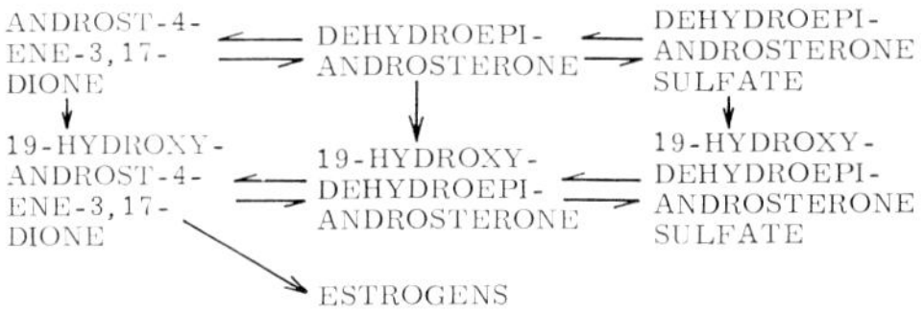

Fig. 14

reactions, indicates a pattern identical to that already suggested for the human testis and ovary. Insert G is related to the C_{19} biosynthetic pathways. Testosterone appears to be formed by at least two pathways, identical to those previously discussed for the androgen pathways in the testis and ovary. Unique relatively weak androgens include 11β-hydroxyandrost-4-ene-3, 17-dione and the 7-keto derivative of dehydroepiandrosterone (Fig. 11).

Figure 12 deals with the biosynthetic routes to androst-4-ene-3, 17-dione, dehydroepiandrosterone and DHS in the human placenta. The biosynthetic routes are a repetition of the previously described pathways for the testis, ovary, and adrenal. Figure 13 indicates the various C_{19} derivatives. Figure 14 deals essentially with the 19-hydroxylated derivatives and the pathway to the estrogens.

PERIPHERAL BIOSYNTHESIS OF TESTOSTERONE

Secretions of the gonads and the adrenals contain testosterone in variable amounts as well as androst-4-ene-3,17-dione, but the effective androgen is testosterone. Testosterone is needed to maintain the effective androgen concentration of the tissues. An important source is the transformation of androst-4-ene-3, 17-dione to testosterone. This point is illustrated by the data in Tables III and IV. In the case of testosterone production in men, the testis does in fact contribute an enormous percentage of the testosterone, perhaps 95% or more (Lipsett *et al.*, 1968). But about 0.3 mg of the total daily production of about 7 mg arises from androst-4-ene-3, 17-dione. Referring to Table III, the entire daily testosterone production in women and in prepuberal children is of the order of 0.3 mg per day and 50% comes from the ovary and about 50% of 0.15 mg from peripheral conversion of androst-4-ene-3, 17-dione.

TABLE III

*Testosterone production**

Source	mg/Day Women (also prepuberal children)	Men
Adrenal	Trace	Trace
Testis	—	6.7
Ovary	0.15	—
Biosynthesis from androst--4-ene-3, 17-dione	0.15	0.3
Total	0.3	7.0

*Lipsett *et al.* (1968).

TABLE IV

*Testosterone production**
in polycystic ovaries and
idiophathic hirsutism

Source	Normal women	mg/Day Polycystic ovaries	Idiopathic hirsutism
Secreted from ovary and/or adrenal	0.15	0.3	0.18
From androst--4-ene-3, 17-dione	0.15	0.9	0.54
Total	0.3	1.2	0.72

*Lipsett *et al.* (1968).

The peripheral contribution to the daily testosterone production is particularly striking in Table IV. The contributions to testosterone production are divided between endocrine glands and the amount arising from androst-4-ene-3,17-dione. In polycystic ovaries the rate of testosterone production is about doubled but the contribution of biosynthesized testosterone from the 17-ketosteroid precursor was increased six-fold (Table IV). In idiopathic hirsutism the increased secretion of testosterone was minimal, while the plasma conversion of androst-4-ene-3,17-dione to testosterone was increased from 0.15 to 0.54 mg/day (Table IV).

BIOSYNTHESIS IN TARGET TISSUE

For a substance to express biological activity there appears to be a requirement of attachment of the substance to an active site. In the case of androgens, it is now visualized that for maximum biological activity there is the need for an endocrine gland which produces a hormone like testosterone or a group of steroids such as dehydroepiandrosterone, dehydroepiandrosterone sulfate and androst-4-ene-3, 17-dione, which are convertible to testosterone in the plasma. But testosterone is still inadequate to trigger off the necessary reactions in certain target tissues. At these sites additional biosynthetic changes are possible and in fact necessary.

After the intravenous administration of testosterone, significant amounts of 17β-hydroxy-5α-androstan-3-one are found within the prostatic nuclei (Bruchovsky and Wilson, 1968; Anderson and Liao, 1968). It has also been demonstrated that the 17β-hydroxy-5α-androstan-3-one and not testosterone is bound to nuclear chromatin within 15 minutes of testosterone administration (Bruchovsky and Wilson, 1968). These observations have been made in the rat and not in man. It is quite likely that this is a factor which must be considered even at this time in the larger context of androgen biosynthesis.

SUMMARY AND CONCLUSIONS

Androgen biosynthesis in man is similar if not identical to that of many species of animals and is identical for all steroid-producing tissues. If the goal for androgen biosynthesis is the formation of the two weak androgens, androst-4-ene-3,17-dione and dehydroepiandrosterone, and the reserve form of androgens, dehydroepiandrosterone sulfate, then the general plan of biosynthesis could be visualized as involving three parallel channels:

The middle channel progresses from cholesterol to pregnenolone to 17α-hydroxypregnenolone to dehydroepiandrosterone. A second parallel channel involves the sulfate esters of the same sequence of reactions leading to the inactive dehydroepiandrosterone sulfate, which is easily convertible to the free compound. At all levels the free and sulfated compounds are interchangeable.

A third channel involves the free steroids with the ring A Δ^4-3-keto configuration. This sequence originates from cholesterol to pregnenolone to progesterone and proceeds to 17α-hydroxyprogesterone and androst-4-ene-3,17-dione, a weak androgen. The free Δ^4-3-keto compounds of this channel are related to the free Δ^5-3β-ol compounds of the middle channel in that the latter are converted to the former in essentially a non-reversible reaction.

Having the weak androgens, androst-4-ene-3,17-dione and dehydroepiandrosterone, the latter is converted to the former, which on reduction at C-17 forms the highly active androgen, testosterone. A second pathway involves the reduction of dehydroepiandrosterone to androst-5-ene-3β, 17β-diol and oxidation of ring A to testosterone.

All the reactions thus far have been related to steroid-producing tissues. The reactions of inactive C_{19} or weakly active androgens to testosterone may and does proceed in peripheral non-endocrine tissue. Thus it is calculated that 50% of testosterone of the daily production of this highly active androgen in women's plasma takes place from androst-4-ene-3,17-dione peripherally.

Another peripheral source of testosterone originates from androst-4-ene-3,17-dione and dehydroepiandrosterone directly and from 17α-hydroxyprogesterone and 17α-hydroxypregnenolone, respectively, indirectly.

Finally, biosynthetic reactions are still operative at the target tissue. Thus at the level of prostate stimulation, the highly active testosterone is not the hormone which triggers the reaction. At least in the rat prostate testosterone is reduced to 17β-hydroxy-5α-androstan-3-one and it is this androgen which acts as the effective androgen.

This androgen biosynthesis occurs in the testis, ovary, adrenal, and placenta at the levels of C_{27} to C_{21} to C_{19} steroids as well as interactions among the C_{19} steroids. Peripherally, biosynthetic reactions involve C_{21} to C_{19} steroids and interaction among the C_{19} steroids and finally even the highly active C_{19} androgen, testosterone, may require an additional biosynthetic step. In the case of the rat prostate, the steroids undergo reduction to 17β-hydroxy-5α-androstan-3-one and then trigger the required reactions.

REFERENCES

AAKVAAG, A. (1969): Pathways in the biosynthesis of androstenedione in the human ovary *in vitro*. *Acta endocr. (Kbh.)*, *60*, 517

ACEVEDO, H. F., AXELROD, L. R., ISHIKAWA, E. and TAKAKI, F. (1961*a*): Steroidogenesis in the human fetal testis: The conversion of pregnenolone-7α-H^3 to dehydroepiandrosterone, testosterone, 4-androstene-3, 17-dione. *J. clin. Endocr.*, *21*, 1611.

ACEVEDO, H. F., AXELROD, L. R., ISHIKAWA, E. and TAKAKI, F. (1961*b*): Steroidogenesis in the human fetal testis. In: *43rd Meeting of the Endocrine Society*, *New York*, p. 22.

ACEVEDO, H. F., AXELROD, L. R., ISHIKAWA, E. and TAKAKI, F. (1963): Studies in fetal metabolism. II. Metabolism of progesterone-4-C^{14} and pregnenolone-7α-H^3 in human fetal testes. *J. clin. Endocr.*, *23*, 885.

ADADEVOH, K. K. and ENGEL, L. L. (1964): Progesterone-4-C^{14} metabolism by hyperplastic human adrenal tissue. In: *Abstracts, 6th International Congress of Biochemistry, New York,* Abstract VII.

ANDERSON, K. M. and LIAO, S. (1968): Selective retention of dihydrotestosterone by prostatic nuclei. *Nature, (Lond.), 219*, 277.

AXELROD, L. R. (1965): Metabolic patterns of steroid biosynthesis in young and aged human testes. *Biochim. biophys. Acta (Amst.)*, *97*, 551.

AXELROD, L. and GOLDZIEHER, J. (1962): Mechanism of biochemical aromatization of steroids. *J. clin. Endocr.*, *22*, 537.

AXELROD, L. R. and GOLDZIEHER, J. W. (1967*a*): The polycystic ovary. VIII. The metabolism of 5-pregnenolone, progesterone, testosterone, 4-androstenedione and oestrone by normal and polycystic ovarian tissues. *Acta endocr. (Kbh.)*, *56*, 255.

AXELROD, L. R. and GOLDZIEHER, J. W. (1967*b*): Steroid biosynthesis by adrenal and ovarian tissue in congenital adrenal hyperplasia. *Acta endocr. (Kbh.)*, *56*, 453.

AXELROD, L. R. and GOLDZIEHER, J. W. (1968): Free steroid biosynthesis from 5[-4-^{14}C-] pregnenolone in normal human adrenal tissue. *Biochim. biophys. Acta (Amst.)*, *152*, 391.

BAULIEU, E.-E., WALLACE, E. and LIEBERMAN, S. (1963): The conversion *in vitro* of Δ^5-androstene-3β, 17β-diol, 17α-H^3 to testosterone-17α-H^3 by human adrenal and placental tissue. *J. biol. Chem.*, *238*, 1316.

BESCH, P. K., BYRON, R. C., BARRY, R. D., TETERIS, N. J., HAMWI, G. J., VORYS, N. and ULLERY, J. C. (1963): Testosterone synthesis by a Brenner tumor. Part II. *In vitro* biosynthetic steroid conversion of a Brenner tumor. *Amer. J. Obstet. Gynec.*, *86*, 1021.

BESCH, P. K., WATSON, D. J., VORYS, N., HAMWI, G. J., BARRY, R. D. and BARNETT, E. B. (1966): *In vitro* biosynthetic studies of endocrine tumors. VI. Malignant granulosa cell tumor. *Amer. J. Obstet. Gynec.*, *96*, 466.

BLOCH, E. (1964): Metabolism of 4-^{14}C-progesterone by human fetal testis and ovaries. *Endocrinology*, *74*, 833.

BLOCH, E. and BENIRSCHKE, K. (1959): Synthesis *in vitro* of steroids by human fetal adrenal gland slices. *J. biol. Chem.*, *234*, 1085.

BLOCH, E. and BENIRSCHKE, K. (1962): Steroidogenic capacity of fetal adrenals *in vitro*. In: *The Human Adrenal Cortex*, pp. 589–595. Editor: A. R. Currie. Livingstone Publ., Edinburgh.

BLOCH, E., DORFMAN, R. I. and PINCUS, G. (1956): The conversion of acetate to dehydroepiandrosterone by human adrenal gland slices. *Arch. Biochem.*, *61*, 245.

BLOCH, E., TISSENBAUM, B. and BENIRSCHKE, K. (1962): The conversion of progesterone to 17α-hydroxyprogesterone, testosterone and Δ^4-androstene-3, 17-dione by human fetal testes *in vitro*. *Biochim. biophys. Acta (Amst.)*, *60*, 182.

BOLTÉ, E., MANCUSO, S., DRAY, F., BAULIEU, E.-E. and DICZFALUSY, E. (1964): Conversion of testosterone-17α-^{3}H into 17β-estradiol-17α-^{3}H by human placentas perfused *in situ*. *Steroids*, *4*, 613.

BRADY, R. O. and GURIN, S. (1951): The synthesis of radioactive cholesterol and fatty acids *in vitro*. *J. biol. Chem.*, *189*, 371.

BRUCHOVSKY, N. and WILSON, J. D. (1968): The intranuclear binding of testosterone and 5α-androstan-17β-ol-3-one by rat prostate. *J. biol. Chem.*, *243*, 5953.

BRYSON, M. J., DOMINGUEZ, O. V., KAISER, I. H., SAMUELS, L. T. and SWEAT, M. T. (1962): Enzymic steroid conversions in a masculinovoblastoma. *J. clin. Endocr.*, *22*, 773.

BRYSON, M. J., KAISER, I. H. and SWEAT, M. L. (1963): Enzymic steroid conversion. *Minnesota Med.*, *46*, 1235.

BURSTEIN, S., KIMBALL, H. L. and GUT, M. (1970): Transformation of labeled cholesterol, 20α-hydroxycholesterol, (22R)-22-hydroxycholesterol, and (22R)-20α-22-dihydroxycholesterol by adrenal acetone-dried preparations from guinea pigs, cattle and man: II. Kinetic studies. *Steroids*, *15*, 809.

CALVIN, H. I. and LIEBERMAN, S. (1964): Evidence that steroid sulfates serve as biosynthetic intermediates. II. *In vitro* conversion of pregnenolone-^{3}H sulfate-^{35}S to 17α-hydroxypregnenolone-^{3}H sulfate-^{35}S. *Biochemistry*, *3*, 259.

CAMERON, E. H. D., BAILLIE, A. H., GRANT, J. K., MILNE, J. A. and THOMSON, J. (1966): Transformation *in vitro* of (7α-^{3}H)-dehydroepiandrosterone to (^{3}H)testosterone by skin from men. *J. Endocr.*, *35*, xix.

CAMERON, E. H. D., JONES, T., JONES, D., ANDERSON, A. B. M. and GRIFFITHS, K. (1969): Further studies on the relationship between C_{19}- and C_{21}-steroid synthesis in the human adrenal gland. *J. Endocr.*, *45*, 215.

CARSTENSEN, H. C. H. (1961): The effect of human interstitial cell-stimulating hormone on the biosynthesis *in vitro* of testosterone from 17α-hydroxy-Δ^5-pregnen-3β-ol, 20-one by human and rat testes. A preliminary report. *Acta Soc. Med. upsalien.*, *66*, 129.

CEDARD, L., FILLMAN, B., KNUPPEN, R., LISBOA, B. P. and BREUER, H. (1964): Metabolism and aromatization of 7-substituted C_{19} steroids in the placenta. *Z. Chem.*, *338*, 89.

CHANG, E., MITTLEMAN, A. and DAO, T. L. (1963): Metabolism of 4-C^{14}-testosterone in normal human adrenal homogenate. *J. biol. Chem.*, *238*, 913.

CHAUDHURI, A. C., HARADA, Y., SHIMIZU, K., GUT, M. and DORFMAN, R. I. (1962): Biosynthesis of pregnenolone from 22-hydroxycholesterol. *J. biol. Chem.*, *237*, 703.

CLEVELAND, W. W., RICE, B. F., SANDBERG, D. H., AHMAD, N. and SAVARD, K. (1965): Testicular function *in vivo* and *in vitro* in male pseudohermaphroditism. In: *Abstracts, VIth Pan-American Congress of Endocrinology*, p. E 166. ICS No. 99. Excerpta Medica, Amsterdam.

COHN, G. L. and MULROW, P. J. (1963): Androgen release and synthesis *in vitro* by human adult adrenal glands. *J. clin. Invest.*, *42*, 64.

COHN, G. L., MULROW, P. J. and DUNNE, V. C. (1963): *In vitro* synthesis of dehydroepiandrosterone sulfate by an adrenal adenoma. *J. clin. Endocr.*, *23*, 671.

COLAS, A., HEINRICHS, W. L. and TATUM, H. J. (1964): The metabolism of 3β, 16α-dihydroxyandrost-5-en-17-one by human placenta. In: *6th Meeting, International Congress of Biochemistry, New York*, p. 569.

COLLA, J. C., COHN, M. L. and UNGAR, F. (1964): Conversion of 4-androstene-3β, 17β-diol-4-C^{14} by human adrenals *in vitro*. *Proc. Soc. exp. Biol. (N.Y.)*, *117*, 717.

COLLA, J. C., LIBERTI, J. P. and UNGAR, F. (1966): Inhibition of 16α-hydroxylation in human testis tissue by SU-9055. *Steroids*, *8*, 25.

DANEZIS, J. M. (1966): Steroidogenesis in mammalian gonads as related to fertility and infertility. *Fertil. and Steril.*, *17*, 488.

DESHPANDE, N., JENSEN, V., BULBROOK, R. D. and DOOUSS, T. W. (1969): Steroid synthesis in human adrenal glands *in vivo*. *Acta endocr. (Kbh.)*, *61 (Supp. 138)*, 47.

DIXON, R., VINCENT, V. and KASE, N. (1965): Biosynthesis of steroid sulfates by normal human testis. *Steroids*, *6*, 757.

DOMINGUEZ, O. V. (1961): Biosynthesis of steroids by testicular tumors complicating congenital adrenocortical hyperplasia. *J. clin. Endocr.*, *21*, 663.

ENGEL, F. L., MCPHERSON, H. T., FETTER, B. F., BAGGETT, B., ENGEL, L. L., CARTER, P., FIELDING, L. L., SAVARD, K. and DORFMAN, R. I. (1964): Clinical, morphological and biochemical studies on a malignant testicular tumor. *J. clin. Endocr.*, *24*, 528.

ENGEL, L. L. and DIMOLINE, A. (1963): The metabolism of 19-hydroxyandrost-4-ene-3, 17-dione and testosterone by human adrenal tissue. *J. Endocr.*, *26*, 233.

ENGEL, L. L., LANMAN, G., SCULLY, R. E. and VILLEE, D. B. (1966): Studies on an interstitial cell tumor of the testis: Formation of cortisol-^{14}C from acetate-1-^{14}C. *J. clin. Endocr.*, *26*, 381.

FAHMY, D., GRIFFITHS, K., TURNBULL, A. C. and SYMINGTON, T. (1967): Testosterone and androstenedione formation from dehydroepiandrosterone sulphate by hilus-cell tumour tissue from a human subject. *Biochem. J.*, *104*, 5P.

FAHMY, D., GRIFFITHS, K. and TURNBULL, A. C. (1968): Oestrogen formation from dehydroepiandrosterone sulphate by tissue from a corpus luteum of early human pregnancy: Some evidence for 19-hydroxydehydroepiandrosterone sulphate synthesis. *Biochem. J.*, *106*, 56P.

FLICKINGER, G. L., WU, C.-H. and TOUCHSTONE, J. C. (1968): Neutral steroid metabolites of dehydroepiandrosterone-7α-^{3}H in human ovarian tissues. *Steroids*, *11*, 398.

FORCHIELLI, E., GUT, M. and DORFMAN, R. I. (1961): A new pathway for the biosynthesis of testosterone. In: *43rd Meeting, The Endocrine Society, New York,* p. 25.

FRENCH, A. P. and WARREN, J. C. (1965): Steroid-3β-sulfatase in fetal and placental tissues. *Steroids*, *6*, 865.

FRENCH, F. S., BAGGETT, B., VAN WYK, J. J. and FORCHIELLI, E. (1965): Studies of testicular feminization. In: *47th Meeting, The Endocrine Society, New York*, p. 26.

FRENCH, F. S., SPOONER, I. and BAGGETT, B. (1967): Metabolism of 17-hydroxyprogesterone in testicular tissue from a patient with the syndrome of testicular feminization. *J. clin. Endocr.*, *27*, 437.

GANIS, F. M., WILDASIN, G. L. and CONNOR, T. B. (1965): *In vitro* production of dehydroepiandrosterone by virilizing Krukenberg tumor of the ovary. *Fed. Proc.*, *24*, 535.

GOLDSTEIN, M., GUT, M. and DORFMAN, R. I. (1960): Conversion of pregnenolone to dehydroepiandrosterone. *Biochim. biophys. Acta (Amst.)*, *38*, 190.

GOLDSTEIN, M., GUT, M., DORFMAN, R. I., SOFFER, L. J. and GABRILOVE, J. L. (1963): Biosynthesis of corticoids and androgens in an adenoma from a Cushing's syndrome patient. *Acta endocr. (Kbh.)*, *42*, 187.

GOLDZIEHER, J. W. and AXELROD, L. R. (1960): Adrenal and ovarian steroidogenesis in the sclerocystic ovary syndrome. *First International Congress of Endocrinology, Copenhagen*, p. 617.

GOWER, D. B. and HASLEWOOD, G. A. (1961): Biosynthesis of androst-16-en-3α-ol from acetate by testicular slices. *J. Endocr.*, *23*, 253.

GRIFFITHS, K., GRANT, J. K. and WHYTE, W. G. (1963): Steroid biosynthesis *in vitro* by cryptorchid testes from a case of testicular feminization. *J. clin. Endocr.*, *23*, 1044.

GRIFFITHS, K., GRANT, J. K., BROWNING, M. C. K., CUNNINGHAM, D. and BARR, G. (1966*a*): Steroid biosynthesis *in vitro* by tissue from granulosa cell multilocular cystadenoma. *J. Endocr.*, *35*, 299.

GRIFFITHS, K., GRANT, J. K., BROWNING, M. C. K., WHYTE, W. G. and SHARP, J. L. (1966*b*): Steroid synthesis *in vitro* by tumor tissue from a dysgenetic gonad. *J. Endocr.*, *34*, 155.

GUAL, C., LEMUS, A. E., KLINE, I. T., GUT, M. and DORFMAN, R. I. (1962*a*): Biosynthesis of dehydroepiandrosterone in a patient with a virilizing adenoma. *J. clin. Endocr.*, *22*, 1193.

GUAL, C., SANCHEZ, J., DORFMAN, R. I. and ROSENTHAL, I. M. (1962*b*): Androgen biosynthesis in an interstitial cell tumor of the testis. *J. clin. Endocr.*, *22*, 1040.

GWINUP, G., BESCH, P. K., WIELAND, R. G. and HAMWI, G. J. (1965): Studies of the mechanism of production of the testicular feminization syndrome. In: *47th Meeting, The Endocrine Society, New York,* p. 92.

GWINUP, G., WIELAND, R. G., BESCH, P. K. and HAMWI, G. J. (1966): Studies on the mechanism of the production of the testicular feminization syndrome. *Amer. J. Med.*, *41*, 448.

HAMMERSTEIN, J., RICE, B. F. and SAVARD, K. (1964): Steroid hormone formation in the human ovary: I. Identification of steroids formed *in vitro* from acetate-1-C^{14} in the corpus luteum. *J. clin. Endocr.*, 24, 597.

HAMWI, G. J., BYRON, R. C., BESCH, P. K., VORYS, N., TETERIS, N. J. and ULLERY, J. C. (1963): Testosterone synthesis by a Brenner tumor. Part I. Clinical evidence of masculinization during pregnancy. *Amer. J. Obstet. Gynec.*, *86*, 1015.

HUANG, W. Y. (1966): Formation of testosterone and 6β-hydroxy-Δ^4-androstene-3,17-dione in human corpus luteum tissue. In: *48th Meeting, The Endocrine Society, Chicago*, p. 132.

HUANG, W. Y. (1967): Studies on the hydroxylation and metabolism of Δ^4-androstene-3, 17-dione-7H^3 in the human corpus luteum tissue. *Steroids*, *9*, 485.

HUSEBY, R. A. and DOMINGUEZ, O. V. (1964): HCG stimulation of androgen production by hyperplastic adrenals of castrated BALB/c mice. In: *46th Meeting, The Endocrine Society, San Francisco,* p. 60.

ICHII, S., FORCHIELLI, E., CASSIDY, C. E., ROSOFF, C. B. and DORFMAN, R. I. (1962): Biosynthesis of androgens by homogenates of normal and abnormal human adrenal glands. *Biochem. biophys. Res. Commun.*, *9*, 344.

JAFFE, R. B., PEREZ-PALACIOS, G., LAMONT, K. G. and GIVNER, M. L. (1968): *De novo* steroid sulfate biosynthesis. *J. clin. Endocr.*, *28*, 1671.

JEFFCOATE, S. L. and PRUNTY, F. T. G. (1968): Steroid synthesis *in vitro* by a hilar cell tumor. *Amer. J. Obstet. Gynec.*, *101*, 684.

KASE, N., FORCHIELLI, E. and DORFMAN, R. I. (1961): *In vitro* production of testosterone and androst-4-ene-3, 17-dione in a human ovarian homogenate. *Acta endocr. (Kbh.)*, *37*, 19.

KASE, N. and KOWAL, J. (1962): *In vitro* production of testosterone in a human adrenal homogenate. *J. clin. Endocr.*, *22*, 925.

KASE, N. and MORRIS, J. M. (1965): Steroid synthesis in the cryptorchid testes of three cases of the 'testicular feminizing syndrome.' *Amer. J. Obstet. Gynec.*, *91*, 102.

KNAPSTEIN, P., WENDLBERGER, F., MENZEL, P. and OERTEL, G. W. (1967*a*): Biosynthese von Steroid-hormonen in menschlichen Gonaden. II. In-vivo-Perfusion eines menschlichen Testis mit (4-^{14}C) Androstenolon und (7α-^{3}H) Androstenolon-(^{35}S) Sulfat. *Hoppe-Seylers Z. physiol. Chem.*, *348*, 990.

KNAPSTEIN, P., WENDLBERGER, F., MENZEL, P., TREIBER, L. and OERTEL, G. W. (1967*b*): Biosynthese von Steroidhormonen in menschlichen Gonaden. IV. In-vivo-perfusion eines Testis mit (7α-^{3}H) Progesteron und (4-^{14}C) Androstenolon. *Hoppe-Seylers Z. physiol. Chem.*, *348*, 1066.

KNAPSTEIN, P., WENDLBERGER, F., MENZEL, P., OERTEL, G. and TOUCHSTONE, J. C. (1968): Biosynthesis of steroid hormones in human gonads. VI. *In vivo* perfusion of the testis with 1-^{14}C-acetate and 7α-^{3}H-cholesterol. *Steroids*, *12*, 191.

KOKHANENKO, E. M. (1965): Estrogen biosynthesis *in vitro* in tissue of polycystic ovaries. *Vop. eksper. Klin. Endokr. Sb.* Moscow, 68. (Ref. *Zh.*, *Biol. Khim.*, 1966, Abstract No. 3F1416.)

KUMARI, L. and GOLDZIEHER, J. W. (1966): *In vitro* steroidogenesis in normal human ovarian tissue. *Acta endocr. (Kbh.)*, *52*, 455.

LANMAN, J. T. and SILVERMAN, L. M. (1957): *In vitro* steroidogenesis in the human neonatal adrenal gland, including observations on human adult and monkey adrenal glands. *Endocrinology*, *60*, 433.

LANTHIER, A. and SANDOR, T. (1960*a*): '*In vitro*' production of androgenic steroids by human normal and 'Stein-Leventhal type' ovarian slices. *Metabolism*, *9*, 861.

LANTHIER, A. and SANDOR, T. (1960*b*): *In vitro* metabolism of 17α-hydroxyprogesterone by slices of normal human ovaries and polymicrocystic ovaries with hyperthecosis. *Laval méd.*, *30*, 624.

LEBEAU, M. C., ALBERGA, A. and BAULIEU, E.-E. (1964): Adrenal biosynthesis of dehydroepiandrosterone sulfate. *Biochem. biophys. Res. Commun.*, *17*, 570.

LEON, N., CASTRO, M. N. and DORFMAN, R. I. (1962): Biosynthesis of testosterone by a Stein-Leventhal ovary. *Acta endocr. (Kbh.)*, *39*, 411.

LEYMARIE, P. and SAVARD, K. (1968): Steroid hormone formation in the human ovary. VI. Evidence for two pathways of synthesis of androgens in the stromal compartment. *J. clin. Endocr.*, *28*, 1547.

LIPSETT, M. B., MIGEON, C. J., KIRSCHNER, M. A. and BARDIN, C. W. (1968): Physiologic basis of disorders of androgen metabolism. (Combined clinical staff conference at the National Institutes of Health). *Ann. intern. Med.*, *68*, 1327.

LITTLE, B. and SHAW, A. (1961): The conversion of progesterone to 17α-hydroxyprogesterone by human placenta *in vitro*. *Acta endocr. (Kbh.)*, *36*, 455.

LITTLE, B., SHAW, A. and PURDY, R. (1963): The conversion of progesterone to 16α-hydroxypregn-4-ene-3, 20-dione and androst-4-ene-3, 17-dione by human placenta *in vitro*. *Acta endocr. (Kbh.)*, *43*, 510

LÖKE, K. H. (1964): Metabolism of testosterone by human placenta. In: *Sixth International Congress of Biochemistry, New York*, 1964, p. 584.

LONGCHAMPT, J. E., GUAL, C., EHRENSTEIN, M. and DORFMAN, R. I. (1960): 19-Hydroxy-Δ^{4}-androstene-3, 17-dione, an intermediate in estrogen biosynthesis. *Endocrinology*, *66*, 416.

LORIAUX, D. L., KAUFMAN, R. H. and NOALL, M. W. (1967): The conversion of dehydroepiandrosterone sulfate to testosterone by human polycystic ovarian tissue. *Europ. J. Steroids*, *2*, 85.

LORIAUX, D. L. and NOALL, M. W. (1967): The metabolism of dehydroepiandrosterone sulfate by normal and polycystic human ovarian tissue. *Europ. J. Steroids*, *2*, 569.

LOUTFI, G. and HAGERMAN, D. D. (1965): Metabolism of progesterone and pregnenolone by an ovarian granulosa cell tumor *in vitro*. In: *47th Meeting, The Endocrine Society, New York*, p. 106.

MCKERNS, K. W. and NORDSTRAND, E. (1964): Simple method for tissue extraction and gas chromatographic separation of estrogens. *Biochim. Biophys. Acta (Amst.)*, *82*, 198.

MENON, K. M. J., DROSDOWSKY. M., DORFMAN, R. I. and FORCHIELLI, E. (1965): Sidechain cleavage of cholesterol-26-^{14}C and 20α-hydroxy-cholesterol-22-^{14}C by rat testis mitochondrial preparations and the effects of gonadotrophin administration and hypophysectomy. *Steroids*, *5 (Supp. 1)*, 95.

MUROTA, S.-I., SHIKITA, M. and TAMAOKI, B.-I. (1966): Androgen formation in the testicular tissue of patients with prostatic carcinoma. *Biochim. biophys. Acta (Amst.)*, *117*, 241.

NEHER, R., KAHNT, F. W., ROVERSI, G. D. and BOMPIANI, A. (1965): Steroid transformations *in vitro* by testicular tissue from two cases of testicular feminisation. *Acta endocr. (Kbh.)*, *49*, 177.

NEVILLE, A. M., ORR, J. C., TROFIMOW, N. D. and ENGEL, L. L. (1969*a*): A time study of the *in vitro* metabolism of 3β-hydroxyandrost-5-en-17-one by human adrenocortical tissue. *Steroids*, *14*, 97.

NEVILLE, A. M. and WEBB, J. L. (1965): The *in vitro* formation of 3β-hydroxyandrost-5-ene-7, 17-dione by human adrenal glands. *Steroids*, *6*, 421.

NEVILLE, A. M., WEBB, J. L. and SYMINGTON, T. (1969*b*): The *in vitro* utilization of (4-^{14}C)-dehydroisoandrosterone by human adrenocortical tumors associated with virilism. *Steroids*, *13*, 821.

NOALL, M. W., ALEXANDER, I. and ALLEN, W. M. (1962): Dehydroisoandrosterone synthesis by the human ovary. *Biochim. biophys. Acta (Amst.)*, *59*, 520.

NOWACZYNSKI, W. and KOIW, E. (1963): Primary hyperaldosteronism. A renal adenoma with 6β-hydroxycorticosterone and its 11-dehydro derivative in the urine. *Un. méd. Can.*, *92*, 248.

O'DONNELL, V. J. and MCCAIG, J. G. (1959): Biosynthesis of steroids by human ovaries. *Biochem. J.*, *71*, 9P.

O'KELLY, D. A. and GRANT, J. K. (1967): Formation of 3β, 19-dihydroxyandrost-5-en-17-one and its sulphate by human placenta *in vitro*. *Europ. J. Steroids*, *2*, 209.

OTA, S. (1963): Biosynthesis of steroid hormones. *Nippon Naibumpi Gakkai Zasshi (Folia Endocr. Jap.)*, *39*, 842.

PÉREZ-PALACIOS, G., PÉREZ, A. E. and JAFFE, R. B. (1968): Conversion of pregnenolone-7α-^{3}H-sulfate to other Δ^5-3β-hydroxysteroid sulfates by the human fetal adrenal *in vitro*. *J. clin. Endocr.*, *28*, 19.

PESONEN, S., IKONEN, M., PROCOPÉ, B. J. and SAURE, A. (1968): Androst-5-ene-3β,17β-diol in ovary of post-menopausal hyperoestrogenic women. *In vitro* metabolism; histological and histochemical studies; clinical data of the patients. *Acta endocr. (Kbh.)*, *58*, 364.

PIERREPOINT, C. G., GRIFFITHS, K., GRANT, J. K. and STEWART, J. S. S. (1966): Neutral steroid sulphation and oestrogen biosynthesis *in vitro* by a feminizing Leydig cell tumour of the testis. *J. Endocr.*, *35*, 409.

PION, R. J., JAFFE, R. B., WIQVIST, N. and DICZFALUSY, E. (1967): Formation of dehydroepiandrosterone sulphate by previable human foetuses. *Biochim. biophys. Acta (Amst.)*, *137*, 584.

PLOTZ, E. J., WIENER, M. and STEIN, A. A. (1966): Steroid synthesis in cystadenocarcinoma of the ovaries. *Amer. J. Obstet. Gynec.*, *94*, 189.

RABINOWITZ, J. L. and OLEKSYSHYN, O. (1956): The biosynthesis of radioactive 17β-estradiol. II. Synthesis by testicular and ovarian homogenates. *Arch. Biochem.*, *64*, 285.

RICE, B. F., HAMMERSTEIN, J. and SAVARD, K. (1964*a*): Gonadotropins and human ovarian steroidogenesis. In: *46th Meeting, The Endocrine Society, San Francisco,* p. 51.

RICE, B. F., HAMMERSTEIN, J. and SAVARD, K. (1964*b*): Steroid hormone formation in the human ovary: III. Action of gonadotropins on testosterone synthesis by normal ovarian stromal tissue. *Steroids*, *4*, 199.

RICE, B. F., HAMMERSTEIN, J. and SAVARD, K. (1964*c*): Steroid hormone formation in the human ovary: II. Action of gonadotropin *in vitro* in the corpus luteum. *J. clin. Endocr.*, *24*, 606.

ROBERTS, K. D., BANDI, L., CALVIN, H. I., DRUCKER, W. D. and LIEBERMAN, S. (1964): Evidence that steroid sulfates serve as biosynthetic intermediates. IV. Conversion of cholesterol sulfate *in vivo* to urinary C_{19} and C_{21} steroidal sulfates. *Biochemistry*, *3*, 1983.

ROSNER, J. M., CONTE, N. F., HORITA, A. and FORSHAM, P. H. (1964): The *in vivo* and *in vitro* production of testosterone by a lipoid ovarian tumor. *Amer. J. Med.*, *37*, 638.

ROSNER, J. M. and MACOME, J. C. (1970): Biosynthesis of 5-androstenediol by human testis *in vitro*. *Steroids*, *15*, 181.

ROVERSI, G. D. and POLVANI, F. (1963): Corticosteroid biosynthesis in the placenta. *Ann. Ostet. Ginec.*, *85*, 1018.

ROVERSI, G. D., POLVANI, F., BOMPIANI, A. and NEHER, R. (1963): Steroid biosynthesis *in vitro* by a virilizing suprarenal tumour. *Acta endocr. (Kbh.)*., *44*, 1.

RYAN, K. J. and PETRO, Z. (1966): Steroid biosynthesis by human ovarian granulosa and thecal cells. *J. clin. Endocr.*, *26*, 46.

RYAN, K. J. and SMITH, O. W. (1961): Biogenesis of estrogens. IV. Formation of neutral steroid intermediates. *J. biol. Chem.*, *236*, 2207.

SAKHATSKAYA, T. S. and BUROVA, E. K. (1965): Corticosteroid biosynthesis by human fetus adrenal glands. I. Transformation of progesterone. *Probl. Endokr. Gormonoter.*, *11*, 68.

SAKHATSKAYA, T. S. and BUROVA, E. K. (1966): The functional state of human fetal adrenals. *Stanov-*

lenie Endokrinnykh Funktsii v Zarodyshevom Razvitii, Materialy Simpoziuma, pp. 82–96. Editor: M. S. Mitskevich. Akademia Nauk SSSR. Institut Morfologii Zhivotnkh. St.

SANDBERG, A. A., SLAUNWHITE, W. R., JACKSON, J. E. and FRAWLEY, T. F. (1962): Androgen biosynthesis by ovarian lipoid cell tumor. *J. clin. Endocr.*, *22*, 929.

SANDBERG, E. C. and JENKINS, R. C. (1965*a*): Steroidal sulfatase and sulfokinase activity in arrhenoblastomatous tissue. *47th Meeting, The Endocrine Society*, New York, 1965, p. 125.

SANDBERG, E. C. and JENKINS, R. C. (1965*b*): Formation of androgens from dehydroisoandrosterone sulfate by virilizing human ovarian tissue *in vitro*. In: *Abstracts, VI Pan-American Congress of Endocrinology*, Mexico City, October, 1965, p. E 167. ICS No. 99. Excerpta Medica, Amsterdam.

SANDBERG, E. C., JENKINS, R. C. and TRIFON, H. M. (1966): Biosynthetic studies of human ovarian arrhenoblastomatous tissue *in vitro*. II. Formation of androgens from dehydroisoandrosterone sulfate. *Steroids*, *8*, 249.

SANDOR, T. and LANTHIER, A. (1960): The *in vitro* transformation of Δ^4-androstene-3, 17-dione to testosterone by surviving human ovarian slices. *Rev. canad. Biol.*, *19*, 445.

SAVARD, K., DORFMAN, R. I., BAGGETT, B. and ENGEL, L. L. (1956): Biosynthesis of androgens from progesterone by human testicular tissue *in vitro*. *J. clin. Endocr.*, *16*, 1629.

SAVARD, K., DORFMAN, R. I. and POUTASSE, E. (1952): Biogenesis of androgens in the human testis. *J. clin. Endocr.*, *12*, 935.

SAVARD, K., GUT, M., DORFMAN, R. I., GABRILOVE, J. L. and SOFFER, L. J. (1961): Formation of androgens by human arrhenoblastoma tissue *(in vitro)*. *J. clin. Endocr.*, *21*, 165.

SAVARD, K. and RICE, B. F. (1965): Biosynthesis of androgenic steroids in the stroma of normal human ovaries *in vitro*. In: *Abstracts Sixth Pan-American Congress of Endocrinology*, p. E 169. ICS No. 99. Excerpta Medica, Amsterdam.

SCHRIEFERS, H., BAYER, J. M. and PITTEL, M. (1963): Vergleichende Untersuchungen zur Biogenese von Steroidhormonen bei Durchströmung überlebender Nebennieren einer Patientin mit Cushing- und einer Patientin mit Conn-Syndrom. *Acta endocr. (Kbh.)*, *43*, 419.

SHAHWAN, M. M., OAKEY, R. E. and STITCH, S. R. (1969): Steroid biosynthesis by adrenal glands from anencephalic infants. *Acta endocr. (Kbh.)*, *61 (Supp., 138)*, 111.

SHARMA, D. C., RACZ, E. A., DORFMAN, R. I. and SCHOEN, E. J. (1967): A comparative study of the biosynthesis of testosterone by human testes and a virilizing interstitial cell tumour. *Acta endocr. (Kbh.)*, *56*, 726.

SHIMIZU, K. (1965): Metabolism of cholest-5-ene-3β,20α-diol-7α-^{3}H and of cholest-5-ene-3β,17, 2α-triol-7α-^{3}H by human adrenal tissue. *J. biol. Chem.*, *240*, 1941.

SHIMIZU, K. (1966): Conversion of 20α-hydroxycholesterol *in vitro* to pregnenolone sulfate by the human adrenal. *J. Biochem.*, *59*, 430.

SHIMIZU, K., DORFMAN, R. I. and GUT, M. (1960): Isocaproic acid, a metabolite of 20α-hydroxycholesterol. *J. biol. Chem.*, *235*, PC25.

SHIMIZU, K., HAYANO, M., GUT, M. and DORFMAN, R. I. (1961): The transformation of 20α-hydroxycholesterol to isocaproic acid and C_{21} steroids. *J. biol. Chem.*, *236*, 695.

SLAUNWHITE, W. R., JR. and SAMUELS, L. T. (1956): Progesterone as a precursor of testicular androgens. *J. biol. Chem.*, *220*, 341.

SLAUNWHITE, W. R., JR., SANDBERG, A. A., STAUBITZ, W. J., JACKSON, J. E. and KOEPF, G. F. (1962): Synthesis of testosterone by subjects with gonadal dysgenesis and XXY chromosome constitution. *J. clin. Endocr.*, *22*, 989.

SMITH, S. W. and AXELROD, L. R. (1969): Studies on the metabolism of steroid hormones and their precursors by the human placenta at various stages of gestation. II. *In vitro* metabolism of 3β-hydroxyandrost-5-en-17-one. *J. clin. Endocr.*, 29, 1182.

SOLOMON, S., LANMAN, J. T., LIND, J. and LIEBERMAN, S. (1958): The biosynthesis of Δ^4-androstenedione and 17α-hydroxyprogesterone from progesterone by surviving human fetal adrenals. *J. biol. Chem.*, *233*, 1084.

STARKA, L., SANDA, V. and STASTNY, J. (1966): The role of 19-hydroxydehydroepiandrosterone in estrogen biosynthesis. *Europ. J. Steroids*, *1*, 309.

UNGAR, F. and DORFMAN, R. I. (1953): Incorporation of C^{14} in the urinary steroids *in vivo*. *J. biol. Chem.*, *205*, 125.

VARANGOT, J., CEDARD, L. and YANNOTTI, S. (1965): Perfusion of the human placenta *in vitro*. *Amer. J. Obstet. Gynec.*, *92*, 534.

VILLEE, C. A. and LORING, J. M. (1964): Δ^5-3β Hydroxysteroid dehydrogenases of human adrenal.

In: *46th Meeting, The Endocrine Society, San Francisco,* p. 60.
VILLEE, C. A. and LORING, J. M. (1965): Synthesis of steroids in the newborn human adrenal *in vitro*. *J. clin. Endocr.*, *25*, 307.
VILLEE, C. A., LORING, J. M. and ROSE, M. (1965): Formation and cleavage of steroid sulfates by human fetal adrenals. In: *47th Meeting, The Endocrine Society, New York,* p. 69.
VILLEE, D. B. (1968): Control of steroid hormone synthesis in human fetal adrenals. *Israel J. med. Sci.*, *4*, 298.
VILLEE, D. B., DIMOLINE, A., ENGEL, L. L., VILLEE, C. A. and RAKER, J. (1962): Formation of 16α-hydroxyprogesterone in hyperplastic adrenal tissue. *J. clin. Endocr.*, *22*, 726.
VILLEE, D. B. and DRISCOLL, S. G. (1965): Pregnenolone and progesterone metabolism in human adrenals from twin fetuses. *Endocrinology*, *77*, 602.
VILLEE, D. B., LORING, J. M. and VILLEE, C. A. (1959): Steroid biosynthesis by human fetal adrenals. *Fed. Proc.*, *18*, 344.
VILLEE, D. B., MACGILLIVRAY, M., CRAWFORD, J. D., SCULLY, R. E. and KLIMAN, B. (1965): Androgen synthesis by testicular tissue from a patient with gonadal insufficiency. *J. clin. Endocr.*, *25*, 506.
VILLEE, D. B. and VILLEE, C. A. (1964): Synthesis of corticosteroids in the fetal-placental unit. In: *Proceedings of the Second International Congress of Endocrinology, Part II, London,* p. 709. ICS No. 83, Excerpta Medica, Amsterdam.
WADE, A. P., WILKINSON, G. S., DAVIS, J. C. and JEFFCOATE, T. N. A. (1968): The metabolism of testosterone, androstenedione and oestrone by testis from a case of testicular feminization. *J. Endocr.*, *42*, 391.
WALLACE, E. Z. and LIEBERMAN, S. (1963): Biosynthesis of dehydroepiandrosterone sulfate by human adrenocortical tissue. *J. clin. Endocr.*, *23*, 90.
WARREN, J. C. and CHEATUM, S. G. (1964): Demonstration of a steroid 17–20 desmolase in the human placenta. *Canad. J. Biochem.*, *42*, 143.
WARREN, J. C. and SALHANICK, H. A. (1961): Steroid biosynthesis in the human ovary. *J. clin. Endocr.*, *21*, 1218.
WELIKY, I. and ENGEL, L. L. (1961): 17-Hydroxypregnenolone as a precursor for cortisol. *Fed. Proc.*, *20*, 179.
WELIKY, I. and ENGEL, L. L. (1963): Metabolism of progesterone-4-C^{14} and pregnenolone-7α-H^3 by human adrenal tissue. Formation of 16α-hydroxyprogesterone-C^{14}, corticosterone-C^{14}, and cortisol-C^{14}-H^3. *J. biol. Chem.*, *238*, 1302.
WEST, C. D., KUMAGAI, L. F., SIMONS, E. L., DOMINGUEZ, O. V. and BERLINER, D. L. (1964): Adrenocortical carcinoma with feminization and hypertension associated with a defect in 11β-hydroxylation. *J. clin. Endocr.*, *24*, 567.
WIEST, W. G., ZANDER, J. and HOLMSTROM, E. G. (1959): Metabolism of progesterone-4-C^{14} by an arrhenoblastoma. *J. clin. Endocr.*, *19*, 297.
WILSON, J. D. and WALKER, J. D. (1969): The conversion of testosterone to 5α-androstan-17β-ol-3-one (dihydrotestosterone) by skin slices of man. *J. clin. Invest.*, *48*, 371.
WOTIZ, H. H., ZISKIND, B. S. and LEMON, H. M. (1960): Studies in steroid metabolism. VIII. Steroidogenesis in a heterologous tumor transplant. *Cancer Res.*, *20*, 34.
YAMAJI, T., MOTOHASHI, K., TANIOKA, T. and IBAYASHI, H. (1968): Androstenediol in canine spermatic vein blood and its significance in testosterone biosynthesis *in vivo*. *Endocrinology*, *83*, 992.

REGULATION OF ANDROGEN SECRETION*

KRISTEN B. EIK-NES

Division of Biochemistry and Physiology of Reproduction and Department of Physiology, University of Southern California Medical School Los Angeles, Calif., U.S.A.,

Since our original observation (Brinck-Johnsen and Eik-Nes, 1957) that increased secretion of the androgens – testosterone and Δ^4-androstenedione – could be measured in spermatic venous blood of the dog 30-60 minutes after i.v. administration of human chorionic gonadotrophin (HCG), much knowledge has accumulated on factors involved in controlling the rates of androgen production and secretion by the male gonad. It is clear that interstitial cell-stimulating hormone (ICSH), pregnant mare serum gonadotrophin (PMS) and follicle-stimulating hormone (FSH) containing ICSH, will all stimulate production and secretion of testosterone by testicular tissue (Eik-Nes, 1962; Hall and Eik-Nes, 1962; Eik-Nes and Hall, 1965). Currently it is not known whether the effect of FSH on testosterone production is due to its contamination with ICSH (Connell and Eik-Nes, 1968). Johnson and Ewing (1970) have recorded that rabbit testes perfused with a combination of ICSH and FSH secrete more testosterone than testes perfused with either gonadotrophin alone.

When HCG is administered via the spermatic artery of the dog, the steroids listed in Figure 1 (except the estrogens) will increase in spermatic venous blood (Eik-Nes, 1970). The canine

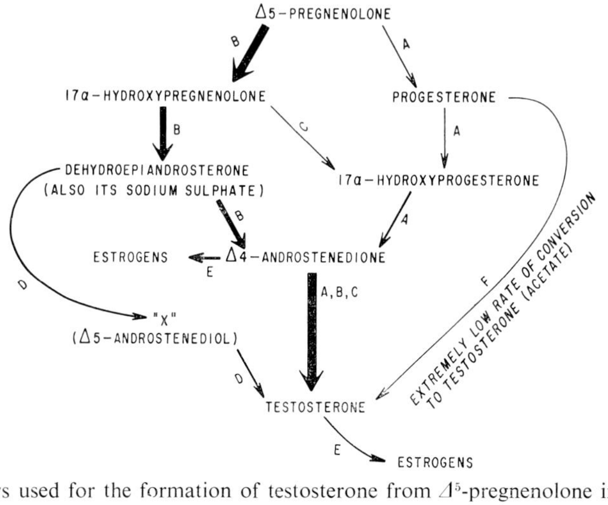

Fig. 1. Pathways used for the formation of testosterone from Δ^5-pregnenolone in the canine testis *in vivo*. The animal preparations used in these experiments are described in detail by Eik-Nes (1969).

* The work reviewed from the author's own laboratory was in part supported by research grant HD 04195–02 from United States Public Health Service, Bethesda, Md., U.S.A.

testis secretes more pregnenolone, 17α-hydroxypregnenolone, 17α-hydroxyprogesterone and dehydroepiandrosterone than progesterone, and one notes with interest that infusion of progesterone via the spermatic artery of the dog is associated with meiotic chromosome changes in the infused organ (Williams *et al.*, 1968). This may be the reason why pathways B, C and D of Figure 1 are the preferred ones for the formation of testosterone in the male dog in experiments *in vivo*. The rates of steroid formation via pathways E and F (Fig. 1) are so small that the end products from such metabolism cannot be measured (Eik-Nes, 1970).

The effects of the gonadotrophins on formation and secretion of testosterone in the dog occur within the first 3-6 minutes during continuous administration via the spermatic artery and the same rapid increment in hormone secretion is observed when cyclic 3′, 5′-AMP is administered via this route (Eik-Nes, 1967). Such data could support the view that the processes leading to augmented secretion of testosterone are almost spontaneously stimulated by the gonadotrophins and that the compound cyclic 3′, 5′-AMP could *in part* or *in toto* be responsible for this rapid effect on secretion of male androgens. Moreover, administration of HCG via the spermatic artery of the dog for 1 minute only is followed by increased rates of testosterone secretion lasting up to 75 minutes (Fig. 2). Therefore, the gonadotrophins show a rapid and relatively prolonged effect on the processes leading to increased secretion of testosterone.

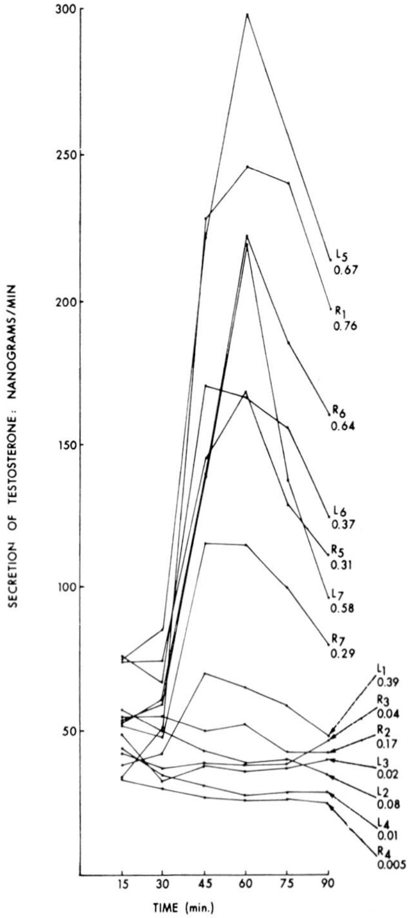

Fig. 2. Secretion of testosterone by the left (L) and right (R) testes of 7 different dogs. The animal preparation used in these experiments is described in detail (animal preparation II) by Eik-Nes (1969). During time 15–16 min, different doses of HCG were administered via the spermatic artery at a constant rate. The doses of HCG (I.U./g testis tissue wet weight) are given on the figure.

All available evidence indicates that the major locus of action for gonadotrophins in the male and female gonads is between cholesterol and Δ^5-pregnenolone (Hall, 1970) and data have been presented on stimulatory effects of ICSH on synthesis of progesterone from cholesterol in the corpus luteum (Hall and Koritz, 1965). ICSH will, moreover, increase the formation of testosterone-^{3}H from cholesterol-^{3}H in slices of rabbit testis (Hall, 1966). Thus, in order to understand mechanisms of action of gonadotrophins on steroidogenesis, detailed knowledge of the metabolism of cholesterol to Δ^5-pregnenolone is needed. In this metabolic pathway 20α-hydroxycholesterol and 20α,22R-dihydrocholesterol are likely intermediates, but only during the last year have data been published on the formation of these intermediates by endocrine tissue synthesizing Δ^5-pregnenolone from cholesterol (Burstein and Gut, 1969). Formation of 20α-hydroxycholesterol was minute in these experiments and if 20α-hydroxycholesterol-^{3}H is incubated with steroid producing tissues, no increment in hormonal end products containing ^{3}H can be measured when the proper trophins are added to the incubation media (Hall and Young, 1968). The trophins could therefore act before the formation of 20α-hydroxycholesterol and in the metabolic pathway cholesterol → Δ^5-pregnenolone, the rate-limiting step sensitive to trophic stimulation could involve formation of either 20α-hydroxycholesterol or 22R-hydroxycholesterol. The central role this latter sterol appears to play in metabolism leading to the formation of Δ^5-pregnenolone in the endocrine tissues (Burstein and Gut, 1970) warrants exact investigations pertaining to trophic effects on bioformation. Such experiments are difficult to perform, particularly in the male gonad where only the cells of Leydig produce Δ^5-pregnenolone from cholesterol. These cells comprise less than 10% of the total testicular cell population in most animal species. Also, the enzymic system converting cholesterol to Δ^5-pregnenolone may be multi-complex in nature (Burstein and Gut, 1970).

If we consider the chemical nature of the known intermediates between cholesterol and Δ^5-pregnenolone, it is evident that hydroxylation reactions requiring TPNH are needed. Side-chain cleavage of cholesterol can be obtained by endocrine tissue fractions in an incubation system containing flavoprotein, nonheme iron and cytochrome P-450 (Simpson and Boyd, 1967). Since side chain cleavage of cholesterol is inhibited by hyperbaric oxygen, and since succinate protects against this inhibition (Hall, 1967), Hall (1970) has postulated that formation of Δ^5-pregnenolone from cholesterol could occur in steroid-forming cells via a separate pool of reduced TPN^+ generated via reversed electron transport. Detailed knowledge on how the trophins promote formation of reduced TPN^+ in restricted pools of cells synthesizing Δ^5-pregnenolone from cholesterol is currently lacking.

Since the work of Haynes and Berthet (1957) on the effects of cyclic 3′,5′-AMP on phosphorylase activity in steroid-forming organs, much work has been done on the formation of cyclic 3′,5′-AMP in the adrenal gland, the testis and the ovary subsequent to stimulation with trophins. Increased phosphorylase activity should lead to release of glucose-1-phosphate from glycogen. Glucose-1-phosphate would then enter the pentose phosphate pathway as glucose-6-phosphate and yield TPNH via oxidation. It is evident from experiments (Murad *et al.*, 1969; Pulsinelli and Eik-Nes, 1970) that the male gonad contains adenyl cyclase activity which can be stimulated with gonadotrophins (Fig. 3). This type of stimulation does not result from decreased activity of the enzyme cyclic 3′,5′-AMP phosphodiesterase, but occurs via augmented synthesis of cyclic 3′,5′-AMP from ATP. Conversion of cholesterol to Δ^5-pregnenolone takes place in the mitochondria of the steroid-forming cells (Hall, 1970). Such organelles do contain adenyl cyclase activity which can be stimulated with the proper trophin (Fig. 3). When cyclic 3′,5′-AMP is added to the mitochondrial fraction of dog testes, formation of Δ^5-pregnenolone from either endogenous or exogenous cholesterol is not stimulated (Pulsinelli and Eik-Nes, 1970). Since the major localization of adenyl cyclase activity in the canine testis is in the nuclear membrane fraction (Fig. 3), our findings raise the question whether initial stimulation with cyclic 3′,5′-AMP occurs outside the mitochondria. Also the lowest testicular cell organization which will augment the production of testosterone

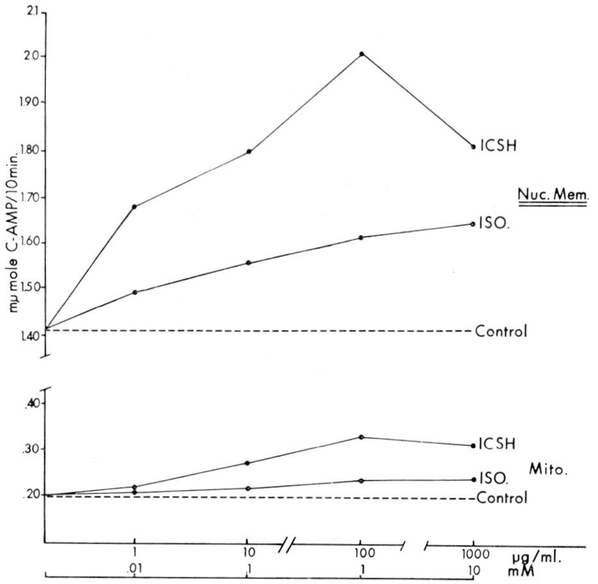

Fig. 3. Conversion of ATP-^{14}C to cyclic 3′,5′-AMP-^{14}C (C-AMP) during 10 minutes of incubation with tissue fractions from canine testis. Incubation of 50 mg equivalent tissue fraction was carried out at 37°C in Tris buffer (40 mM, pH 7.4) containing .25 M sucrose, .02 M theophylline and .1 M magnesium sulfate. Cyclic 3′,5′-AMP-^{3}H was added at end of incubation to determine recovery through isolation method and conversion of ATP-^{14}C to cyclic 3′,5′-AMP-^{14}C stopped by boiling (5 min). Isolation of radioactively pure cyclic 3′,5′-AMP-^{14}C was accomplished by successive chromatography on: Dowex 50 ion exchange resin, paper (ethanol: .5 M ammonium acetate, 5 : 2) and thin-layer plates (90% aqueous ethanol).

Nuc.: nuclear membrane fraction
Mito.: mitochondrial fraction
ICSH: N.I.H. preparation of interstitial cell-stimulating hormone (doses used in μg/ml incubation medium)
Iso.: isoproterenol (doses used in mM)
Control: no addition of ICSH or isoproterenol
Addition of synthetic ACTH has no effect on cyclic 3′,5′-AMP-^{14}C formation in this system. The data are from an investigation by Pulsinelli and Eik-Nes (1970).

in the presence of gonadotrophins is the testicular slice (Hall, 1970). One notes with interest that addition of Ca^{2+} to testis mitochondria will stimulate the formation of Δ^5-pregnenolone from cholesterol (Pulsinelli and Eik-Nes, 1970). It is therefore tempting to postulate that the first phase of trophic action in the testis could be associated with changes in Ca^{2+} distribution within membrane structures of the cells of Leydig.

In a review of gonadotrophic action on steroidogenesis written in 1963 (Eik-Nes, 1964), the question was posed: can cyclic 3′, 5′-AMP stimulate protein formation in the gonads? At that time it was known that when compounds, known to inhibit protein formation *de novo* in mammalian tissues, were added to adrenal or testicular slices, no effect on steroidogenesis could be determined when these slices were exposed to specific trophins (Eik-Nes, 1964). Admittedly, the doses of the different antimetabolites used to obtain these effects were high, and the experimental data were open to the serious criticism of studying steroid formation by tissues 'intoxicated' with such antimetabolites. During the last year, however, information has been collected on effects of cyclic 3′,5′-AMP on enzyme synthesis in mammalian (Jost *et al.*, 1970) as well as in non-mammalian (DeCrombrugghe *et al.*, 1969) cells, and recently the possibility has been discussed (Garren *et al.*, 1970) that ACTH could promote specific protein synthesis at the level of translation in the adrenal gland. Whether an adrenal protein kinase which can be stimulated with cyclic 3′,5′-AMP (Garren *et al.*, 1970) alone is responsible for the effect of cyclic 3′,5′-AMP on steroidogenesis in this tissue remains to be determined. It would also be of interest to investigate whether the steroid-forming organs contain a specific binding protein for cholesterol and whether such a binding principle is influenced by cyclic 3′,5′-AMP or by a 'protein' sensitive to cyclic 3′,5′-AMP stimulation (Garren *et al.*, 1970). The relationship between trophic-induced formation of *free* TPNH and trophic-induced protein formation in steroid-secreting tissues must not be forgotten during our current enthusiasm about a possible 'third factor' of 'protein' nature directing steroidogenesis via cyclic 3′,5′-AMP. Moreover, since a trophin will promote growth of its target organ, data on the growth-promoting effect of cyclic 3′,5′-AMP on the adrenal gland and on the gonads must be forthcoming. Finally, conclusive experiments must be conducted on the ability of cyclic 3′,5′-AMP or of a cyclic 3′,5′-AMP sensitive 'protein' (formed in a steroid-producing tissue) to remove Δ^5-pregnenolone from the mitochondria of the steroid-secreting cells. Δ^5-Pregnenolone appears to inhibit its own formation from cholesterol in adrenal mitochondria

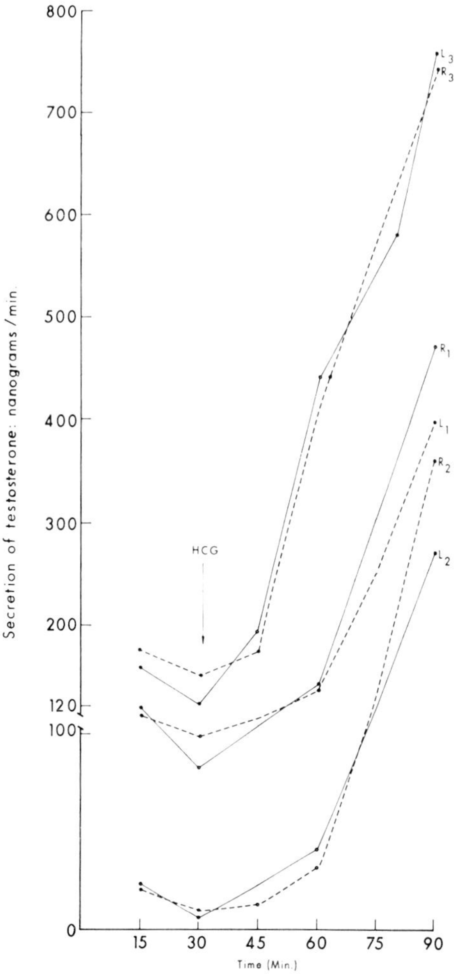

Fig. 4. Rates of secretion of testosterone by left (L) and right (R) testes of 3 different dogs. The animal preparation used in these experiments (animal preparation II) is described by Eik-Nes (1969). During time 0–90 min, one testis (dotted line) was infused with 5.5 μg propranolol/min via the spermatic artery while the other testis (solid line) served as control. During time 30–90 min both testes were infused with 26 I.U. HCG/min via the spermatic arteries.
L_1 and R_1, L_2 and R_2: testes infused with a mixture of 0.38 ml 0.9% sodium chloride solution and 3.87 ml oxygenated Krebs-Ringer bicarbonate buffer (pH 7.4) containing 70 mg% glucose/min. L_3 and R_3: testes infused with a mixture of 0.38 ml 0.9% sodium chloride solution and 3.87 ml oxygenated arterial blood/min.

(Koritz and Hall, 1964) probably via inhibition of 20α-hydroxylation of cholesterol. It should be kept in mind that when data on ACTH-induced secretion of adrenal hormones are subjected to system analysis (Urquhart, 1970), release of hydroxylation inhibition by Δ^5-pregnenolone removal is a highly probable answer.

Over the years several workers have suggested that the gonadotrophins could promote their effect on steroidogenesis via increased tissue permeability. Data have also been published on cyclic 3′,5′-AMP-induced increment in cell permeability (Orloff and Handler, 1962). We have, however, been unable to determine an increase in total cell permeability of testes slices producing testosterone under the influence of gonadotrophins (Hall and Eik-Nes, 1962). A marked change in permeability of the cells of Leydig would, however, be so diluted by tubular elements in these experiments that specific permeability changes of the steroid-producing cells would be difficult to measure.

Variation of blood flow in the ovary (Romanoff *et al.*, 1962) and in the testis (Eik-Nes, 1964) will alter steroid secretion. We have observed that when isoproterenol is infused via the spermatic artery in our volume-controlled animal preparation *in vivo*, the secretion of testosterone in spermatic venous blood increases (Eik-Nes, 1969). Moreover, testes infused with a β-cell inhibitor via the spermatic artery will not augment the secretion of testosterone in a normal fashion when subjected to isoproterenol stimulation (Eik-Nes, 1969). Testes infused with an α-cell inhibitor via the spermatic artery, however, show normal response patterns in rates of testosterone secretion when stimulated with catecholamines (Eik-Nes, 1969). It is clear (Fig. 3) that isoproterenol will stimulate formation of cyclic 3′,5′-AMP in the canine testis. Testes treated with a β-cell inhibitor will not increase the formation of cyclic 3′,5′-AMP when exposed to catecholamines (Murad *et al.*, 1969) and testes producing cyclic 3′,5′-AMP in the presence of maximal doses of gonadotrophins will increase the production of this nucleotide further when stimulated with epinephrine (Murad *et al.*, 1969). We have made similar observations on the canine testis using a combined treatment of gonadotrophins and isoproterenol. Finally, testes infused with a β-cell inhibitor via the spermatic artery (dog) will augment the secretion of testosterone in a normal fashion when HCG is infused via this route (Fig. 4). Such data suggest that the male gonad either contains different adenyl cyclases or also that the receptor sites for the gonadotrophins are different from those of the catecholamines in this organ. A receptor-stimulation interaction results in increased production of cyclic 3′,5′-AMP (Fig. 3), but where in the testis these receptors are located (Leydig cells, germinative epithelium, Sertoli cells) is not known. It is currently our working theory that the isoproterenol-sensitive receptor site in the canine testis shares the properties of a β-receptor cell and that this receptor influences the microcirculation of the male gonad, probably via the compound cyclic 3′,5′-AMP (Eik-Nes, 1970).

REFERENCES

BRINCK-JOHNSEN, T. and EIK-NES, K. B. (1957): Effect of human chorionic gonadotrophin on the secretion of testosterone and 4-androstene-3,17-dione by the canine testis. *Endocrinology, 61*, 676.

BURSTEIN, S. and GUT, M. (1969): A preliminary report on the intermediates in the conversion *in vitro* of cholesterol to pregnenolone in adrenal preparations. *Steroids, 14*, 207.

BURSTEIN, S. and GUT, M. (1970): Biosynthesis of pregnenolone. *Recent Progr. Hormone Res.* In press.

CONNELL, G. M. and EIK-NES, K. B. (1968): Testosterone production by rabbit testis slices. *Steroids, 12*, 507.

DECROMBRUGGHE, B., PERLMAN, R. L., VARMUS, H. E. and PASTAN, I. (1969): Regulation of inducible enzyme synthesis in *Escherichia coli* by cyclic adenosine 3′, 5′-monophosphate. *J. biol. Chem., 244*, 5828.

EIK-NES, K. B. (1962): Secretion of testosterone in anesthetized dogs. *Endocrinology, 71*, 101.

EIK-NES, K. B. (1964): On the relationship between testicular blood flow and the secretion of testosterone in anesthetized dogs stimulated with human chorionic gonadotrophin. *Canad. J. Physiol. Pharmacol., 42*, 671.

EIK-NES, K. B. (1964): The effects of gonadotrophins on the secretion of steroids by the ovary and the testis. *Physiol. Rev.*, *44*, 609.
EIK-NES, K. B. (1967): Factors regulating the secretion of steroids by the canine testis. *Ciba Foundation Colloquia on Endocrinology*, *16*, 120.
EIK-NES, K. B. (1969): Patterns of steroidogenesis in vertebrate gonads. *Gen. comp. Endocr. Supp.*, *2*, 87.
EIK-NES, K. B. (1969): An effect of isoproterenol on rates of synthesis and secretion of testosterone. *Amer. J. Physiol.*, *217*, 1764.
EIK-NES, K. B. (1970): Synthesis and secretion of androstenedione and testosterone. In: *The Androgens of the Testis*, Chapter 1, pp. 8–10. Editor: K. B. Eik-Nes. Marcel Dekker, New York.
EIK-NES, K. B. (1970): Production and secretion of testicular steroids. *Recent Progr. Hormone Res.*, *27*, 517.
EIK-NES, K. B. and HALL, P. F. (1965): Action of pregnant mare serum on the production of testosterone *in vivo* and *in vitro*. *J. Reprod. Fertil.*, *9*, 233.
GARREN, L. D., GILL, G. N., MASUI, H. and WALTON, G. M. (1970): On the mechanism of action of adrenal corticotropic hormone. *Recent Progr. Hormone Res.*, *27*.
HALL, P. F. (1966): On the stimulation of testicular steroidogenesis in the rabbit by interstitial cell-stimulating hormone. *Endocrinology*, *78*, 690.
HALL, P. F. (1967): Electron transport in relation to steroid biosynthesis. Inhibition of side-chain cleavage of cholesterol by hyperbaric oxygen. *Biochemistry*, *6*, 2794.
HALL, P. F. (1970): Gonadotrophic regulation of testicular function. In: *The Androgens of the Testis*, Chapter 3, pp. 81–94. Editor: K. B. Eik-Nes. Marcel Dekker, New York.
HALL, P. F. and EIK-NES, K. B. (1962): The action of gonadotrophic hormones upon rabbit testis *in vitro*. *Biochim. biophys. Acta, (Amst.)*, *63*, 411.
HALL, P. F. and EIK-NES, K. B. (1962): Interstitial cell-stimulating hormone and penetration of D-xylose-1-C^{14} and α-aminoisobutyric acid-1-C^{14} into slices of testis. *Proc. Soc. exp. Biol. (N.Y.)*, *110*, 148.
HALL, P. F. and KORITZ, S. B. (1965): Influence of interstitial cell-stimulating hormone on the conversion of cholesterol to progesterone by bovine corpus luteum. *Biochemistry*, *4*, 1037.
HALL, P. F. and YOUNG, D. G. (1968): Site of action of trophic hormones upon the biosynthetic pathways to steroid hormones. *Endocrinology*, *82*, 559.
HAYNES, R. C. and BERTHET, L. (1957): Studies on the mechanism of action of the adrenocorticotropic hormone. *J. biol. Chem.*, *225*, 115.
JOHNSON, B. H. and EWING, L. L. (1970): Testosterone secretion by rabbit testis perfused *in vitro* with an artificial media. Abstract No. 55, Third Annual Meeting of the Society for the Study of Reproduction, Ohio State University, Columbus, O., p. 28.
JOST, J.-P., HSIE, A., HUGHES, S. D. and RYAN, L. (1970): Role of cyclic adenosine 3′,5′-monophosphate in the induction of hepatic enzymes. *J. biol. Chem.*, *245*, 351.
KORITZ, S. B. and HALL, P. F. (1964): End-product inhibition of the conversion of cholesterol to pregnenolone in an adrenal extract. *Biochemistry*, *3*, 1298.
MURAD, J., STRUACH, B. S. and VAUGHAN, M. (1969): The effects of gonadotrophins on testicular adenyl cyclase. *Biochim. Biophys. Acta (Amst.)*. *177*, 591.
ORLOFF, J. and HANDLER, J. S. (1962): The similarity of effects of vasopressin, adenosine-3′,5′-phosphate (cyclic AMP) and theophylline on the toad bladder. *J. clin. Invest.*, *41*, 702.
PULSINELLI, W. A. and EIK-NES, K. B. (1970): Adenyl cyclase activity in subcellular fractions of dog testis. *Fed. Proc.*, *29*, 918.
PULSINELLI, W. A. and EIK-NES, K. B. (1970): Regulation of cyclic 3′,5′-AMP activity in the canine testis. In press.
ROMANOFF, E. B., DESHPANDE, N. and PINCUS, G. (1962): Rate of ovarian progesterone secretion in the dog. *Endocrinology*, *70*, 532.
SIMPSON, E. R. and BOYD, G. S. (1967): Partial resolution of the mixed-function oxidase involved in the cholesterol side-chain cleavage reaction in bovine adrenal mitochondria. *Biochem. biophys. Res. Commun.*, *28*, 945.
URQUHART, H. (1970): Blood-borne signals. The measuring and modelling of humoral communication and control. *Physiologist*, *13*, 7.
WILLIAMS, D. L., RUNYAN, J. W. and HAGEN, A. A. (1968): Meiotic chromosome alterations produced by progesterone. *Nature (Lond.)*, *220*, 1145.

IN VITRO METABOLISM OF ANDROGENS IN NON-ENDOCRINE TISSUE

TOMÁS MORATO, FERNANDO FLORES and GREGORIO PÉREZ-PALACIOS

Hormone Research Laboratories, Department of Endocrinology, Instituto Nacional de la Nutrición, México 22, D.F., Mexico

The metabolic pathways for androgen biosynthesis have been well established in the testes, ovary and adrenal. The effects of these hormones on tissues such as prostate, seminal vesicles, skin, muscle and others considered as end organs are well recognized in the human and in several animal species. Such hormones are transported in the blood by specific proteins (Mercier, 1966) whose physical and chemical properties have been described recently (Kato and Horton, 1968). Regulatory mechanisms involved in hormone transport are not known at present and remain to be elucidated.

Interest in the relationship between androgens and target tissues has become a matter of intense research during the past few years. Previous studies have shown that after intravenous administration of radiolabeled testosterone to rats which had been either castrated (Anderson and Liao, 1968; Tveter and Attramadal, 1968), or castrated and hepatectomized (Bruchovsky and Wilson, 1968) there is an accumulation of radioactive material in male accessory genital organs. The subcellular distribution of ^{3}H-testosterone and its metabolites was studied in the rat by Bruchovsky and Wilson (1968) who demonstrated that most of the radioactivity was found in the prostatic cell nuclei. In addition, an important amount of tritium was located in the cytosol fraction. Ninety percent of this material was identified as testosterone, 5α-androstanediol and 5α-dihydrotestosterone. The nuclei and cytoplasm of prostatic cells are capable of converting testosterone to 5α-dihydrotestosterone, which has been suggested to be a more potent androgen than testosterone in some species (Dorfman and Shipley, 1956).

Recent work has shown the presence of two specific cytoplasmic proteins, one that binds testosterone and another that binds 5α-dihydrotestosterone (Fang *et al.*, 1969).

During the past few months we have studied the *in vitro* metabolism of androgens in several non-endocrine tissues that have been considered as targets of androgen action. During the course of this presentation we will give data obtained in rat bone marrow, preputial gland and kidney tissues, canine central nervous system tissues and normal human skin.

METABOLISM OF ANDROGENS IN RAT BONE MARROW, KIDNEY AND PREPUTIAL SKIN TISSUES

The erythropoietic effect of androgens has been demonstrated in animals (Steinglas *et al.*, 1941) and in man (Kennedy and Gilbertson, 1957). It has been proposed that its action is mediated by erythropoietin production which in turn activates bone marrow tissue (Mirand *et al.*, 1965). However, a direct effect of androgens on bone marrow cells has also been suggested (Reisner, 1966; Jacobson *et al.*, 1968). Recent work has shown that heme formation is increased by etiocholanolone, a metabolite of testosterone, in human bone marrow tissue *in vitro* (Necheles and Rai, 1969). We investigated the capacity of bone marrow tissue (BMT) to metabolize androgens in several *in vitro* experiments. During the first one, rat bone marrow tissue obtained from femoral bones was incubated with 7-^{3}H-testosterone (s.a. 10 Ci/mM) in Krebs Ringer bicarbonate fortified with an NADPH-generating system under an atmosphere of 95% oxygen and 5% carbon dioxide during 6 hours. Isolation of metabolites was accomplished by means of partition chromatography on Celite 545 columns using systems of increasing polarity (Fig. 1). Identification was achieved by isotope dilution techniques until constant specific activity was obtained. The results show the formation of 5α-androstanedione

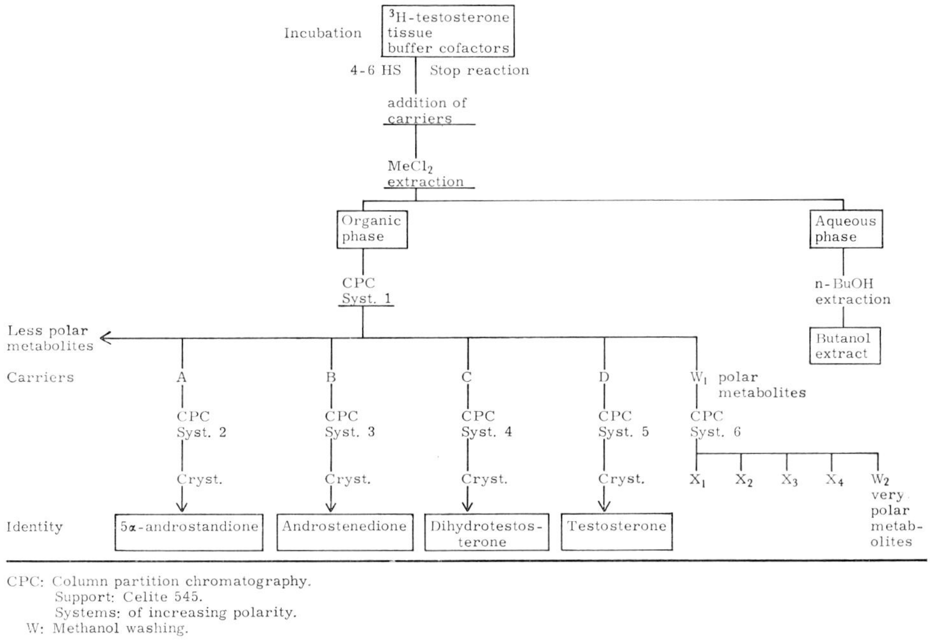

Fig. 1. Isolation of metabolites by partition chromatography.

(5α-A), 4-androstenedione (Δ^4) and 5α-dihydrotestosterone (DHT) as well as several radioactive areas more polar than testosterone, one with less polarity than the 5-androstenedione which was the less polar metabolite identified. Unchanged testosterone was found to be 50.8% of the starting amount. The radioactivity content of the polar areas is a minimal estimate since losses were not corrected during the experimental procedures. This also applies to the less polar radioactive area, which was less than 1%. These results have been published elsewhere (Morato *et al.*, 1970). To our knowledge this is the first evidence of a steroid metabolic capacity for erythropoietic tissues. The metabolic pathway suggested by these results is shown in Figure 2.

When 7-^{3}H-dehydroepiandrosterone sulfate (s.a. 2.5 Ci/mM) was incubated with rat bone marrow tissue, without addition of cofactors, two free metabolites were isolated following preliminary purification procedures. They were identified as dehydroepiandrosterone (DHA) and 5-androstene-3β,17β-diol (Δ^5-diol) by crystallization to constant specific activity. Additionally, two radioactive areas were isolated from the aqueous (conjugated) fraction. They were solvolized, and repurified by paper chromatography. Finally, one was identified as DHA and the other as Δ^5-diol.

When 4-^{14}C-DHA (s.a. 27.5 mCi/mM) was incubated under identical conditions with BMT used for the above-described experiment only a more polar radioactive area was found

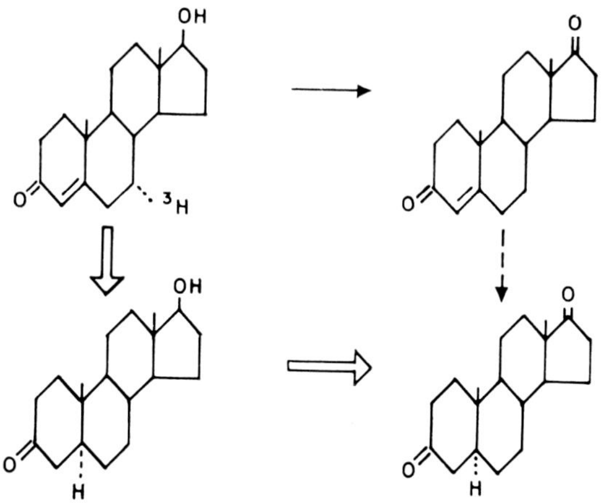

Fig. 2. Metabolism of ³H-testosterone by bone marrow tissue *(in vitro)*. Isolated metabolites.

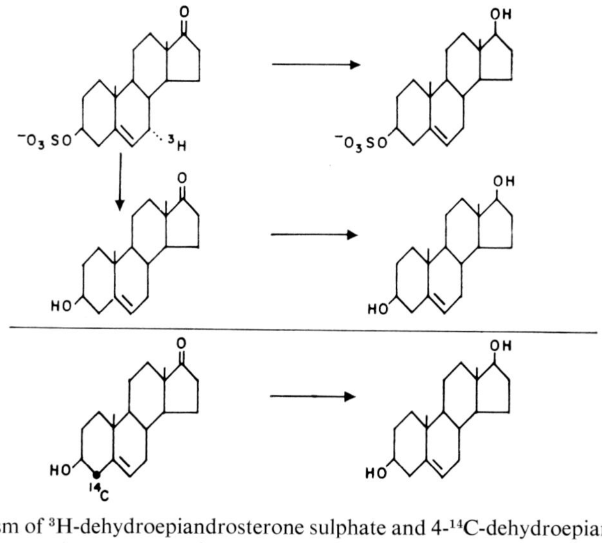

Fig. 3. Metabolism of ³H-dehydroepiandrosterone sulphate and 4-¹⁴C-dehydroepiandrosterone by rat bone marrow tissue *(in vitro)*. Isolated metabolites.

as a metabolic conversion product and further identified as Δ^5-diol (Fig. 3). These studies show the capacity of the bone marrow tissue to metabolize either free or sulfoconjugated androgens. Several enzymatic systems were demonstrated in this tissue: Of these oxido-reductases acting upon C-17 oxygenated functions were observed for free or sulfoconjugated steroid, Δ^5-steroid reductase and sulfatase activities among others that have not been established. From the results presented here for this particular tissue, we can assume that testosterone may be metabolized when available to the bone marrow cell but this latter is unable to transform precursors with a Δ^5-3β-ol-hydroxy-structure, due to an apparent lack of 3β-ol-dehydrogenase and Δ^5-isomerase systems.

Since DHT was the major product of testosterone from BMT it was felt of interest to investigate its effects on erythropoiesis. For this purpose, DHT propionate was administered subcutaneously to male rats at different doses. Testosterone propionate and untreated rats were used as controls following previous work (Duarte *et al.*, 1967). The erythrocytemic effect was evaluated by incorporation of ^{59}Fe in red blood cells on the fourth day of treatment. The results showed a definitive erythropoietic effect that was even higher than that observed with testosterone propionate which has been shown to be a good erythropoietic agent in rats and mice (Duarte *et al.*, 1967).

Several anabolic-androgenic steroids with low virilizing activity, such as metholone (1α-methyl-17β-hydroxy-5α-androstan-3-one), oxymetholone (2-hydroxy-methylene-17α-methyl-17β-hydroxy-5α-androstan-3-one) or methenolone (1α-methyl-17β-hydroxy-1-androsten-3-one), were demonstrated as efficient erythropoietic agents in either the rat (Duarte *et al.*, 1967) or man with aplastic anemia (Sánchez-Medal *et al.*, 1969). It is interesting to note that such anabolic compounds are 5α-reduced modified androgens.

The erythropoietic effect observed by the *in vivo* therapy with DHT propionate opens the question as to whether DHT acts directly on BMT or has an indirect action; also, whether this effect is produced by DHT itself or whether DHT requires to be metabolized further. The work of Necheles and Rai (1969) suggests the last possibility. In addition, recent work has shown that other testosterone metabolites, particularly 5α-androstan-3β-17β-diol, is active and responsible for some of the activities known for testosterone as demonstrated in other target organs (Baulieu *et al.*, 1968; 1969).

Rat kidney tissue was capable of producing several changes in the testosterone molecule when this was used as substrate. A minced preparation of medullary portion of kidney was incubated with 7-^{3}H-testosterone, in Krebs Ringer bicarbonate during 4 hours. No co-factors were added. After preliminary purification procedures, several radioactive areas were noted. Using a reverse isotope dilution technique the identity of 5α-androstanedione, 4-androstenedione and 5α-dihydrotestosterone could be established. The extent of these reactions is shown in Table I. As can be seen, testosterone was extensively metabolized, since only 5.0% of the starting radioactivity was found as unconverted testosterone. Both reduced androgens (5α-A and DHT) were formed in a similar proportion, these compounds having a higher tritium content than 4-androstenedione.

In order to compare the *in vitro* metabolism of testosterone with a well-known androgen-dependent target tissue, we incubated rat preputial skin with ^{3}H-testosterone under identical conditions as described for bone marrow. The enzymatic activity found in this tissue was higher than in the other rat tissues studied, as reflected by the increased formation of iden-

TABLE I

Metabolism of ^{3}H-testosterone by rat tissues. mμM formed/mg

Tissue	Metabolites		
	5α-androstanedione	androstenedione	dihydrotestosterone
BMT, NL	8.5×10^{-6}	89.0×10^{-6}	287.4×10^{-6}
PG, C	292.8×10^{-5}	314.3×10^{-5}	1028.5×10^{-5}
PG, Rx	87.8	56.1	300.0×10^{-5}
K, NL	166.5×10^{-6}	54.9×10^{-6}	187.2×10^{-6}

BMT = Bone Marrow Tissue
PG = Preputial Gland
K = Kidney
Rx = Cyproterone Treated Rat

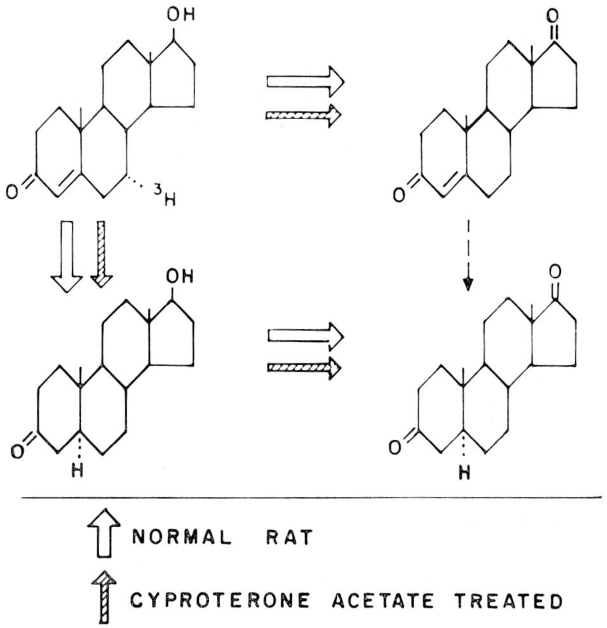

Fig. 4. Metabolism of ^{3}H-testosterone by preputial gland *(in vitro)* – isolated metabolites.

tified metabolites on the basis of tissue weight. The results are shown in Table I. 5α-Dihydrotestosterone was formed to the greatest extent, but 5α-androstanedione and androstenedione yields were also higher as compared with bone marrow and kidney tissues. Unmetabolized ^{3}H-testosterone contained 22.0% of the initial amount.

Preputial skin of rats treated during 21 days with 12.5 mg of cyproterone acetate (1,2-methylene-6-chloro-17β-hydroxy-1,4-pregnadiene-3,20-dione-17β-yl-acetate) administered subcutaneously was incubated with ^{3}H-testosterone under conditions identical to those already described. A decrease in the formation of 5α-A, Δ^4 and DHT was observed (Fig. 4). Unchanged testosterone accounted for 44.9% of the amount of tritium incubated.

The antiandrogenic effect of cyproterone acetate was noted on the rat skin. This compound interferes with testosterone metabolism – probably by competing with the protein that binds testosterone (Stern and Eisenfeld, 1969). There is no evidence that 5α-steroid reductase activity is altered by cyproterone acetate treatment.

METABOLISM OF ANDROGEN IN DOG HYPOTHALAMUS, PITUITARY, AND LIMBIC SYSTEM

Since the central nervous system plays an important role in controlling the production and secretion of androgens by specific endocrine tissues and also acts as a target organ for androgens, it was of interest to study the enzymatic capacity of the hypothalamus and pituitary for biotransformation of testosterone, particularly since both structures are involved on the feed-back mechanisms regulating LH (ICSH) or FSH biosynthesis and secretion. In addition, the limbic system was also included in this study since it participates in the regulation of sexual behavior (Bajusz, 1967) and might be considered as a point of action of androgens. These experiments were reported recently (Pérez-Palacios *et al.*, 1969*a*). Tissues from the canine central nervous system were obtained by surgery. Immediately after removal minced preparations were made separately from the pituitary, the hypothalamus, and the hippocampus (limbic area), and incubated either with 7-^{3}H-testosterone or 4-^{14}C-androstenedione. Following preliminary partition of the crude extracts from hypothalamus, pituitary and limbic area incubates, more than 90% of the radioactive material was found in the methanol fraction. Identification of several formed metabolites was then accomplished by reverse isotope dilution techniques which included identical chromatographic behavior with the steroid carrier under study and recrystallization to constant specific activity. With this criterion it was possible to demonstrate the transformation of testosterone to 5α-dihydrotestosterone, androstenedione and 5α-androstanedione (5α-A). When androstenedione was used as substrate, the following metabolites were identified: 5α-androstanedione, testosterone and 5α-dihydrotestosterone. The dog pituitary tissue effected the conversion of Δ^4 to T, 5α-A and 5α-DHT to the greatest extent (33.7×10^{-9} mμmol/mg, 12.1×10^{-9} mμmol/mg and 2.6×10^{-9} mμmol/mg respectively). The hypothalamus was also capable of effecting these conversions but to a lesser extent than the pituitary (16.8×10^{-9} mμmol/mg, 4.4×10^{-9} mμmol/mg, and 1.33×10^{-9} mμmol/mg), whereas in the limbic area, the metabolic conversions were lower than in the two other tissues (3.9×10^{-9} mμmol/mg, 4.1×10^{-9} mμmol/mg, and 0.8×10^{-9} mμmol/mg, respectively). In the experiment in which testosterone served as substrate, again the pituitary had the greatest enzymatic conversion to Δ^4, 5α-DHT, and 5α-A (116.0×10^{-9} mμmol/mg, 69.9×10^{-9} mμmol/mg, and 69.9×10^{-9} mμmol/mg respectively). The hypothalamus gave metabolic conversions to a lesser extent than the pituitary (37.8×10^{-9} mμmol/mg, 16.2×10^{-9} mμmol/mg, and 16.2×10^{-9} mμmol/mg respectively), but higher than those effected by the limbic area. In addition we demonstrated the failure of these tissues to utilize testosterone sulfate due to absence of a 17β-ol sulfatase (Cabeza and Pérez-Palacios, 1970).

Whether these small *in vitro* conversions relate to the situation in the living dog brain, remains to be elucidated. However, it has been demonstrated very recently that 5α-DHT enhanced the incorporation of cytidine into RNA in rat pituitary (Charreau *et al.*, 1970) suggesting the participation of the 5α-reduced metabolite in the process of protein biosynthesis.

Our results confirm and extend those of Jaffe (1969), who demonstrated the presence of a testosterone 5α-reductase system in the rat and human fetal pituitary and hypothalamus with enzymatic activity very similar to our findings, and support the concept that metabolic interaction may occur between brain and androgenic steroids, as has been suggested in the rat (Sholiton *et al.*, 1966).

STUDIES ON HUMAN SKIN

We have been interested in some metabolic aspects of the testicular feminization syndrome, a particular form of male pseudo-hermaphroditism. Pérez-Palacios *et al.* (1968*a*) reported -a ultrastructural and biochemical correlation study on the gonads of these patients demonn strating the *de novo* biosynthesis of androgens, and Morato and Gual (1967), using both free and conjugated C_{21} and C_{19} steroid substrates, reported androgen formation by gonadal tissue from a patient with the so-called 'complete' form of the syndrome.

Very recently it was suggested that the defect in this genetic abnormality is located at the cellular level of target tissues and it has been proposed that the absence of the 5α-steroid reductase may explain the non-response to androgens observed in these patients.

In this regard we reported recently (Pérez-Palacios *et al.*, 1970) that at least in the incomplete form of the syndrome there is no enzymic impairment. We compared the activity of pubic skin from two patients with both normal male and normal female pubic skin when incubated *in vitro* with ^{3}H-testosterone and 4-^{14}C-androstenedione. Both 5α-reduced androgens were found as metabolic conversion products and no difference was noted between normal and 'abnormal' pubic skin. Furthermore during this congress one of us (Pérez-Palacios *et al.*, 1970) will report the presence of testosterone and androstenedione 5α-reductase in the pubic skin of a patient with the complete form of the syndrome. In addition, the metabolic response to testosterone and 5α-dihydrotestosterone propionate was studied in this patient and in a normal subject. The parameters used were urinary nitrogen and phosphorus during a constant diet. No effect was noted in the patient with TFS, whereas a marked anabolic effect was observed in the normal control. This last study confirms and extends that of Strickland and French (1969) who used free dihydrotestosterone and obtained the same results. The use of the propionate ester does not modify the metabolic response. Our studies suggest that the concept of an enzymic defect in this syndrome must betaken with caution and that individual variations may occur.

Several investigators have demonstrated the presence of a 5α-reductase system that converts testosterone to 5α-dihydrotestosterone in prostate, seminal vesicle and preputial glands among other tissues. There is recent evidence that indicates that 5α-reduced androgens influence biochemical processes that lead to protein synthesis in target tissues (Bashirelaki *et al.*, 1969; Charreau *et al.*, 1970). Our data confirm the presence of 5α-reductases and demonstrate the capability of other tissues to effect this reaction. Although there may be a correlation between 5α-reduction and androgen dependency in the so-called androgen target tissues, this reaction has been demonstrated in many mammalian tissues. The actual biological significance of these events remains to be elucidated.

ACKNOWLEDGMENT

The experimental part of these studies was supported partially by a Ford Foundation Grant.

REFERENCES

ANDERSON, K. M. and LIAO, S. (1968): Selective retention of dihydrotestosterone by prostatic nuclei. *Nature (Lond.) 219*, 277.

BAJUSZ, E. (1967): Modern trends in neuroendocrinology with special reference to clinical problems. A concluding review. In: *An Introduction to Clinical Neuroendocrinology*, p. 428. Editor: E. Bajusz. Williams and Wilkins, Baltimore.

BASHIRELAKI, N., CHADER, G. J. and VILLEE, C. A. (1969): Effects of dihydrotestosterone on the synthesis of nucleic acid and ATP in prostate nuclei. *Biochem. biophys. Res. Commun. 37*, 976.

BAULIEU, E. E., LASNITZKI, I. and ROBEL, P. (1968): Metabolism of testosterone and action of metabolites on prostate glands grown in organ culture. *Nature (Lond.)*, *219*, 1155.

BAULIEU, E. E., LASNITZKI, I. and ROBEL, P. (1969): Metabolism of testosterone and activity of metabolites in prostate organ culture. In: *Abstracts, 51st Meeting of the U.S. Endocrine Society.*

BRUCHOVSKI, N. and WILSON, J. D. (1968): The conversion of testosterone to 5α-androstan-17β-ol-3-one by rat prostate *in vivo* and *in vitro*. *J. biol. Chem.*, *243*, 2012.

CABEZA, A. and PEREZ-PALACIOS, G. (1970): Unpublished data.

CHARREAU, E. H. BALDI, A., BLAQUIER, J. and WASSERMAN, G. (1970): Studies on the mechanism of action of testosterone and dihydrotestosterone Uptake and effects on RNA-metabolism in castrated rats. *Acta endocr. (Panam.)*, *1*, 39.

DORFMAN, R. I. and SHIPLEY, R. A. (1956): Androgens: biochemistry, physiology and clinical significance, p. 118. Wiley, New York.

DUARTE, L., SANCHEZ-MEDAL, L., LABARDINI, J. and ARRIAGA, L. (1967): The erythropoietic effects of anabolic steroids. *Proc. Soc. exp. Biol. (N.Y.)*, *125*, 1030.

FANG, S., ANDERSON, K. M. and LIAO, S. (1969): Receptor proteins for androgens. On the role of specific proteins in selective retention of 17β-hydroxy-5α-androstan-3-one by rat ventral prostate *in vivo* and *in vitro*. *J. biol. Chem.*, *244*, 6584.

JACOBSON, W., SIDMAN, R. L. and DIAMOND, L. K. (1968): The effect of testosterone on the uptake of tritiated thymidine by the bone marrow of children. *Ann. N.Y. Acad. Sci.*, *149*, 389.

JAFFE, R. B. (1969): Testosterone metabolism in target tissues: Hypothalamic and pituitary tissues of the adult rat and human fetus, and the immature rat epiphysis. *Steroids*, *14*, 483.

KATO, T. and HORTN, R. (1968): Studies of testosterone binding globulin. *J. clin. Endocr. 28*, 1160.

KENNEDY, B. J. and GILBERTSON, A. S. (1957): Increased erythropoiesis induced by androgenic hormone therapy. *New Engl. J. Med., 256*, 719.

MAINWARNIG, W. I. P. (1969): The binding of 1,2-^{3}H testosterone within nuclei of the rat prostate. *J. Endocr. 44*, 323.

MERCIER, C. (1966): Specificity of a plasma testosterone binding globulin. In: *Abstracts, II International Congress on Hormonal Steroids,* Milan, 1966, p. 269. ICS No. 111. Excerpta Medica, Amsterdam.

MIRAND, E. A., GORDON, A. S. and WENIG, J. (1965): Mechanism of testosterone action on erythropoiesis. *Nature (Lond.), 206*, 270.

MORATO, T., FLORES, F. and PEREZ-PALACIOS, G. (1970): In vitro metabolism of testosterone in rat bone marrow tissue. In: *Abstracts, 52nd Meeting of the U.S. Endocrine Society.*

MORATO, T. and GUAL, C. (1968*a*): Metabolism of free and sulfoconjugated dehydroisoandrosterone by feminizing testicular tissue. In: *Abstracts, III International Congress of Endocrinology,* p. 105. Editor: C. Gual. ICS No. 157, Excerpta Medica, Amsterdam.

MORATO, T. and GUAL, C. (1968*b*): Biosíntesis de andrógenos y estrógenos por tejido testicular feminizante, *Mem. Soc. Mex. Nut. Endocr. 8*, 47.

NECHELES, T. F. and RAI, U. S. (1969): Studies on the control of hemoglobin synthesis: The in vitro stimulatory effect of a 5β-H steroid metabolite on heme formation in human bone marrow cells. *Blood, 34*, 380.

PEREZ-PALACIOS, G., CASTAÑEDA, E., GOMEZ-PEREZ, F., PEREZ, A. E. and GUAL C. (1969*a*): In vitro metabolism of androgens in dog hypothalamus, pituitary and limbic system. *Mem. Soc. Mex. Nutr. Endocr., 9*, 129.

PEREZ-PALACIOS, G., LAMONT, K. G., PEREZ, A. E., JAFFE, R. B. and PIERCE, B. G. (1969*b*): De novo formation and metabolism of steroid hormones in feminizing testes: Biochemical and ultrastructural studies. *J. clin. Endocr., 29*, 786.

PEREZ-PALACIOS, G., PEREZ, A. E., CASTAÑEDA, E. and MORATO, T., (1970): Presence of testosterone and androstenedione 5α-reductase in two cases of the incomplete testicular feminization syndrome. In: *Abstracts, 52nd Meeting of the U.S. Endocrine Society,*

PEREZ-PALACIOS, G., PEREZ, A. E., CASTAÑEDA, E., RAMIREZ, S., GUILLEN, M. A. and GULA, C. (1970): In vitro biotransformation of androgens in the skin from a case of complete testicular feminization syndrome. In: *Abstracts, VIII Pan-American Congress of Endocrinology*, São Paulo, Brasil.

REISNER, E. H., Jr. (1966): Tissue of culture bone marrow. II. Effect of steroid hormones on hematopoiesis in vitro. *Blood, 27*, 460.

SANCHEZ-MEDAL, L., GOMEZ-LEAL, A., DUARTE, L. and RICO, M. G. (1969): Anabolic androgenic steroids in the treatment of acquired aplastic anemia. *Blood, 34*, 283.

SHOLITON, L. J., MARNELL, R. T. and WERK, E. E. (1966): Metabolism of testosterone-4-^{14}C by rat brain homogenates and subcellular fraction. *Steroids, 8*, 265.

STEINGLAS, P., GORDON, A. S. and CHARIPPER, H. A. (1941): Effect of castration and sex hormones on the blood of rats. *Proc. Soc. exp. Biol. (N.Y.), 48*, 169.

STERN, J. M. and EISENFELD, A. J. (1969): Androgen accumulation and binding to macromolecules in seminal vesicles: Inhibition by cyproterone. *Science, 166*, 233.

STRICKLAND, A. L. and FRENCH, F. S. (1969): Absence of response to dihydrotestosterone in the syndrome of testicular feminization. *J. clin. Endocr. 29*, 1284.

TVETER, K. J. and ATTRAMADAL, A. (1968): Selective uptake of radioactivity in rat ventral prostate following administration of testosterone, 1,2-^{3}H. *Acta endocr. (Kbh.), 59*, 218.

INTRA-TESTICULAR INCLUSIONS OF ADRENAL-CORTICAL TISSUE; CLINICAL, HISTOLOGICAL AND HORMONAL OBSERVATIONS IN THREE CASES

H. BRICAIRE, M. H. LAUDAT, J. P. LUTON and G. TURPIN

Centre de Recherches Endocrinologiques, Hôpital Cochin, Paris XIV, France

Intra-testicular inclusions of adrenal-cortical tissue occur very rarely. But because the similarity between suprarenal and Leydig tissue is so close from the structural and functional points of view, even the existence of ectopic adrenal-cortical tissue in the gonads is disputed by some investigators.

We have had the opportunity to observe, over a period of a few years, three patients presenting with the above condition. They seemed to us to pose, schematically, major nosological and diagnostic problems and we therefore felt that it was important to record all the clinical, histological and hormonal findings associated with intra-testicular inclusions gathered during this study.

With regard to these findings, we will recapitulate the arguments and counter-arguments which one uses to substantiate or reject a possible adreno-cortical origin of this tissue.

MATERIAL AND METHODS

The following methods were used: urinary 17-hydroxycorticoids (Porter and Silber); pregnanediol (PG); pregnanetriol (PGT) (Bongiovanni-Eberlein); tetrahydro 11-deoxycortisol (TH_4 S) (Henke-Doe); tetrahydroaldosterone (Legrand); normal: 40-60 μg/day (24 hours on normal (salt) diet); total urinary gonadotropins (biological method); plasma ACTH (biological method of Lipscomb-Nelson, modified by Girard-Binoux); normal: 0.21 milli-units per 100 ml $\pm$ 0.09; plasma testosterone (Dray); normal: male 0.80 $\pm$ 0.12 μg%, female 0.045 $\pm$ 0.02 μg%; plasma corticosterone (Eechaute); normal: 0.8 μg%; plasma cortisol (De Moor); prolan B (biological method).

Our studies are based on the following 3 observations.

OBSERVATION I:

Pierre Far . . ., male, 17 years old, hospitalized in 1965.

(1) *History*: 4 years – spurt of growth and BP = 140/80 mm Hg; 7 years – onset of signs of puberty with appearance of 2 large testes; 12 years – cessation of growth, final height 147 cm; 13 years – BP = 150 mm Hg (systolic).

(2) *Examination in 1965*: A boy of 17 years, measuring 147 cm, and having a characteristic build: head very large, muscularly well developed; BP = 190/140 mm Hg. Both testes increased in volume and multinodular, particularly the left one. Epididymis was difficult to palpate. Spermatic cord and prostate normal. The rest of clinical examination was normal, including mental development.

(3) *A review of the family history revealed several cases of congenital hyperplasia of the adrenal gland.*

(4) *Main examinations*: The routine biochemical tests were normal (urea, glucose, cholesterol, ESR, CBC, blood and urinary electrolytes). The diagnosis of congenital hyperplasia of the adrenal gland with a deficiency of 11β-hydroxylation was confirmed by clinical and pathological data.

TABLE I

Far . . ., Pierre (observation I)

	Stimulation			Metyrapone		Dexamethasone		
	75 I.U. ACTH i.v.			4 g orally		3 mg × 5 days		
	0	1st day	2nd day	1st day	2nd day	0	3rd day	5th day
17-ketosteroids (mg/day)	57.8	108.6	82	52.8	79.2	59.2	4.8	4.6
DHEA (mg/day)	8							
17-hydroxycorticosteroids (mg/day)	44.1	48.3	40	41.6	39.9	23.8	2.8	1.5
Estrone + estradiol (μg/day)	48							
Estriol (μg/day)	85							
Pregnanediol (mg/day)						13.5	1.4	
Pregnanetriol (mg/day)	6					2.7	0.1	
Tetrahydro compound 'S' (mg/day)	35					18.8		
Urinary aldosterone (μg/day)	4							
Urinary gonadotrophins	–3							

There was a closure of growing cartilage. A testicular biopsy was performed (Dr. Steg) (see Histology).

(5) *Progress*: Treatment by dexamethasone (1 mg/24 hr) resulted in a total regression of the intra-testicular nodules on clinical examination, a normalization of the BP at 130/80 mm Hg, and a significant decrease of urinary steroids: 17-ketosteroids – 3.6 mg/24 hr; 17 hydroxycorticoids – 1.6 mg/24 hr.

When 0.5 mg dexamethasone was given per 24 hr, excretion of urinary steroids was normal, but the intra-gonadal nodules reappeared. The disappearance of the intra-testicular nodules was thus only obtained at the price of a fairly significant inhibitory effect on the hypothalamic-hypophyseal-adrenal axis.

OBSERVATION II:

Denis Fou . . ., male 19 years old, hospitalized in February 1968, when 2 testicular tumours were discovered at routine medical examination for military service.

(1) *The pathological history developed by various stages*:

1st phase: At 2 years of age, appearance of pubic hair and erection. In 1953, at 4 years of age, the child was hospitalized in a pediatric unit, with the diagnosis of precocious pseudo-puberty. Height: 111.5 cm; weight: 19.5 kg; presence of signs of puberty: significant pubic hair, penile development; small infantile testes (normal for a 4-year-old child); bone age: 8 years; sella turcica normal; 17-ketosteroids excretion was 18.5 mg/24 hr.

In view of a doubtful shadow apparent on induction of a retropneumoperitoneum, surgical exploration of the left suprarenal was performed. This revealed a general hyperplasia of the suprarenal gland (the suprarenal was not removed). Post-operatively, there had been an episode of acute renal insufficiency, well controlled by the use of deoxycorticosterone.

One month later a right adrenalectomy was performed; precise histological examination revealed a considerable hyperplasia of the adrenal cortex involving the zona fasciculata.

After excision of the right suprarenal: gonadotrophins – less than 3 U.S.; 17-ketosteroids – 35 mg/day (remember that the left suprarenal had simply been explored and left in place).

At 6 years, the genital development was that of a pubescent child; height: 130 cm; weight: 29 kg.

2nd phase: 1955–1968; no other medical examination was performed or treatment given. It appeared that arrest of growth had occurred at the age of 12 years (161 cm). One particular pathological feature demonstrated by the patient was the need to take an abundant amount of salt with his food.

(2) *Examination in 1968*: Height: 161 cm; weight: 55.8 kg. Morphologically android, with the muscle mass well developed. The pilosity was that of an adult, and he had been shaving 3 times weekly since the age of 13. Examination of the genital organs revealed a penis of adult dimensions, a large right testis (6.5 cm × 3.5 cm) with 2 nodules at the level of the 2 poles and a small nodule between the epididymis and the testis; a large, hard, irregular left testis (4.5 cm × 2.5 cm) with a midline mass; epididymis and vas deferens appeared normal; the prostate was not palpated; there was no gynaecomastia. No evidence of erection or ejaculation.

The rest of the examination was absolutely normal. BP = 110/60 mm Hg.

(3) *Family history*: There was no known precocious puberty in the family, nor any of the toxicoses of childhood, nor death at an early age of brother or sister.

(4) *Principal examinations*: Routine pathological tests were normal (urea, sugar, cholesterol, ESR, CBC). The diagnosis of congenital hyperplasia of the adrenals with a deficiency of 21-hydroxylation was confirmed by the following biochemical data.

A testicular biopsy was performed (Dr. Steg) (the results are documented in the section on Histology).

The day after this procedure, all therapy having been previously stopped, the syndrome of suprarenal insufficiency became apparent, clinically and biochemically (hyponatraemia). This was rapidly controlled by intramuscular cortisone.

(5) *Progress*: From the end of the post-operative phase, prolonged inhibition of the hypothalamic-pituitary-adrenal axis was undertaken for 15 days, using dexamethasone (3 mg/day). This produced a progressive and spectacular shrinkage of the testicular nodules (4.5 × 2.5 cm on the right, and 3.5 × 2 cm on the left). In parallel with this, the biochemical abnormalities improved (Table II). At this time, the patient was treated with 0.5 mg dexamethasone/day (at midnight) and 20 mg hydrocortisone/day (10 mg at 8.00 a.m. and 10 mg at 8.00 p.m.). The hydrocortisone had to be stopped a month later, because of the appearance of hypercortisolism.

In 1970, the testis had a normal volume. The biochemical data (with 0.5 mg dexamethasone and then 1 mg of dexamethasone/24 hr, because of a rise in 17-ketosteroid excretion) are summarized in Table II.

OBSERVATION III:

Joël Duv . . ., 14 years old.

(1) *Pathological history*:

1st phase: At the age of 6½ years, medical examination for precocious puberty revealed a large right testis (having the same volume as that of pubertal child) and an ectopic left testis. Height: 135 cm; weight: 29.5 kg; total 17-ketosteroids: 8.1 mg/day; 17 hydroxycorticoids: 2.4 mg/day; urinary gonadotrophins: less than 6 U.S.

TABLE II

Fou . . ., Denis (observation II)

	February 1968			March 1968				May 1968	November 1968	July 1969	
	Depot Synacthen (0.5 mg/day)			Dexamethasone (3 mg/day)				Dexamethasone (0.5 mg/day)	Dexamethasone (0.5 mg/day)	Dexa-methasone	
	0	1st day	2nd day	0	3rd day	5th day	12th day			0.5/mg day	3mg 3rd, 5th d
sma											
tosterone 8 a.m. (μg/100 ml)	0.40			0.40		0.089	0.052				
rtisol 8 a.m. (μg/100 ml)	7.6										
rticosterone 8 a.m. (μg/100 ml)	6.6										
TH 9 a.m. mU/100 ml	0.7										
ne											
ketosteroids (mg/day)	61.6	128	89.5	61	20.3	6.1	6.5	4.8	25.7	37.7	9.8
IEA (mg/day)	9.8			9.8		0.5	0.6				
hydroxycorticosteroids mg/day)	1.4	1.3	2.5	1.4	2	3.2	3.2	1.3		0.9	0.4
rone + estradiol + striol (μg/day)	11			11							
gnanediol (mg/day)	25.2	41.4		25.2	4.8	5.4		6.6	51.4	47.6	4.8
gnanetriol (mg/day)	23.4	46		23.4	3.3	0.9		0.3	4.6	20.5	0.4
trahydro compound S' (mg/day)										<0.5	<0.5
trahydroaldesterone μg/day)	116		120			55					
tal urinary gonadotrophins (u/day)	+5	—30									

The ectopic left testis, the size of a small bean, was brought down surgically and a right testicular biopsy revealed the histological appearance of a testis at puberty, without any other cytological abnormality. A diagnosis of true precocious puberty was made at the time and neurological examinations, including air encephalogram, were normal.

2nd phase: At 8 years, puberty was completed and the appearance of the testes unchanged. Height: 148 cm; weight: 35.3 kg. An adult-type hirsutism was evident (17-ketosteroids: 24.7 mg/24 hr; gonadotrophins: less than 3 U.S.). The growth rate slowed down, until in 1966 a final height of 165 cm was reached. At 11 years of age, the child was shaving every day.

(2) *Examination in 1969*: Height: 165 cm; weight: 55.4 kg. Android morphology; adult-sized penis; scrotum wrinkled and pigmented; right testis measuring 6.5 cm × 4.5 cm, with a hard, regular and homogeneous nodule covering the superior pole; left testis atrophic and firm, measuring 2 cm × 1 cm and insensitive. Epididymis, vas deferens and prostate normal. No gynaecomastia. The libido was difficult to assess accurately, but erection with ejaculation was present. BP: 150/80 mm Hg.

The rest of the examination was normal, except for the presence of a flushed face and genuine vasomotor attacks of sweating alternating with flushing and pallor (normal levels

TABLE III

Duv . . ., Joël, 1 (observation III)

		Dexamethasone (3 mg/day)				Depot Synacthen (0.5 mg i.m.)		
	0	5th day	7th day +10000 U HCG	9th day +10000 U HCG	11th day +10000 U HCG	0	1st day	2nd day
Plasma								
Testosterone 8 a.m. (μg/100 ml)	1.43	1.37			1.37			
Cortisol 8 a.m. (μg/100 ml)	30							
ACTH 9 a.m. mU/100 ml	<0.13							
Urine								
17-ketosteroids (mg/day)	93.8	120	115	96.3	154.3	144	108.3	118
DHEA (mg/day)	7.9	21						
17-hydrocorticosteroids (mg/day)	3.7	0.9	0.8	1.6	1.9	2.4	4.6	2.8
Estrone+estradiol+estriol (μg/day)	24.2				21.1			
Pregnanediol (mg/day)		10.4						9
Pregnanetriol (mg/day)	1.5	3.6						3.5
Tetrahydro compound 'S' (mg/day)	0.5						0.5	
Tetrahydroaldesterone (μg/day)	68.5							
Urinary gonadotrophins (U/day)	—3							
Prolan B (U/day)	<5							

of VMA, catecholamines and 5-HIAA). There was no adenopathy. Chest X-ray normal.

(3) *Main biochemical investigations*: The principal biochemical data have been recorded in Table III which shows essentially an elevation of the plasma testosterone, 17-ketosteroids and estrogens.

The abnormalities were not very responsive to the usual dynamic tests of stimulation and inhibition. The data were not suggestive of congenital hyperplasia of the suprarenals. Prolan B levels were normal.

Surgical exploration (Dr. Steg) revealed right testis with increased volume, hypervascular and having the macroscopic appearance of a seminoma. Beneath the head of the epididymis a very firm, nodular area was present. After opening the tunica albuginea, a multilobulated tumour with a cystic appearance was enucleated, but the contents were not liquid. This tumour involved the whole testis. The testis was surgically removed, removing en bloc the testis and only the proximal part of the cord. A right testicular prosthesis was inserted.

During the course of the surgical exploration, catheterization of the right spermatic vein was carried out. The levels of the plasma testosterone during surgery were 25.8 μg% in the spermatic vein, and 1.07 μg% in a peripheral vein (of the elbow (anteriorly)) respectively. (See the histological examination.)

(4) *Progress*: Since the operation, the patient has not had any treatment. Clinically, the

testicular prosthesis has been well tolerated and the left testis increased progressively in volume, to attain in June 1970 the dimensions of a normal adult testis. No adenopathy was apparent. BP: 110/80 mm Hg. The rubrosity and the sudden vasomotor attacks ceased. Chest X-ray normal.

The new biochemical tests are summarized in Table IV.

There is essentially normalization of the excretion of steroid breakdown products, and a normal level of urinary gonadotrophins.

Principal comments on the above 3 observations

In 2 of our cases, the diagnosis was almost certainly intra-testicular suprarenal inclusion (observations I and II), with congenital adrenal hyperplasia as well. This is shown by the deficiency in 11β-hydroxylase (observation I), and the deficiency in 21-hydroxylase (observation II).

In these 2 observations, the diagnosis rests on impressive clinical, biochemical and developmental data.

On the other hand, the diagnostic problem is much more difficult in observation III, characterized by a precocious pseudo-puberty, and a right testicular tumor.

A Leydig-cell tumor is a possibility: unilateral tumor, precocious pseudo-puberty, gonadotrophins less than 3 U.S., hyperandrogenism, hyperestrogenism, with a predominance of

TABLE IV

Duv . . ., Joël, 2 (observation III)

	Orchid-ectomy at 8 days	Depot Synacthen 3 months later			8 months later			14 months later Dexamethasone	
	0	0	1st day	2nd day	0	1st day	2nd day	0	(3 mg/day)
sma									
tosterone 8 a.m. (μg/100 ml)	0.004	0.259			0.274				
rtisol 8 a.m. (μg/ml)	18	16							
TH 9 a.m. (mU/100 ml)		<0.13							
ne									
ketosteroids (mg/day)	5.5	12.8	14	9.4	7.8	9.7	7.8	9.4	5.8
EA (mg/day)	0.6	0.9	1.6					2.8	
hydroxycorticosteroids mg/day)	3.7	6.4	11.9	4.4	4.2	12.2	3.6	3.2	3.2
rone + estradiol + striol (μg/day)		6			8				
gnanediol (mg/day)		0.7	1.6		0.9			1.5	
gnanetriol (mg/day)		0.3	0.6		0.5			0.5	
rahydro compound S' (mg/day)		<0.1			1			0.4	
rahydroaldosterone μg/day)		92							
nary gonadotrophins U/day)		+10 —25			+10 —25				

estradiol, elevation of the level of pregnanediol, absence of abnormal excretion of pregnanetriol and of tetrahydro-S, unresponsiveness to the dynamic tests, and finally, the appearance of true puberty with elevation of gonadotrophins and increase in the remaining testicular volume, a few months after excision of the tumoral testis.

However, since the histological studies were not very conclusive and urinary androgen excretion was very high, we should also consider the possibility of an autonomous intratesticular tumor arising from the intra-gonadal suprarenal tissue.

HISTOLOGICAL, HISTOCHEMICAL AND ULTRASTRUCTURAL STUDIES AND INCUBATION OF TISSUE SECTIONS

Histological study by light microscopy

Technique:

Different fixatives were used for each case: Bouin, Baker's formal-calcium chloride, 10% formol saline. After placing the tissue in paraffin and sectioning at 5 μ, the following dyes were used systematically: H and E, Masson's trichrome, silver impregnation of the reticulin following the technique of Gordon-Sweet and MacManus, Alcian blue. The methods of Fontana and of Schmorl were also used to try to show up some of the intra-cytoplasmic granulations.

Results:

1st observation: The histological pattern of this neoplasm, composed of strictly monomorphic, eosinophilic-like elements with an endocrine structure had, in spite of the absence of crystalloids of Reinke, rather the nature of Leydig cells. The appearance of this proliferation, which did not contain any trace of testicular tissue, was more that of a true adenoma than a simple hyperplastic phenomenon. However, a suprarenal origin is not incompatible with such an appearance (Fig. 1).

2nd observation: The structure of this tumor, composed, in part, of small eosinophilic-type cells, was frankly endocrine and had a glomerular and trabecular structure. Microscopic examination was more in favor of a suprarenal origin, without however being able to exclude the possibility of a Leydig-cell tumor. This impression was based on the general structure of the growth, on the clarified spongiocytic appearance of some of the cells and their mode of arrangement (Fig. 2).

3rd observation: The macroscopic appearance of the tissue was typified by its brown-black color, similar to that which one observes in suprarenal adenomas. A significant cellular proliferation was apparent, occupying nearly the whole gland. Its interpretation was difficult because, while the general structure was typically that of an endocrine tumor, the appearances were neither entirely those of a Leydig adenoma (cells too large, proliferation too dense, cytoplasm too heterogeneous) nor entirely those of suprarenal tissue; the characteristic spongiocytes were only very poorly marked (Fig. 3).

In this case it is impossible to draw a conclusion from the light microscopy alone.

The examination by classical light microscopy seems to us to be inadequate to define precisely the origin of these cellular growths.

Histoenzymological study:

This study has been summarized in observations II and III.

(1) *Technique*: The histological study was made on fresh sections stored at –70° and cut with a cryostat. 3β-Hydroxysteroid dehydrogenase and 17β-hydroxysteroid dehydrogenase levels were studied by the techniques of Wattenberg (1958) and Davies *et al.* (1966).

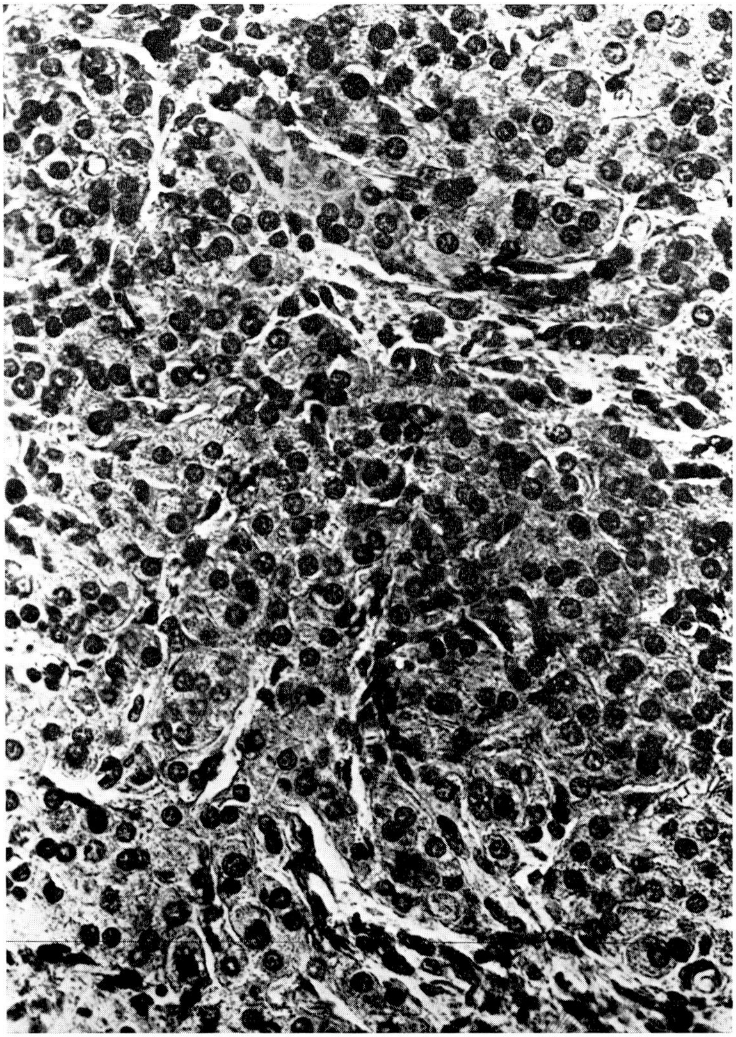

Fig. 1. Histological pattern (× 410, reduced for reproduction 10%) observation I (Far. . ., Pierre) (see text).

(2) *Description*: The cells of the 2 tumors examined possessed a rich enzymatic content, closely comparable to that which we have observed in normal human suprarenal tissue. We noticed, in particular, the high activity of 2 enzymes involved in the formation of the steroid hormones, 3β-hydroxy-dehydrogenase and 17β-hydroxy-dehydrogenase.

(3) *Commentary*: Histoenzymology has established categorically that the tumorous cells of the 2 cases studied actively produce steroid hormones. The distribution of the formazan which demonstrates this activity morphologically is uniform and is seen in all the cells with, at the very most, some variations in intensity; it shows that all the tumorous cells are capable of elaborating some steroid hormones.

The histoenzymological study does permit one to settle the problem of the precise nature of the tumorous cells and of their significance (suprarenal remnants or Leydig cells): the two enzymatic activities disclosed, are, in fact, found in both the suprarenal tissue and in normal

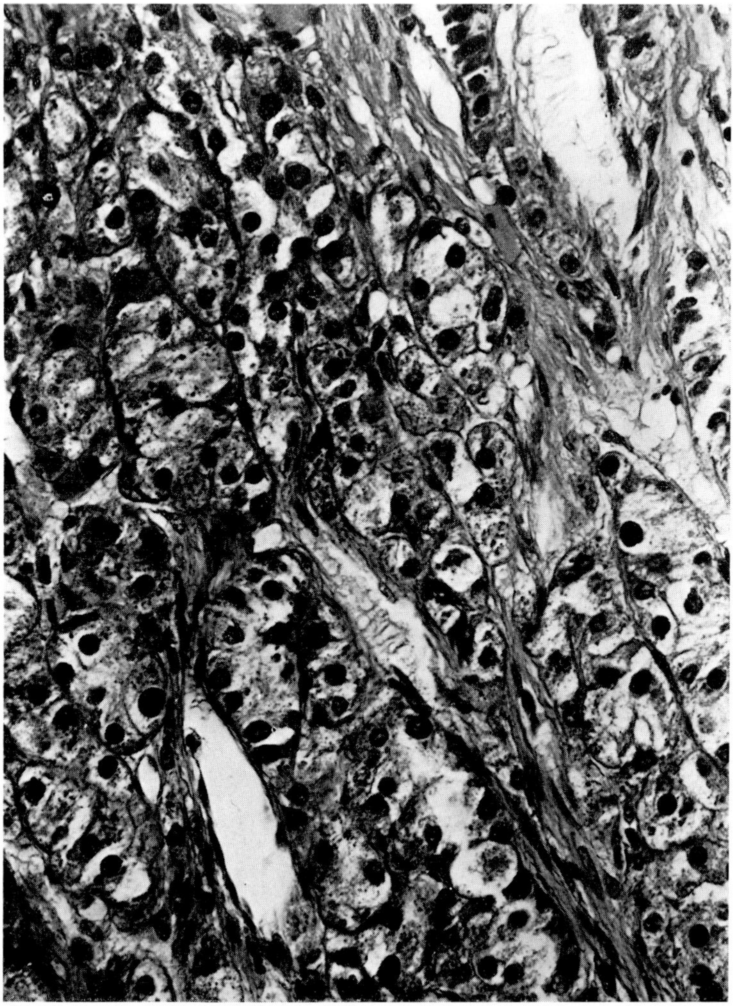

Fig. 2. Histological pattern ($\times$ 410, reduced for reproduction 10%) observation II (Fou. . ., Denis).

Leydig tissue, as our studies and those of others on normal suprarenal and testis have confirmed. Nevertheless, the general physiognomy of the group of enzymatic activities, and especially the intensity of the reactions of the 3β-hydroxy-dehydrogenase persuade us in favor of a suprarenal origin. The 3β-hydroxy-dehydrogenase reaction is much weaker when using Leydig tissue, than when using suprarenal tissue, when utilizing the substrate employed here (dehydroepiandrosterone).

These arguments are however insufficient to enable us to draw a firm conclusion about the nature of the tumorous nodules.

Ultrastructural studies:

Ultrastructured studies of the second and third observations were carried out.

(1) *Technique*: The tissues sectioned for this study were immediately fixed in glutaraldehyde, then in osmium tetroxide and enclosed in epon. The contrast in the ultrafine sections

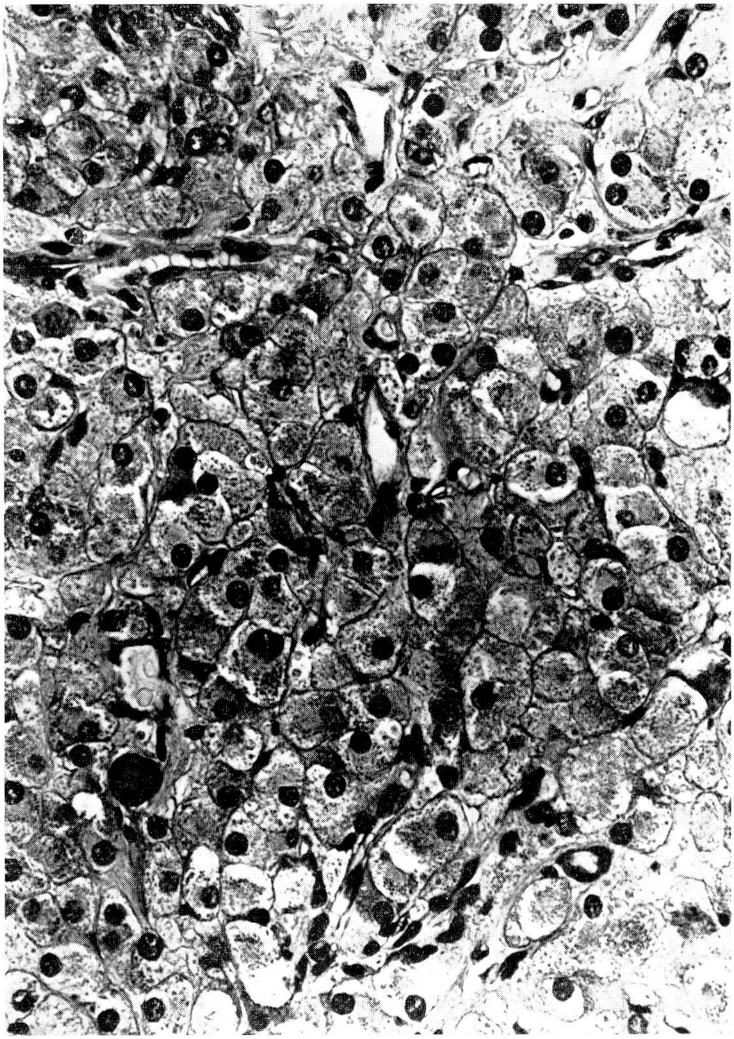

Fig. 3. Histological pattern ($\times$ 410, reduced for reproduction 10%) observation III (Duv. . ., Joël).

was effected with the aid of lead citrate associated with alcoholic uranyl acetate. The examination was performed with the Siemens Elmiskop I microscope. Histological checks were made on sections from the original sample and on some semi-fine sections dyed with silver nitrate.

(2) *Results*: In the 2 observations, the ultrastructural study turned out to be identical. The cells were tightly packed together, so much so that it was difficult to discern the cellular outlines.

The results of the electron microscopy confirmed those of light microscopy (Fig. 4). The cellular elements frequently had an eosinophilic or spongiocytic appearance. In certain areas of the cytoplasm, the mitochondria or some dense bodies formed compact accumulations, whereas in other areas there was only endoplasmic reticulum. The cells had an agranular endoplasmic reticulum, vesicular or with open spaces, some mitochondria with tubular crests and Golgi apparatuses secreting very little.

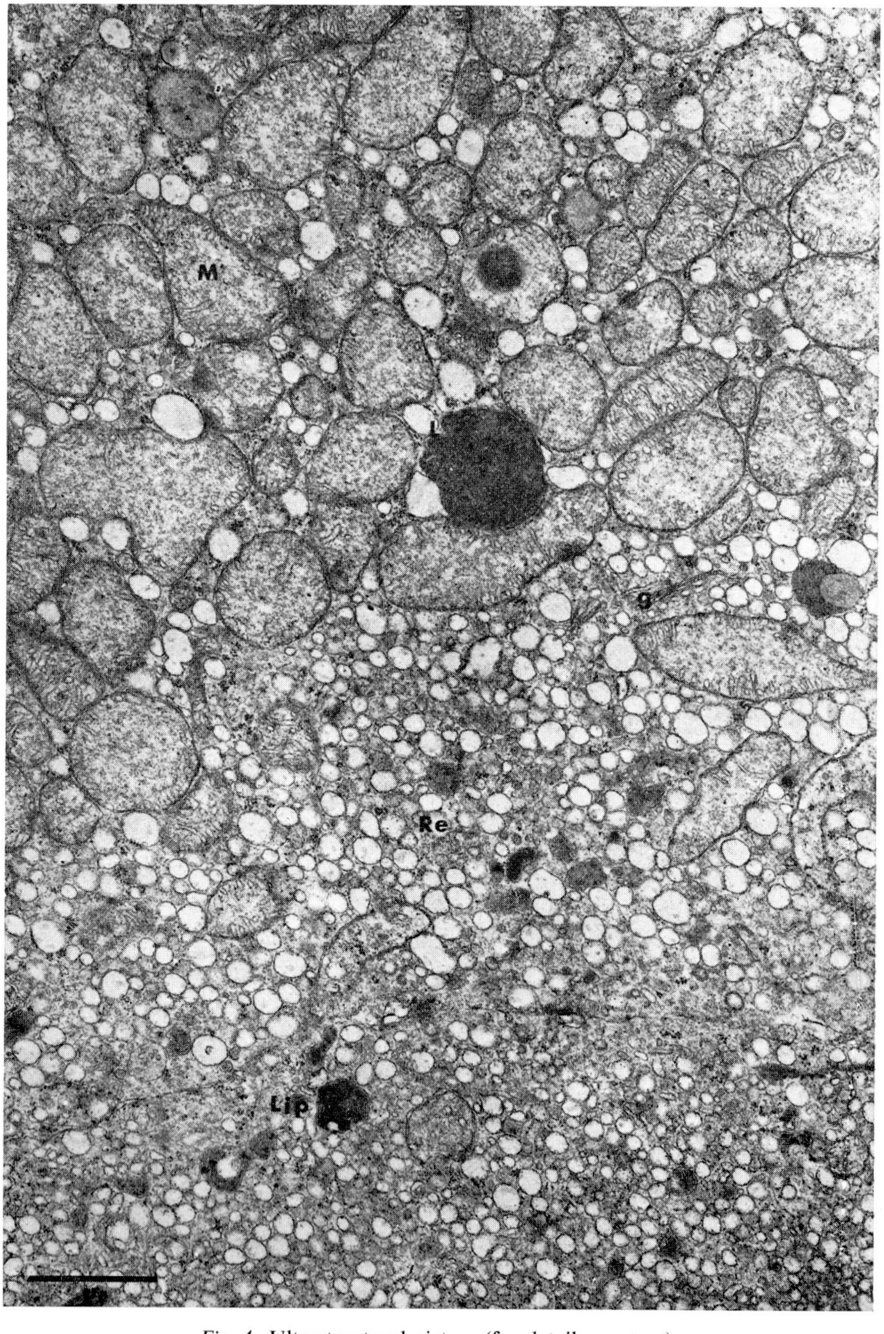

Fig. 4. Ultrastructural picture (for details, see text).

L = Liposomes
re = Reticulum
M = Mitochondris
g = Golgi
Lip = Lipofuscin

This appearance is entirely characteristic of cells which are actively producing steroids. The large, distended vacuoles of the reticulum conferred on these proliferations a spongiocytic appearance, but are not, for all that, solely the characteristic of suprarenal cells, because a Leydig-cell hyperplasia is not exempt from this appearance.

Finally, there are the dense bodies, some of which closely resemble liposomes, while some other, smaller, heterogeneous bodies resemble more closely the lipofuscins. The presence of lipofuscins is in favor of a Leydig-type cell, while the absence of myelinated forms is against this hypothesis.

In none of these preparations have we seen myelinated figures or crystalloids of Reinke.

INCUBATION OF TISSUE FRAGMENTS WITH RADIOACTIVE STEROID PRECURSORS

As soon as the required tissue had been cut, it was taken dry at 4°C to the laboratory. The tissue was cut into thin sections of about 100 mg with the aid of a razor-blade, and incubated at 37°C for 3 hr, in a Warburg apparatus containing a gaseous mixture of $CO_2 + O_2$, in 10 ml of Krebs-Ringer bicarbonate at pH 7.5, in the presence of 0.04 M nicotinamide, 0.4 mM ATP, 0.4 mM NAD, and 1 mM fumaric acid, 0.1 mM NADP, 0.5 mM glucose-6-phosphate, 0.1 mM glucose-6-phosphate-dehydrogenase per vial incubated.

The radioactive substrate utilized was C^{14}-17-hydroxy-progesterone (0.5 μCi/incubation) and H^3-5-pregnenolone (5 μCi/incubation). The incubation was stopped by the addition of N-HCl, 1 ml/vial. The tissue was then crushed in a Teenbroeck potter.

The steroids were extracted by organic solvents, and purified by chromatography on florisil. The extracts were then chromatographed on plates of silica gel (HF 254 Merck) with addition of appropriate cold steroids. The solvents used for the separation of the steroids were the following:

1. $CHCl_3$ – EtOH (99-1) – 1 x
   $CHCl_3$ – acetone (90-10) – 3 x

(progesterone, 17-hydroxyprogesterone, 21-deoxycortisol, 4-androstenedione, 4-androstenediol, dehydroepiandrosterone (DHEA), 5-pregnenolone, 17-hydroxy-5-pregnenolone, testosterone);

2. $CHCl_3$ – acetone (7-3) – 1 x
   $CHCl_3$ – MEOH – H_2O (90-9) – 1 x

(cortisol, cortisone, corticosterone, 11-deoxycorticosterone, 11-deoxycortisol, 17-hydroxyprogesterone, 5-pregnenolone).

Method of identification:

The different spots were detected either by their absorption in UV light (2660 A) or after revelation with the aid of a sulphuric-ethanolic mixture (1 : 2). The different spots on the plates were then cut out, and the radioactivity measured with a scintillation counter (Packard 3375) in presence of PPO, POPOP, methanol and toluene. The portions of silica gel found between the spots revealed by the methods mentioned above were likewise cut out and counted.

The results have been expressed in the following manner:

The quantity of radioactivity found in the different steroids isolated from the chromatography plates has allowed us to establish the percentage of the original precursor substance utilized (Table V).

We have then taken this percentage as 100% utilized for calculating the distribution of the radioactivity in the different steroids.

Discussion of the results:

The interpretation of the results shown in Tables V-VII can only be made on a hypothetical

TABLE V

Patient Precursors:	C^{14}-17-OH-progesterone	H^3-5-pregnenolone
Duv. .	22%	79%
Fou. .	31%	63%

TABLE VI

Incorporation of radioactivity into various steroids after incubation in the presence of H^3-5-pregnenolone

	Fou. . .	Duv. . .
Testosterone	15.9%	6 %
DHEA	22.1%	71 %
17-hydroxyprogesterone	30 %	10.9%
17-hydroxy-5-pregnenolone	30 %	12.6%

TABLE VII

Incorporation of radioactivity into various steroids after incubation in the presence of C^{14}-17-OH-progesterone

	Fou. . .	Duv. . .
21-deoxycortisol	11.2%	28 %
11-deoxycortisol	48.2%	16.3%
Cortisol	1.5%	7.1%
4-androstendione	23.4%	22.2%
Testosterone	(not determined)	22 %

basis, since strictly they relate only to the *in vitro* system in which the incorporation of radioactivity into the different steroids is unquestionably conditioned in part by the quality and the quantity of the diverse co-factors used in the system and by the duration of the incubation.

(1) *Incubations in presence of C^{14}-17-OH-progesterone*:

(a) *Patient Fou . . .*: Hydroxylation of 17-OH-progesterone at C-21 yielding compound S seems to have been adequate, since 48.2% of the radioactivity was found in this product. (In the same conditions, a normal suprarenal gives 42%.) However, conversion of S to cortisol was deficient since only 1.5% of the radioactivity is found in the isolated cortisol, demonstrating inadequate 11-hydroxylation of compound S.

It is worth noting that 11-hydroxylation of 17-OH-progesterone proceeded satisfactorily since 11.2% of the radioactivity was found in the 21-deoxycortisol (7% in normal tissue).

(b) *Patient Duv . . .*: As in the preceding case, little radioactivity was found in the cortisol, indicating that 11-hydroxylation of compound S proceeded with difficulty. Biosynthesis of compound S was very clearly inferior to that in the preceding case (16.3% against 48.2%).

Conversely, the production of 21-deoxycortisol was increased in comparison to the preceding case (28% against 11.2%), whereas less cortisol was formed (7.1% against 1.5% previously). This is clearly less than 'normal' tissue (15.5%).

(2) *Incubations in the presence of H^3-5-pregnenolone*:

An important fact to notice is the extremely significant quantity of radioactivity found in DHEA (with patient Duv . . .) compared to Fou . . . (71 % against 22.1 %).

The enzymatic systems required for steroid biosynthesis (17-hydroxylase and 17-dehydrogenase) seemed to function perfectly, considering the amount of substrate utilized.

The incorporation of the radioactivity into testosterone was 15.9 % with Fou . . ., against only 6 % with Duv . . .

Analysis of these results, taking into account the experimental conditions described and the reservations stated, *shows the preponderant role of the substrate in studies of biosynthesis carried out 'in vitro'*. In fact, it seems that the action of a particular enzyme depends on the initial availability of precursor.

The classical terminology of the suprarenal enzymatic disorders, by reference to various deficiencies should, in our opinion, be modified to take note of the above considerations. In the majority of cases, the enzyme deficiencies are incomplete and only relate, strictly, to the particular substrate investigated.

COMMENT

Most authors believe that intragonadal inclusions of suprarenal tissue are functional; others (Landing and Gold, 1951) consider that the tissue is Leydig in origin, but has deviated metabolically during its development, and is then subjected to the action of ACTH (although the sensitivity of the primitive Leydig cells to ACTH has never been demonstrated). Finally, others (Shanklin *et al.*, 1963) think that these hyperplastic nodules may be constituted from a third type of undifferentiated cell, similar to the preceding two, but having an unusual functional potential.

It is difficult to form an opinion of the exact incidence of these inclusions, because a number of earlier observations only give very incomplete clinical, biological and histological information; furthermore, to confirm this diagnosis is always difficult. If one considers only those observations where one is certain of the diagnosis, there is a total of 20 observations (Table VIII) (included in this number is the first observation of this paper).

In these 20 observations (from 1 to 19), there were 12 cases of a uniform or multinodular growth of variable size (obs. 3, 4, 5, 7, 8, 9, 10, 13, 14, 17, 18, 20) in newborn or children (10 cases) and only twice in adults, whereas the 8 other cases comprise true tumors, compressing the normal testicular structures which were not invaded at the periphery. The testis was always immature, without spermatogenesis (except obs. 18) and without Leydig cells.

By contrast, the cells of the intragonadal inclusions were hyperplastic, having the histological appearance of intense functional activity, but without the cytological characteristics of malignancy. These testicular nodules were situated mostly at the level of the rete testis and were always bilateral. In a certain number of cases, there was associated some paratesticular nodules of unquestionable suprarenal origin, and of identical appearance to the testicular nodules (epididymal and funicular: obs. 6, 8 and 13) or some pararenal nodules (obs. 1).

The biological results are interpreted with difficulty, because they are very variable and incomplete, especially the older observations: in all cases where they have been determined, the 17-ketosteroids have been shown to be very elevated (with a predominance of the DHA fraction: obs. 15, 17, 19, 20), as were the levels of pregnanetriol (obs. 15, 16, 17, 19, 20). 17-Hydroxycorticosteroids were elevated in 3 cases (obs. 16, 17, 19). An ACTH test carried out in 5 cases (obs. 15, 16, 18, 19 and 20) was positive in 4. A suppression test using dexamethasone in 6 cases (obs. 15, 16, 17, 18, 19 and 20) produced each time a considerable reduction in the level of 17-ketosteroids (except in the observation where the inhibition was incomplete, but was effective with prednisone). Complete regression of the intratesticular nodules has followed the biochemical data in observation 16 (where the result has been confirmed by a new biopsy) and in the observations 11 and 19. In observation 17, by contrast, the

TABLE VIII

1. Wilkins (1940)	3½ yr	C.A.H. + salt losing
2. Cohen (1946)	20 yr	Virilizing syndrome
3. Thelander (1946)	6 yr	C.A.H. + salt losing
4. Allibone-Barr-Cant (1947)	2 yr	Virilizing syndrome
5. Fassbender (1949)	6 yr	Virilizing syndrome
6. Gardner-Sniffen (1950)	11 yr	C.A.H. + salt losing
7. Sobel-Sniffrn-Talbot (1951)	14 mth	C.A.H. + salt losing
8. Landing-Gold (1951)	14 mth	C.A.H. + salt losing
9. Landing-Gold	10 wk	C.A.H. + salt losing
10. Landing-Gold	3 wk	C.A.H. + salt losing
11. Hedinger (1954)	37 yr	C.A.H.
12. Larson-Reberger (1954)	40 yr	C.A.H.
13. Piyaratn-Rosahn (1957)	2½ yr	C.A.H. + salt losing
14. Shanklin (1963)	3½ yr	C.A.H. + salt losing
15. Glenn-Boyce (1963)	19 yr	Bilateral testicular tumour
16. Glenn-Boyce	15 yr	C.A.H.
17. Schoen-Di Raimondo-Dominguez (1961)	14 yr	C.A.H. + salt losing
18. Kaplan (1966)	9 yr	C.A.H.: 21-hydroxylase deficiency
19. Bricaire-Luton (1966)	17 yr	C.A.H. + hypertensive state: 11-hydroxylase deficiency
20. Earll-Newman-Di Raimondo (1969)	40 yr	C.A.H.

C.A.H.: Congenital adrenal hyperplasia.

biochemical and clinical inhibition, which was immediately apparent, became ineffective little by little, as if the aberrant tissue was autonomous, which necessitated orchidectomy.

Only observations 17 and 18 have been the object of more exhaustive biological studies: in observation 17, the steroid constituents in the spermatic vein show the presence of 17-hydroxy-progesterone and 5-pregnenolone. The level of 17-hydroxy-progesterone clearly increased in response to ACTH. These results tally with those obtained with the incubations where the predominant enzymatic activity was 17α-hydroxylase, even though 21- and 11-hydroxylation were very feeble (this suggests a partial block in 21-hydroxylation). In observation 18, the estimation of steroids in the spermatic vein shows the presence of testosterone, 17-hydroxy-progesterone, and 4-androstenedione. The different levels were not increased by ACTH (but the patient was, at the time, subjected to supplementary corticosteroid therapy).

The light microscopy study showed that the testicular nodules were histologically similar to the hyperplastic suprarenal in 10 cases (obs. 1, 2, 3, 4, 5, 7, 11, 12, 13, 19) but histologically different to adrenocortical hyperplasia and close to Leydig-cell morphology in the other observations.

In fact, the diagnosis of intragonadal inclusions of functional adrenal tissue is difficult, the principal differential diagnosis being a testicular Leydig-cell tumor.

(1) ARGUMENTS IN FAVOR OF THE DIAGNOSIS: It is known that embryologically adrenal cortex and gonads are both derived from the celomic epithelium between the root of the mesentery and the Wolffian body. This explains the frequency with which one finds suprarenal inclusions in the testis of newborn: Dahl and Bahn (1962), employing serial sections of testis and adjacent structures of 100 infants of 1 year or thereabouts, noticed the presence of suprarenal tissue in 15 of the 200 testes (11 children); 12 of the 15 nodules had a diameter of more than 1 mm; most of them were situated at the level of the rete testis, 4 at the level of the hilus of the testis and not buried in the testicular parenchyma; the histological appearance of these nodules bears a very small resemblance to the suprarenals. In 4 newborns, in whom the suprarenals

still contained a significant fetal cortex, the aberrant tissue had a ratio identical to that of the fetal cortex.

The morphological modifications, which were noticed at the time of the replacement of fetal cortex by an adult-type cortex, were exactly reproduced by some other, older nodules. The frequency of such inclusions has been found by other authors to be between 7.5 and 14.8%.

(a) *Nosological arguments*: It is possible to observe such intratesticular growths in some pathological conditions other than congenital suprarenal hyperplasia, where there exists an increased level of ACTH. The literature contains 3 observations of Cushing's syndrome of hypothalamic-hypophyseal origin: Rose *et al.* (bilateral, micro-adenomatous suprarenal hyperplasia); Hamwi *et al.* (increased ACTH and a macroscopic hypophyseal tumor); and Engel *et al.*; and one observation of Addison's disease by Zandanell.

(b) *Biological arguments*: The basal biochemical data are in support of congenital-suprarenal hyperplasia (nearly always a deficit in 21-hydroxylation, very rarely a deficit in 11-hydroxylation as in our obs. 1). The ACTH test was in general positive and the inhibition test with dexamethasone reduced the level of the 17-ketosteroids and pregnanetriol (and/or tetrahydro 'S') to normal.

(c) *Evolutive arguments*: These are very important and it is very evident that the true shrinkage of the intratesticular nodules with dexamethasone is an almost decisive argument. This argument can however be faulted when the testicular tumors are autonomous.

(2) INCONCLUSIVE ARGUMENTS

(a) *Anatomical data:* The argument based on the premise that the suprarenal inclusions are bilateral is not absolute, seeing that one finds in the literature some exceptional observations of bilateral Leydig cell tumors; it occurs in certain cases of diagnostic error (like the observation of Garvey and Daniel in 1951, which was taken up again as congenital suprarenal hyperplasia by Miller and Murray, 1962). The other cases (Staubitz *et al.*, 1953; Ostergaard, 1947; Martelli and Torchi, 1965; Tokuna and Egami, 1967) appear eminently suspect.

(b) *Histological data*: All authors at the present time recognize that the distinction between adrenocortical and Leydig cells is impossible; in both cases they are endocrine cells, of average size (15 to 25 μ) having a slightly acidophilic and granular cytoplasm and possessing a central or excentric nucleolar nodule. The arrangement in strands, surrounded by a capsule, of the adrenocortical cells, can be reproduced by the Leydig tissue. This can also assume the spongiocytic appearance of the suprarenal cells. Finally, the crystalloids of Reinke are particularly rare in the Leydig tumor (moreover, they appear only at puberty).

Even examination with the electron microscope does not permit an absolute distinction between these two cell-types, characterized equally by an agranular endoplasmic reticulum, well developed, a poorly developed ergastoplasm (rough endoplasmic reticulum), a non-secreting Golgi apparatus, and some variable lipid-like inclusions. In no case were secretory granules found. However, the same author puts emphasis on some special modification of the mitochondria and vacuoles in the Leydig cell tumors.

(c) *Biochemical data*: Enzymatic studies are unable to confirm the diagnosis. Indeed,the adrenal is capable of secreting testosterone in certain pathological conditions; congenital adrenal hyperplasia in particular (Burger *et al.*, 1964; Hudson *et al.*, 1967; Migeon and Baulieu, 1965), and in the physiological state (Cameron *et al.*, 1969; Baird *et al.*, 1969). Baird, studying the concentration of androstenedione and testosterone in the suprarenal venous blood before and after ACTH, found that the concentrations of these steroids were elevated after injection of ACTH into 2 normal females and into a female suffering from congenital suprarenal hyperplasia due to a disorder of 11-hydroxylation.

This work confirms the earlier studies of Kase and Kowall (1962).

In another connection, the testicle in certain pathological conditions, and the Leydig cell tumor in particular, is capable of secreting some cortisol (Besch *et al.*, 1964; Engel *et al.*, 1966; Inano *et al.*, 1968). The latter has been obtained from pregnenolone and progesterone labelled with C^{14}, and after incubation with sections of interstitial tumor from a mouse, deoxycorticosterone and corticosterone were found which supports our conclusion in the third observation.

All this indicates that the pathological testis is capable of carrying out biosynthetic functions entirely similar to the suprarenal gland and in particular 21- and 11-hydroxylation, as was demonstrated by Savard *et al.* in 1960. The only special point is that the major pathway of biosynthesis would pass through 17-hydroxyprogesterone and 4-androstenedione, 'short-circuiting' the 5-pregnenolone and dehydroepiandrosterone route, agreeing with the results of Axelrod (1965), since only 6.4% of DHA is formed. The fact that we found in our third observation a very significant level of DHA (71%) is perhaps the only argument which pleads, on the whole, rather in favor of an intratesticular suprarenal inclusion than of an interstitial Leydig cell tumor.

SUMMARY

Intra-testicular inclusions of adrenal cortical tissue occur very rarely. We report the study of 3 patients presenting such a syndrome. The first 2 cases are congenital adrenal hyperplasia (one is 21-hydroxylase deficiency, the other is an 11-hydroxylase lack), with bilateral intra-testicular inclusions. The third observation is characterized by a precocious pseudo-puberty and a right testicular tumor. We have compared these cases with those reported in the literature.

The differential diagnosis between intra-gonadal inclusions of functional adrenal tissue and testicular Leydig-cell tumor is very difficult, due to the great similarity of these tissues. Biochemical, histological, histochemical and ultrastructural studies are not sufficient to ascertain the diagnosis. From these studies, the best arguments for diagnostic purposes seem to us the nosological and evolutive arguments.

ACKNOWLEDGEMENTS

We wish to express our thanks to Dr. Steg for surgical studies, Dr. Galian (histological studies), Dr. Ganter (histoenzymological studies) and Dr. Dadoune for ultrastructural pictures. We thank also Dr. L. Novis and Mrs. F. Victor for translating this article.

REFERENCES

Aimez, P. (1968): *Contribution à l'Étude des Inclusions de Tissu Cortico-surrénalien dans les Gonades* Thesis (Paris).

Allibone, E. C., Barr, H. S. and Cant, N. H. (1947): The interrenal syndrome in children. *Arch. Dis. Childh.*, *22*, 210.

Axelrod, L. R. (1965): Metabolic patterns of steroid biosynthesis in young and aged human testes. *Biochim. biophys. Acta (Amst.)*, *97*, 551.

Baird, D. T., Uno, A. and Melby, J. C. (1969): Adrenal secretion of androgens and oestrogens. *J. Endocr.*, *45*, 135.

Besch, P. K., Barry, R. D., Miller, R. R. and Watson, D. J. (1964): *In vitro* biosynthetic studies of endocrine tumors. III. Cortisol production by a testicular tumor. *J. clin. Endocr.*, *24*, 1339.

Birman, M. (1966): *Hyperplasie Surrénale Congénitale avec Gros Testicules par Nodules Tumoraux Intra-testiculaires*. Thesis (Paris).

Bricaire, H. and Luton, J. P. (1966): Les inclusions de tissu surrénalien fonctionnel dans les gonades. In: '*Actualités Endocrinologiques*'. *Journées de la Pitié*, pp 79–101. Expansion Scientifique, Paris.

Burger, H. G., Kent, J. R. and Kellie, A. E. (1964): Determination of testosterone in human peripheral and adrenal venous plasma. *J. clin. Endocr.*, *24*, 432.

CAMERON, E. H., JONES, T., JONES, D., ANDERSON, A. B. and GRIFFITHS, K. (1969): Further studies on the relationship between C19 and C21 steroid synthesis in the human adrenal gland. *J. Endocr.*, *45*, 215.

COHEN, H. (1946): Hyperplasia of the adrenal cortex associated with bilateral testicular tumors. *Amer. J. Path.*, *22*, 157.

DADOUNE, J. P., GALIAN, P. and ABELANET, R. (1969): Observations sur l'ultrastructure des inclusions surrénaliennes intra-testiculaires. *C.R. Soc. Biol. (Paris)*, *7*, 1488.

DADOUNE, J. P., GALIAN, P., STEG, A., GANTER, P. and ABELANET, R. (1967): Adénome du testicule à cellules de Leydig. Etude histologique, ultrastructurale, histo-enzymatique et biochimique d'un cas. *Arch. Anat. path.*, *15*, 322.

DAHL, E. V. and BAHN, R. C. (1962): Aberrant adrenal cortical tissue near the testis in human infants. *Amer. J. Path.*, *40*, 587.

DAVIES, J., DAVENPORT, G. R., NORRIS, J. L. and RENNIE, P. I. C. (1966): Histochemical studies of hydroxysteroid deshydrogenase activity in mammalian reproductive tissues. *Endocrinology*, *78*, 667.

DRAY, F. (1965): Mesure de la testostérone du plasma veineux périphérique chez l'homme adulte par une technique de double dilution isotopique. *Bull. Soc. Chim. Biol. (Paris)*, *47*, 2145.

EARLL, J. M., NEWMAN, S. G. and DI RAIMONDO, V. C. (1969): Bilateral testicular tumors in untreated congenital adrenocortical hyperplasia. *J. Amer. med. Ass.*, *209*, 937.

EECHAUTE, W. (1966): A simple method for the separate determination of cortisol and corticosterone in plasma. *Clin. chim. Acta*, *13*, 785.

ENGEL, L. L., LANMAN, G., SCULLY, R. E. and VILLEE, D. B. (1966): Studies of an interstitial cell tumor of the testes. Formation of cortisol C^{14} from acetate C^{14}. *J. clin. Endocr.*, *26*, 381.

ENGEL, F. L., MCPHERSON, H. T., FETTER, B. F., BAGGET, B., ENGEL, L. L., CARTER, P., FIELDING, L. L., SAVARD, K. and DORFMAN, R. I. (1964): Clinical, morphological and biochemical studies on a malignant testicular tumor. *J. clin. Endocr.* *24*, 528.

FASSBENDER, M. (1949): Pseudopubertas praecox bei doppelseitiger diffuser Nebennierenrinden Hyperplasia und ektopischen Nebennierenrinden Knötchen im Hoden. *Zbl. allg. Path. path. Anat.*, *85*, 110.

GARDNER, L. I. and SNIFFEN, R. C. (1950): Follow-up studies in a boy with mixed adrenal cortical disease. *Pediatrics*, *5*, 808.

GARVEY, F. K. and DANIEL, T. B. (1951): Bilateral interstitial cell tumors of the testis. *J. Urol. (Baltimore)*, *66*, 173.

GIRARD, F., BINOUX, M., PHAM HUU TRUNG, M. T. (1966): Méthode d'estimation de l'activité corticotrope du plasma. *Rev. franç. Etud. clin. biol.*, *II*, 732.

GLENN, J. F. and BOYCE, W. H. (1963): Adrenogenitalism with testicular adrenal rests stimulating interstitial cell tumors. *J. Urol. (Baltimore)*, *89*, 456.

HAMWI, J., GWINUP, G., MOSTOW, J. H. and BESCH, P. K. (1963): Activation of testicular adrenal rest tissue by prolonged excessive ACTH production. *J. clin. Endocr.*, *23*, 861.

HEDINGER, C. H. (1954): Beidseitige Hodentumoren und kongenitales adrenogenitales Syndrom (Leydig-Zellen oder Nebennierenrindengewebe?). *Schweiz. Z. allg. Path.*, *17*, 743.

HENKE, W. J., DOE, R. P. and JACOBSON, M. E. (1960): A test of pituitary reserve utilizing intravenous SU 48 85 with a new method for extraction of 11 desoxycorticosteroids. *J. clin. Endocr.*, *20*, 1527.

HUDSON, B., COGHLAN, J. P. and DULMANIS, A. (1967): Testicular function in man. In: *Endocrinology of the Testis: Ciba Found. Coll. Endocr., Vol. 16.* Editors: G. E. W. Wolstenholme and M. O'Connor. Churchill, London.

INANO, M., MACHINO, A., TAMAOKI, B. I. and TSUBURA, Y. (1968): Steroid biosynthesis *in vitro* by transplantable interstitial cell tumor of mice. I. Identification and quantitative determination of the metabolites and intra-cellular distribution of the enzymes related to testosterone formation. *Endocrinology*, 83, 659.

KAPLAN, M., GRUMBACH, R., BRIMAN, M. and COMBOURIEU, M. (1966): Hyperplasie surrénale congénitale avec gros testicules. A propos d'une nouvelle observation. *Ann. Pédiat.*, *2340*, 608.

KASE, N. and KOWAL, J. (1962): *In vitro* production of testosterone in a human adrenal homogenate. *J. clin. Endocr.*, *22*, 9.

LANDING, B. H. and GOLD, E. (1951): The occurrence and significance of Leydig cell proliferation in familial adrenal cortical hyperplasia. *J. clin. Endocr.*, *11*, 1436.

LARSON, C. P. and REBERGER, C. C. (1954): Macrogenitosomia praecox with adrenal hyperplasia and heterotopic adrenal cortical tissue in the testis. *West. J. Surg.*, *62*, 602.

LEGRAND, J. C., LEGRAND, S. and ZOGBI, F. (1967): Détermination quantitative de la tétrahydroaldostérone urinaire. *Ann. Biol. clin.*, *25*, 1199.

LUTON, J. P., LAUDAT, PH. and BRICAIRE, H. (1969): L'emploi de la bêta 1–24 corticotrophine retard dans l'exploration fonctionnelle du cortex surrénal. *Ann. Endocr. (Paris)*, *30*, 456.

MARTELLI, A. and TORCHI, B. (1965): Tumore a cellule interstiziali del testicolo a sede bilaterale. *Minerva Chir.*, *20*, 860.

MILLER, E. C. and MURRAY, H. L. (1962): Congenital adrenocortical hyperplasia: case previously reported as 'bilateral interstitial cell tumor of the testicle'. *J. clin. Endocr.*, *22*, 655.

MIGEON, C. J. and BAULIEU, F. F. (1965): Hyperplasie congénitale des surrénales. Etude biologique. In: *'Troubles Congénitaux de l'Hormonogénèse'*. VIII Réunion des Endocrinologistes de Langue Française, juin 1965, pp 153–173.

OSTERGAARD, E. (1947): Feminizing tumor of the testis. Presumably aberrant adrenocortical tumor. *J. clin. Endocr.*, *7*, 438.

PIYARATN, P. and ROSAHN, P. D. (1957): Congenital adrenocortical hyperplasia associated with hyperplasia of aberrant (intratesticular) adrenal tissue. *J. clin. Endocr.*, *17*, 1245.

ROSE, E. K., ENTERLINE, H. T., RHOADS, J. E. and ROSE, E. (1952): Adrenal cortical hyperfunction in childhood. Report of a case with adrenocortical hyperplasia and testicular adrenal rests. *Pediatrics*, *9*, 475.

SAVARD, K., DORFMAN, R. I., BAGGETT, B., FIELDING, L. L., ENGEL, L. L., MCPHERSON, H. T., LISTER, L. M., JOHNSON, D. S., HAMBLEN, E. C. and ENGEL, F. L. (1960): Clinical, morphological and biochemical studies of a virilizing tumor in the testis. *J. clin. Invest.*, *39*, 534.

SCHOEN, E. J., DI RAIMONDO, V. and DOMINGUEZ, O. V. (1961): Bilateral testicular tumors complicating congenital adrenocortical hyperplasia. *J. clin. Endocr.*, *21*, 518.

SHANKLIN, D. R., RICHARDSON, A. P., ROTHSTEIN, G. and GAINESVILLE, A. (1963): Testicular hilar nodules in adrenogenital syndrome. *Amer. J. Dis. Child.*, *106*, 243.

SOBEL, E. H., SNIFFEN, R. C. and TALBOT, N. B. (1951): Use of testicular biopsy in the differential diagnosis of precocious puberty. *Pediatrics*, *8*, 701.

STAUBITZ, W. J., UBERKIRCHER, O. S. and OLICK, M. (1953): Precocious puberty in a case of bilateral interstitial cell tumors of the testis. *J. Urol. (Baltimore)*, *69*, 562.

THELANDER, H. E. (1946): Congenital adrenal cortical insufficiency associated with macrogenitosomia. *J. Pediat.*, *29*, 213.

TOKUNAGA, Y. and EGAMI, T. (1967): Case of bilateral interstitial cell tumor of the testis. *Surg. Ther. (Osaka)*, *16*, 712.

WATTENBERG, L. W. (1958): Microscopic histochemical demonstration of steroid-3 beta-ol deshydrogenase in tissue sections. *J. Histochem. Cytochem.*, *6*, 225.

WILKINS, L., FLEISCHMANN, W. and HOWARD, J. E. (1940): Macrogenitosomia praecox associated with hyperplasia of the androgenic tissue of the adrenal and death from cortico-adrenal insufficiency. *Endocrinology*, *26*, 385.

ZANDANELL, E. (1953): Hyperplasie akzessorischer Nebennieren bei Morbus Addison. *Frankfurt. Z. Path.*, *64*, 100.

ABNORMALITIES OF ANDROGEN METABOLISM IN VIRILIZED WOMEN

C. WAYNE BARDIN

Department of Medicine, Milton S. Hershey Medical Center, Pennsylvania State University, Hershey, Pa., U.S.A.

Androgens are defined as substances which stimulate growth of the male reproductive tract. Testosterone was first quantified in human plasma in 1961 (Finkelstein *et al.*, 1961) and in the intervening years there have been many studies in man to indicate that this is the most important androgen. In men it or its metabolites are responsible for genital development, beard growth, muscle development and sexual drive. In normal women the role of androgens is less well defined but in pathological conditions increased androgen production results in virilization. Investigation of a large number of women has indicated that virilization is usually associated with increased testosterone production. Recent studies have suggested that other potent androgens such as dihydrotestosterone; 3α, 17β-dihydroxy-5-androstane; and 3β, 17β-dihydroxyandrost-5-ene are also present in blood. However, as yet there is no instance where any one of these steroids has appeared to be primarily responsible for virilism. Therefore while these hormones along with testosterone may contribute to the total blood androgen load their role in androgen pathophysiology remains to be established.

It has been assumed, with some justification, that androgens reach their active sites in most target tissues through the blood or plasma. Therefore, in this review only the production of testosterone and other androgenic steroids into the plasma will be discussed. We shall first consider the origin of plasma and androgens in normal women in an effort to define the biologic plasma androgen pool. The origin of plasma testosterone in several types of virilism will be discussed in an effort to illustrate the sites of abnormal androgen production. Then, certain aspects of androgen metabolism will be examined in an effort to delineate factors which influence the biological activity of androgens in plasma. Finally, we shall not be able to refer to all relevant references in the extensive field of androgen metabolism, but have selected key studies for discussion.

THE ORIGIN OF PLASMA ANDROGENS IN NORMAL AND VIRILIZED WOMEN

Testosterone

The origin of plasma testosterone is illustrated in Figure 1. There is considerable evidence to indicate that this steroid is secreted by both the adrenals and the ovaries. In addition to the direct secretion from endocrine glands, plasma testosterone is also synthesized in non-endocrine tissues from relatively non-androgenic plasma steroid precursors or prehormones.

Testosterone Prehormones: A prehormone is a substance with little or no inherent biologic potency, which is converted to a more active product that contributes significantly to an overall biologic activity (Baird *et al.*, 1966). The conversion of prehormones to active androgens can occur in many organs, including target tissues. Although a prehormone may contribute to the intracellular active androgen activity within the tissue where the conversion

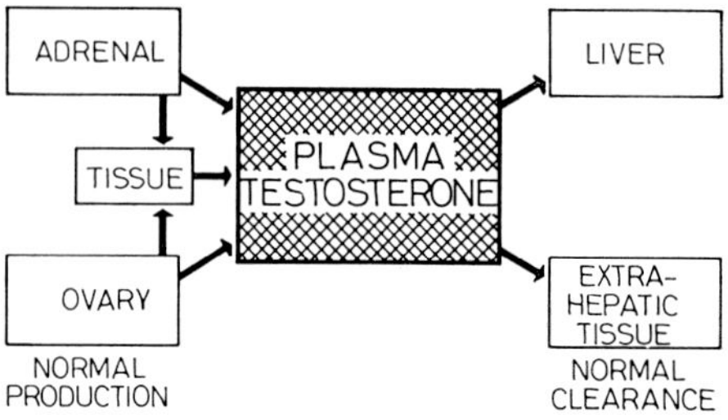

Fig. 1. The origin of plasma testosterone in women (from Bardin and Kirschner (1970)). The plasma level is determined by both production and clearance.

occurs, a portion of the product may re-enter the plasma and exert a biologic effect on other tissues. Since in practice only a small fraction (usually less than 10%) of any steroid precursor is converted to an active plasma androgen product, only those prehormones with production rates which are much higher than those of the product can contribute significantly to total androgenic activity. The theoretical and practical approaches used by many investigators for estimating the fraction of a prehormone converted to a product steroid in plasma have been detailed in several reviews (Baird *et al.*, 1968; Tait and Horton, 1966).

Androstenedione is by far the most important prehormone for plasma androgens. Although only 3–4% of this steroid is converted to plasma testosterone, this accounts for 120–160 μg per day or about 50% of the testosterone in normal women (Bardin and Lipsett, 1967; Horton and Tait, 1966). In virilized patients, androstenedione may contribute a variable fraction of plasma testosterone. For example, in women with polycystic ovaries only 25% of testosterone is from this precursor; whereas in women with congenital adrenal hyperplasia 50% of testosterone is from this source. Since only 5% of plasma androstenedione in men

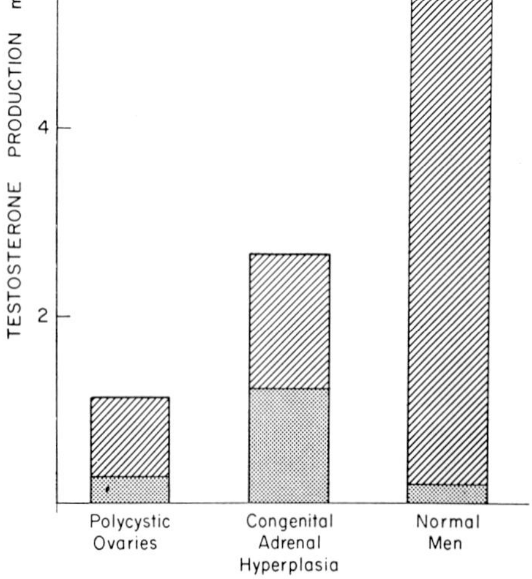

Fig. 2. The contribution of plasma androstenedione to plasma testosterone. The lower portion of each bar gives the fraction of the testosterone production rate derived from androstenedione. In normal women (not shown) 50% of testosterone arises from this source.

is converted to plasma testosterone, this prehormone accounts for only a small fraction ($0.05 \times 2000 = 100$ µg/day) of the total blood androgen load (Fig. 2).

Adrenal: Wieland *et al.* (1965) were the first to study testosterone secretion by the adrenal in conscious patients. Baird *et al.* (1969) subsequently found evidence for adrenal secretion of testosterone in one postmenopausal woman and in one hirsute woman by demonstrating a gradient between adrenal and peripheral venous blood. Similarly, Burger *et al.* (1964) and Kirschner and Jacobs (1970) found variable adrenal testosterone secretion (from adrenals of normal size) in hirsute women studied by retrograde adrenal vein catheterization. Despite the limited number of these studies, they do indicate that the adrenal can secrete a significant but variable amount of testosterone in virilized women. More studies are required to determine the contribution of the normal adrenal gland to plasma testosterone.

In some virilized subjects the adrenals may contribute to plasma testosterone both directly and indirectly. Testosterone secretion has been demonstrated from adrenal neoplasms (Saez *et al.*, 1967) and from hyperplastic adrenals in patients with congenital C-21-hydroxylase deficiency (Baird *et al.*, 1969). In addition increased androstenedione secretion and thus increased testosterone production from this prehormone also occurs in both these conditions (Bardin *et al.*, 1968) (Fig. 2).

Ovary: Ovarian venous testosterone has been measured in a few women by several groups of investigators (Gandy and Peterson, 1968; Rivarola *et al.*, 1967; Horton *et al.*, 1966). Although these laboratories reported different ovarian to peripheral vein gradients, it is none the less clear that the normal ovary does secrete some testosterone. By assuming an ovarian blood flow of 25 ml per minute one can estimate, from the available data on ovarian venous testosterone levels, that the ovaries secrete from 5 to 20% of plasma testosterone in normal women (Lipsett and Bardin, 1970).

In virilized patients with obvious ovarian pathology, testosterone may be derived from multiple sources. This is illustrated by the three patients summarized in Table I: The woman

TABLE I

Sites of testosterone production in women with ovarian virilism

Sites	Hyperthecosis	Ovarian carcinoma	Leydig cell hyperplasia
Production rate mg/day	3.0	5.0	1.0
From ovary	95%	—	30%
From androstenedione	—	95%	30%
From adrenal and other precursors	—	—	40%

with hyperthecosis had an elevated plasma testosterone which was primarily of ovarian origin (Bardin *et al.*, 1967). By contrast, in another woman an ovarian lipid cell tumor produced predominantly androstenedione which served as a precursor for 90% of plasma testosterone (Lipsett *et al.*, 1970) and finally in a woman with Leydig cell hyperplasia testosterone was produced in almost equal quantities from the gonad, from plasma androstenedione and from the adrenal (Bardin *et al.*, 1969).

It is apparent from the above considerations that testosterone production in virilized women may be extremely complex. A detailed study of these patients must assess not only the ovarian and adrenal but also the prehormone contribution to plasma testosterone.

Dihydrotestosterone (17β-hydroxy-5α-androstan-3-one)

Dihydrotestosterone is a more potent androgen than testosterone in many bioassay systems. Interest in this steroid has recently been stimulated by the observations that testosterone is metabolized to dihydrotestosterone in several target tissues and by the possibility that this steroid could exert an androgenic action in tissues other than where it was synthesized (Farnsworth and Brown, 1963; Chamberlain *et al.*, 1966; Bruchovsky and Wilson, 1968; Wilson and Walker, 1969). The production rate of dihydrotestosterone in normal women is about 1/3 that of testosterone so that it does comprise a significant fraction of the plasma androgen pool (Ho and Horton, 1970). Plasma testosterone serves as precursor for 10 μg and androstenedione for 65 μg of plasma dihydrotestosterone each day (Ho and Horton, 1970; Mahoudeau *et al.*). Therefore, since its entire production rate can arise from plasma precursors, there is little evidence at present to suggest that appreciable quantities of this steroid are secreted by endocrine glands. If the major fraction of plasma dihydrotestosterone arises from plasma androstenedione, women with certain pathological conditions associated with increased androstenedione production (congenital adrenal hyperplasma, adrenal tumors, ovarian tumor) will have increased dihydrotestosterone levels. However, in these women the production rate of testosterone will probably be greater than that of dihydrotestosterone since in patients in whom the estimates have been made, the androstenedione conversion to the former exceeded that of the latter steroid (Mahoudeau *et al.*).

Androstandiol (3α, 17β-dihydroxy-5α-androstane)

Even though androstandiol is a potent androgen in man, its plasma levels and production rates have not been measured. There are several studies of testosterone metabolism which suggest that this 'diol' could contribute to the plasma androgen pool (Farnsworth and Brown, 1963; Chamberlain, 1966; Bruchovsky and Wilson, 1968). That androstandiol made *in vivo* from testosterone can re-enter the blood was suggested by a study in which urinary diol excretion was examined after both percutaneous and intravenous administration of radioactive testosterone (Mauvais-Jarvis *et al.*, 1970). In recent studies from this laboratory, tritiated androstandiol has been isolated from plasma following infusions of testosterone-^{3}H and dihydrotestosterone-^{3}H (Mahoudeau *et al.*). If we assume that the MCR is the same as that for dihydrotestosterone, then both these precursors will account for only 4.5 μg of androstandiol per day in normal women. This would be greater in virilized women. Whether plasma androstenedione contributes significantly to androstandiol remains to be established.

Androstenediol (3β, 17β-dihydroxyandrost-5-ene)

Peripheral blood levels and production rate of androstenediol have not been determined. The presence of an adrenal venous androstenediol level of about 0.5 μg/100 ml plasma indicates that the adrenal gland actively secretes this steroid into the blood of women (Wieland *et al.*, 1965). Although there is no direct evidence for gonadal secretion of androstenediol, its role as a possible testosterone precursor suggests that the ovary may also contribute to the plasma levels of this steroid. Plasma dehydroepiandrosterone (DHA) is another possible source of plasma androstenediol. If DHA and androstenedione undergo reduction of their 17-ketones at the same rate in peripheral tissues, then at least 200 μg of androstenediol would be derived from 7 mg of plasma DHA.

It should again be emphasized that the information concerning the production of plasma androgens other than testosterone is fragmentary. Thus the relative importance and the individual contribution of each steroid to the plasma androgen pool and to the androgenic activity on the end organ must await further study.

FACTORS WHICH DETERMINE THE PLASMA LEVEL AND THE BIOLOGIC ACTIVITY OF TESTOSTERONE

Production Rate

The total amount of testosterone which enters the blood per day from all sources is defined as the production rate. In men 95% of testosterone arises from the testicular Leydig cells which are maintained in a steady secretory state by pituitary LH. The plasma level of testosterone is maintained within narrow limits by a reciprocal feed-back relationship with LH from the pituitary. With this type of regulation the plasma levels of testosterone will remain fairly constant regardless of the rate of testosterone metabolism (Fig. 3). By contrast, the

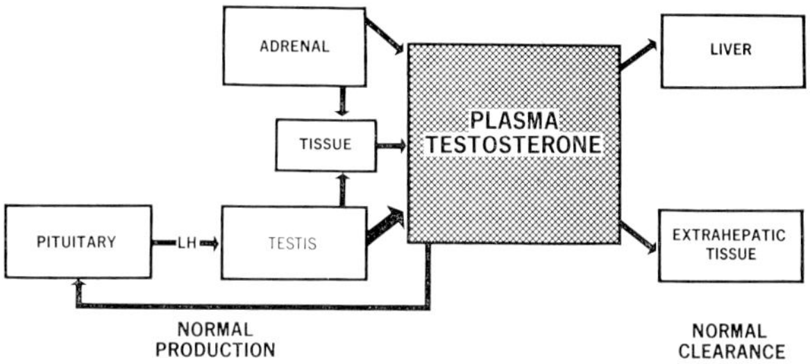

Fig. 3. The origin of plasma testosterone in men. About 95% of testosterone is secreted by the testes and the plasma level is maintained by feedback control of plasma LH.

minute to minute control of testosterone production in women is poorly understood and there is no evidence to suggest that circulating testosterone regulates its own production in a fashion analogous to the feedback inhibition of testosterone on the pituitary Leydig cell axis. It is obvious that the production rate in large measure determines the plasma concentration in women (as it does in men); however, since there is no mechanism for maintaining fixed concentration, the testosterone level is also influenced by the rate of steroid metabolism (Fig. 1).

Metabolic Clearance Rate

A useful way of expressing the rate of steroid metabolism is the metabolic clearance rate which is defined as the volume of blood or plasma irreversibly cleared of steroid per unit time. The plasma level of testosterone (T) is related to the production rate (PR) and the metabolic clearance rate (MCR):

$$T = \frac{PR}{MCR}$$

From this expression we see that a decrease in clearance without a change in production would result in an increased plasma concentration, and similarly an increase in clearance may result in a lower plasma level. Recent studies from a number of investigators have indicated that the metabolic clearance rate of testosterone may increase or decrease by 50–100% in a variety of clinical conditions (Table II). It follows from these considerations that when disease or drugs alter the metabolic clearance rate in women, the plasma level of testosterone may be a poor index of the production rate. The best studied example of this phenomenon is the hirsute woman: About one-third of hirsute patients with polycystic ovaries and idiopathic hirsutism had normal plasma testosterone levels even though the production rates were elevated. This was explained by an increase in the metabolic clearance

TABLE II

Conditions associated with changes in the testosterone metabolic clearance rate

Increased clearance	Reference	Decreased clearance	Reference
Hypothyroidism	Gordon *et al.*, 1969	Hyperthyroidism	Gordon *et al.*, 1969
Virilization	Bardin and Lipsett, 1967 Southren *et al.*, 1969	Aging	Kent and Acone, 1966
Androgen treatment	Southren *et al.*, 1968	Estrogen treatment	Kirschner *et al.*, 1970 Migeon *et al.*, 1968 Bird *et al.*, 1969
Medroxyprogesterone acetate treatment	Gordon *et al.*, 1970*b*	Barbiturate treatment (S)	Southren *et al.*, 1969
Dexamethasone treatment (S)*	Bardin *et al.*, 1968*a*	Erect posture (S)	Southren *et al.*, 1968 Lipsett *et al.*, 1966
Large adrenal, ovarian and testicular tumors	Bardin *et al.*, 1968*b* Lipsett *et al.*, 1970 Lipsett *et al.*, 1966		

* (S) = Changes small but significant.

of testosterone in women with increased testosterone production (Bardin and Kirschner, 1970).

Since the metabolic clearance rate can influence the plasma level of testosterone it is apparent that factors which change the clearance could profoundly influence its overall biologic activity. The control of the testosterone metabolic clearance rate is poorly understood but ultimately it will depend upon testosterone interaction with both plasma proteins and tissues which extract and metabolize this steroid.

Testosterone-Estradiol Binding Globulin

In human plasma, testosterone is bound with high affinity to a β-globulin (Mercier-Bodard *et al.*, 1970) which also binds estradiol: testosterone-estradiol binding globulin (TeBG) (Fig. 4). From the previous studies of cortisol and cortisol-binding globulin (CBG) one might assume that TeBG would retard the metabolism of testosterone (Sandberg *et al.*, 1966). The studies which support this assumption have recently been reviewed (Bardin and Ma-

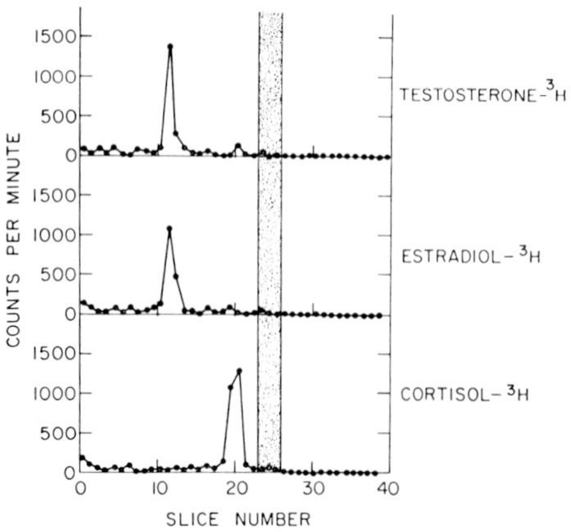

Fig. 4. Polyacrylamide gel electrophoresis of steroid binding proteins. Plasma incubated with ^{3}H-steroids was submitted to electrophoresis at pH 10.2. The anode is at the right. After electrophoresis the gels were cut into 1.3 mm slices and counted. Testosterone-estradiol binding globulin is shown on the upper panels and cortisol binding globulin on the lower panel.

houdeau, 1970). Suffice it to say that in many clinical conditions the testosterone metabolic clearance rate is inversely correlated with the TeBG binding capacity. For example when TeBG increases during estrogen treatment the metabolic clearance rate of testosterone decreases (Bardin and Mahoudeau, 1970). Recent studies have further emphasized the importance of this plasma protein by demonstrating that the testosterone metabolic clearance rate was directly correlated with non-TeBG bound testosterone (Vermeulen *et al.*, 1969). However, this same study demonstrated that factors in addition to plasma protein binding influenced the clearance rate of testosterone as men have higher testosterone clearances than women even with the same non-TeBG bound testosterone levels (Vermeulen *et al.*, 1969).

Tissue Extraction and Metabolism

There are few studies in which changes in tissue metabolism of a steroid have been correlated with the rate of steroid removal from plasma. In one such study patients treated with medroxyprogesterone acetate had a 50-100% increase in the testosterone metabolic clearance rate associated with a 3-fold increase in hepatic steroid A-ring reductase (Gordon *et al.*, 1970*a*; *b*). It should be noted, however, that all drugs which alter steroid metabolism in man do not necessarily procuce a change in the rate of steroid removal from blood. The barbiturate Phetbarbital unexpectedly produced a small decrease in the testosterone clearance in spite of the increased activity of several steroid metabolizing enzymes (Southren *et al.*, 1969).

In the rat, testosterone and other drugs increase both the activity of a variety of hepatic oxidative enzymes and the rate of steroid metabolism from blood (Gillette, 1967). Although there are no studies in man which correlate hepatic enzyme activity and testosterone clearance, Southren *et al.* (1968) have clearly demonstrated that the testosterone metabolic clearance rate in women was increased to that of men by chronic testosterone administration. These studies suggested (*a*) that testosterone increased its own tissue extraction and (*b*) that the increased testosterone clearance rates observed in hirsute women were due primarily to a

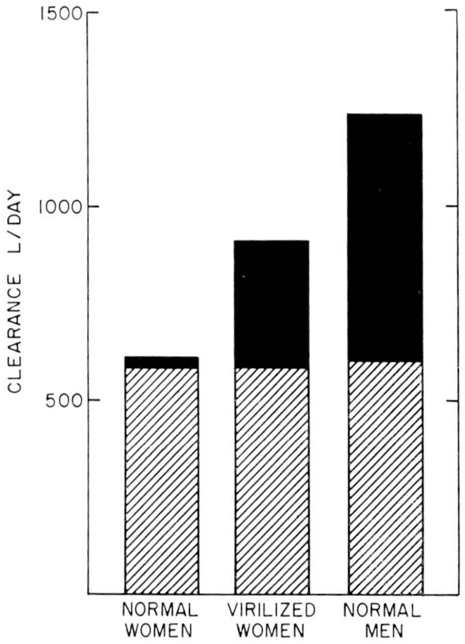

Fig. 5. The metabolic clearance rates are given by the height of the bars. The upper (black) portion of each bar is the extra hepatic clearance and the lower (shaded) portion the hepatic clearance.

change in testosterone metabolism rather than just a decrease in TeBG. That the testosterone clearance rates for men, virilized women and normal women can be normalized by dividing by the log of the testosterone production rate is consistent with the concept that the rate of testosterone metabolism is dependent upon androgen action (Bardin and Lipsett, 1967).

One of the changes occurring in testosterone metabolism as a result of increased androgen production was demonstrated in a study in which the testosterone metabolic clearance, hepatic clearance and extrahepatic clearance rates were determined (Bardin and Kirschner, 1970). In normal women hepatic clearance was essentially equal to metabolic clearance so that the liver could account for almost all of testosterone metabolism. By contrast, in virilized women 32% and in men 50% of plasma testosterone was metabolized in extrahepatic tissue (Fig. 5). The estimated hepatic clearances in the 3 groups were the same even though the metabolic clearance rates were higher in men and hirsute women. If testosterone metabolism in target tissues is required for biologic activity, then it follows that very little testosterone in normal women will be active on tissues other than the liver. In virilized women, however, a larger fraction is available for extraction and metabolism by target tissues such as the skin.

REFERENCES

BAIRD, D. T., HORTON, R., LONGCOPE, C. and TAIT, J. F. (1968): Steroid prehormones. *Perspect. Biol. Med., 11*, 384.

BAIRD, D. T., HORTON, R., LONGCOPE, C. and TAIT, J. F. (1969): Steroid dynamics under steady-state conditions. *Recent Progr. Hormone Res., 25*, 611.

BAIRD, D. T., UNO, A. and MELBY, J. C. (1969): Adrenal secretion of androgens and oestrogens. *J. Endocr., 45*, 135.

BARDIN, C. W., HEMBREE, W. C. and LIPSETT, M. B. (1968): Suppression of testosterone and androstenedione production rates with dexamethasone in women with idiopathic hirsutism and polycystic ovaries. *J. clin. Endocr., 28*, 1300.

BARDIN, C. W. and KIRSCHNER, M. A. (1970): The clinical usefulness of testosterone measurements in virilizing syndromes in women. In: *The Laboratory Diagnosis of Endocrine Disease.* Editor: F.W. Sunderman, Assoc. of Clinical Scientists. In press.

ARDIN, C. W. and LIPSETT, M. B. (1967): Testosterone and androstenedione blood production rates in normal women and women with idiopathic hirsutism or polycystic ovaries. *J. clin. Invest., 46*, 891.

BARDIN, C. W., LIPSETT, M. B., EDGCOMB, J. H. and MARSHALL, J. R. (1967): Studies of testosterone metabolism in a patient with masculinization due to stromal hyperthecosis. *New Engl. J. Med., 277*, 399.

BARDIN, C. W., LIPSETT, M. B. and FRENCH, A. (1968*b*): Testosterone and androstenedione production rates in patients with metastatic adrenal cortical carcinoma. *J. clin. Endocr., 28*, 215.

BARDIN, C. W. and MAHOUDEAU, J. A. (1970): Dynamics of androgen metabolism in women with hirsutism. *Ann. clin. Res.* In press.

BARDIN, C. W., ROSEN, S., LEMAIRE, W. J., TJIO, J. H., GALLUP, J., MARSHALL, J. and SAVARD, K. (1969): *In vivo* and *in vitro* studies of androgen metabolism in a patient with pure gonadal dysgenesis and Leydig cell hyperplasia. *J. clin. Endocr., 29*, 1429.

BIRD, C. E., GREEN, R. N. and CLARK, A. F. (1969): Effect of the administration of estrogen on the disappearance of ^{3}H-testosterone in the plasma of human subjects. *J. clin. Endocr., 29*, 123.

BRUCHOVSKY, N. and WILSON, J. R. (1968): The conversion of testosterone to 5α-androstan-17β-ol-3-one by rat prostate *in vivo* and *in vitro*. *J. biol. Chem., 243*, 2012.

BURGER, H. G., KENT, J. R. and KELLIE, A. E. (1964): Determination of testosterone in human peripheral and adrenal venous plasma. *J. clin. Endocr. 24*, 432.

CHAMBERLAIN, J., JAGARINEC, N. and OFNER, P. (1966): Catabolism of 4-^{14}C testosterone by subcellular fractions of human prostate. *Biochem. J., 99*, 610.

FARNSWORTH, W. E. and BROWN, J. R. (1963): Testosterone metabolism in the prostate. In: *Biology of the Prostate and Related Tissues*, p. 323. Editor: E. P. Vollmer. *Nat. Cancer. Inst. Monogr.*

FINKELSTEIN, M., FORCHIELLI, E. and DORFMAN, R. I. (1961): Estimation of testosterone in human plasma. *J. clin. Endocr., 21*, 98.

GANDY, H. M. and PETERSON, R. E. (1968): Measurement of testosterone and 17-ketosteroids in plasma by the double isotope dilution derivative technique. *J. clin. Endocr., 28*, 949.

GILLETTE, J. R. (1967): Individually different responses to drugs according to age, sex and functional or pathological state. In: *Ciba Foundation Symposium on Drug Responses in Man*. Editors: G. E.W. Wolstenholme and R. Porter. Churchill, London.

GORDON, G. G., ALTMAN, K. and SOUTHREN, A. L. (1970*a*): Induction of hepatic steroid A-ring reductase by medroxyprogesterone acetate in the human and its effect on the metabolism and biological activity of testosterone. In: *Program of the Endocrine Society*, p. 71.

GORDON, G. G., SOUTHREN, A. L., TOCHIMOTO, S., OLIVO, J., ALTMAN, K., RAND, J. and LEMBERGER, L. (1970*b*): Effect of medroxyprogesterone acetate (Provera) on the metabolism and biological activity of testosterone. *J. clin. Endocr.*, *30*, 449.

GORDON, G. G., SOUTHREN, A. L., TOCHIMOTO, S., RAND, J. J. and OLIVO, J. (1969): Effect of hyperthyroidism and hypothyroidism on the metabolism of testosterone and androstenedione in man. *J. clin. Endocr.*, *29*, 164.

HORTON, R., ROMANOFF, E. and WALKER, R. (1966): Androstenedione and testosterone in ovarian venous and peripheral plasma during ovariectomy for breast cancer. *J. clin. Endocr.*, *26*, 1267.

HORTON, R. and TAIT, J. E. (1966): Androstenedione production and interconversion rates measured in peripheral blood and studies on the possible site of its conversion to testosterone. *J. clin. Invest.*, *45*, 301.

ITO, T. and HORTON, R. (1970): Dihydrotestosterone dynamics in human plasma. In: *Abstract of the 52nd Meeting of the Endocrine Society*, p. 73.

KENT, J. R. and ACONE, A. B. (1966): Plasma testosterone levels and aging in males. In: *Androgens in Normal and Pathological Conditions*. Editors: A. Vermeulen and D. Exley. ICS No. 101, Excerpta Medica, Amsterdam.

KIRSCHNER, M. A., BARDIN, C. W., HEMBREE, W. C. and ROSS, G. T. (1970): Effect of estrogen administration on androgen production and plasma luteinizing hormone in hirsute women. *J. clin. Endocr.*, *30*, 727.

KIRSCHNER, M. A. and JACOBS, J. B. (1970): Determining the site of androgen overproduction in hirsute women. In: *Program of the Endocrine Society*, p. 76.

LIPSETT, M. B. and BARDIN, C. W. (1970): Production and metabolism of androgens in man. In: *International Encyclopedia of Pharmacology and Therapeutics: Androgen and Related Substances*. Editor: Z. Laron, Pergamon Press, London.

LIPSETT, M. B., KIRSCHNER, M. A., WILSON, H. and BARDIN, C. W. (1970): Malignant lipid cell tumor of the ovary: Clinical, biochemical and etiologic considerations. *J. clin. Endocr.*, *30*, 336.

LIPSETT, M. B., WILSON, H., KIRSCHNER, M. A., KORENMAN, S. G., FISHMAN, L. M., SARFATY, G. A. and BARDIN, C. W. (1966): Studies of Leydig cell physiology and pathology: Secretion and metabolism of testosterone. *Recent. Progr. Hormone Res.*, *22*, 245.

MAHOUDEAU, J. A., BARDIN, C. W. and LIPSETT, M. B.: Studies of the metabolism of 5α-dihydrotestosterone in human plasma. *Steroids*.

MAUVAIS-JARVIS, P., BERCOVICI, J. P., CREPY, O. and GAUTHIER, F. (1970): Studies on testosterone metabolism in subjects with testicular feminization syndrome. *J. clin. Invest.*, *49*, 31.

MERCIER-BODARD, C., ALFSEN, A. and BAULIEU, E. E. (1970): Sex steroid binding plasma protein (SBP). *Acta endocr. (Kbh.)*, Suppl. 147.

MIGEON, C. J., RIVAROLA, M. A. and FOREST, M. G. (1968): Studies of androgens in transsexual subjects: effects of estrogen therapy. *Bull. Johns Hopk. Hosp. 123*, 128.

RIVAROLA, M. A., SAEZ, J. M., JONES, H. W., JONES, G. S. and MIGEON, C. J. (1967): Secretion of androgens by the normal, polycystic and neoplastic ovaries. *Johns Hopk. med. J.*, *121*, 82.

SAEZ, J. M., RIVAROLA, M. A. and MIGEON, C. J. (1967): Studies of androgens in patients with adrenocortical tumors. *J. clin. Endocr.*, *27*, 615.

SANDBERG, A. A., ROSENTHAL, H., SCHNEIDER, S. L. and SLAUNWHITE, W. R. (1966): Protein-steroid interactions and their role in the transport and metabolism of steroids. In: *Steroid Dynamics*. Editors: G. Pincus, T. Nakao and J. F. Tait. Academic Press, New York.

SOUTHREN, A. L., GORDON, G. G. and TOCHIMOTO, S. (1968): Further study of factors affecting the metabolic clearance rate of testosterone in man. *J. clin. Endocr.*, *28*, 1105.

SOUTHREN, A. L., GORDON, G. G., TOCHIMOTO, S., KRIKUN, E., KRIEGER, D., JACOBSON, M. and KUNTZMAN, R. (1969*a*): Effect of N-phenylbarbital (Phetharbital) on the metabolism of testosterone and cortisol in man. *J. clin. Endocr.*, *29*, 251.

SOUTHREN, A. L., GORDON, G. G., TOCHIMOTO, S., OLIVO, J., SHERMAN, D. H. and PINZON, G. (1969*b*): Testosterone and androstenedione metabolism in the polycystic ovary syndrome: Studies of the percentage binding of testosterone in plasma. *J. clin. Endocr.*, *29*, 1356.

TAIT, J. F. and HORTON, R. (1966): The *in vivo* estimation of blood production and interconversion rates of androstenedione and testosterone and the calculation of their secretion rates. In: *Steroid Dynamics*. Editors: G. Pincus, T. Nakao and J. F. Tait. Academic Press, New York.

VERMEULEN, A., VERDONCK, L., VAN DER STRAETEN, M. and ORIE, N. (1969): Capacity of the testosterone-binding globulin in human plasma and influence of specific binding of testosterone on its metabolic clearance rate. *J. clin. Endocr.*, *29*, 1470.

WIELAND, R. G., DECOURCY, C., LEVY, R. P., ZALA, A. P. and HIRSCHMANN, H. (1965): $C_{19}O_2$ steroids and some of their precursors in blood from normal human adrenals. *J. clin. Invest.*, *44*, 159.

WILSON, J. D. and WALKER, J. D. (1969): The conversion of testosterone to 5α-androstan-17β-ol-3-one (DHT) by skin slices of man. *J. clin. Invest.*, *48*, 371.

CLINICAL CORRELATIONS OF ANDROGEN EXCESS*

J. LESTER GABRILOVE

The Endocrine Research Laboratory of the Department of Medicine, Mount Sinai School of Medicine and The Mount Sinai Hospital, New York, N.Y., U.S.A.

The biosynthesis of androgens and estrogens is illustrated in Figure 1. Since embryologically the gonads and adrenal cortex arise together on the urogenital ridge, it is not surprising that the biosynthetic pathways to androgen and estrogen in these organs are similar if not identical. In general one may view the problem of virilization or androgenicity as resulting from the inappropriate elaboration of androgen either because of excessive production of androgen from precursors and/or inadequate conversion into estrogen (Gabrilove, 1964). Little is known about excessive end-organ sensitivity to androgen although in a diametric view it seems likely, at present, that an important, if not the chief defect seen in the syndrome of the feminizing testis is end-organ refractoriness to the action of androgen.

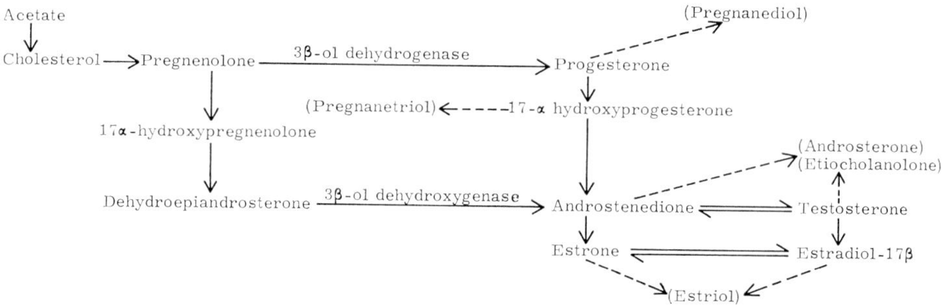

Fig. 1. Biosynthetic pathway of androgens and estrogens and some of the important urinary metabolites

The undifferentiated gonad evolves into an ovary (cortex) or testis (medulla) in the fetus presumably under the influence of the genetic sex or karyotype (XY → testis; XX → ovary). It seems likely that normally the ratio of conversion of androgen into estrogen is also primarily under the influence of (or controlled by) the genetic sex or karytotype (i.e. XX facilitating the conversion of androgen to estrogen) (Gabrilove, 1964).

Although a host of disorders have been associated with virilism and/or hirsutism (Table I), clinically virilization is most frequently a reflection of gonadal or adrenal disease. For example, mild degrees of virilism are seen in pituitary disorders such as acromegaly, but here, too, the intermediacy of the gonads or adrenal seems to be essential.

* Aided by Grant HD-02764 from the National Institutes of Health.

TABLE I

Disorders associated with virilism or hirsutism in women (after Brooksbank (1961) and Greenblatt (1968))

Pituitary (via adrenal cortex or gonad)	*Genetic*
(1) Cushing's disease	(1) Androgen sensitivity
(2) Achard-Thiers	(2) Racial or familial
(3) Acromegaly	(3) Male pseudohermaphroditism
(4) Chiari-Frommel	(4) Gonadal dysgenesis with androgenic manifestations
(5) Syndrome of excess LH	(5) ?Atavism
Adrenal Cortex	*Central Nervous System Defects*
(1) Tumor	Morgagni syndrome
a. Cushing's syndrome	Encephalitis
b. Adrenogenital syndrome	Multiple sclerosis
(2) Hyperplasia	Concussion
a. Adrenogenital	Schizophrenia
1. congenital	
2. acquired	
b. Cushing's syndrome	*Miscellaneous*
	Menopause
Ovary	Pregnancy
(1) Tumor	Stress
Arrhenoblastoma	Anorexia nervosa
Leydig (hilus) cell tumor	Drugs
(Luteoma)	Mumps
(Lipoid cell)	Dermatomyositis
(2) Stein-Leventhal (non-tumorous)	Teratomas, etc.
	Idiopathic Hirsutism

It has been customary to correlate virilizing disorders of the adrenal or gonad, or in a wider perspective feminizing disorders as well, with anatomic or pathologic abnormalities of a tumorous or non-tumorous nature (Table I). It is probably more satisfactory, however, to view these pathophysiologic disorders in a more functional or biochemical view as abnormalities in the ratio of conversion of androgen to estrogen (Gabrilove, 1964). Table II reveals such a tentative classification.

The clinical criteria for virilization are given in Table III. It will be noted that virilization in the male is also included although detection in the adult male is often difficult (Gabrilove, 1958). Not all of the clinical criteria are necessarily encountered in any given patient and it is a tribute to our increasing clinical diagnostic acumen and our advancing technology that milder and milder forms of the virilizing syndrome are being detected and treated. However, the question is still to be resolved as to whether isolated hirsutism is in itself indicative of virilism.

The biochemical hallmark of virilism is a demonstrable increase in androgenic hormones in the blood or urine or, more elegantly, an increase in the production rate. It is on these criteria that isolated hirsutism may be termed a virilizing or non-virilizing manifestation. It is on the basis of high titers of testosterone that the clinical investigator often discards 'idiopathic' hirsutism for a diagnosis of adrenal or gonadal induced hirsutism. However, recent papers have still categorized patients with high plasma androgen titers as having 'idiopathic' hirsutism because of an inability to localize the source of the excessive androgen (Aakvaag *et al.*, 1970).

TABLE II

	Increased androgen (? conversion normal)	Increased conversion androgen → estrogen (with or without increased androgen)	Decreased conversion androgen to estrogen
Male			
Adrenal cortex	Adrenogenital virilism tumor hyperplasia {congenital, acquired}	Prepuberal castration (functional) Adrenogenital feminizing syndrome due to tumor or hyperplasia	
Testis	Interstitial cell tumor (child)	Klinefelter's syndrome Interstitial cell tumor in adult (?Sertoli cell tumor)	
Etiology?		?Puberal gynecomastia	
Female			
Adrenal cortex	Adrenogenital virilism tumor hyperplasia {congenital, acquired}	Adrenogenital feminizing syndrome tumor ?hyperplasia	?Post-menopausal hirsutism
	Stein-Leventhal ovary	?Sexual precocity	
Ovary	Arrhenoblastoma and virilizing ovarian tumors	Tumor granulosa cell	Stein-Leventhal syndrome
	Stein-Leventhal syndrome	theca cell	?Arrhenoblastoma

TABLE III

Virilization

Prepuberal Male
- Precocious pseudosexual precocity
- Enlarged penis
- Muscular development
- Pubic hair
- Facial hair
- Testes enlarged but usually no spermatogenesis
- Acne
- Accelerated bone age
- True precocious (isosexual) precocity

Prepuberal Female
- Pseudohermaphroditism – plus features seen in adult female
- Accelerated bone age

Adult Male
- Maturation arrest (Gabrilove, 1958) of testis

Adult Female
- Hirsutism
- Amenorrhea
- Masculine body build
- Enlarged clitoris
- Atrophy of the breasts
- Frontal balding
- Acne

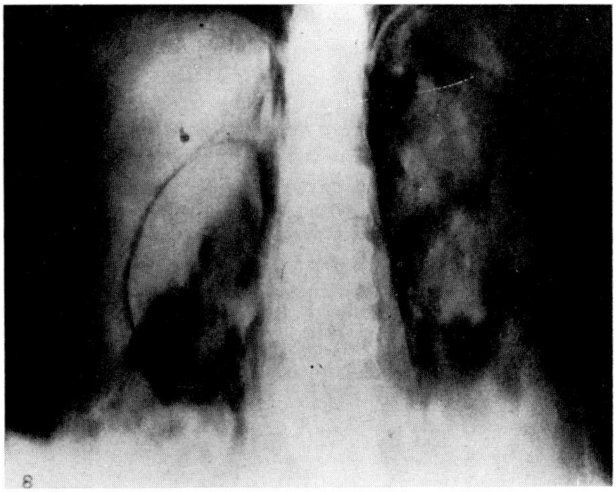

A1

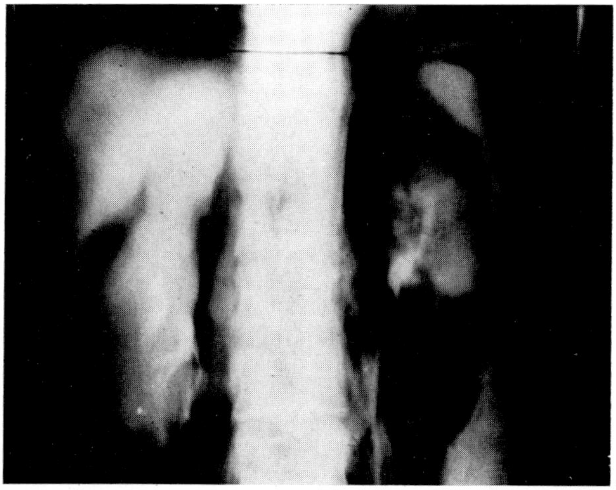

A2

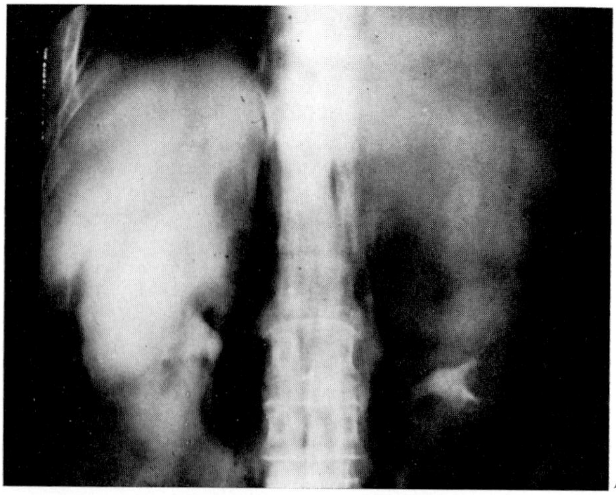

A3

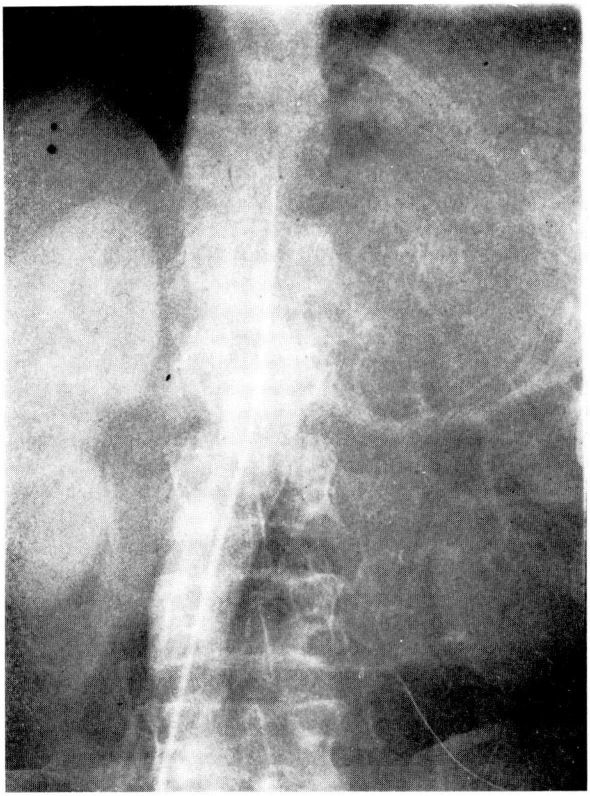

B1

Fig. 2. A. Presacral gas insufflation
(1) normal adrenal
(2) adenoma (Cushing)
(3) carcinoma (Cushing)
B. Arteriogram
(1) carcinoma (feminizing)

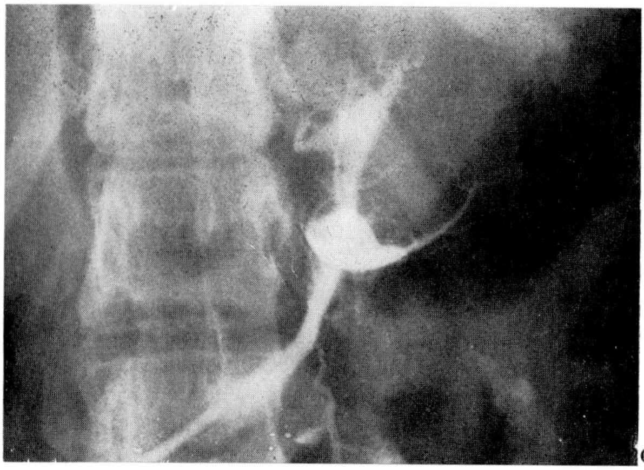

C1

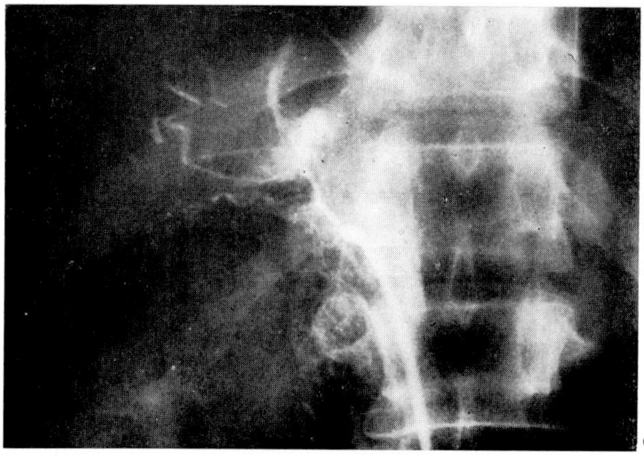

C2

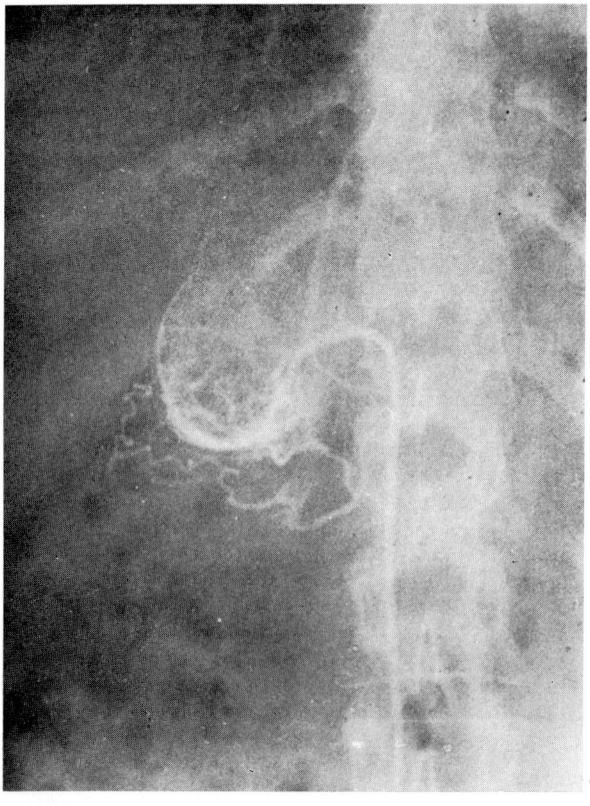

C3

C. Venogram
(1) adenoma (virilizing)
(2) adenoma (aldosterone)
(3) adenoma (Cushing)

TABLE IV

Urinary and plasma titers in various virilizing syndrome

	Adrenal Cortex			Testis	Ovary		
	Congenital adrenocortical hyperplasia (21-hydroxylase)	Acquired adrenogenital syndrome non-tumorous	Adrenal tumor malignant	Interstitial cell tumor child (Lipsett *et al.*, 1966; Wegienka and Kolb, 1967)	Virilizing tumor (arrhenoblastoma) (hilus cell) (Sato *et al.*, 1969; Mori *et al.*, 1970; Prunty, 1967)	Lipoid cell tumor (Lipsett *et al.*, 1970; Prunty, 1967)	Stein-Leventhal (Prunty, 1967, Shearman and Cox, 1966; Thomas and Steinbeck, 1966; Lawrence, 1968)
Urinary neutral 17-KS	↑	→ ↑	↑	↑	→ ↑ (occ.)	→ ↑	→ ↑
Urinary testosterone	↑	↑	↑	↑	↑	→ ↑	↑
Plasma testosterone	↑	↑	↑	↑ →?	↑	↑	↑
Urinary 17-OH	↓ →	→	→ ↑	→	→	→ ? ↑ ?	→
Urinary pregnanediol	↑		↑	↑	→ ↑	→	→
Urinary pregnenetriol	? ↑		↑	↑		↑	↑
Urinary pregnanetriol	↑	↑ ?	↑ →	↑	? ↑ →	↑	→
Urinary pregnenetriolone	↑ (3β-ol)*						↑
Urinary pregnanetriolone	↑		↑				↑
Urinary dehydroepiandrosterone	↑ (3β-ol)*	↑ ?	↑	↑	↑ →	↓ →	↑
Urinary THS	→ (↑ : 11β-OH)**		↑				→
Urinary estrogens	↑		↑ →	→	→		→
Urinary gonadotropin				↓	↓	↓	→ ↑ (? LH)
Plasma corticotropin	↑		→	→			

↓ decreased
→ normal
↑ increased
* In 3β-ol dehydrogenase defect
** In 11β-hydroxylase defect LH: luteinizing hormone occ: occasional

The underlying cause of virilism is delineated essentially by (1) roentgenographic (anatomical) demonstration of a tumor and its site or on (2) biochemical data (Fig. 2 and Table IV). In more recent times, biochemical data based on selective venous angiography have been of particular help.

Adequate understanding of the approach to diagnosis and treatment requires some comment in regard to some of the pathologic lesions encountered and the biochemical abnormalities.

(1) Congenital adrenocortical hyperplasia (Bongiovanni, 1966; Gabrilove, 1961) is essentially due to a single or possibly occasionally to a multiple enzymic defect in the biosynthetic pathway to cortisol. There is a consequent impairment of cortisol production and an increased corticotropin secretion. Since corticotropin increases the quantity of precursors, these precursors are driven into the other available pathways, particularly the one to androgen and estrogen with resultant clinical syndromes that have been well delineated. These include, depending on the defect (21-hydroxylase, 11β-hydroxylase, 3β-ol-dehydrogenase, 17-hydroxylase, 20–22 desmolase), pseudohermaphroditism, virilization, hypertension, gonadal insufficiency and salt wastage. The former two enzymic defects, 21-hydroxylase and 11β-hydroxylase, are for practical purposes unique for the adrenal, the others are important in both adrenal and gonads. Basically the hallmark of congenital adrenocortical hyperplasia is the increased urinary titer of the metabolite of the steroid proximal to the block and its suppression following the administration of cortisol.

(2) Adult adrenocortical hyperplasia appears to be either a mild form of congenital adrenocortical hyperplasia in which the enzymic defect may not be demonstrable with our current technology or a congenital or acquired facilitation of the androgen pathway at the expense of the other adrenocortical biosynthetic pathways. Here, too, the criteria are (*a*) increased urinary or plasma androgens, more particularly testosterone, (*b*) a clinical picture of virilism, and (*c*) suppression of androgen production by cortisone administration and possibly improvement of the clinical picture, especially the return of ovulatory menses if they are absent.

Although virilization appears at present to be more common in the female, similar considerations apply to the prepuberal male in whom pseudosexual precocity is the feature and in the adult male in whom the sole manifestation may perhaps be an impairment of spermatogenic maturation (Gabrilove, 1958).

(3) Adrenocortical tumors of a virilizing nature, benign or malignant, are characterized by a virilizing syndrome, high urinary and plasma titers of androgen (including testosterone), lack of suppression by cortisone, frequently high titers of precursors or their metabolites, particularly tetrahydro S derived from the corticoid pathway (especially with carcinoma), and anatomical demonstration of tumor by adrenal venography or presacral gas insufflation.

It is thus important to note that in adrenal tumors varying amounts of various androgen or cortisol precursors may be released by the adrenal and found as their metabolites in the urine as the result of impaired enzymic conversion in the biosynthetic pathway at various sites (Fukushima and Gallagher, 1963; Lipsett and Wilson, 1962; Hutter and Kayhoe, 1966; Lipsett *et al.*, 1963). For example, the impairment of 11β-hydroxylation in malignant adrenal tumors results in high secretory rates of 11-deoxycortisol and high urinary titers of THS, an important diagnostic aid (Nicolis and Gabrilove, 1969). Data for benign adrenal virilizing tumors are relatively scant (Guinet, 1966; Osborn *et al.*, 1969).

GONADS

Testis

(1) Non-tumorous hyperfunction of the testis resulting in virilization has not been delineated. Logic would dictate that the disorder exists. Whether some instances of sexual precocity are indeed examples of this must be considered.

(2) Interstitial cell tumors in the prepuberal child are rare and are associated with pseudosexual precocity and virilism. The tumor is apparent on clinical examination. Histologic examination of the non-involved testis reveals the lack of full spermatogenic maturation. Savard *et al.* (1960) as well as Sharma and his associates (1967) demonstrated the *in vitro* formation of androstenedione and testosterone by tissue from such tumors and correlated it with the high urinary excretion of testosterone and neutral 17-ketosteroids (Lipsett *et al.*, 1966; Wegienka and Kolb, 1967).

It is of particular interest, on the other hand, to note that interstitial tumors in the adult often result in gynecomastia and feminization (Gabrilove *et al.*, 1965). It is also of note that occasionally hilus cell tumors of the ovary are estrogenic rather than androgenic (Dunihoo *et al.*, 1966).

Ovary

(1) Arrhenoblastomas and hilus cell tumors result in virilization. The former rarely occur before the age of 16 and most generally are found between 20 and 35 years of age. Perhaps 5–20% are malignant (De Costa, 1969; Prunty, 1967). Approximately 250 were reported by 1966 (Sato *et al.*, 1969).

Only about 50 hilus cell tumors have been reported (Mori *et al.*, 1970; Dunihoo *et al.*, 1966). They are slightly more frequent premenarchally than arrhenoblastomas but in large measure occur in the 45–75 year age group. Only about 2% are malignant (De Costa, 1969).

The clinical picture of virilism associated with a pelvic (ovarian) mass demonstrable by pelvic examination, gynecography, culdoscopy, or perhaps by selective venography, is confirmatory. The latter affords a method of demonstrating a localized high plasma level of androgen coming directly from the tumor. Urinary titers of neutral 17-ketosteroids are usually normal but may be high. Plasma and urinary titers of testosterone are increased.

The studies of Savard *et al.* (1961) demonstrated the production of androstenedione and testosterone and lack of production of estrogen by an arrhenoblastoma (Sato *et al.*, 1969). Similar findings were reported by Corral-Gallardo *et al.* for hilus cell tumor (Fahmi *et al.*, 1968; Gabrilove, 1961; Mori *et al.*, 1970).

Lipoid cell (adrenal-like) tumors are rare. Over 100 such tumors have been reported (Osborn *et al.*, 1969; Hughesdon, 1966; Dunihoo *et al.*, 1966). The incidence of malignancy is said to be about 21% (De Costa, 1969). Lipsett *et al.* (1970) believe they are not truly adrenocortical rest in origin but derive from the ovarian stroma, and thus in a sense can biochemically behave like the other virilizing ovarian tumors (Prunty, 1967; Hughesdon, 1966). Theoretically they should manifest evidence of 21- and 11β-hydroxylation if they are truly adrenocortical in origin.

(2) Non-tumorous hyperfunction of the ovary with respect to androgen is seen in the Stein-Leventhal syndrome. This syndrome is characterized by infertility, oligo- or amenorrhea, and enlarged cystic ovaries, as well as hirsutism, obesity, and, less commonly, enlargement of the clitoris (Brooksbank, 1961; Greenblatt and Caniff, 1968; Aakvaag *et al.*, 1970; Shearman and Cox, 1966).

Presumably the mechanism is a defective conversion of androgen, particularly androstenedione and dehydroepiandrosterone, into estrogen (Mahesh, 1966; Shearman, 1966; Jeffcoate, 1964).

Clinically, the large white ovaries may be demonstrated by culdoscopy and/or gynecography if not by pelvic examination.

Treatment may be carried out by wedge resection, the administration of clomiphene, suppression with corticoids or contraceptive pills or both, or with the use of gonadotropins. Very little is known as to the mechanism by which wedge resection, clomiphene and the gonadotropins exert their beneficial effects (Prunty, 1967; Shearman and Cox, 1966).

The problem of isolated (idiopathic) hirsutism is presently under intensive study in many laboratories. In some instances it seems clearly to be part of one of the aforementioned syndromes on clinical grounds. In other instances it may be associated with high plasma levels or increased production rates of testosterone, and the hirsutism may thus also be a reflection of adrenal or ovarian abnormalities. Selective catheterization of the adrenal or ovarian veins may be the preferred method of delineating the site or sites of the abnormality. The use of selective ovarian or adrenal suppression by estrogens or corticoids has also been advocated as a means of localizing the site of abnormality, but further experience has shown these measures to be lacking in specificity in that both the adrenal and ovary may simultaneously be providing excessive androgen. Practically it may therefore be useful, as has been suggested, to utilize combined estrogen and glucocorticoid for the suppression of hirsutism particularly in patients with elevated plasma levels of testosterone (Prunty, 1967; Korenman *et al.*, 1965; Aakvaag *et al.*, 1970).

Since we have shown that in the monkey the adrenal cortex behaves like the gonad in respect to the conversion of androgen into estrogen, XY minimizing it and XX facilitating it (Sharma and Gabrilove, 1970), it would seem likely that in some clinical disorders similar considerations might apply. A logical deduction from this should be that in Klinefelter's syndrome where we have shown that there is an increased conversion of androgen to estrogen in the testes (Gabrilove *et al.*, 1970), similar findings should be noted in the adrenal. Contrariwise if in the Stein-Leventhal syndrome there is an impaired conversion of androgen to estrogen in the ovary, does this also occur in the adrenal? Looking at it in still another light, it should be kept in mind that in congenital adrenocortical hyperplasia, the usual enzymic defects are in the cortisol pathway, *i.e.* 21-hydroxylase, 11β-hydroxylase, enzymes that are believed to be almost unique to the adrenal. Consequently, in these disorders no direct effect of their absence is seen in the gonad. On the other hand, in adrenal 17-hydroxylase defects, 3β-ol defects and desmolase impairments, clinical reflection is also seen in the gonad since these enzymes are necessary for the androgen-estrogen biosynthetic pathway. Accordingly, it seems logical to presume that in the non-tumorous virilizing syndromes of the gonads, if there is a biosynthetic defect, a similar defect in the adrenal may accompany that in the gonad. These considerations would explain the superior effectiveness of combined suppression of estrogens and dexamethasone in so-called idiopathic hirsutism (and the Stein-Leventhal syndrome), both of which may truly be a combined congenital gonadal-adrenal disease.

In summary, the virilizing syndromes appear to be in large measure, if not exclusively, mediated via the adrenal cortex or gonads. They are due to tumor or non-tumorous hyperfunction, the latter on a congenital or acquired basis. They are associated usually with increased production and high titers of plasma and urinary androgen. It is possible that virilization may result from impaired conversion of androgen to estrogen.

The defects in the biosynthetic pathway have been delineated by *in vitro* (incubation) and *in vivo* studies of the production and excretion of the various precursors as well as end products and their metabolites. Further aid clinically has been afforded by roentgenographic demonstration of tumors and selective venous catheterization and analysis of the venous effluent. These latter should be of increasing importance in future studies.

So-called idiopathic hirsutism has been found to be frequently associated with high titers of androgen, particularly plasma testosterone. It is thus possible that many of these patients have true virilizing syndromes.

REFERENCES

AAKVAAG, A., VOGT, J. H. and FYLLING, P. (1970): Plasma and urinary androgens in hirsute women during adrenal and ovarian suppression. *Acta endocr. (Kbh.)*, *64*, 103.

BONGIOVANNI, A. M. (1966): The adrenogenital syndrome due to congenital adrenocortical hyperplasia. In: *Abstracts, II International Congress on Hormonal Steroids Milan*, p. 8. Editors: E. B. Romanoff and L. Martini. ICS 111. Excerpta Medica, Amsterdam.

BROOKSBANK, B. W. L. (1961): Endocrinologic aspects of hirsutism. *Physiol. Rev.*, *41*, 623.

CORRAL-GALLARDO, J., ACEVEDO, H. A., PEREZ DE SALAZAR, J. L., LORIA, M. and GOLDZIEHER, J. W. (1966): The polycystic ovary: VI: A hilus cell tumour of the ovary associated with polycystic ovarian disease. *In vivo* and *in vitro* studies. *Acta endocr. (Kbh).*, *52*, 425.

DE COSTA, E. J. (1969): Ovarian tumors with endocrine activity and related problems. *Surg. Clin. N. Amer.*, *19*, 105.

DUNIHOO, D. R., GRIENE, D. L. and WOOLF, R. B. (1966): Hilar-cell tumors of the ovary. Report of two cases and review of the literature. *Obstet. Gynec. (N.Y.)*, *27*, 703.

FAHMY, D., GRIFFITH, K., TURNBULL, A. C. and SYMINGTON, T. (1968): A comparison of the metabolism of ($7\alpha^3$-)dehydroepiandrosterone sulphate and (4-^{1}C) pregnenolone by tissue from a hilus cell tumor of the ovary. *J. Endocr.*, *41*, 61.

FUKUSHIMA, D. K. and GALLAGHER, T. F. (1963): Steroid production in 'non-functioning' adrenal cortical tumors. *J. clin. Endocr.*, *23*, 923.

GABRILOVE, J. L. (1958): Spermatogenic maturation arrest and the male adrenogenital syndrome. *Lancet*, *2*, 902.

GABRILOVE, J. L. (1961): A biologic concept of adrenocortical function. *Acta endocr. (Kbh.)*, *36*, 281.

GABRILOVE, J. L. (1964): Diseases associated with some enzymic defects in the gonads and adrenal cortex. A classification based on a theory of the biogenesis of the feminizing and virilizing syndromes. *J. Mt Sinai Hosp.*, *31*, 449.

GABRILOVE, J. L., NICOLIS, G. L. and HAUSKNECHT, R. U. (1970): Urinary testosterone, oestrogen production rate and urinary oestrogen in chromatin positive Klinefelter's syndrome. *Acta endocr. (Kbh.)*, *63*, 499.

GABRILOVE, J. L., SHARMA, D. C., WOTIZ, H. H. and DORFMAN, R. I. (1965): Feminizing adrenocortical tumors in the male. *Medicine (Baltimore)*, *44*, 37.

GREENBLATT, R. B. and CANIFF, R. F. (1968): Hirsutism and Stein-Leventhal syndrome. *Fertil. and Steril.*, *19*, 661.

GUINET, P. (1966): Androgenic tumors of the adrenal. *Rev. lyon. Méd.*, *15*, 275.

HUGHESDON, P. E. (1966): Ovarian lipoid and theca cell tumors. Their origins and interrelationships. *Obstet. gynec. Surv.*, *21*, 245.

HUTTER, A. M. and KAYHOE, D. E. (1966): Adrenal cortical carcinoma. *Amer. J. Med.*, *41*, 572.

JEFFCOATE, T. N. A. (1964): The androgenic ovary with special reference to the Stein-Leventhal syndrome. *Amer. J. Obstet. Gynec.*, *88*, 143.

KORENMAN, S. G., KIRSCHNER, M. A. and LIPSETT, M. B. (1965): Testosterone production in normal and virilized women and in women with the Stein-Leventhal syndrome or idiopathic hirsutism. *J. clin. Endocr.*, *25*, 798.

LAWRENCE, D. M. (1968): Steroid excretion in the Stein-Leventhal syndrome. *J. Obstet. Gynaec. Brit. Cwlth.*, *75*, 922.

LIPSETT, M. B., HERTZ, R. and ROSS, G. T. (1963): Clinical and pathologic aspects of adrenocortical carcinoma. *Amer. J. Med.*, *35*, 374.

LIPSETT, M. B., KIRSCHNER, M. A., WILSON, H. and BARDIN, C. W. (1970): Malignant lipid cell tumors of the ovary: clinical, biochemical and etiologic considerations. *J. clin. Endocr.*, *30*, 336.

LIPSETT, M. B., SARFATY, G. A., WILSON, H., BARDIN, C. W. and FISHMAN, L. M. (1966): Metabolism of testosterone and related steroids in metastatic interstitial cell carcinoma of the testis. *J. clin. Invest.*, *45*, 1700.

LIPSETT, M. B. and WILSON, H. (1962): Adrenocortical cancer: steroid biosynthesis and metabolism evaluated by urinary metabolites. *J. clin. Endocr.*, *22*, 906.

MAHESH, V. B. (1966): Androgen secretion in the Stein-Leventhal syndrome. *Proc. roy. Soc. Med.*, *59*, 1289.

MAHESH, V. B. and GREENBLATT, R. B. (1964): Urinary steroid patterns in hirsutism. II. Effect of ovarian stimulation with human pituitary FSH on urinary 17-ketosteroids. *J. clin. Endocr.*, *24*, 1293.

MORI, T., YOSHIDA, Y., NISHIMURA, T., KONO, T., YAMADA, S. and TATSUMI, S. (1970): Clinical and biochemical studies of a patient with a hilus cell tumor. *J. Endocr.*, *47*, 13.

NICOLIS, G. L. and GABRILOVE, J. L. (1969): Studies on the efficiency of adrenocortical 11β-hydroxylation in the human subject. *J. clin. Endocr.*, *29*, 831.

OSBORN, R. H., BRADBURY, J. J. and YANNONE, M. E. (1969): Androgen studies in a patient with lipoid-cell tumor of the ovary. *Obstet. and Gynec.*, *33*, 666.

OSBORN, R. H., YANNONE, M. E. and BRADBURY, J. J. (1969): Androgen studies in virilism secondary to an adrenal adenoma and to congenital adrenal hyperplasia. *Obstet. and Gynec.*, *33*, 658.

PRUNTY, F. T. G. (1967): Hirsutism, virilism and apparent virilism and their gonadal relationship. *J. Endocr.*, *38*, 85; 203.

SATO, J., SHINADA, T. and MATSUMOTO, S. (1969): A clinical and metabolic study of masculinizing arrhenoblastoma. *Amer. J. Obstet. Gynec.*, *104*, 1124.

SAVARD, K., DORFMAN, R. I., BAGGETT, B., FIELDING, L. L., ENGEL, L. L., MCPHERSON, H. T., LISTER, L. M., JOHNSON, D. S., HAMBLEN, E. C. and ENGEL, F. L. (1960): Clinical morphological and biochemical studies of a virilizing tumor in the testis. *J. clin. Invest.*, *39*, 534.

SAVARD, K., GUT, M., DORFMAN, R. I., GABRILOVE, J. L. and SOFFER, L. J. (1961): Formation of androgens by human arrhenoblastoma tissue *in vitro*. *J. clin. Endocr.*, *21*, 165.

SHARMA, D. C. and GABRILOVE, J. L. (1969): Difference in steroid metabolism *in vitro* by the adrenal cortex from male and female monkeys, *Macaca mulatta*. *Comp. Biochem. Physiol.*, *31*, 379.

SHARMA, D. C., RACZ, E. A., DORFMAN, R. I. and SCHOEN, E. J. (1967): A comparative study of the biosynthesis of testosterone by human testes and a virilizing interstitial cell tumor. *Acta endocr. (Kbh.)*, *56*, 726.

SHEARMAN, R. P. (1966): The diagnosis and treatment of the Stein-Leventhal syndrome. *Proc. roy. Soc. Med.*, *59*, 1285.

SHEARMAN, R. P. and COX, R. I. (1966): The enigmatic polycystic ovary. *Obstet. gynec. Surv.*, *21*, 1.

THOMAS, F. J. and STEINBECK, A. W. (1969): Semiquantitative estimation of urinary pregnanetriol, pregnanetriolone, tetrahydro S and Δ5-pregnenetriol in the investigation of adrenocortical function. *Acta endocr. (Kbh.)*, *60*, 657.

THOMAS, J. P. (1968): Adrenocortical function in Stein-Leventhal syndrome. *J. clin. Endocr.*, *28*, 1781.

WEGIENKA, L. C. and KOLB, F. (1967): Hormonal studies of a benign interstitial cell tumor of the testis producing androstenedione and testosterone. *Acta endocr. (Kbh.)*, *56*, 481.

NEUROENDOCRINOLOGY

CONTENTS

RECENT ADVANCES IN HYPOTHALAMIC HORMONES REGULATING PITUITARY FUNCTION*

ANDREW V. SCHALLY, A. ARIMURA, ABBA J. KASTIN, CYRIL Y. BOWERS, TOMMIE W. REDDING, I. WAKABAYASHI, Y. BABA, R. M. G. NAIR and JERRY J. REEVES

Endocrine and Polypeptide Laboratories and Endocrinology Section, Veterans Administration Hospital and Department of Medicine, Tulane University School of Medicine, New Orleans, La., U.S.A.

INTRODUCTION

The concept that the hypothalamus controls the secretions of the pituitary gland by releasing regulatory substances into the portal blood flowing from the hypothalamus to the pars distalis was firmly established by the brilliant work of Professor Geoffrey Harris (1955) in England. Even so, the existence of the hypothalamic neurohormones (then called factors) responsible for this control was for many years held to be more of a myth than a reality, and the search for them was associated with tremendous efforts (Guillemin, 1964; McCann and Ramirez, 1964; Mittler and Mittes, 1966; Schally *et al.*, 1968*a*). However, during the past few years, the hypothalamic neurohormones have blossomed into a family of 7 well-established substances as well as a few of a doubtful status (Schally *et al.*, 1968*a*). The evidence of their physiological role became so strong that we have suggested a change in nomenclature from factors to hormones (Schally *et al.*, 1968*a*). This presentation summarizes recent biochemical, physiological and clinical studies on hypothalamic substances controlling the release of thyrotropin, growth hormone, and luteinizing hormone as well as follicle-stimulating hormone from the pituitary gland.

THYROTROPIN-RELEASING HORMONE (TRH)

There is now convincing evidence that the hypothalamus is involved in the control of the secretion of thyrotropic hormone from the anterior pituitary gland through a neurohormone designated thyrotropin-releasing hormone (TRH). The release of thyrotropin from the pituitary gland is regulated by both TRH and a feedback from the thyroid gland. The hypothalamo-pituitary-thyroid relationship is such that TRH exerts a stimulatory effect and thyroid hormones an inhibitory one. Large doses of T_3 and T_4 will block the pituitary responses to TRH *in vivo* and *in vitro* (Bowers and Schally, 1970; Reichlin, 1966; Schally *et al.*, 1968*a*). This is an important difference from other releasing hormones. During the past few years potent TRH preparations were obtained from hypothalami of sheep (Burgus and Guillemin,

* Supported by grants from Research Service, Veterans Administration; grants AM-07467, NS-07664 and AM-09094 from NIH; The Population Council, New York, N.Y. and NIH Fellowship FO2 AM-43308.

1970), cattle (Schally *et al.* 1968*a*), pigs (Schally *et al.*, 1968*a*; Schally *et al.*, 1969*a*) and humans. These preparations were shown to induce the release of TSH *in vivo* in rats and mice (Bowers and Schally, 1970; Schally *et al.*, 1968*a*) and to stimulate the release and synthesis of TSH *in vitro* (Mittler *et al.*, 1969; Schally and Redding, 1967). Some typical responses to TRH *in vivo* are shown in Figure 1. It can be seen that a log dose-response relationship to

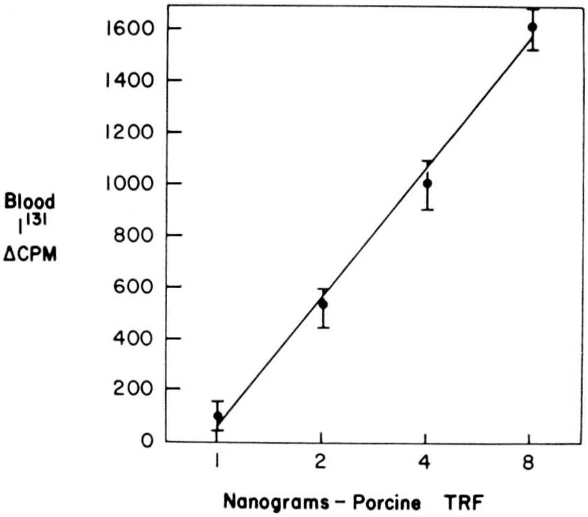

Fig. 1. Dose response curve to porcine TRH *in vivo* in mice given 0.1 μg L-T_2 and 4 μc ^{131}I, 24 hours before the assay. From Schally *et al.* (1968*a*). By courtesy of Academic Press (New York).

porcine TRH was readily obtained between 1 and 9 ng in mice placed on a low iodine diet and treated with 0.1 μg L-T_3 and 4 μc ^{131}I 24 hours before the experiment. Similarly *in vitro* TRH is active in doses as low as 0.01 ng and as the doses of TRH are increased, greater amounts of TSH are found in the incubation media (Table I). When tritium-labeled TRH was injected into rats, the highest concentration of radioactivity was found in the pituitary and the kidneys (Redding and Schally, 1971). The accumulation of labeled TRH in the pituitary indicates that TRH probably acts on this organ (Redding and Schally, 1971).

The structure of thyrotropin-releasing hormone of porcine origin has been systematically investigated by a series of degradation reactions (Nair *et al.*, 1970). Cleavage with N-bromosuccinimide followed by the 'dansyl' reaction and Edman degradation revealed a C-terminal prolyl end group, preceded by the histidyl moiety. Mild alkaline hydrolysis and subsequent 'dansyl' reaction proved the N-terminal residue to be (pyro)-glutamic acid. The fragmentation patterns in the mass spectra of free as well as permethylated thyrotropin-releasing hormone supported the Glu-His-Pro sequence for the constituent amino acids (Nair *et al.*, 1970; Schally *et al.*, 1969*a*). The results obtained support L-(pyro)Glu-L-His-L-Pro-NH_2 or 2-pyrolidone-5-carboxylyl (PCA)-His-Pro-amide as being the structure of the porcine thyrotropin-releasing hormone (Nair *et al.*, 1970). Figure 2 shows this structural formula of porcine TRH. Burgus *et al.* showed that the structure of ovine TRH is also (pyro)Glu-His-Pro-amide (Burgus *et al.*, 1970). L-(pyro)-Glu-L-His-L-Pro-NH_2 has been synthesized recently (Bøler *et al.*, 1969; Gillessen *et al.* 1970; Schally *et al.*, 1970*c*). The R_f values of natural TRH of porcine origin and synthetic L-(pyro)Glu-His-Pro-amide were identical in 17 chromatographic systems (Bøler *et al.*, 1969). On thin layer electrophoresis at pH 4, 6.3 and 8 synthetic (pyro)Glu-His-Pro-amide and natural porcine TRH showed the same mobility. Gel filtration on Sephadex G-25 in 0.2 M acetic acid revealed that synthetic and natural TRH displayed an identical migration rate (Fig. 3) (Schally *et al.*, 1970*e*). The biological activity

TABLE I

Effect of porcine TRH on release of TSH from rat pituitaries in vitro

Dose TRH added to experimental ng	TSH assay, change in blood ^{131}I (cpm) at 2 hr ± S.E. Control		Exp		Mean Δ cpm	P
.01	− 3	±12	47	± 11	40	.05
.01	1	±16	31	± 11		'05
.03	− 18	±13	70	± 9	77	.01
.03	− 5	± 9	61	± 9		.01
.09	98	±28	178	± 17	82	.01
.09	− 23	±21	62	± 19		.05
.27	130	±15	456	± 98	340	.01
.27	142	±15	457	±116		.01
.27	− 11	± 8	369	±124		.01
.54	65	±14	741	±163	653	.01
.54	47	±32	727	±154		.01
.54	4	±34	653	±117		.01
.54	60	±25	668	±117		.01
1.08	20	±20	1,390	±198	1,174	.01
1.08	− 43	±21	944	±239		.01

From Schally and Redding (1967). By Courtesy of Proc. Soc. exp. Biol. (N.Y.).

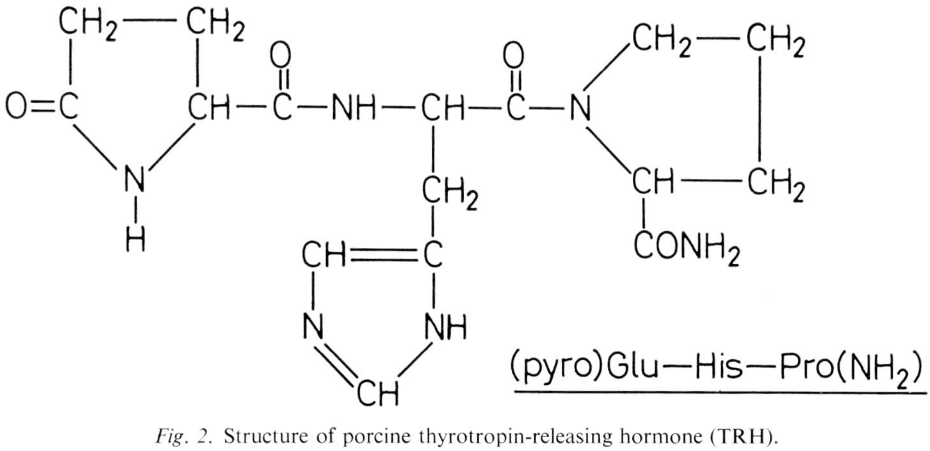

Fig. 2. Structure of porcine thyrotropin-releasing hormone (TRH).

of the synthetic L-(pyro)Glu-L-His-L-Pro-NH_2 of Bøler *et al.* (Bøler *et al.*, 1969) and Flouret (unpublished) was determined to be equivalent to that of natural porcine TRH (Schally *et al.*, 1970*e*). A comparison of the effects of natural porcine TRH and synthetic (pyro)glu-His-Pro-amide on ^{125}I release in mice is shown in Table II (Bøler *et al.*, 1969). Synthetic TRH was also found to increase plasma TSH levels in rats and to stimulate the release of TSH *in vitro* from isolated rat pituitaries.

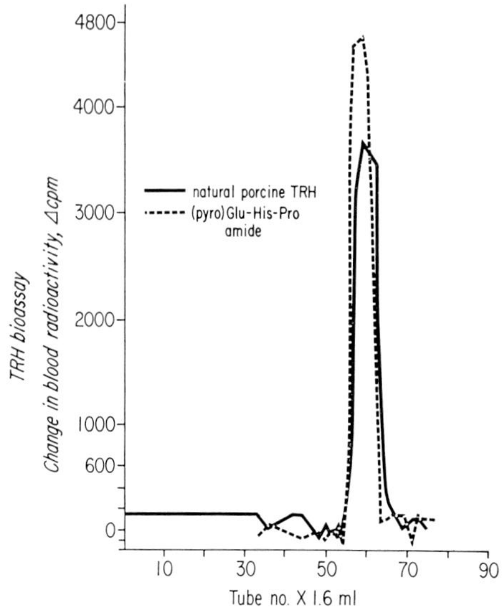

Fig. 3. Gel filtration of natural porcine TRH (160 μg) and synthetic (pyro) Glu-His-Pro amide (200 μg) on Sephadex G-25. Column 1.1 × 123 cm. Solvent 0.2 M acetic acid. Fraction size 1.6 ml. The biological activity of effluents was followed by bioassay for TRH. From Enzmann *et al.* (1971), *J. med. Chem.*, 14, 469. By courtesy of the American Chemistry Society.

Previously we have shown that natural porcine TRH stimulates TSH release in cretins as evidenced by bioassay and radioimmunoassays (Bowers *et al.*, 1968). The effect of synthetic TRH ((pyro)Glu-His-Pro (NH_2)) was studied in 12 normal males (Bowers *et al.*, 1970). Blood was taken at various intervals during a 3-hour period after a quick single i.v. injection of 100, 200, 400 and 800 μg of synthetic TRH. Measurements of serum TSH, FSH, LH and GH levels were carried out by radioimmunoassays. Serum TSH levels rose significantly after injection of TRH. When the dose of TRH was increased, the TSH levels rose higher. In each instance levels of TSH were significantly elevated at 10 minutes after injection of TRH and at 2 minutes in a patient given 800 μg TRH. The highest TSH levels occurred at 30 minutes (range 60–370%). Except in one patient given 800 μg pf TRH, levels were lower at 60 minutes. Pretreatment of 4 patients with 100 μg T_3 orally 5–7 hours before injection of 400 or 800 μg of TRH, partially or completely inhibited the response to TRH in 3 of these patients. GH,

TABLE II

Comparison of biological activity of porcine TRH and *synthetic (pyro) Glu-His-Pro (NH_2) by the T_3-TRH method in mice*

Dose ng	I^{125} Δ cpm TRH	I^{125} Δ cpm I**	p-value†	Dose ng	I^{125} Δ cpm TRH	I^{125} Δ cpm I**	p-value†
Control	24	—		Control	280	—	—
1	582*	825*	ns	2	1450*	1605*	ns
3	2834*	2746*	ns	6	4011*	4243*	ns
9	4015*	4664*	ns	18	5401*	5205*	ns

* All highly significant vs saline.
** (pyro) Glu-His-Pro (NH_2)
† Significance of difference between natural and synthetic TRH.
Modified from Bøler *et al.* (1969). By courtesy of Academic Press and *Biochem. biophys. Res. Commun.*

LH and FSH levels did not significantly change in the patients given TRH. These results summarized in Table III demonstrate that synthetic TRH is active in man and specifically elevates serum levels of TSH (Bowers *et al.*, 1970).

TABLE III

Summary of preliminary studies on the effect of synthetic TRH in man*

Subjects: 13 normal men
Dose: 100, 200, 400 and 800 μg synthetic TRH.
Assay: Plasma TSH, FSH, LH and GH measured by RIA's

Results:

(1) Elevation of plasma TSH, initially significant at 2–10 min after TRH.
(2) ,, ,, ,, ,, maximal at 30 min after TRH.
(3) % ,, ,, ,, ,, after TRH = 60–670%
(4) Range of plasma TSH 100–500 μU TSH**/100 ml
(5) No rise in plasma LH, FSH and GH.

* (Pyro)Glu-His-Pro-amide
** In terms of MRC human TSH standard.

GROWTH HORMONE-RELEASING HORMONE (GH-RH)

There is now good evidence that the release of growth hormone from the anterior pituitary gland is controlled by a hypothalamic neurohormone designated growth hormone-releasing hormone (GH-RH). This hormone has been demonstrated in hypothalamic extracts from 9 mammals including man as well as some birds and amphibia (Schally *et al.*, 1968*a*; Schally *et al.*, 1968*b*). It is interesting that kittens with bilateral lesions in the region of the paraventricular nuclei show retardation of growth. No GH-RH can be found in their hypothalami (Sawano, 1968). We have also reported that an injection of 1 mg cortisone or cortisol given to rats during the first post-natal day results in retardation of growth. When GH-RH activity was measured in their hypothalami at 5 or 6 weeks of age, none was found (Sawano, 1968). GH-RH activity was also found in the blood of hypophysectomized rats (Muller *et al.*, 1970).

We have reported the isolation of GH-RH on a large scale from porcine hypothalami and some of its physiological and biochemical properties (Schally *et al.*, 1969*b*; Schally *et al.*, 1970*b*). Thus, porcine GH-RH was purified by gel filtration on Sephadex G-25, free-flow electrophoresis, ion exchange chromatography on CMC, DEAE, TEAE and finally partition chromatography (Schally *et al.*, 1969*b*; Schally *et al.*, 1970*b*). GH-RH prepared according to these methods was active at the dose of 1 ng *in vivo* and at the levels of 0.1 pg *in vitro*. GH-RH activity was abolished after digestion with trypsin, chymotrypsin and papain (Schally *et al.*, 1970*b*). The amino acid composition of GH-RH is shown in Table IV. The results indicate that GH-RH is an acidic peptide (Schally *et al.*, 1971*c*).

Structural studies on GH-RH were based on preliminary splitting with trypsin and papain and were followed by the 'Edman-Dansyl' degradation of fragments. GH-RH appears to be straight chain decapeptide with valine at the N-terminus and alanine at C-terminus (Schally *et al.*, 1971*c*). However, the final structure has to be confirmed by synthesis.

The effects of porcine GH-RH were investigated by measuring the GH content of medium and tissue in 5-day rat pituitary organ culture systems (Mittler *et al.*, 1970*b*). The results illustrated in Table V demonstrated that rat pituitary tissue can release appreciable amounts of GH activity in an organ culture system during 5 days and that GH-RH can produce significant increases in GH in both medium and tissue relative to the control. The experi-

TABLE IV

*Amino acid composition of porcine growth hormone releasing hormone (GRH)**

Amino acid	Molar ratio***	Probable residues**
Lysine	0.99	1
Histidine	0.83	1
Ammonia	2.07	2
Serine	0.95	1
Glutamic acid	3.36	3
Aspartic acid	0.15	–
Glycine	0.12	–
Alanine	1.78	2
Valine	0.82	1
Leucine	1.0	1

* Amino acids account for 98% dry weight.
** To the nearest integer, assuming 10 amino acid residues.
*** Accepting leucine as 1.0.

From Schally *et al.* (1970). By courtesy of *J. biol. Chem.* and the American Society for Biological Chemists.

TABLE V

Effects of GH-RH on medium and tissue GH contents

Treatment	Total of 10 doses of GH-RH/mg tissue	GH (as μg NIH-GH-S7/mg of pituitary tissue)	
		Medium[1]	Tissue[1]
Control	—	41 (31–51)	43 (27–59)
Stimulated[2]	0.81 μg	100 (80–126)[3]	80 (54–116)[4]
Control	—	84 (60 – 118)	27 (21–36.8)
Stimulated[2]	2.90 μg	228 (163–309)[3]	50 (36.9–70)[3]
Control	—	141 (93–213)	38 (32–48)
Stimulated[2]	21.7 pg	312 (297–401)[3]	48 (40–60)[4]
Control	—	34 (20–39)	24 (16–36)
Stimulated[2]	225 pg	64 (50–107)[3]	28 (19–41)

[1] Data presented as means and 95% fiducial limits.
[2] GH-RH code numbers: AVS 35–73 # 111-123 (expts. 1 and 2), GH-RH purified by CMC and AVS 11-83 # 185-210, GH-RH at final purity stage (in experiments 3 and 4).
[3] P<.01 *vs.* controls (when 95% fiducial limits of both experimentals and controls failed to overlap).
[4] P<.05 *vs.* controls (when 95% fiducial limit of the relative potency estimate of the experimental sample failed to overlap the potency for the control and *vice versa*).

From Mittler *et al.* (1970). By courtesy of *Proc. Soc. exp. Biol. (N.Y.)* and Academic Press.

mental means averaged 231% of the controls for the media and 151% for the tissues. In these experiments, the weight of GH activity produced, expressed as NIH-GH-S7, was 8,400,000 times greater than the dose of GH-RH added. Thus a significant multiplier ratio was obtained (Mittler *et al.*, 1970*b*).

The results of tissue culture experiments presented in Table VI show the radioactivity associated with the electrophoretically separated GH bands. The data are presented as cpm per mg tissue after correction for quenching. The amount of radioactive amino acid incor-

TABLE VI

Effect of GH-RH on incorporation of labeled amino acids into medium and tissue GH zones

Sample	Total of 10 doses of GH-RH/mg tissue	CPM per mg tissue		Total increase over control medium and tissue
		Medium	Tissue	
Control	—	1,050 ± 110	3,190 ± 40	
Stimulated	2.5 ng	2,540 ± 130*	7,640 ± 760*	5,940
Control	—	620 ± 70	5,920 ± 380	
Stimulated	1.4 ng	1,670 ± 80*	6,590 ±1,940	1,720
Control	—	—	10,200 ± 810	
Stimulated	673 ng	—	13,100 ±2,300	—
Control	—	18,000 ±1,040	7,500 ± 200	
Stimulated	545 ng	26,800 ±1,230*	17,100 ±2,040*	18,400
Control	—	18,400 ± 30	18,200 ± 40	
Stimulated	579 ng	32,500 ±1,100*	16,800 ±6,030	12,700
Control	—	33,100 ±5,400	—	—
Stimulated	5.6 ng	66,200 ±6,450	—	—
Control	—	16,800 ±1,210	34,000 ±2,490	
Stimulated	4.6 ng	51,700 ± 160*	70,000 ±1,840*	71,300
Control	—	19,900 ±1,720	5,900 ± 130	
Stimulated	6.1 ng	35,600 ±4,310*	17,700 ±5,220	27,500

* P .05 *vs* matched control.

From Mittler *et al.* (1970). By courtesy of *Proc. Soc. exp. Biol. (N.Y.)* and Academic Press.

poration was increased in both medium and tissue GH bands after stimulation with GH-RH. Calculations show an average increased incorporation into GH in the experimental medium of 218% and in the stimulated tissue of 186% as compared with the controls. This increased radioactivity associated with GH bands after stimulation of the pituitaries by GH-RH is additional evidence for stimulation of GH synthesis by GH-RH (Mittler *et al.*, 1970*b*).

Electron microscope studies of pituitary somatotrophs of female Sprague-Dawley rats were conducted following intracarotid injection of 2 μg of purified pig GH-RH (Couch *et al.*, 1969). Animals were sacrificed by decapitation 0.5, 1, 2.5, 5 and 15 min after GH-RH injection. Saline-injected control animals were sacrificed according to the same schedule. Tissues were fixed in phosphate-buffered osmium tetroxide. A marked increase in the number of secretory granules undergoing extrusion into the perivascular space from the somatotroph, as compared to controls, was found to occur as early as 2.5 min after GH-RH injection (Couch *et al.*, 1969). Some of these results can be seen in Figure 4. These observations provide direct evidence that GH-RH acts on somatotrophs (Couch *et al.*, 1969).

LUTEINIZING HORMONE-RELEASING HORMONE (LH-RH) AND FOLLICLE-STIMULATING HORMONE-RELEASING HORMONE (FSH-RH)

There is now excellent evidence that the secretion of luteinizing hormone (LH) and follicle-stimulating hormone (FSH) from the anterior pituitary gland is controlled principally by the hypothalamus and a feedback system, involving sex steroids (Guillemin, 1964; Harris, 1955; McCann and Ramirez, 1964; Schally and Kastin, 1964; Schally *et al.*, 1968*a*). This control is mediated by FSH-releasing hormone (FSH-RH) and LH-releasing hormone (LH-RH) whose

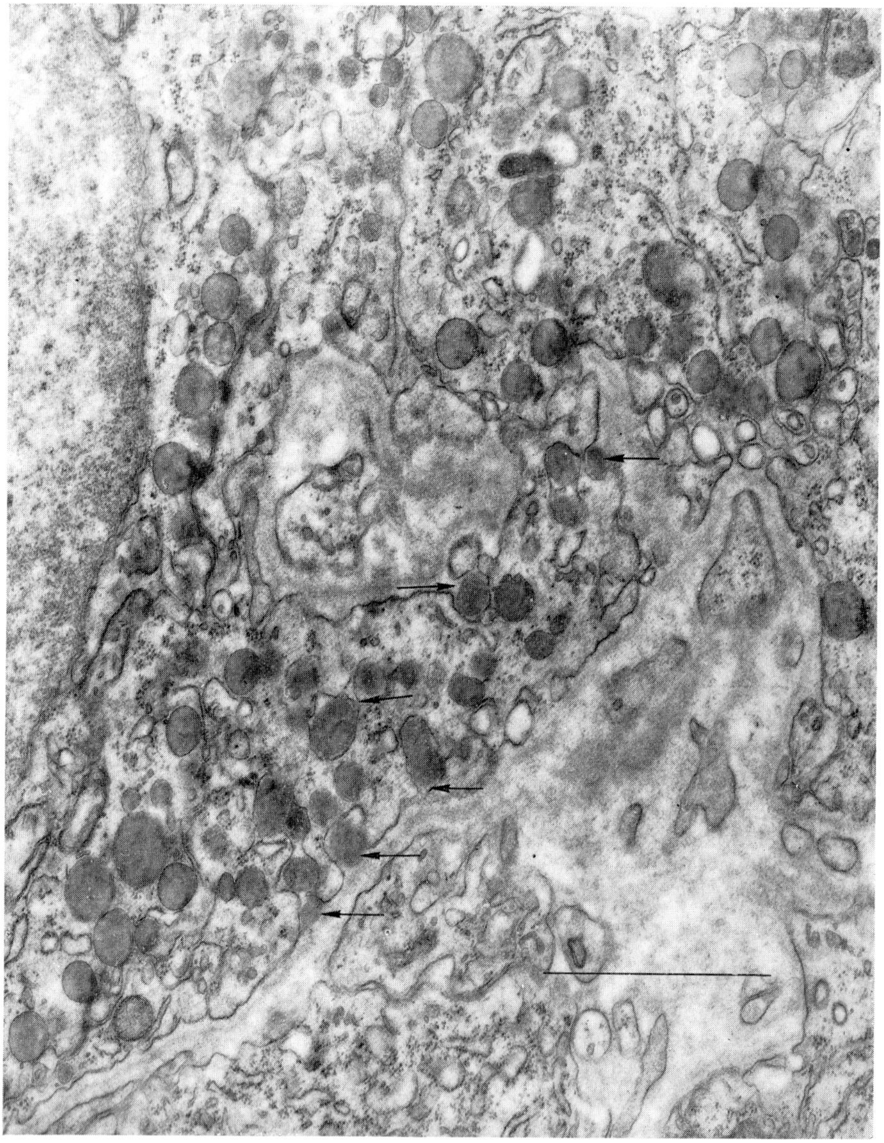

Fig. 4. Electron micrograph of a portion of a somatotroph (× 49,600, reduced for reproduction 30 %) from a rat sacrificed 2½ min following CRF injection. Numerous areas of granule extrusion (arrows) can be seen. Coalescence of granules can be seen. From Couch *et al.* (1969). By courtesy of *Endocrinology* and Lippincott (Philadelphia).

function is to augment the secretion of FSH and LH. The sex steroids derived from the ovary and the testes exert mainly an inhibitory influence called a 'negative feedback' by acting principally on the hypothalamus (Schally and Kastin, 1970). However, there is some evidence suggesting that estrogen and progesterone can exert some direct effect on the pituitary gland as well (Arimura and Schally, 1970; Hilliard *et al.*, 1970).

The remainder of this presentation will cover some of our latest studies on LH-releasing hormone (LH-RH) and FSH-releasing hormone (FSH-RH). We will also mention our work with some compounds affecting fertility, by reporting some recent results concerning the actions of clomiphene and the oral contraceptive steroids on the hypothalamo-pituitary axis in rats. In addition, we will describe the effects of administration of LH-RH to humans.

LH-RH used in these physiological and human studies was prepared from pig hypothalamic extracts. The purification steps included gel filtration on Sephadex G-25, extraction of the LH-RH active fractions with phenol, chromatography and rechromatography on carboxymethylcellulose (CMC), free flow-electrophoresis, countercurrent distribution (CCD) and partition chromatography (Schally *et al.*, 1967; 1970*a*).

Thin-layer chromatography (TLC) of LH-RH purified according to this procedure, revealed only one spot in the system 1-butanol : acetic acid : water = 4 : 1 : 5 positive to chlorine/o-tolidine. This spot had all the LH-RH activity. There was no LH-RH activity in other areas of the TLC plate (Fig. 5) (Schally *et al.*, 1970*a*). The preparations of porcine and human

TLC OF HIGHLY PURIFIED PIG LH-RH

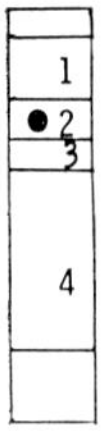

	Zone	LH-RH Activity Plasma LH ng/ml mean ± SE	P
Solvent Front			
	1	8.5 ± 2.93	NS
	2	88.2 ± 8.6	< 0.001
	3	9.5 ± 2.6	NS
	4	11.0 ± 2.9	NS
	Saline	12.6 ± 2.5	----

Fig. 5. Thin layer chromatography of porcine LH-RH in 1-butanol: acetic acid: water = 4 : 1 : 5. From Schally *et al.* (1970*a*). By courtesy of Springer (Berlin).

LH-RH also contained FSH-RH activity, which may be intrinsic to LH-RH or due to contamination with FSH-RH. Recent results indicate that LH-RH activity is abolished following incubation with chymotrypsin, subtilisin, amino peptidase M and papain (Schally *et al.*, 1970*b*) (Table VII). This supports the concept that LH-RH may be a polypeptide. The molecular weight of LH-RH is of the order of several hundred (Schally *et al.*, 1970*a*; 1971*b*). The biological activity of materials at various purification stages is described below.

Porcine LH-RH, at doses as low as 0.5 ng, induced an elevation of plasma LH in ovariectomized rats pre-treated with estrogen (50 μg) and progesterone (25 mg) (Schally *et al.*, 1970*a*) (Table VIII) as measured by bioassay and radioimmunoassays (Schally *et al.*, 1970*a*; 1971*a*). LH-RH also increased plasma LH in intact rats and castrated, testosterone-pretreated male rats (Schally *et al.*, 1968*a*; 1970*a*). Preliminary studies of the kinetics of the response to LH-RH *in vivo* indicate that the response to LH-RH in rats is rapid with maximal levels of LH being reached in 10–12 minutes (Schally *et al.*, 1970*a*). (Fig. 6) Log-dose responses to LH-RH were readily obtained *in vivo* and *in vitro* (Schally *et al.* 1968*a*; 1970*a*). Stimulation of FSH-release *in vitro* from pituitaries of rats (6 hr incubation) was obtained with 1 ng/ml of LH-RH, but not with putrescine, cadaverine, spermine or spermidine (Schally *et al.*, 1970*d*). These results are shown in Tables IX and X. In tissue cultures of rat pituitaries (3 days), addition of LH-RH significantly increased the release and synthesis of LH and FSH as measured by bioassay and radioimmunoassays (Mittler *et al.*, 1970*a*). Some of these results are illustrated in Tables XI and XII.

Massive doses (1–20 mg/rat) of 12 oral contraceptive preparations administered to ovariec-

TABLE VII

Effects of various treatments on the biological activity of LH-RH and FSH-RH

Treatment	LH-RH			FSH-RH		
		Inactivation			Inactivation	
	No effect	Partial	Complete	No effect	Partial	Complete
Trypsin*, pH 8.1	+			+		
Pepsin*, pH 2	+			+		
Chymotrypsin*, pH 8.1			+			+
Subtilisin*, pH 8.1			+			+
Papain*, pH 5.1			+			+
Amino peptidase M, pH 8.1	+			+		
Carboxypeptidase* A, pH 8.1	+					
Carboxypeptidase* B, pH 8.1	+					
Neuraminidase*, pH 5.1	+			+		
pH 8.1*	+			+		
pH 2*	+			+		
pH 5.1*	+			+		
HCl IM – 60 min 100° C			+			+
Ninhydrin		+			+	
N-bromosuccinimide			+			+
Diazotized sulfanilic acid			+			+
Nitrous acid	+			+		
Periodate oxidation		+			+	+
Performic acid			+			

E : S = 1 : 10 for all enzymes.
* Incubations at 37° C for 20 hr.

From Schally *et al.* (1970*b*). By courtesy of the *J. biol. Chem.* and the American Society for Biological Chemists.

TABLE VIII

Effect of highly purified porcine LH-RH on LH release in vivo

Group	LRH dose ng dry wt. per rat	Plasma LH activity OAA change μg/100 mg ± S.E.	P Group	P	Radioimmuno-assay for rat LH serum LH* mμg/ml
1. Saline	—	− 3.0 ±0.5	—	—	< 131
2. LRH	0.5	− 8.2 ±0.9	2 *vs* 1	0.001	243
3. LRH	5	−15.6 ±1.2	3 *vs* 1	0.001	1090
			3 *vs* 2	0.01	
4. LRH	25	−22.0 ±1.7	4 *vs* 1	0.001	2460
			4 *vs* 3	0.05	

* Expressed in terms of NIAMD rat LH-RP-1.

Modified from Schally *et al.* (1970*b*); Schally and Kastin (1970); Schally *et al.*, 1970*c*). By courtesy of Academic Press (New York), *Endocrinology*, Lippincott (Philadelphia), Williams and Wilkins (Baltimore) and Springer (Berlin).

tomized rats lowered plasma LH to 1/5 of its basal concentration, but did not suppress the stimulatory effect of 0.1 μg LH-RH on LH and FSH release (3–10-fold increase) (Schally *et al.*, 1970*f*) (Table XIII). This suggests that the contraceptive steroids act mainly on the

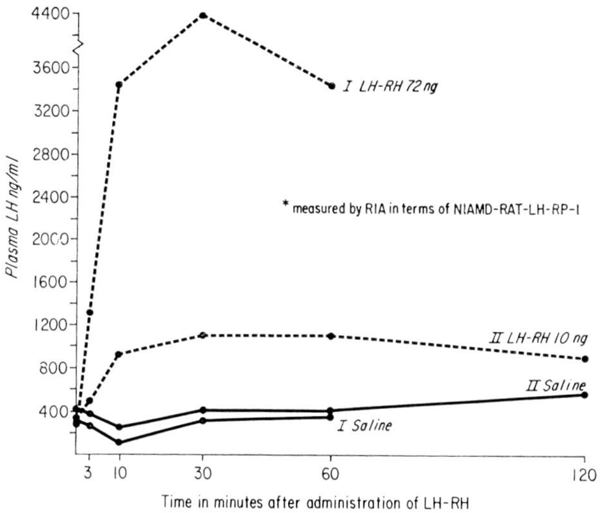

Fig. 6. Time study of the elevation of plasma LH in ovariectomized, estrogen progesterone-treated urethane-anesthetized rats after administration of 10 and 72 ng of porcine LH-RH. From Schally *et al.* (1970*a*). By courtesy of Springer (Berlin).

TABLE IX

Lack of effect of some polyamines histamine on FSH release in vitro *from pituitaries of normal male rats*

Exp. No.	Group of pituitaries	Addition	Dose μg/ml	FSH content of medium, ovarian wt mg ±SE	P *vs* control
1	Control	—	—	65.3 ±4.1	—
	Experimental	Putrescine	0.01	77.9 ±6.7	N.S.
2	Control	—	—	65.2 ±5.4	—
	Experimental	Putrescine	0.01	68.8 ±4.8	N.S.
3	Control	—	—	49.0 ±4.2	—
	Experimental	Spermidine	1.0	60.2 ±6.5	N.S.
	Experimental	Cadaverine	0.2	54.8 ±7.1	N.S.
	Experimental	Putrescine	0.2	53.4 ±5.4	N.S.
	Experimental	Spermine	1.0	67.0 ±8.8	N.S.
4	Control	—	—	61.6 ±4.2	—
	Experimental	Sperimine	1.0	53.4 ±4.0	N.S.
	Experimental	Cadaverine	0.2	58.0 ±4.1	N.S.
5	Control	—	—	68.0 ±6.1	—
	Experimental	Agmatine	1.5	73.6 ±7.2	N.S.
6	Control*	—	—	73.5 ±5.9	—
	Experimental*	Histamine	0.2	71.1 ±6.0	N.S.

* Pituitaries from ovariectomized rats pre-treated with estrogen and progesterone.

Modified from Schally *et al.* (1970*d*). By courtesy of *Endocrinology* and Lippincott (Philadelphia).

TABLE X

Effect of porcine FSH-RH-preparations at various stages of purity on FSH release in vitro from rat pituitaries

Group of pituitaries	Dose μg/ml	FSH content of medium ovarian wt ± SE	P *vs* control
Control, normal male pits.	—	59.6 ± 4.4	—
Exp. ,, ,, ,,	0.0006	69.2 ± 7.4	N.S.
Exp. ,, ,, ,,	0.0025	87.4 ± 6.2	0.01
Exp. ,, ,, ,,	0.01	105.2 ±17.6	0.05
Exp. ,, ,, ,,	0.04	196.2 ±17.9	0.001
Control ,, ,, ,,	—	47.8 ± 3.8	—
Exp. ,, ,, ,,	0.001	61.6 ± 2.8	0.02
Exp. ,, ,, ,,	0.003	82.4 ± 5.1	0.001
Control, O.E.P. pits*	—	74.8 ±11.6	—
Exp. ,, ,,	0.01	152.0 ±17.3	0.01
Control castrated T.P. pits*	—	59.5 ± 4.6	—
Exp. ,, ,, ,,	0.075	67.8 ± 7.2	N.S.
Exp. ,, ,, ,,	0.37	92.0 ± 7.8	0.01

* Pituitaries from ovariectomized, estrogen- and progesterone-treated rats.
** Pituitaries from castrated, testosterone propionate-treated male rats.

Modified from Schally *et al.* (1970*d*). By courtesy of *Endocrinology* and Lippincott (Philadelphia).

TABLE XI

Effects of porcine LH-RH preparations on medium and tissue LH contents in rat pituitary cultures

Treatment	Total of six doses of LH-RH per pituitary in μg	LH content as mμg NIH-LH-S_{14} per pituitary by radioimmunoassay			
		Medium	Tissue	Total	Increase
Control	—	846	1,444	2,290	
Stimulated	0.46	2,166	468	2,634	344
Control	—	682	1,006	1,688	
Stimulated	1,25	1,925	383	2,258	570
Control	—	472	1.027	1,499	
Stimulated	0.25	1,208	445	1,653	154
Control	—	440	748	1,188	
Stimulated	6.25	1,705	165	1,870	682
Control	—	600	2,152	2,752	
Stimulated	0.31	2,625	315	2,940	188
Tissue cultured	—	—	730	—	—
for 2 days only	—	—	560	—	—

From Mittler *et al.* (1970). By courtesy of *Proc. Soc. exp. Biol. (N.Y.)* and Academic Press.

hypothalamus or another brain center (Schally and Kastin, 1970; Schally *et al.*, 1970*f*). However, progesterone also may exert some direct effect on the pituitary. This is indicated by the following data: (*a*) administration of 2 mg progesterone induced partial blockade of ovulation in estrous rabbits in response to the pituitary infusion of threshold doses of LH-RH

TABLE XII

Effects of porcine LH-RH preparations on medium and tissue FSH contents in rat pituitary cultures

Experiment No.	Treatment	Total of 6 doses of LH-RH per pituitary in μg	FSH by radioimmunoassay (as μg NIAMD rat FSH RP-1 per pituitary)			
			Medium	Tissue	Total	Increase
1	Control	—	2.03	2.49	4.52	
	Stimulated	0.46	6.23	0.77	7.00	2.48
2	Control	—	1.76	1.73	3.49	
	Stimulated	1.25	10.53	0.87	11.40	7.91
3	Control	—	3.94	1.20	5.14	
	Stimulated	0.25	10.08	1.39	11.47	6.33

From Mittler *et al.* (1970). By courtesy of *Proc. Soc. exp. Biol. (N.Y.)* and Academic Press.

(Hilliard *et al.*, 1970); (*b*) administration of 25 mg progesterone decreased the responses to small doses of LH-RH in normal rats (Arimura and Schally, 1970).

In analogy to steroidal contraceptive preparations, clomiphene also seems to act principally on the hypothalamus (Schally *et al.*, 1970*c*). Clomiphene appears to exert a dual, dose-dependent effect. Large doses of clomiphene (10 mg/rat/day) or its trans- and cis-isomers, which lowered plasma LH in rats (Tables XIV and XV), did not suppress the response to LH-RH (Table XV). Small doses of clomiphene (15–50 μg/rat), especially the cis-isomer, which raised plasma LH and FSH (Table XIV), seemed to potentiate the effect of LH-RH (Schally *et al.*, 1970*c*).

Clinical studies showed that porcine LH-RH preparations (administered intravenously or subcutaneously) induced an elevation of plasma LH (2–8 fold) and FSH (2–5 fold) in normal or sex steroid-treated men and women, or women with secondary amenorrhea (Kastin *et al.*, 1969; Kastin *et al.*, 1970). Four post-menopausal women responded to LH-RH regardless of whether their normally elevated serum LH had been suppressed by an oral contraceptive (Lyndiol) (Kastin *et al.*, 1970). In 6 men in whom LH levels had been elevated by pretreatment for 8 or 16 days with clomiphene (200 mg/day), LH-RH caused an additional sharp increase in plasma LH (Schally *et al.*, 1970*a*). This work demonstrates that species specificity in man is not a problem with porcine LH-RH and suggests the possible clinical usefulness of LH-RH in the control of fertility.

TABLE XIII

Effect of large doses of 8 oral contraceptive preparations on plasma LH and FSH levels and on the response to LH-RH in ovariectomized rats as measured by the RIA

Group No.	Treatment	Dose* mg mg	LH-RH Dose μg	Plasma LH mμg/ml**	Plasma FSH mμg/ml
1	Ovariectomized control	—	—	653	3900
2	Oracon (dimethisterone + ethinyl estradiol)	 20 0.08	—	153	1800
3	Oracon (dimethisterone + ethinyl estradiol)	 20 0.08	0.1	2338	2525
4	Ovral (norgestrel + ethinyl estradiol)	1 1 0.1	—	137	2775
5	Ovral (norgestrel + ethinyl estradiol)	 1 0.1	0.1	905	2150
6	Ortho Novum (norethindrone +mestranol)	 5 0.25	—	130	1500
7	Ortho Novum (norethindrone + mestranol)	 5 0.25	0.1	1610	2650
8	Ovulen (ethynodiol diacetate + mestranol)	 2	—	199	2150
9	Ovulen (ethynodiol diacetate + mestranol)	 2	0.1	1860	2100
10	Provest (medroxyprogesterone acetate + ethinyl estradiol)	 2 0.01	—	142	2200
11	Provest (medroxyprogesterone acetate + ethinyl estradiol	 2 0.01	0.1	1313	2750
12	Enovid (norethinodrel + mestranol	 10	—	156	1500
13	Enovid (norethinodrel + mestranol	 10	0.1	1485	2325
14	C-Quens (chlormadinone acetate + mestranol)	 10 0.4	—	172	1850
15	C-Quens (chlormadinone acetate + mestranol	 10 0.4	0.1	1843	1850
16	Norlestrin (norethindrone acetate + ethinyl estradiol)	 5 0.16	—	135	2575
17	Norlestrin (norethindrone acetate + ethinyl estradiol)	 5	0.1	1778	2650

* Daily for 5 days.

** Mean of 2 replicate RIA.

Reference preparations for LH and FSH in RIA were NIAMD Rat LH-RP-1 and R817B respectively. From Schally *et al.* (1970*c*). By courtesy of *Endocrinology* and Lippincott (Philadelphia).

TABLE XIV

Effect of clomiphene and its isomers on plasma LH and FSH levels of ovariectomized rats determined by radioimmunoassay

Group number	Treatment	Dose* (μg/rat)	Serum FSH Assay number	Serum FSH (mμg/ml)**	Serum FSH mean	Serum LH Assay number	Serum LH (mμg/ml)***	Serum LH mean
1	Control	—	1	2800	2700	1	1031	1056
			2	2600		2	1081	
2	Clomiphene	5	1	4200	4100	1	1125	1122
			2	4000		2	1119	
3	Clomiphene	15	1	4300	4150	1	875	897
			2	4000		2	919	
4	Clomiphene	45	1	3500	3850	1	1375	1407
			2	4200		2	1438	
5	Clomiphene	135	1	4250	3925	1	844	904
			2	3600		2	963	
6	Clomiphene	10,000	1	2900	2950	1	288	304
			2	3000		2	319	
7	Cisclomiphene	5	1	3600	3500	1	1375	1238
			2	3400		2	1100	
8	Cisclomiphene	15	1	3900	3950	1	1563	1482
			2	4000		2	1400	
9	Cisclomiphene	45	1	5500	4750	1	1188	1276
			2	4000		2	1363	
10	Cisclomiphene	135	1	4350	3975	1	1125	1053
			2	3600		2	981	
11	Cisclomiphene	10,000	1	4500	4150	1	531	547
			2	3800		2	563	
12	Transclomiphene	5	1	3600	3800	1	1219	1241
			2	4000		2	1263	
13	Transclomiphene	15	1	2650	2725	1	844	813
			2	2800		2	781	
14	Transclomiphene	45	1	3950	3875	1	844	963
			2	3800		2	1081	
15	Transclomiphene	135	1	4800	4200	1	813	766
			2	3600		2	719	
16	Transclomiphene	10,000	1	1750	1775	1	181	197
			2	1800		2	213	

* Given subcutaneously in oil daily for 3 days.
** Expressed in terms of a rat FSH reference preparation 1.4 x NIH-FSH-S1 in biologic potency.
*** Expressed in terms of a rat LH preparation 0.03 x NIH-LH-S1 in biologic potency.

From Schally *et al.* (1970*f*). By courtesy of *Amer. J. Obstet. Gynec.* and Mosby (St. Louis).

TABLE XV

*Effect of LRH on plasma LH levels (OAA assay) of ovariectomized rats pretreated with large doses of clomiphene, its isomers and/or estrogen plus progesterone (E.P.**)*

Group number	Treatment	Dose* (μg/rat)	Dose of LRH μg/rat	Plasma LH activity OAA change (μg/100 mg ± S.E.)	P group	P
1	Control	—	—	−14.4 ±0.9	—	—
2	Control	—	0.25	−20.6 ±1.6	—	—
3	E.P. (control)	—	—	− 2.7 ±3.3	3 vs 1	0.001
4	E.P.	—	0.25	−18.7 ±2.1	4 vs 3	p.01
5	Clomiphene	500	—	−11.8 ±1.1	5 vs 1	N.S.
6	Clomiphene	500	0.25	−14.0 ±1.4	6 vs 5	N.S.
7	Clomiphene	2,500	—	−11.8 ±0.7	7 vs 1	N.S.
					7 vs 3	0.01
8	Clomiphene	2,500	0.25	−18.6 ±0.8	8 vs 7	0.01
9	Clomiphene	10,000	—	−10.0 ±1.1	9 vs 1	N.S.
10	Clomiphene	10,000	0.25	−17.0 ±1.1	10 vs 9	0.01
11	Clomiphene	10,000	—	− 6.8 ±2.2	11 vs 1	0.01
					11 vs 3	N.S.
12	Clomiphene	10,000	0.25	−17.6 ±0.8	12 vs 11	0.01

* Clomiphene or isomers given subcutaneously in oil daily for 3 days except for groups No. 11 and 12 given as single dose 72 hours before sacrifice.

** Single dose of 50 μg estradiol benzoate and 25 mg progesterone per rat 72 hours before sacrifice.

From Schally *et al.* (1970*f*). By courtesy of *Amer. J. Obstet. Gynec.* and Mosby (St. Louis).

REFERENCES

ARIMURA, A. and SCHALLY, A. V. (1970): Progesterone suppression of LH-releasing hormone-induced stimulation of LH release in rats. *Endocrinology, 87*, 653.

COUCH, E. F., ARIMURA, A., SCHALLY, A. V., SAITO, M. and SAWANO, S. (1969): Electron microscope studies of somatotrophs of rat pituitary after injection of purified growth hormone releasing factor (GRF). *Endocrinology, 85*, 1084.

BØLER, J., ENZMANN, F., FOLKERS, K., BOWERS, C. Y. and SCHALLY, A. V. (1969): The identity of chemical and hormonal properties of the thyrotropin releasing hormone and pyroglutamyl-histidyl-proline amide. *Biochem. biophys. Res. Commun., 37*, 705.

BOWERS, C. Y. and SCHALLY, A. V. (1970): Assay of thyrotropin-releasing hormone. In: *Hypophysiotropic Hormones of the Hypothalamus: Assay and Chemistry*, Chapter 6, pp. 74–89. Editor: J. Meites. Williams and Wilkins, Baltimore, Md.

BOWERS, C. Y., SCHALLY, A. V., HAWLEY, W. F., GUAL, C. and PARLOW, A. F. (1968): Effect of thyrotropin-releasing factor in man. *T. J. clin. Endocr. 28*, 978.

BOWERS, C. Y., SCHALLY, A. V., SCHALCH, D. S., GUAL, C., KASTIN, A., CASTANEDA, E. and FOLKERS, K. (1970). Synthetic thyrotropin releasing hormone (TRH): Effect in man. In: *Program of the Fifty-Second Meeting of the Endocrine Society*, p. 41.

BURGUS, R., DUNN, T. F., DESIDERIO, D., WARD, D. N., VALE, W. and GUILLEMIN, R. (1970): Characterization of ovine hypothalamic hypophysiotropic TSH-releasing factor. *Nature (Lond.), 226*, 321.

BURGUS, R., and GUILLEMIN, R. (1970): Chemistry of thyrotropin-releasing factor (TRF). In: *Hypophysiotropic Hormones of the Hypothalamus: Assay and Chemistry*, Chapter 15, pp. 227–241. Editor: J. Meites. Williams and Wilkins, Baltimore, Md.

GILLESSEN, D., FELIX, A. M., LERGIER, W. and STUDER, R. O. (1970): Synthese des thyrotropin-releasing Hormons (TRH) (Schaf) und verwandter Peptide. *Helv. chim. Acta 53*, 63.

GUILLEMIN, R. (1964): Hypothalamic factors releasing pituitary hormones. *Rec. Progr. Hormone Res. 20*, 89.

HARRIS, G. W. (1955). In: *Neural Control of the Pituitary Gland*,. Arnold, London.

HILLIARD, J., SCHALLY, A. V. and SAWYER (1970): Progesterone blocks ovulation in rabbits in response to intrapituitary infusion of purified LH-RH. In: *III International Congress on Hormonal Steroids* p. 224. Editor: V. T. H. James. ICS No. 210. Excerpta Medica, Amsterdam.

KASTIN, A. J., SCHALLY, A. V., GUAL, C., MIDGLEY, A. R., JR., BOWERS, C. Y. and DIAZ-INFANTE, A., JR. (1969): Stimulation of LH release in men and women by LH-releasing hormone purified from porcine hypothalami. *J. clin. Endocr*, *29*, 1046.

KASTIN, A. J., SCHALLY, A. V., GUAL, C., MIDGLEY, A. R., JR., BOWERS, C. Y. and GOMEZ-PEREZ, E. (1970): Administration of LH-releasing hormone to selected subjects. *Amer. J. Obstet. Gynec.*, *108*, 177.

MCCANN, S. M. and RAMIREZ, V. D. (1964): Neuroendocrine regulation of hypophyseal luteinizing hormone secretion. *Recent. Progr. Hormone Res.*, *20*, 131.

MITTLER, J. C. and MEITES, J. (1966): Effects of hypothalamic extract and androgen on pituitary FSH release *in vitro*. *Endocrinology*, *78*, 500.

MITTLER, J. C., REDDING, T. W. and SCHALLY, A. V. (1969): Stimulation of thyrotropin (TSH) secretion by TSH-releasing factor (TRF) in organ cultures of anterior pituitary. *Proc. Soc. exp. Biol. (N.Y.)*, *130*, 406.

MITTLER, J. C., ARIMURA, A. and SCHALLY, A. V. (1970*a*): Release and synthesis of luteinizing hormone and follicle-stimulating hormone in pituitary cultures in response to hypothalamic preparations. *Proc. Soc. exp. Biol. (N.Y.)*, *133*, 1321.

MITTLER, J. C., SAWANO, S., WAKABAYASHI, I., REDDING, T. W. and SCHALLY, A. V. (1970*b*): Stimulation of release and synthesis of growth hormone (GH) in tissue cultures of anterior pituitaries in response to GH-releasing hormone (GH-RH). *Proc. Soc. exp. Biol. (N.Y.)*, *133*, 890.

MULLER, E. E., ARIMURA, A., SAITO, T. and SCHALLY, A. V. (1967): Growth hormone-releasing activity in plasma of normal and hypophysectomized rats. *Endocrinology*, *80*, 77.

NAIR, R. M. G., BARRETT, J. F., BOWERS, C. Y. and SCHALLY, A. V. (1970): Structure of porcine thyrotropin releasing hormone. *Biochemistry*, *9*, 1103.

REDDING, T. W. and SCHALLY, A. V. (1971): The distribution of labeled thyrotropin releasing hormone (TRH) in rats and mice. *Endocrinology*, October issue.

REICHLIN, S. (1966): Control of thyrotropic hormone secretion. In: *Neuroendocrinology*, *Vol. 1*, Chapter 12, pp. 445–536. Editors: L. Martini and W. F. Ganong. Academic Press, New York.

SAWANO, S., ARIMURA, A., SCHALLY, A. V., SAITO, T., BOWERS, C. Y., O'BRIEN, C. P. and BACK, L. M. N. (1968): Growth hormone-releasing activity in the hypothalamus of kittens with lesions of the region of the paraventricular nuclei. *Acta endocr. (Kbh.)*, 59, 317.

SAWANO, S., ARIMURA, A., SCHALLY, A. V., REDDING, T. W. and SCHAPIRO, S. (1969): Neonatal corticoid administration: Effects upon adult pituitary growth hormone and hypothalamic growth-hormone-releasing hormone activity. *Acta endocr. (Kbh.)*, *61*, 57.

SCHALLY, A. V. and KASTIN, A. J. (1970): The role of sex steroids, hypothalamic LH-releasing hormone in the regulation of gonadotropin secretion from the anterior pituitary gland. In: *Advances in Steroid Biochemistry*, *Vol. 2*, pp. 41–64. Editor: M. H. Briggs. Academic Press, New York.

SCHALLY, A. V. and REDDING, T. W. (1967): *In vitro* studies with thyrotropin releasing factor. *Proc. Soc. exp. Biol. (N.Y.)*, *126*, 320.

SCHALLY, A. V., BOWERS, C. Y., WHITE, W. F. and COHEN, A. I. (1967): Purification and *in vivo* and *in vitro* studies with porcine luteinizing hormone-releasing factor (LRF). *Endocrinology*, *81*, 77.

SCHALLY, A. V., ARIMURA, A,. BOWERS, C. Y., KASTIN, A. J., SAWANO, S. and REDDING, T. W. (1968*a*): Hypothalamic neurohormones regulating anterior pituitary function. *Recent. Progr. Hormone Res.*, *24*, 497.

SCHALLY, A. V., SAWANO, S., MULLER, E. E., ARIMURA, A., BOWERS, C. Y., REDDING, T. W. and STEELMAN, S. L. (1968*b*): Hypothalamic growth hormone-releasing hormone (GRH). Purification and *in vivo* and *in vitro* studies. In: *Growth Hormone*, Session IV, pp. 185–203. Editors: A. Pecile and E. Muller. ICS No. 158. Excerpta Medica, Amsterdam.

SCHALLY, A. V., REDDING, T. W., BOWERS, C. Y. and BARRETT, J. F. (1969*a*): Isolation and properties of porcine thyrotropin releasing hormone. *J. biol. Chem.*, *244*, 4077.

SCHALLY, A. V., SAWANO, S., ARIMURA, A., BARRETT, J. F., WAKABAYASHI, I., and BOWERS, C. Y. (1969*b*): Isolation of growth hormone-releasing hormone (GRH) from porcine hypothalami. *Endocrinology*, 84, 1493.

SCHALLY, A. V., ARIMURA, A., KASTIN, A. J., REEVES, J. J., BOWERS, C. Y., and BABA, Y. (1970)a): Hypothalamic LH-releasing hormone: chemistry, physiology and effect in humans. In: *Mamma-*

lian Reproduction pp. 45–83. Editors: H. Gibian and E. J. Plotz. Springer-Verlag, Berlin.

SCHALLY, A. V., ARIMURA, A., WAKABAYASHI, I., SAWANO, S., BARRETT, J. F., BOWERS, C. Y., REDDING, T. W., MITTLER, J. C. and SAITO, M. (1970*b*): The chemistry of hypothalamic growth hormone-releasing hormone (GRH). In: *Hypophysiotropic Hormones of the Hypothalamus: Assay and Chemistry*, Chapter 14, pp 208–222. Editor: J. Meites. Williams and Wilkins, Baltimore, Md.

SCHALLY, A. V., CARTER, W. H., PARLOW, A. F., SAITO, M., ARIMURA, A., BOWERS, C. Y. and HOLTKAMP, D. E. (1970*c*): Alteration of LH and FSH release in rats treated with clomiphene or its isomers. *Amer. J. Obstet. Gynec.*, *107*, 1156.

SCHALLY, A. V., MITTLER, J. C. and WHITE, W. F. (1970*d*): Failure of putrescine and other polyamines to promote FSH release *in vitro*. *Endocrinology*, *86*, 903.

SCHALLY, A. V., NAIR, R. M. G., BARRETT, J. F., BOWERS, C. Y. and FOLKERS, K. (1970*e*): The structure of hypothalamic thyrotropin-releasing hormone. *Fed. Proc.*, *29*, 470.

SCHALLY, A. V., PARLOW, A. F., CARTER, W. H., SAITO, M., BOWERS, C. Y. and ARIMURA, A. (1970*f*): Studies on the site of oral contraceptive steroids. II. Plasma LH and FSH levels after administration of antifertility steroids and LH-releasing hormone (LH-RH). *Endocrinology*, *86*, 530.

SCHALLY, A. V., ARIMURA, A., BABA, Y., NAIR, R. M. G., MATSUO, H., REDDING, T. W., DEBELJUK, L. and WHITE, W. F. (1971*a*): Purification and properties of the LH and FSH-releasing hormone from porcine hypothalami. In: *Program of the Fifty-Third Meeting of the Endocrine Society*, 'in press'.

SCHALLY, A. V., BABA, T., ARIMURA, A., REDDING, T. W. and WHITE, W. F. (1971*b*): Evidence for peptide nature of LH and FSH-releasing hormones. *Biochem. biophys. Res. Commun.*, *42*, 50.

SCHALLY, A. V., BABA, Y., NAIR, R. M. G. and BENNETT, C. (1971*c*). Amino acid sequence of growth hormone releasing hormone from porcine hypothalami. *J. biol. Chem.*

CONTROL OF MSH RELEASE IN MAMMALS*

ABBA J. KASTIN and ANDREW V. SCHALLY

Endocrinology Section of the Medical Service, Endocrine and Polypeptide Laboratories, Veterans Administration Hospital, and Department of Medicine, Tulane University School of Medicine, New Orleans, La., U.S.A.

Melanocyte-stimulating hormone (MSH), a hormone with no clearly established role in mammals, has an intricate system of control for its release from the pituitary gland. The principal regulation of MSH release occurs at the hypothalamic level and is predominantly of an inhibitory nature. It is exerted primarily by a substance present in hypothalamic tissue which has been named MSH-release inhibiting factor (MIF or MRIH) (Schally *et al.*, 1968). This review will summarize evidence accumulated during the last few years which has resulted in establishing (Leading article, 1970) MIF as one of the hypothalamic substances controlling hormonal release from the pituitary. In connection with these studies, we shall also describe some of the extra-pigmentary effect(s) of MSH.

The idea that the hypothalamus inhibits the release of MSH in mammals originates in work performed with amphibians. It was found that removal of the pituitary gland of a frog from its close anatomical proximity to the hypothalamus, either by transplantation or destruction of the hypothalamus, results in darkening of the frog. This was interpreted as evidence for an inhibitory influence of the hypothalamus on MSH release in the frog (Etkin, 1962), although no measurements of MSH activity were made.

Embarking upon a series of experiments designed to investigate the control of MSH release in mammals, Kastin and Ross decided to measure MSH in the darkened frogs whose hypothalami had been destroyed. They found that the pituitaries of frogs with hypothalamic lesions contained less MSH activity than the pituitaries in frogs in which the hypothalamus was intact (Kastin and Ross, 1965). Since there are many dangers involved in interpreting hormonal release from inspection of only pituitary content, attempts were made to measure circulating levels of MSH. This was not possible at that time, but the question was answered indirectly by experiments in which lesioned frogs or suitable controls were linked in parabiosis with hypophysectomized frogs. The light-colored hypophysectomized parabionts turned dark to a significant extent only when physically attached to the black frogs with hypothalamic lesions (Kastin and Ross, 1965). This essentially proved Etkin's interpretation (Etkin, 1962) that the hypothalamus inhibits MSH release in amphibians.

There is now evidence that this inhibition may be due to a substance, MIF, present in hypothalamic tissue of amphibians (Bercu and Brinkley, 1967; Kastin and Schally, 1967*b*; Ralph and Sampath, 1966). How MIF reaches the pituitary gland from the hypothalamus has not been demonstrated. Many studies have been reported concerning neural control of the intermediate lobe and the possible role of neurotransmitter systems. Some of the able investigators studying this problem in amphibians include Jorgensen, Larsen and Spies,

* Supported in part by grants from NIH Ns-07664 (AJK) and AM-07467 (AVS) and Veterans Administration.

Iturriza, Oshima and Gorbman, Enemar and Falck, Dierickx, Goos, Dierst-Davies, and Sawyer. Others have been working mostly with mammals (Vincent and Kumar, 1969). In some mammals, such as the rat and monkey, there is evidence that only a few cells of the intermediate lobe are in direct contact with nerve fibers (Vincent and Kumar, 1969). None of the work on neural control of MSH release, however, is incompatible with the concept that a substance, MIF, which can be extracted from hypothalamic tissue, controls MSH release in mammals.

The first demonstration of the existence of such a substance in the mammalian hypothalamus was provided by Kastin in 1965. Addition of crude rat hypothalamic extracts to pituitary glands incubated for 96 hours resulted in a decreased release of MSH into the tissue culture medium as compared to groups of controls (Kastin, 1965). Unfortunately, the MSH content of these incubated pituitaries was not measured in this *in vitro* study.

Pituitary MSH content was measured, however, in an earlier *in vivo* study in which direct hypothalamic control of MSH release was minimized by transplantation of the pituitary gland beneath the renal capsule (Kastin and Ross, 1964*a*). There was much less MSH activity in the transplanted pituitaries no matter whether expressed per whole pituitary gland, per mg pituitary tissue, or per mg of pituitary protein. This experiment was analogous to that described in frogs (Etkin, 1962; Kastin and Ross, 1965). In each experiment the pituitary was removed from direct hypothalamic control either by destruction of the hypothalamus (frog) or by transplantation (rat), and in each experiment less MSH activity remained in the pituitary. Studies in which the pituitary stalk was transected (Hamori, 1960) or the median eminence destroyed (Bal and Smelik, 1967; Kastin and Ross, 1965) also resulted in a decreased pituitary content of MSH, although the synthesis of MSH may also be affected (Howe and Thody, 1969).

Investigations of the hypothalamic control of MSH release which are based on techniques involving pituitary transplantation or hypothalamic lesions can only indicate an influence of the hypothalamus. That this influence is due to a substance present in hypothalamic tissue was shown *in vivo* by intravenous injection of crude rat hypothalamic extracts into normal albino rats which were decapitated 20 minutes later. If the rate of MSH synthesis remained the same, or increased, then it would be expected that an elevated pituitary content of MSH would be found after such injections. This indeed occurred (Kastin and Schally, 1966*a*). Using this test system, we demonstrated MIF activity in hypothalamic extracts from seven species of mammals, including the human being (Kastin and Schally, 1967*b*). MIF was then purified 11,000-fold from bovine hypothalamic tissue (Schally and Kastin, 1966).

The demonstration of increased pituitary MSH content following injection of MIF would be more meaningful if blood levels of MSH were determined at the same time. When a method of measuring MSH levels in the circulation of a rat became available (Geschwind and Huseby, 1966; Kastin *et al.*, 1969*b*) such a study was performed. As expected, injection of MIF resulted in a decrease in plasma MSH activity accompanied by an increase in pituitary MSH activity (Kastin *et al,* 1969*b*). This strongly supported the concept that in mammals, as well as amphibians, MIF inhibits the release of MSH from the pituitary. Additional evidence for this concept is provided by injecting hypothalamic extracts into frogs in which the inhibitor of MSH release has been eliminated by destruction of the hypothalamus. These frogs lighten (Kastin and Schally, 1967*b*).

Thus, evidence for the existence of MIF in mammals is based upon tests made in the following types of preparations:

1. Pituitary glands
   a. MSH activity decreased after removal from direct hypothalamic control (Kastin and Ross, 1964*a*).
   b. MSH activity increased after injection of hypothalamic extracts (Kastin and Schally, 1966*a*; 1967*b*; Schally and Kastin, 1966).

2. Incubation medium
   a. MSH activity decreased after addition of hypothalamic extracts (Kastin, 1965).
3. Darkened frogs
   a. Lightened after injection of hypothalamic extracts (Kastin and Schally, 1967*b*).
4. Plasma
   a. MSH activity decreased after injection of hypothalamic extracts (Kastin *et al.*, 1969*b*).

In addition to MIF, another hypothalamic factor-MRF (MSH-releasing factor) (Kastin and Schally, 1966*a*; Kastin *et al.*, 1970; Taleisnik and Orias, 1965) may modify MSH release in mammals. Thus, MSH is the first pituitary hormone for which a dual hypothalamic control (Kastin and Schally, 1966*a*) has been suggested to exist. Apparently our concept that MIF exerts the predominant control of MSH release in mammals is now generally accepted (see Kastin and Schally, 1971).

It has been presumed that most of the other conditions (Kastin and Schally, 1971; Kastin *et al.*, 1970) which are known to affect MSH-release act through the hypothalamus and probably via MIF, even though little effort has been made to document this. For example, phenothiazine drugs have been shown to decrease pituitary content of MSH (Kastin and Schally, 1966*b*) and increase plasma levels (Kastin *et al.*, 1969*b*). They also release prolactin (Danon *et al.*, 1963; Meites *et al.*, 1963; Ratner *et al.*, 1965), the only other pituitary hormone whose release is primarily controlled by a hypothalamic inhibitor. The tranquilizers exert their effect on prolactin release through the hypothalamus, not the pituitary (Danon *et al.*, 1963; Ratner *et al.*, 1965). These drugs probably release MSH through a similar hypothalamic mechanism.

One of the first indications that the pineal may affect the pituitary was the change in pituitary MSH content observed after injection of the pineal product melatonin (Kastin and Schally, 1967*a*). A similar change in pituitary MSH content was observed after exposure of rats to darkness (Kastin *et al.*, 1967*c*). Since darkness also results in increased melatonin synthesis (Wurtman *et al.*, 1963) it seemed possible that the effect of darkness was mediated through the pineal gland. Experiments involving pinealectomy showed this assumption to be correct (Kastin *et al.*, 1967*b*). Although this supported the concept of a relationship between the pineal and pituitary glands, a role for the hypothalamus and MIF was only inferred.

Rust and Meyer, in an elegant experiment (Rust and Meyer, 1969), provided evidence that the action of melatonin upon MSH release was exerted at the hypothalamic level. They treated both brown weasels and white weasels (undergoing the spring change to a brown pelage) with melatonin. The melatonin caused a new white coat to appear, whereas controls retained or acquired the brown coat. Did this mean that melatonin had a direct effect on the skin or an effect mediated through the release of MSH? If MSH was involved, was the effect at the pituitary or hypothalamic level?

These questions appear to have been answered by the use of hypophysectomized weasels with pituitary autografts. Weasels with pituitary grafts had been shown to grow brown hair even when exposed to a decreased amount of light (which induced the growth of white hair in intact controls). This effect was probably due to increased MSH release which was reversed by removal of the graft (Rust and Meyer, 1968). In such weasels with transplanted pituitaries, melatonin failed to induce the growth of white hair. This observation indicated not only that melatonin did not exert its effect directly upon the skin, but that it also did not affect MSH release from the transplanted pituitary. Consequently, Rust and Meyer postulated that melatonin affects hair color in the weasel by releasing MIF from the hypothalamus (Rust and Meyer, 1969).

It has also been suggested that MSH modifies its own release, possibly via the hypothalamus (Kastin and Schally, 1967*a*). This autoregulation constitutes a type of short feedback.

More recent evidence, however, indicates that at least some of this feedback may be at the pituitary level (Kastin *et al.*, 1971*a*). A direct effect of a pituitary hormone upon its own release at the pituitary level has never been clearly demonstrated previously, although it had been suggested. (Muller *et al.*, 1967). This mass-action type of direct feedback control was shown *in vitro* in three ways (Kastin *et al.*, 1971*a*): (1) Pituitary glands were incubated for 15 minutes. Groups in which the medium was changed every five minutes for the 15 minutes released significantly more MSH than groups in which the medium was either sham-changed or not changed at all. (2) Incubation of pituitaries in a larger volume resulted in significantly increased total MSH release. (3) Addition of highly purified MSH significantly reduced the release of MSH from the incubated pituitaries.

Although the other conditions which have been shown to affect MSH release probably act mainly through the hypothalamus and MIF, it remains to be seen whether part of their effect is also exerted at the pituitary level. A discussion of these other treatments, which include morphine, Nembutal, stress, vasopressin, hypertonic saline, dehydration, copulation, suckling, pregnancy, and estrogen can be found in two recent review articles (Kastin and Schally, 1971; Kastin *et al.*, 1970).

One of these reviews (Kastin *et al.*, 1970) is concerned primarily with the assay(s) of MIF. In brief, the main assay involves pretreatment of rats with Nembutal and morphine (Kastin *et al.*, 1968*c*). Although neither drug by itself changes pituitary MSH content, together they result in a marked decreased hormonal content of the pituitary. A gland with an initially lowered MSH content appears to be more responsive to MIF. Rats pretreated with Nembutal and morphine also have increased plasma levels of MSH (Kastin *et al.*, 1969*b*), a condition which tends to magnify the decrease observed after injection of MIF.

Almost all of the investigations described up to this point have involved determination of MSH activity. The method used for its measurement in blood has been indicated (Geschwind and Huseby, 1966; Kastin *et al.*, 1969*a*). Pituitary content of MSH is assayed after injection of the material into the dorsal lymph sac of a hypophysectomized frog (Kastin and Ross, 1964*b*). This simple and precise method gives the same results as the *in vitro* assay (Shizume *et al.*, 1954) for all samples except some stereoisomers and analogues of MSH (Kastin *et al.* 1965).

Since ACTH has intrinsic MSH-like activity, due to shared amino acid sequences, it is also necessary to measure ACTH in experiments involving control of MSH release. In all the experiments discussed in this review, both calculation (Kastin *et al.*, 1967*a*) and measurement of ACTH reveal that it cannot fully account for the changes observed in MSH activity. However, it is important to keep in mind that the intermediate lobe of the pituitary, the presumed site of MSH synthesis, also affects ACTH synthesis (Gosbee *et al.*, 1970). A complete understanding of the mechanism involved in this phenomenon may also have implications for hypothalamic substances like MIF.

Since extra-adrenal actions of ACTH have been known for years, it should not be surprising that there are extra-pigmentary effects of MSH. It is likely, moreover, that some of the extra-adrenal effects of ACTH are due to its MSH-like component. The central nervous system (CNS) appears to be a site for both the extra-adrenal effects of ACTH and the extra-pigmentary effects of MSH. Both compounds cause a similar effect upon the electroencephalogram of the human being (see Kastin *et al.*, 1968*b*) and certain behavior in rats (see DeWied *et al.*, 1968). DeWied and associates found that the full effect of ACTH on conditioned avoidance behavior can be elicited by a heptapeptide sequence of ACTH (4–10) which is shared with the MSHs.

Together with Sandman, we have recently extended these investigations by showing that MSH affects other types of behavior. Hungry rats were tested for maintenance of an appetitive response by determining whether they would continue to run to the chamber of a T-maze which had previously contained food. Rats injected with MSH ran faster and persisted in this behavior to a significantly greater extent than the controls (Sandman *et al.*, 1969). This implied that MSH had a positive effect on (*a*) memory, (*b*) the inability to inhibit a response, or (*c*) general motivational factors.

The last two possibilities were essentially ruled out by testing the ability of a rat to inhibit a response in a passive avoidance situation which minimized the influence of motivational components (Sandman *et al.*, 1971). Each rat was placed in one chamber of a two-chamber box and the time required for entry into the second chamber was measured. A shock was administered after entry into the second chamber. On subsequent days, the rats receiving MSH took significantly longer to enter the second chamber than the controls, when tested during the peak of activity (darkness). This showed that the effect of MSH in the T-maze experiment (Sandman *et al.*, 1969), testing appetitive behavior, was not due to the inability of the recipient rats to inhibit a response. It indicates the possibility that MSH exerts an effect on memory and the expression of fear which may be beneficial to the animal.

If, during the course of evolution, MSH has acquired an extra-pigmentary function in mammals, is there any similarity in this function between the behavioral changes in rats described above and the color changes of frogs? Certainly MSH is important in the camouflage of amphibians. The melanocytes, which are derived embryologically from the neural crest, are affected by MSH so that a change of skin color results. This has obvious survival value to the amphibian. It is interesting to speculate that the behavioral changes (*e.g.*, avoidance of shock) observed in the rat after injection of MSH may indicate that MSH has a corresponding 'survival' role in mammals. In each class of vertebrates, MSH might act to facilitate 'survival' by affecting tissue of neural origin.

There are, however, indications that MSH may have other extra-pigmentary functions in mammals, especially the human being (Kastin *et al.*, 1968*b*). Perhaps the most intriguing of these possible actions of MSH is that of inducing menstrual bleeding, probably anovulatory. Unfortunately, it has not been definitely established whether this effect is solely due to MSH or to the procedure itself (Kastin *et al.*, 1968*b*; Kastin *et al.*, 1971*b*). Whatever the role(s) of MSH, it is available to the human fetus at an early age (Kastin *et al.*, 1968*a*).

Studies concerning the extra-pigmentary effect(s) of MSH may help the investigations of the control of MSH release. Those functions which are affected by MSH are quite likely to be accompanied by changes in the mechanisms controlling the release of MSH. This review has indicated that the most important of these controlling influences is hypothalamic MIF.

ACKNOWLEDGMENTS

The authors appreciate the assistance of Dr. John Coury, Miss Carol Garvin, Mrs. Sharon Viosca, Mrs. Beverly LeBlanc and Miss Linda Hasenkampf.

REFERENCES

Bal, H. and Smelik, P. G. (1967): Effect of hypothalamic lesions on MSH content of the intermediate lobe of the pituitary gland in the rat. *Experientia (Basel)*, *23*, 759.

Bercu, B. B. and Brinkley, H. J. (1967): Hypothalamic and cerebral cortical inhibition of melanocyte-stimulating hormone secretion in the frog, *Rana pipiens*. *Endocrinology*, *80*, 399.

Danon, A., Dikstein, S. and Sulman, F. G. (1963): Stimulation of prolactin secretion by perphenazine in pituitary-hypothalamus organ culture. *Proc. Soc. exp. Biol. (N.Y.)*, *114*, 366.

DeWied, D., Bohus, B. and Greven, H. M. (1968): Influence of pituitary and adrenocortical hormones on conditioned avoidance behaviour in rats. In: *Endocrinology and Human Behaviour*, pp. 188–196. Editor: R. P. Michael. Oxford University Press, London.

Etkin, W. (1962): Hypothalamic inhibition of pars intermedia activity in the frog. *Gen. comp. Endocr. Suppl.*, *1*, 148.

Geschwind, I. I. and Huseby, R. A. (1966): Melanocyte-stimulating activity in a transplantable mouse pituitary tumor. *Endocrinology*, *79*, 97.

GOSBEE, J. L., KRAICER, J., KASTIN, A. J. and SCHALLY, A. V. (1970): Functional relationship between the pars intermedia and ACTH secretion in the rat. *Endocrinology*, *86*, 560.

HAMORI, J. (1960): Gewebsreaktionen und Funktionsänderungen des Hypophysenmittellappens der Albinoratte nach Hypothalamus-und Hypophysenstielläsion. *Acta morph. Acad. Sci. hung.*, *9*, 155.

HOWE, A. and THODY, A. J. (1969): The effect of hypothalamic lesions on the melanocyte-stimulating hormone content and histology of the pars intermedia of the rat pituitary gland. *J. Physiol. (Lond.)*, *203*, 159.

KASTIN, A. J. (1965): Effect of hypothalamic extracts on MSH release *in vitro* (Abstract). In: *Program of the 47th Endocrine Society Meeting*, 98.

KASTIN, A. J., ARIMURA, A., SCHALLY, A. V. and MILLER, M. C. (1971*a*): Mass-action type direct feed-back control of pituitary MSH release. *Nature (Lond.)*, *231*, 29.

KASTIN, A. J., BARRETT, L., VIOSCA, S., ARIMURA, A. and SCHALLY, A. V. (1967*a*): MSH activities in pituitaries of rats exposed to stress. *Neuroendocrinology*, *2*, 200.

KASTIN, A. J., GENNSER, G., ARIMURA, A., MILLER, M. C. and SCHALLY, A. V. (1968*a*): Melanocyte-stimulating and corticotrophic activities in human foetal pituitary glands. *Acta endocr. (Kbh.)*, *58*, 6.

KASTIN, A. J., KULLANDER, S., BORGLIN, N. E., DYSTER-AAS, K., DAHLBERG, B., INGVAR, D., KRAKAU, C. E. T., MILLER, M. C., BOWERS, C. Y. and SCHALLY, A. V. (1968*b*): Extrapigmentary effects of melanocyte-stimulating hormone in amenorrheic women. *Lancet*, *1*, 1007.

KASTIN, A. J., MILLER, M. C. and SCHALLY, A. V. (1968*c*): MSH activity in the rat pituitary after treatment with Nembutal and morphine: a new bioassay for MSH-release inhibiting factor. *Endocrinology*, *83*, 137.

KASTIN, A. J., MILLER, M. C. and SCHALLY, A. V. (1969*a*): Modified *in vitro* assay for melanocyte-stimulating hormone. *Experientia (Basel)*, *25*, 192.

KASTIN, A. J., REDDING, T. W. and SCHALLY, A. V. (1967*c*): MSH activity in rat pituitaries after pinealectomy. *Proc. Soc. exp. Biol. (N.Y.)*, *124*, 1275.

KASTIN, A. J. and ROSS, G. T. (1964*a*): Melanocyte-stimulating hormone (MSH) and ACTH activities of pituitary homografts in albino rats. *Endocrinology*, *75*, 187.

KASTIN, A. J. and ROSS, G. T. (1964*b*): Modified *in vivo* assay for MSH. *Experientia (Basel)*, *20*, 461.

KASTIN, A. J. and ROSS, G. T. (1965): Melanocyte-stimulating hormone activity in pituitaries of frogs with hypothalamic lesions. *Endocrinology*, *77*, 45.

KASTIN, A. J. and SCHALLY, A. V. (1966*a*): MSH activity in pituitaries of rats treated with hypothalamic extracts. *Gen. comp. Endocr.*, *7*, 452.

KASTIN, A. J. and SCHALLY, A. V. (1966*b*): MSH activity in pituitary glands of rats treated with tranquilizing drugs. *Endocrinology*, *79*, 1018.

KASTIN, A. J. and SCHALLY, A. V. (1967*a*): Autoregulation of release of melanocyte-stimulating hormone from the rat pituitary. *Nature*, *213*, 1238.

KASTIN, A. J. and SCHALLY, A. V. (1967*b*): MSH activities in pituitaries of rats treated with hypothalamic extracts from various animals. *Gen. comp. Endocr.*, *8*, 344.

KASTIN, A. J. and SCHALLY, A. V. (1969*b*): MSH activity in plasma and pituitaries of rats after various treatments. *Endocrinology*, *84*, 20.

KASTIN, A. J., SCHALLY, A. V., VIOSCA, S., BARRETT, L. and REDDING, T. W. (1967*c*): MSH activity in the pituitaries of rats exposed to constant illumination. *Neuroendocrinology*, *2*, 257.

KASTIN, A. J., SCHALLY, A. V. VIOSCA, S. and MILLER, M. C. (1971): MSH release in mammals. In: *Pigmentation: Its Genesis and Biological Control*, Editor: V. Rily. Appleton, Century and Crofts New York.

KASTIN, A. J., SCHALLY, A. V., YAJIMA, H. and KUBO, K. (1965): Melanocyte-stimulating hormone activity of synthetic MSH and ACTH peptides *in vivo* and *in vitro*. *Nature (Lond.)*, *207*, 978.

KASTIN, A. J., VIOSCA, S. and SCHALLY, A. V. (1970): Assay of mammalian MSH-release regulating factor(s). In: *Hypophysiotropic Hormones of the Hypothalamus*, pp. 171–183. Editor: J. Meites. Williams and Wilkins, Baltimore, Md.

KASTIN, A. J., ZARATE, A., MILLER, M. C., HERNANDEZ-AYUP, S., DYSTER-AAS, K., GUAL, C. and SCHALLY, A. V. (1971*b*): Anovulatory uterine bleeding after administration of MSH to women with secondary amenorrhea. *J. reprod. Fertil.* (in press).

Leading Article (1970): Thyrotropin-releasing hormone. *Brit. med. J.*, *2*, 249.

MEITES, J., NICOLL, C. S. and TALWALKER, P. K. (1963): The central nervous system and the secretion and release of prolactin. In: *Advances in Neuroendocrinology*, Chapter 8, pp. 238–277. Editor: A. V. Nalbandov. University of Illinois Press, Urbana, Ill.

MULLER, E. E., SAWANO, S., ARIMURA, A. and SCHALLY, A. V. (1967): Mechanism of action of growth hormone in altering its own secretion rate: comparison with the action of dexamethasone. *Acta endocr. (Kbh.)*, *56*, 499.

RALPH, C. L. and SAMPATH, S. (1966): Inhibition by extracts of frog and rat brain of MSH release by frog pars intermedia. *Gen. comp. Endocr.*, *7*, 370.

RATNER, A., TALWALKER, P. K. and MEITES, J. (1965): Effect of reserpine on prolactin-inhibiting activity of rat hypothalamus. *Endocrinology*, *77*, 315.

RUST, C. C. and MEYER, R. K. (1968): Effect of pituitary autografts on hair color in the short-tailed weasel. *Gen. comp. Endocr.*, *11*, 548.

RUST, C. C. and MEYER, R. K. (1969): Hair color, molt, and testis size in male, short-tailed weasels treated with melatonin. *Science*, *165*, 921.

SANDMAN, C., KASTIN, A. J. and SCHALLY, A. V. (1969): Melanocyte-stimulating hormone and learned appetitive behavior. *Experientia (Basel)*, *25*, 1001.

SANDMAN, C., KASTIN, A. J. and SCHALLY, A. V. (1971): Behavioral inhibition as modified by melanocyte-stimulating hormone (MSH) and light-dark conditions. *Physiol. Behav.*, *6*, 45.

SCHALLY, A. V., ARIMURA, A., BOWERS, C. Y., KASTIN, A. J., SAWANO, S. and REDDING, T. W. (1968): Hypothalamic neurohormones regulating anterior pituitary function. *Recent Progr. Hormone Res.*, *24*, 497.

SCHALLY, A. V. and KASTIN, A. J. (1966): Purification of a bovine hypothalamic factor which elevates pituitary MSH levels in rats. *Endocrinology*, *79*, 768.

SHIZUME, K., LERNER, A. and FITZPATRICK, T. B. (1954): *In vitro* bioassay for the melanocyte-stimulating hormone. *Endocrinology*, *54*, 553.

TALEISNIK, S., DEOLMOS, J., ORIAS, R. and TOMATIS, M. E. (1967): Effect of hypothalamic lesions on pituitary melanocyte-stimulating hormone. *J. Endocr.*, *39*, 485.

TALEISNIK, S. and ORIAS, R. (1965): A melanocyte-stimulating hormone-releasing factor in hypothalamic extracts. *Amer. J. Physiol.*, *208*, 293.

VINCENT, D. S. and KUMAR, T. C. A. (1969): Electron microscopic studies on the pars intermedia of the ferret. *Z. Zellforsch. Abt. Histochem.*, *99*, 185.

WURTMAN, R. J., AXELROD, J. and PHILLIPS, L. (1963): Melatonin synthesis in the pineal gland: control by light. *Science*, *142*, 1071.

ADDENDUM

MIF has now been isolated from bovine hypothalamic extracts and its structure determined to be Pro-Leu-Gly-NH_2 (Nair, R.M.G., Kastin, A. J. and Schally, A. V., (1971): *Biochem. biophys. Res. Comm. 43,* 1376). It has also been shown that a tripeptide with this structure and MIF activity can be split from oxytocin by an exopeptidase (Celis, M.E., Taleisnik, S., Schwartz, I. L. and Walter, R. (1971): *Biophysical Soc. Abstr.* TPM-K 12, p. 98a).

CONTROL OF LH AND FSH SECRETION*

S. M. McCANN

Department of Physiology, University of Texas Southwestern Medical School at Dallas, Dallas, Texas, U.S.A.

INTRODUCTION

An imposing array of evidence indicates that the hypothalamus regulates the secretion of the adenohypophyseal hormones. It is also clear that the anterior pituitary is a gland under neural control, but lacking a secretomotor innervation. Instead there is a specialized vascular link between the hypothalamus and the pituitary, the hypophyseal portal system of veins. These take origin in the median eminence and stalk and carry capillary blood from these regions to the sinusoids of the anterior lobe. Hinsey (1937), Green and Harris (1949) and others suggested that hypothalamic control over the pituitary might be mediated by means of specific neurohormones which are liberated into the primary capillary plexus of the hypophyseal portal vessels and pass down the pituitary stalk to reach the sinusoids of the anterior lobe, there to trigger release of particular pituitary hormones. This prophetic suggestion has borne fruit, and it is now evident as a result of many investigations over the past ten to fifteen years that a whole new family of neurohormones called hypophysiotropic hormones or hypothalamic-releasing and -inhibiting factors governs the secretion of each hormone from the adenohypophysis. There appears to be at least one neurohormone for each pituitary hormone and, in some instances, both releasing and inhibiting factors appear to exist, thereby providing a dual control over the pituitary hormone (McCann and Porter, 1969). The nomenclature used is to specify the pituitary hormone affected and follow this by releasing factor. Corticotrophin-releasing factor (CRF) was the first such factor to be described. Shortly thereafter an LH-releasing factor (LRF), an FSH-releasing factor (FRF), a TSH-releasing factor (TRF) and a growth hormone releasing factor (GRF) were discovered. In contrast to these pituitary hormones which are under the influence of a stimulatory factor from the hypothalamus, prolactin is under inhibitory hypothalamic control which is mediated by a prolactin-inhibiting factor (PIF). More recently, evidence has accrued to suggest the presence of dual factors influencing MSH discharge, an MSH-releasing factor (MRF), and an MSH-inhibiting factor (MIF). There is evidence also for an inhibitor of growth hormone release, growth hormone inhibiting factor (GIF). In this article we will restrict our consideration to the FRF and LRF since they trigger release of gonadotropins responsible for ovulation.

EVIDENCE FOR EXISTENCE OF LRF AND FRF

Ten years after its discovery there can be no doubt of the existence of a specific LRF in

* This study was supported by Public Health Service research grant AM 10073–04, by a grant from the Ford Foundation, and by a grant from the Texas Population Crisis Foundation.

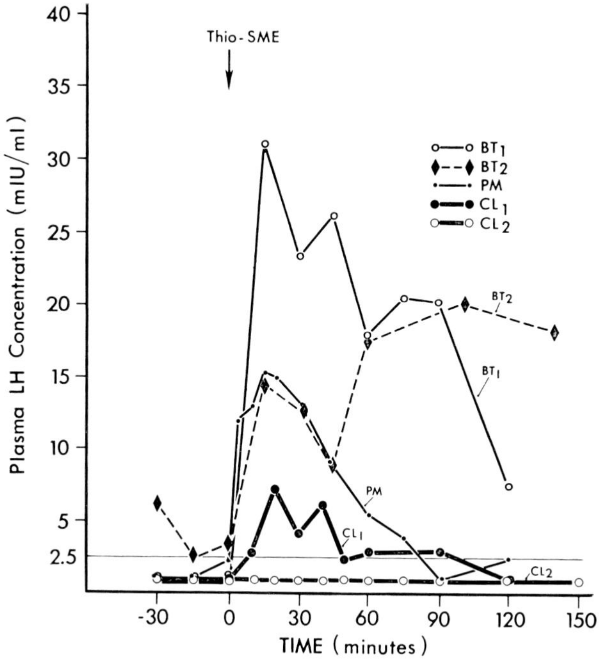

Fig. 1. Effect on LH release in human infants of i.v. injection of ovine hypothalamic extract treated with thioglycollate to inactivate neurohypophyseal polypeptide hormones. All patients responded with an increase in plasma LH. There was no response in one patient to a lower dose of extract (CL2), and none of the patients responded to an injection of equivalent amounts of a cerebral cortex extract.

hypothalamic extracts from a number of mammalian species including man (McCann, 1970; McCann and Porter, 1969; Schally *et al.*, 1968).

There appears to be no species specificity of FRF and LRF since crude and purified extracts from sheep, beef and pig have been shown to increase FSH and LH release in man (Igarashi *et al.*, 1968; Root *et al.*, 1969; Kastin *et al.*, 1969). One recent example of the effect of hypothalamic extracts on release of pituitary hormones in man is provided by the observation that these extracts will increase the radio-immunoassayable LH in plasma of children with chromosomal abnormalities within a few minutes of their intravenous injection (Fig. 1) (Root *et al.*, 1969). Extracts derived from the cerebral cortex were ineffective.

Both the FRF and LRF act directly on the pituitary gland to evoke release of their respective pituitary tropins. The factors are active in rats with median eminence lesions which eliminate neural control of the gland (McCann, 1962) when injected directly into the adenohypophysis (Nikitovitch-Winer, 1962; Campbell *et al.*, 1964), or on injection directly into individual cannulated portal vessels (Porter and Mical, 1969). Addition of hypothalamic extracts to the incubation medium leads to a dose-related increase in FSH and LH release by anterior pituitaries incubated *in vitro* (Watanabe and McCann, 1968; McCann, 1970).

LOCALIZATION OF LRF AND FRF

These factors are not distributed widely in the CNS but are localized to discrete regions in the medial basal hypothalamus. LRF activity was observed as far forward as the optic chiasm and extended caudally into the pituitary stalk (McCann, 1962; Crighton *et al.*, 1970). Lesions in the suprachiasmatic region lowered the LRF activity on measurement some weeks later (Schneider *et al.*, 1969). These results were interpreted to mean that some of the neurons presumed to secrete LRF had cell bodies as far rostrally as the optic chiasm with relatively long axons which ran superficially along the medial basal hypothalamus to end in juxtaposition to the portal vessels. Since some releasing activity persisted in the stalk-median eminence after these lesions, some of these neurons are thought to have cell bodies which lie more caudally in the arcuate nuclear-median eminence region.

FRF could only be detected more caudally in a region including the arcuate nucleus, median eminence and pituitary stalk (Watanabe and McCann, 1968). The distribution of FRF-secreting neurons appears to be similar to that for LRF except that the neurons appear to originate somewhat more caudally in the arcuate-median eminence region.

THE PHYSIOLOGICAL SIGNIFICANCE OF GONADOTROPIN-RELEASING FACTORS

The mere demonstration of these activities in hypothalami does not constitute proof of their physiological significance. Several lines of investigation indicate that these factors are probably of prime significance in conveying information from the hypothalamus to the pituitary gland. One type of experiment has been to impose a physiological condition in the animal which would alter the release of the pituitary hormone effected by a particular hypothalamic factor. Then the effect of this intervention on the hypothalamic content of the hypothalamic hormone is assessed. This type of experiment has been carried out extensively and the results indicate that in general acute or chronic alterations in the release of pituitary hormone can result in alterations in the content of stored hypothalamic factor. Some examples of this type of experiment are shown for LH and LRF in Table I. This type of experiment although implicating the hypothalamic factor in the regulation of pituitary hormone secretion leaves a good bit to be desired since it is impossible to be sure whether the change in hypothalamic content of the factor is due to altered synthesis or release of the factor or a combination of the two (McCann and Porter, 1969).

If one could demonstrate the releasing factors in peripheral blood and show that the blood

TABLE I

Conditions in which an alteration in hypothalamic LRF has been reported in rats

Sex	Condition	Effect on LH release	Effect on hypothalamic LRF
Male	Castration	+	+
	Testosterone, inj.	—	—
	Testosterone, hypothalamic implant	—	—
Female	Spaying	+	—
	Estrogen, inj.	—	—
	Estrogen, hypothalamic implant	—	—
	Enovid	—	—
	Proestrus	+	—
	Puberty	+	—
	Suckling	—	—
	Light	?	+ (sheep)

+ = increase — = decrease

level of the factors varied in situations which alter pituitary hormone release, then strong evidence for the physiological significance of these factors would be at hand. To date it has not been possible to demonstrate releasing factors in peripheral blood of animals with intact pituitaries; however, after hypophysectomy a number of the factors appear in peripheral blood in sufficient quantities to be measurable. These activities have been reported to disappear after lesions in the median eminence which should eliminate the source of the releasing factor. CRF activity was first reported in blood of hypophysectomized rats; this was followed by reports of LRF, GRF and FRF activity in this blood (McCann and Porter, 1969). Most reports indicate that the level is not measurable immediately after hypophysectomy, but rises after a period of time to detectable albeit rather low levels. There is some evidence that these levels of circulating releasing factors can be altered in the hypophysectomized animals by imposition of stimuli which alter pituitary hormone secretion in intact animals (Table II).

TABLE II

Releasing factors observed in blood of hypophysectomized rats

Factor	Stimuli which alter its level	Response to stimulus
CRF	Corticoids[1]	—
LRF	LH, gonadal steroids[2]	—
FRF	light[3]	+
	testosterone[4]	—
	reserpine	—
GRF	hypoglycemia[5], cold[6]	+

[1] Brodish, A. (1962): *Endocrinology*, *71*, 298.
[2] Preliminary experiments only of Nallar and Antunes-Rodrigues.
[3] Negro-Vilar, A., Dickerman, E. and Meites, J. (1968): *Endocrinology*, *82*, 939.
[4] Negro-Vilar, A., Dickerman, E. and Meites, J. (1968): *Endocrinology*, *83*, 1349.
[5] Krulich, L. and McCann, S. M. (1966): *Proc. Soc. exp. Biol. (N.Y.)*, *122*, 668.
[6] Müller, E. E., Arimura, A., Saito, T. and Schally, A. V. (1967): *Proc. Soc. exp. Biol. (N.Y.)*, *125*, 874.

For example, insulin-induced hypoglycemia, which is a stimulus for growth hormone release, caused the appearance of increased levels of GRF in the blood of hypophysectomized rats. Stimuli which alter FSH release have been shown to alter the level of circulating FRF in blood of chronically hypophysectomized animals.

Considerable gonadotropin secretion occurs when multiple pituitary grafts are placed into hypophysectomized hosts; the degree of maintenance is proportional to the number of such grafts (Gittes and Kastin, 1966). Recent studies indicate that the residual function of the grafted gland is at least in part caused by circulating gonadotropin-releasing factors since median eminence lesions in the hypophysectomized-grafted animals led to regression of testicular and accessory organ weight (Beddow and McCann, 1969). Earlier it had been observed in a small series of animals that implants of testosterone in the basal tuberal region of hypophysectomized-grafted rats inhibited gonadotropin secretion, presumably because the androgen blocked the release from the hypothalamus of gonadotropin-releasing factors (Smith and Davidson, 1967).

Why does LRF (and a number of other releasing factors) appear in the blood of chronically hypophysectomized rats? The answer is not available, but in this situation there is reduction in output of target gland hormones. Thus negative feedback of gonadal steroids would be reduced, which should stimulate LRF release and synthesis. Furthermore, if a negative feedback of LH on its own secretion also exists (McCann *et al.*, 1968; Martini *et al.*, 1968), then this would also be eliminated by hypophysectomy which could augment LRF discharge.

Conclusive proof for the physiological significance of releasing factors would be available if their content in hypophyseal portal vessel blood could be shown to be higher than that in peripheral blood and to vary under conditions which vary the output of the target pituitary hormone. Porter was the first to show that CRF activity could be obtained in blood dripping from the cut stalk of the dog, and that this activity was higher in stalk blood than in peripheral blood (Porter and Rumsfeld, 1956). More recently there have been reports of LRF (Fink, 1967) activity in blood collected from the cut stalk of the rat.

INTERACTION BETWEEN RELEASING FACTORS AND TARGET GLAND HORMONES

If one accepts the significance of these hypothalamic releasing factors, it is important to examine the interplay between these new hormones and the target gland hormones which feedback to modify pituitary secretion (McCann *et al.*, 1968; McCann and Porter, 1969). Although all the evidence is not at hand, it appears now that most target gland hormones feedback both at the hypothalamic and at the pituitary level to modify release of pituitary hormones. The relative importance of these two sites for feedback seems to vary depending on the pituitary hormone in question. In the case of thyroxin the principal feedback appears to be at the pituitary level, and it is possible to block the response to TRF by infusion of thyroxin. In the case of the gonadal steroids the principal feedback actions appear to lie at the hypothalamic level, where both positive and negative feedback are operative. Even in this situation some action of gonadal steroids directly at the pituitary level is demonstrable; however, it has been difficult to block the response of the pituitary gland to LRF or FRF by the administration of gonadal steroids, either *in vivo* or *in vitro*.

Recently, considerable attention has been focused on the possibility that pituitary hormones themselves feed back, in an autofeedback, to alter the secretion of the pituitary hormone in question (Martini *et al.*, 1968; McCann *et al.*, 1968). These autofeedbacks may occur at least in part at the hypothalamic level, since implants of the pituitary hormones in the hypothalamus will suppress pituitary hormone secretion and also alter the content of stored releasing factor in the hypothalamus. As in the case of target gland hormones, it is also possible that the autofeedback action may occur at least in part at the pituitary level.

CHARACTERISTICS OF ACTION OF RELEASING FACTORS

It has been considered axiomatic that at least one of the primary actions of the releasing factors is to stimulate release of a particular pituitary hormone from its cellular storage site. This view is supported by the very rapid release of hormone which follows injection of releasing factors into the circulation. For example, ACTH release occurs within a minute or two after application of stressful stimuli or injection of CRF, whereas LH and FSH release occur within five or ten minutes or less of administration of LRF and FRF, respectively (Fig. 1).

Since depletion of pituitary content of GH and FSH has been reported to occur shortly after giving the appropriate releasing factor (Martini *et al.*, 1968; McCann and Porter, 1969), it would appear that in some instances release exceeds new synthesis of hormone leading to a depletion of stores. Conversely, suckling-induced depletion of pituitary prolactin is blocked by PIF (Grosvenor *et al.*, 1965). These are strong arguments for a primary action of these agents on the release of hormone.

The major mechanism for release of hormone appears to be the discharge of secretory granules from the cell. The limiting granular membrane fuses with the cell membrane and the granular core is extruded to the extracellular space. This process has been studied most thoroughly in somatotrophs which are readily recognizable and abundant but extends to other cell types including the gonadotrophs (Coates *et al.*, 1970). Dramatic release of granules can be observed within a few minutes of injection of hypothalamic extract.

There is now little doubt that these neurohormones also influence synthesis of pituitary hormones, either by another primary action or secondary to accelerated release of stored hormone. Evans and Nikitovitch-Winer (1969) were able to maintain target organs and cause return of secretory granules in grafted pituitaries following chronic treatment with hypothalamic extracts and similar observations have been made in our laboratory (Beddow, Dhariwal, McCann, unpub.). On the other hand, it has been difficult to demonstrate increased synthesis of LH or FSH in short term incubation experiments (Samle and Geschwind, 1970; Wakabayashi and McCann, 1970; Watanabe and McCann, 1968), which might argue that the effects observed *in vivo* were secondary to enhanced release. By contrast short term enhancement of GH synthesis has been observed *in vitro* (Krulich *et al.*, 1968).

LACK OF INTERACTION BETWEEN LRF AND OTHER RELEASING FACTORS

One additional important characteristic of the action of the releasing factors appears to be their specificity of action. For example, in the case of the LH-secreting cell, its release of hormone *in vitro* is uninfluenced by the addition of GRF, GIF, CRF, or FRF (unless contaminated with LRF). These other releasing factors also fail to alter the release of LH which is stimulated by the LRF (Crighton *et al.*, 1969). If this specificity holds for each pituitary cell, it means that release of a given pituitary tropin is controlled primarily by the rate of discharge of its releasing factor into hypophyseal portal blood and is uninfluenced by discharge of other factors. This would provide a means by which the hypothalamus could selectively alter output of individual tropins.

MECHANISM OF ACTION OF RELEASING FACTORS

There are two hypotheses to explain the rapid releasing action of these neurohormones. The first hypothesis is an extension of the hypothesis of Douglas and Poisner (1964) to explain the release of neurohypophyseal hormones. According to this view the releasing factors modify the permeability of pituitary cell membranes which leads to depolarization of the cell membrane, and uptake of calcium which then activates the release process. Elevated medium (K^+), which presumably depolarizes cell membranes, enhances release of both FSH and LH from pituitaries incubated *in vitro* (Samli and Geschwind, 1967; Wakabayashi *et al.*, 1969), whereas elimination of Ca^{++} from the medium blocks the response to both high medium (K^+) and to FRF and LRF (Samli and Geschwind, 1967; Wakabayashi *et al.*, 1969). Conversely, high medium (Mg^{++}) has an inhibitory effect on resting and stimulated release (Wakabayashi *et al.*, 1969).

According to the second hypothesis, releasing factors activate adenyl cyclase in the cell membrane and this results in elevation of cyclic AMP which in turn activates hormone release. In favor of this hypothesis are the ability of dibutyryl cyclic AMP and aminophyllin to enhance ACTH (Fleisher *et al.*, 1969) and GH release (Wilbur *et al.*, 1968) and of hypothalamic extracts to elevate rapidly adenyl cyclase and cyclic AMP levels in the pituitary (Zor *et al.*, 1970). The effect of hypothalamic extract was specific to the adenohypophysis since there was no effect on neural lobe, thyroid or adrenal cortical levels. Furthermore, cerebral cortical extracts had little or no effect on anterior pituitary adenyl cyclase or cyclic AMP.

It is possible that both theories may be linked together. According to this view releasing factors would activate adenyl cyclase and this would elevate cyclic AMP levels. Cyclic AMP would alter membrane permeability which would cause uptake of Ca^{++} as suggested by Rasmussen and Tenenhouse (1968). Ca^{++} would be required for activation of granular extrusion. Obviously much more work must be done before the cellular mode of action of the RF's will be completely elucidated.

THE SYNAPTIC TRANSMITTER WHICH RELEASES GONADOTROPHIN-RELEASING FACTORS

Influences from the rest of the central nervous system impinge on the secretory neurons which secrete LRF. A variety of drugs which might be expected to interfere with transmission across adrenergic synapses are capable of blocking ovulation (Everett, 1964). Alterations in hypothalamic catecholamine content and turnover and monamine oxidase concentrations with the states of the estrous cycle or following altered titers of gonadal steroids have recently been observed (Anton-Tay and Wurtman, 1968; Donoso *et al.*, 1967; McCann *et al.*, 1968). Furthermore, drugs which deplete brain stores of catecholamines block pregnant mares' serum-induced ovulation in the rat (Coppola *et al.*, 1966). Therefore it is possible that adrenergic synapses are involved at certain points in the transmission of information from the central nervous system to the pituitary. At one time it was thought that acetylcholine or epinephrine might be the transmitter agent released into the portal vessels to trigger gonadotropin release; however, current evidence renders this view untenable. The presence of serotonin and noradrenaline-containing neurons in the hypothalamus has recently been demonstrated by fluorescence microscopy (Hillarp *et al.*, 1966). In particular, dopamine-containing neurons originate in the vicinity of the arcuate nucleus and end near the primary plexus of the hypophyseal portal vessels in the median eminence (Fuxe and Hökfelt, 1967). The content of dopamine in these neurons is altered in situations associated with altered gonadotropin secretion (Fuxe *et al.*, 1967). Thus, the possibility was raised that dopamine might be LRF or FRF. Recent evidence indicates that this is not the case since dopamine failed to augment FSH (Kamberi and McCann, 1969) or LH release (Schneider and McCann, 1969) by pituitaries incubated *in vitro*. At high doses the amount of FSH and LH recovered from the medium was reduced, but this was caused by destruction of the hormone. Similarly, dopamine fails to alter gonadotropin release when perfused into a portal vessel (Kamberi *et al.*, 1969).

Although dopamine is not a gonadotropin-releasing factor, it appears likely that it may play a role as a synaptic transmitter to stimulate release of FRF and LRF from their secretory neurons. This possibility has been revealed by incubating median eminence tissue together with pituitaries *in vitro*. The addition of dopamine increased the release of LH from the combined tissue, whereas serotonin, epinephrine or norepinephrine in equivalent doses were ineffective (Schneider and McCann, 1969) (Fig. 2). Control studies revealed that dopamine failed to potentiate the action of LRF in releasing LH from pituitaries incubated alone, so the conclusion drawn was that dopamine evoked a release of LRF from the hypothalamic fragments. Dopamine appears to act on modified α-adrenergic receptors in evoking LRF release since the response to the drug was blocked by α-receptor-blocking drugs such as phentolamine and phenoxybenzamine, but not by the β blocker, pronethalol. The releasing action of dopamine was also blocked by haloperidol, which appears to be a specific dopamine blocker (Schneider and McCann, 1969).

Recent experiments in which dopamine was infused directly into the third ventricle of rats indicate that it has an LH-releasing action *in vivo* as well. Dopamine elevated plasma LH as determined by radioimmunoassay in normal females during most of the estrous cycle. It was most effective on the second day of diestrus and in proestrus, less effective in estrus and

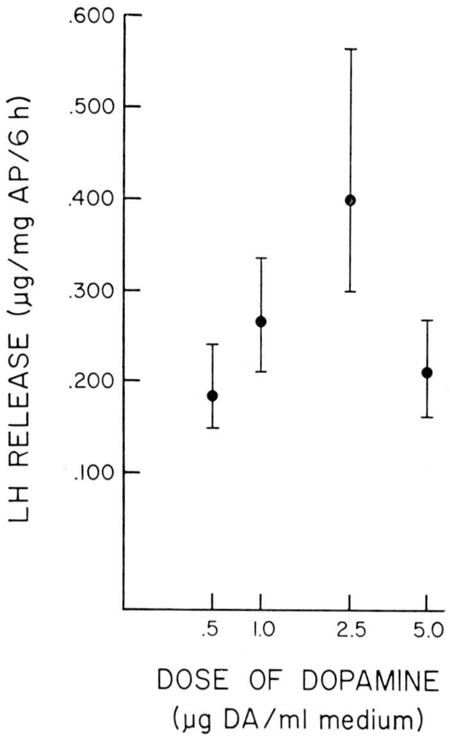

Fig. 2. Dose-response relationship between dose of dopamine and LH released into the medium of anterior pituitaries incubated with SME. The dose of dopamine is on a logarithmic scale. Vertical bars give the 95% confidence limits. From Schneider and McCann, 1969.

almost totally ineffective on the first day of diestrus. No consistent changes were observed in ovariectomized rats with initially high levels of plasma LH, but when LH levels were lowered by pre-treatment of the rats with estrogen and progesterone, a dramatic rise in plasma LH followed intraventricular dopamine. These rats were particularly sensitive to dopamine as they have been previously observed to be supersensitive to LRF itself. Dopamine acts centrally to evoke LH release since similar doses were completely ineffective when administered intravenously. There is very little lag in response to dopamine; an elevation in plasma LH was observable as early as three minutes after the intraventricular injection of the amine (Schneider and McCann, 1970*a*) (Fig. 3).

The cause of the altered sensitivity to dopamine during different stages of the cycle is not known, but it may reflect either altered hypothalamic stores of LRF or an altered sensitivity of the LRF-secreting neurons to dopamine. The failure of ovariectomized rats to respond to dopamine may be an expression of the failure of these animals to respond to LRF itself, presumably because of high rates of release of endogenous LRF. Furthermore plasma LH fluctuates wildly in ovariectomized rats (Fay and Midgely, 1969) and this might obscure a response. Normal male rats also respond to intraventricular dopamine with a discharge of LH (Schneider and McCann, 1970*a*).

That dopamine is acting *in vivo* as *in vitro* to provoke LRF release has been demonstrated clearly. A rise in peripheral circulating LRF in hypophysectomized rats occurred when dopamine was injected into the third ventricle. Norepinephrine had a much smaller effect and epinephrine was inactive even at a much higher dose (Schneider and McCann, 1970*b*; 1970*c*).

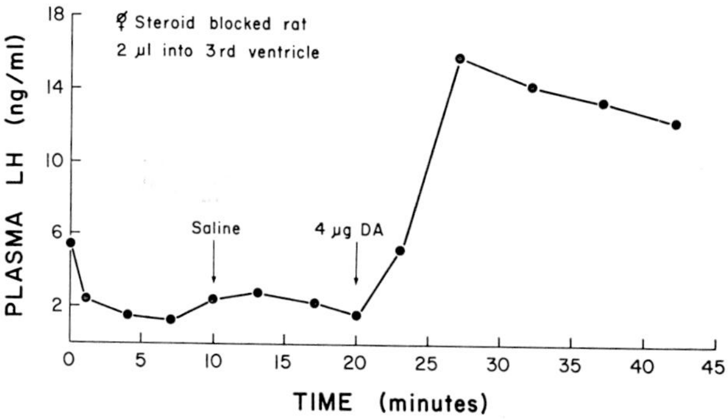

Fig. 3. Effect of dopamine (DA) injected into the third ventricle on plasma-LH in ovariectomized, steroid-blocked rats. Note that intraventricular saline was without effect.

Furthermore, third ventricular injection of dopamine elevated LRF in portal vessel blood (Kamberi *et al.*, 1969).

By contrast to the stimulatory effect of dopamine, serotonin dramatically lowered plasma LH in ovariectomized rats which suggests a possible role for this amine as an inhibitory transmitter (Schneider and McCann, 1970*a*).

We have also shown that dopamine can enhance the release of FRF from median eminence incubated *in vitro* (Kamberi *et al.*, 1970). Consequently, dopamine may be the synaptic transmitter for release of FRF as well as LRF. It can also depress blood prolactin levels in lactating rats (Kuhn *et al.*, 1970) and appears to play a role in regulation of prolactin secretion either by a stimulation of PIF discharge or by a direct inhibitory action at the pituitary level.

One of the sites of feedback of estrogen to inhibit LH release may involve the dopaminergic link in LRF discharge, for estradiol has been observed to block the dopamine-induced discharge of LRF both *in vitro* (Schneider and McCann, 1970*c*) and *in vivo* (Schneider and McCann, 1970*d*).

CHEMISTRY OF RELEASING FACTORS

We will attempt to summarize very briefly the progress to date in this important area (for refs. see Fawcett, 1970; Meites, 1970; McCann and Porter 1969; Root *et al.*, 1969).

Considerable progress has been made in purification of releasing factors with the utilization of hypothalamic tissue as the starting material. Since most factors appear to be concentrated in the stalk-median eminence region, the use of stalk-median eminence rather than whole hypothalamic extracts gives an advantage in subsequent attempts at purification.

Most workers have defatted the frozen or lyophilized tissue prior to extraction, and nearly all workers employ extraction with dilute acid as the initial step. Little data can be found to indicate whether or not these methods are effective in extracting all of the activity.

Several chromatographic procedures have been used to accomplish further purification of the releasing factors and to separate them from each other. The most widely used initial step is gel filtration on Sephadex G-25, a technique introduced to separate substances according to their molecular size. There is a characteristic pattern of elution of the factors from Sephadex columns. The gonadotropin-releasing factors are the last releasing factors eluted from Sephadex. FRF is first eluted and this is followed by LRF. It has been difficult to separate PIF from LRF by gel filtration; however, PIF tends to emerge just prior to LRF. Vasopressin, which is also found in stalk-median eminence extracts, emerges just after LRF. Gel filtration provides a good separation of the early emerging CRF and GRF from the later emerging gonadotrophin-releasing factors.

Further purification has been obtained by ion-exchange chromatography on carboxy-methyl cellulose, but unless the fractions are desalted, either by extraction with glacial acetic acid and by a preliminary pass through the column, or by the use of phenol or by chromatography on Dowex and Amberlite Cg4B columns, some of the releasing factor activity will appear at the void volume of the column. Following desalting, all of the factors are well retained on carboxy-methyl cellulose. Chromatography on carboxy-methyl cellulose has been used successfully to purify the factors and to separate them from residual contaminating activities.

A variety of other procedures have been employed in several laboratories for further purification and most of the factors have now been obtained in a highly purified state.

Methods of isolation were adapted from those in use to purify peptides and most of the factors have been shown to be inactivated by proteolytic enzymes. Consequently, it was reasonable to postulate that the releasing factors were polypeptide hormones. On the basis of their migration rates on Sephadex, molecular weights were estimated to lie between 1000 and 2500. It is now realized that factors other than molecular size affect mobility on Sephadex, so that these estimates of molecular weight should be viewed with caution. Amino acid compositions of the purified factors were published and they were all thought to be basic peptides.

Although CRF was originally thought to be related to vasopressin, it now appears unlikely that any of these hypothalamic hormones has a similar structure to that of vasopressin or oxytocin. Hypothalamic CRF and LRF are not inactivated by treatment with thioglycollate under conditions which inactivate both vasopressin and oxytocin by reduction of the disulfide bond (McCann and Porter, 1969).

What then can we say about the chemical nature of these factors? First, they can be purified and separated from each other. It appears quite likely that each is a distinct chemical entity. This is certainly an important first step. All of the factors appear to be heat stable, at least to 100°C for 10 minutes in crude or partially purified extracts. Most of the factors are inactivated by proteolytic digestion. They appear to be relatively small molecules.

Recently, in an important breakthrough, two laboratories (Folkers *et al.*, 1969; Burgus *et al.*, 1970, 1968) have announced that a synthetic tripeptide, pyroglutamyl, histidyl, proline amide, has TRF activity and corresponds in structure to isolated natural TRF. FRF and LRF may well be related small peptides and it is anticipated that their structure may soon be elucidated. The availability of synthetic LRF should provide an important clinical tool for inducing ovulation and for testing pituitary reserve for LH in man. Quite possibly analogues of the synthetic factors might have anti-FRF or anti-LRF activity and be useful as antifertility agents.

CONCLUDING REMARKS

As a result of the work of many investigators during the past fifteen years, it is now clear that the final common pathway between hypothalamus and anterior pituitary gland is bridged by a family of neurohormones. These agents are secreted into the hypophyseal portal vessels and act directly, and specifically on the adenohypophysis, to increase or decrease the release of each pituitary tropic hormone. Admittedly fragmentary evidence suggests that variations in the rate of secretion of the factors is responsible in large part for variations in secretion rate of anterior pituitary hormones in response to stimuli. The major site of feedback action of target gland hormones and the pituitary hormones themselves appears to be at the hypothalamic level to alter the rate of release of releasing factors; however, it is clear that this feedback of target gland hormones is also exerted at the pituitary level. If an animal is hypophysectomized for a period of time, releasing factors appear in the peripheral circulation which may be responsible at least in part for the residual function of the pituitary grafted to a site distant from the median eminence. Recent evidence indicates that dopamine may be the synaptic transmitter involved in the release of FRF and LRF from neuro-secretory neurons. Although the precise chemical nature of the gonadotropin-releasing factors remains elusive, they have been prepared in highly purified form. It is thought that they are small peptides.

REFERENCES

ANTON-TAY, F. and WURTMAN, R. J. (1968):Norepinephrine: Turnover in rat brains after gonadectomy. *Science*, *159*, 1245.

BEDDOW, D. G. and MCCANN, S. M. (1969): The effect of median eminence lesions on the function of multiple pituitary homografts with particular reference to the secretion of gonadotrophins and growth hormone. *Endocrinology*, *84*, 595.

BURGUS, R., DUNN, T. F., DESIDERIO, D. M., WARD, D. M., VALE, W. and GUILLEMIN, R. (1970): Biological activity of synthetic polypeptide derivatives related to the structure of hypothalamic TRF. *Endocrinology*, *86*, 573.

CAMPBELL, H. J., FEUER, G. and HARRIS, G. W. (1964): The effect of intrapituitary infusion of median eminence and other brain extracts on anterior pituitary gonadotrophic secretion. *J. Physiol. (Lond.)*, *170*, 474.

COATES, P. W., ASHBY, E. A., KRULICH, L., DHARIWAL, A. P. S. and MCCANN, S. M. (1970): Morphologic alterations in somatotrophs of the rat adenohypophysis following administration of hypothalamic extracts. *Amer. J. Anat.*, *128*, 389.

COPPOLA, J. A., LEONARDI, R. and LIPPMAN, W. (1966): Ovulatory failure in rats after treatment with brain norepinephrine depletors. *Endocrinology*, *78*, 225.

CRIGHTON, D. B., SCHNEIDER, H. P. G. and MCCANN, S. M. (1969): Possible interaction of luteinizing hormone-releasing factor with other hypothalamic releasing factors at the level of the adenohypophysis. *J. Endocr.*, *44*, 405.

CRIGHTON, D. B., SCHNEIDER, H. P. G. and MCCANN, S. M. (1970): Localization of LH-releasing factor in the hypothalamus and neurohypophysis as determined by an *in vitro* method. *Endocrinology*, *87*, 323.

DONOSO, A. O., STEFANO, F. J. E., BISCARDI, A. M. and CUKIER, J. (1967): Effects of castration on hypothalamic catecholamines. *Amer. J. Physiol.*, *212*, 737.

DOUGLAS, W. W. and POISNER, A. M. (1964): Stimulus-secretion coupling in a neurosecretory organ: the role of calcium in the release of vasopressin from the neurohypophysis. *J. Physiol. (Lond.)*, *172*, 1.

EVANS, E. S. and NIKITOVITCH-WINER, M. B. (1969): Functional reactivation and cytological restoration of pituitary grafts by continuous local intravascular infusion of median eminence extracts. *Neuroendocrinology*, *4*, 83.

EVERETT, J. W. (1964): Central neural control of reproductive functions of the adenohypophysis. *Physiol. Rev.*, *44*, 373.

FAWCETT, C. P. (1970): The present status of the chemistry of PIF, FRF, and LRF. In: *Hypophysiotropic Hormones of the Hypothalamus: Assay and Chemistry, 1st ed.*, Chapter 16, pp. 242–253. Editor: J. Meites. Williams and Wilkins, Baltimore, Md.

FINK, G. (1967): Nature of luteinizing hormone releasing factor in hypophysial portal blood. *Nature, (Lond.)* *215*, 159.

FLEISHER, N., DONALD, R. A. and BUTCHER, R. W. (1969): Involvement of adenosine 3′, 5′-monophosphate in release of ACTH. *Amer. J. Physiol.*, *217*, 1287.

FOLKERS, K., BØLER, J., ENZMANN, F., BOWERS, C. Y. and SCHALLY, A. V. (1969): The identity of chemical and hormonal properties of the thyrotrophin releasing hormone and pyroglutamylhistidylproline amide. *Biochem. biophys. Res. Commun.*, *37*, 705.

FUXE, K. and HÖKFELT, T. (1967): The influence of central catecholamine neurons on the hormone secretion from the anterior and posterior pituitary. In: *Proceedings of the 4th International Symposium on Neurosecretion*, p. 165.

FUXE, K., HÖKFELT, T. and NILSSON, O. (1967): Activity changes in the tuberoinfundibular dopamine neurons of the rat during various states of the reproductive cycle. *Life Sci.*, *6*, 2057.

GAY, V. L. and MIDGLEY, A. R., JR. (1969): Response of the adult rat to orchidectomy and ovariectomy as determined by LH radioimmunoassay. *Endocrinology*, *84*, 1359.

GITTES, R. F. and KASTIN, A. J. (1966): Effects of increasing numbers of pituitary transplants in hypophysectomized rats. *Endocrinology*, *78*, 1023.

GREEN, J. D. and HARRIS, G. W. (1949): Observation of the hypophysio-portal vessels of the living rat. *J. Physiol. (Lond.)*, *108*, 359.
GROSVENOR, C. E., MCCANN, S. M. and NALLAR, R. (1965): Inhibition of nursing-induced and stress-induced fall in pituitary prolactin concentration in lactating rats by injection of acid extracts of bovine hypothalamus. *Endocrinology*, *76*, 883.
HARRIS, G. W., REED, M. and FAWCETT, C. P. (1966): Hypothalamic releasing factors and the control of anterior pituitary function. *Brit. med. Bull.*, *22*, 266.
HILLARP, N-Å., FUXE, K. and DAHLSTRÖM (1966): Demonstration and mapping of central neurons containing dopamine, noradrenaline, and 5-hydroxytryptamine and their reactions to psychopharmaca. *Pharmacol. Rev.*, *18*, 727.
HINSEY, J. C. (1937): The relation of the nervous system to ovulation and other phenomena of the female reproductive tract. *Cold Spr. Harb. Symp. quant. Biol.*, *5*, 269.
IGARASHI, M., YOKOTA, N., EHARA, Y., MAYUZUMI, R., HIRANO, T., MATSUMOTO, S. and YAMASAKI, M. (1968): Clinical effects with partially purified beef hypothalamic FSH-releasing factor. *Amer. J. Obstet. Gynec.*, *100*, 867.
KAMBERI, I. A. and MCCANN, S. M. (1969): Effect of biogenic amines, FSH-releasing factor (FRF) and other substances on the release of FSH by pituitaries incubated *in vitro*. *Endocrinology*, *85*, 815.
KAMBERI, I. A., MICAL, R. and PORTER, J. C. (1969): Luteinizing hormone-releasing activity in hypophysial stalk blood and elevation by dopamine. *Science*, *166*, 388.
KAMBERI, I. A., MICAL, R. S. and PORTER, J. C. (1970*a*): Follicle stimulating hormone releasing activity in hypophysial portal blood and elevation by dopamine. *Nature (Lond.)*, *227*, 714.
KAMBERI, I. A., SCHNEIDER, H. P. G. and MCCANN, S. M. (1970*b*): Action of dopamine to induce release of FSH-releasing factor (FRF) from hypothalamic tissue *in vitro*. *Endocrinology*, *86*, 278.
KASTIN, A. J., SCHALLY, A. V., GAUL, C., MIDGLEY, A. R., BOWERS, C. Y. and DIAZ-INFANTE, A. (1969): Stimulation of LH release in men and women by LH-releasing hormone purified from porcine hypothalami. *J. clin. Endocr.*, *29*, 1046.
KRULICH, L., DHARIWAL, A. P. S. and MCCANN, S. M. (1968): Stimulatory and inhibitory effects of purified hypothalamic extracts on growth hormone release from rat pituitary *in vitro*. *Endocrinology*, *83*, 783.
KUHN, E., KRULICH, L., QUIJADA, M., ILLNER, P., KALRA, P. S. and MCCANN, S. M. (1970): Effect of oxytocin and adrenergic agents on prolactin release *in vivo* and *in vitro*. In: *Program of the 52nd Endocrine Society Meeting*, p. 126.
MARTINI, L., FRASCHINI, F. and MOTTA, M. (1968): Neural control of anterior pituitary functions. *Rec. Progr. Hormone Res.*, *24*, 439.
MEITES, J. (1970): Direct studies of the secretion of the hypothalamic hypophysiotropic hormones (HHH). In: *Hypophysiotropic Hormones of the Hypothalamus: Assay and Chemistry, 1st ed.*, Chapter 18, pp. 261–281. Editor: J. Meites. Williams and Wilkins, Baltimore, Md.
MCCANN, S. M. (1957): The ACTH-releasing activity of extracts of the posterior lobe of the pituitary *in vivo*. *Endocrinology*, *69*, 664.
MCCANN, S. M. (1962): A hypothalamic luteinizing hormone-releasing factor (LH-RF). *Amer. J. Physiol.*, *202*, 395.
MCCANN, S. M. (1970): Bioassay of luteinizing hormone-releasing factor. In: *Hypophysiotropic Hormones of the Hypothalamus: Assay and Chemistry, 1st ed.*, Chapter 7, pp. 90–102. Editor: J. Meites. Williams and Wilkins, Baltimore, Md.
MCCANN, S. M., DHARIWAL, A. P. S. and PORTER, J. C. (1968): Regulation of the adenohypophysis. *Ann. Rev. Physiol.*, *30*, 589.
MCCANN, S. M. and PORTER, J. C. (1969): Hypothalamic pituitary stimulating and inhibiting hormones. *Physiol. Rev.*, *49*, 240.
MOTTA, M., PIVA, F., FRASCHINI, F. and MARTINI, L. (1970): 'Pituitary depletion methods' for the bioassay of hypothalamic releasing factors. In: *Hypophysiotropic Hormones of the Hypothalamus: Assay and Chemistry, 1st ed.*, Chapter 4, pp. 44–59. Editor: J. Meites. Williams and Wilkins, Baltimore, Md.
NEGRO-VILAR, A., DICKERMAN, E. and MEITES, J. (1968*a*): FSH-releasing factor activity in plasma of rats after hypophysectomy and continuous light. *Endocrinology*, *82*, 939.
NEGRO-VILAR, A., DICKERMAN, E. and MEITES, J. (1968*b*): Removal of plasma FSH-RF activity in hypophysectomized rats by testosterone propionate or reserpine. *Endocrinology*, *83*, 1349.
NIKITOVITCH-WINER, M. B. (1962): Induction of ovulation in rats by direct intrapituitary infusion of median eminence. *Endocrinology*, *70*, 350.

PORTER, J. C. and MICAL, R. S. (1969): Description of a method for the microcannulation and perfusion of a hypophysial portal vessel in the rat. *Fed. Proc.*, *28*, 317.
PORTER, J. C. and RUMSFELD, H. W., JR. (1956): Effect of lyophilized plasma and plasma fractions from hypophyseal-portal vessel blood on adrenal ascorbic acid. *Endocrinology*, *58*, 359.
ROOT, A. W., SMITH, G. P., DHARIWAL, A. P. S. and MCCANN, S. M. (1969): Luteinizing hormone releasing activity of crude ovine hypothalamic extract in man. *Nature (Lond.)*, *221*, 570.
SAMLI, M. H. and GESCHWIND, I. I. (1967): Some effects of the hypothalamic luteinizing hormone releasing factor on the biosynthesis and release of luteinizing hormone. *Endocrinology*, *81*, 835.
SAMLI, M. H. and GESCHWIND, I. I. (1968): Some effects of energy-transfer inhibitors and of Ca^{++} -free or K^{+}-enhanced media on the release of luteinizing hormone (LH) from the rat pituitary gland *in vitro*. *Endocrinology*, *82*, 225.
SCHALLY, A. V., ARIMURA, A., BOWERS, C. Y., KASTIN, A. J., SAWANO, S. and REDDING, T. W. (1968): Hypothalamic neurohormones regulating anterior pituitary function. *Rec. Progr. Hormone Res.*, *24*, 497.
SCHNEIDER, H. P. G., CRIGHTON, D. B. and MCCANN, S. M. (1969): Suprachiasmatic LH-releasing factor. *Neuroendocrinology*, *5*, 271.
SCHNEIDER, H. P. G. and MCCANN, S. M. (1969*a*): Possible role of dopamine as transmitter to promote discharge of LH-releasing factor. *Endocrinology*, *85*, 121.
SCHNEIDER, H. P. G. and MCCANN, S. M. (1969): Dopaminergic pathways and gonadotropin releasing factors. In: *Aspect of Endocrinology,* p. 177. Editors: W. Bargmann and B. Scharrer. Springer-Verlag, Berlin.
SCHNEIDER, H. P. G. and MCCANN, S. M. (1970*a*): Mono- and indolamines and control of LH secretion. *Endocrinology*, *86*, 1127.
SCHNEIDER, H. P. G. and MCCANN, S. M. (1970*b*): Luteinizing hormone-releasing factor discharge by dopamine in rats. *J. Endocr.*, *46*, 401.
SCHNEIDER, H. P. G. and MCCANN, S. M. (1970*c*): Release of LH-releasing factor (LRF) into the peripheral circulation of hypophysectomized rats by dopamine and its blockage by estradiol. *Endocrinology*, *87*, 249.
SCHNEIDER, H. P. G. and MCCANN, S. M. (1970*d*): Estradiol and the neuroendocrine control of LH release *in vitro*. *Endocrinology*, *87*, 330.
SMITH, E. R. and DAVIDSON, J. M. (1967): Testicular maintenance and its inhibition in pituitary-transplanted rats. *Endocrinology*, *80*, 725.
WAKABAYASHI, K., KAMBERI, I. A. and MCCANN, S. M. (1969): *In vitro* response of the rat pituitary to gonadotrophin-releasing factors and to ions. *Endocrinology*, *85*, 1046.
WAKABAYASHI, K. and MCCANN, S. M. (1970): *In vitro* responses of anterior pituitary glands from normal, castrated and androgen-treated male rats to LH-releasing factor (LRF) and high potassium medium. *Endocrinology*, *87*, 771.
WATANABE, S. and MCCANN, S. M. (1968): Localization of FSH-releasing factor in the hypothalamus and neurohypophysis as determined by *in vitro* assay. *Endocrinology*, *82*, 664.
WILBER, F. J., PEAKE, G. T., MARIZ, I., UTIGER, R. and DAUGHADAY, W. (1968): Theophylline and epinephrine effects upon the secretion of growth hormone (GH) and thyrotropin (TSH) *in vitro*. *Clin. Res.*, *16*, 277.
WILBER, F. J. and PORTER, J. C. (1970): Thyrotropin and growth hormone releasing activity in hypophysial portal blood. *Endocrinology*, *87*, 807.
ZOR, W., KANEKO, T., SCHNEIDER, H. P. G., MCCANN, S. M., LOWE, I. P., BLOOM, G., BORLAND, B. and FIELD, J. B. (1969): Stimulation of anterior pituitary adenyl cyclase activity and adenosine 3′:5′-cyclic phosphate by hypothalamic extract and prostaglandin E_1. *Proc. nat. Acad. Sci.*, *63*, 918.

THE NEUROVASCULAR LINK OF THE HYPOTHALAMIC-HYPOPHYSIAL SYSTEM AND THE ROLE OF MONOAMINES IN THE CONTROL OF GONADOTROPIN RELEASE*

JOHN C. PORTER, IBRAHIM A. KAMBERI and RENON S. MICAL

Department of Physiology, University of Texas Southwestern Medical School at Dallas, Dallas, Texas, U.S.A.

INTRODUCTION

The essential anatomical features of the hypothalamic-hypophysial portal vasculature were described by Popa and Fielding (1930; 1933), but they concluded erroneously that blood in this portal system flowed toward the hypothalamus. Although Houssay *et al.* (1935) subsequently observed that flow in the portal vessels was from the hypothalamus to the anterior pituitary, it was primarily the work of Wislocki (1936; 1937; 1938) that won acceptance of the notion that the anterior pituitary did in fact receive portal blood. A unique feature of this vascular system is that capillaries draining into the portal vessels are contained in the pituitary stalk and the median eminence of the hypothalamus, providing a vascular interface between the brain and the anterior pituitary.

The importance of this vascular link was first recognized by Friedgood. (For a belated account of his proposal, see Friedgood (1970).) He proposed the view that the brain might control function of the anterior pituitary by way of a neurohumoral mechanism, *i.e.*, by means of a substance(s) which was elaborated by the brain, diffused into the primary capillaries of the portal system, and then carried to the anterior pituitary in portal blood. It was presumed that the hypothetical neurohumor(s) stimulated the anterior pituitary to release one or more of its trophic hormones. Subsequently, results of many experiments have been reported which were believed to support indirectly this concept. It must be admitted, however, that experiments providing direct support of the neurohumoral hypothesis are less plentiful. Reasons why the hypothesis has not been tested directly heretofore are, first, the fact that the ventromedial hypothalamus and the hypophysial portal vasculature are not readily accessible to the investigator and, second, the fact that a test substance injected into the systemic circulation must pass first through primary capillaries in the diencephalon before reaching the anterior pituitary. For example, it was difficult to say with certainty that a substance given via the systemic circulation did not cause the hypothalamus to release a hypophysiotropic substance which in turn stimulated the anterior pituitary.

These complexities have been overcome in part by recent advances. Porter and Smith (1967) described a procedure for the collection of all the blood passing down the pituitary stalk of rats during a period of several hours. Stalk blood collected by their procedure was uncontaminated by extraneous blood and cerebrospinal fluid. More recently, workers from

* This investigation was supported by a research grant AM01237 from the National Institut Health, Bethesda, Md., and a grant from the Population Council, New York, N.Y.

the same laboratory reported a method for the microcannulation of a hypophysial portal vessel (Porter *et al.*, 1970), making it possible to perfuse the anterior pituitary by way of its affluent blood supply while simultaneously bypassing the hypothalamus. We will now discuss recent findings of investigations in which these new experimental methods were used. The results provide direct support of the neurohumoral hypothesis.

ANTERIOR PITUITARY PERFUSION

Hypothalamic extracts. A crude extract of hypothalamic tissue was prepared by homogenizing fragments of hypothalamic tissue in 0.1 N hydrochloric acid. The supernatant fluid, obtained following centrifugation at 14,000 × g at 0°C, was neutralized to pH 7.2 and passed sequentially through millipore filters having nominal pore diameters of 8, 3, 0.8 and 0.3 μ to remove particulate matter. The filtrate was infused into a portal vessel of anesthetized, adult male rats for 30 minutes at the rate of 2 μl/min (Porter *et al.*, 1970). The concentration of the infusate was such that a solution equivalent to 1/60, 1/180 or 1/360 of a hypothalamic fragment or 131, 43 or 22 μg (wet weight) hypothalamic tissue was infused per minute. For control purposes, a similarly prepared extract of cerebrocortical tissue was infused into a portal vessel. The rate of infusion was equivalent to 135 μg (wet weight) cortical tissue per minute (Kamberi *et al.*, 1970*a*).

The infusion of cerebrocortical tissue into the anterior pituitary via a cannulated portal vessel caused no significant change in the concentration in plasma of luteinizing hormone (LH), follicle-stimulating hormone (FSH) or prolactin during the 30 minutes of the infusion period or during the 60-minute period immediately following the infusion. The solution containing the extract of hypothalamic tissue had a pronounced stimulatory effect on the release of LH and FSH and an inhibitory effect on the release of prolactin during the period of the infusion. After 10 minutes of infusion at the rate of 1/60 of a hypothalamic fragment per minute, the concentration of LH and FSH in plasma was twofold greater than the pre-infusion level. In contrast to these findings, the concentration of prolactin after 10 minutes of infusion was only 65% of the pre-infusion level. The peak concentration of LH in plasma occurred at the end of the 30-minute infusion period. At this time, the level of LH in plasma was fivefold greater than the control level. The maximal concentration of FSH in plasma occurred 10 minutes after the infusion was stopped and was threefold greater than the FSH concentration in the plasma of the animals given the cerebrocortical extract. The minimal concentration of prolactin, which was found at the end of the period of infusion, was less than 25% that seen in the control animals. The infusion of the extract of hypothalamic tissue at slower rates, *viz.*, 1/180 or 1/360 hypothalamic fragment per minute, caused correspondingly smaller releases of LH and FSH and inhibition of prolactin release. Shortly after cessation of the infusion via a portal vessel, the concentrations of FSH and LH in plasma began to fall and that of prolactin began to rise. These results are consistent with the view that hypothalamic tissue contains one or more substances which can stimulate the anterior pituitary to release FSH and LH and to inhibit the release of prolactin (Kamberi *et al.*, 1970*a*).

Catecholamines. It was shown by Heape (1905) that rabbits ovulate following coitus and it has long been suspected that the catecholamines may have a role in the control of release of the gonadotropins causing ovulation. Markee *et al.* (1948) found that the intravenous injection of certain adrenergic blocking agents into the rabbit shortly after coitus can prevent ovulation.

When epinephrine bitartrate or norepinephrine bitartrate was infused at the rate of 2 μg/min for 30 minutes directly into the anterior pituitary via a cannulated portal vessel, no change in the plasma level of LH, FSH or prolactin was observed. Similarly, the infusion of dopamine hydrochloride into a portal vessel at the rate of 0.002, 0.02, 0.2 or 2 μg/min for 30 minutes had no effect on LH (Kamberi *et al.*, 1969*a*; 1970*b*), FSH (Kamberi *et al.*, 1970*c*; 1971*a*) or prolactin (Kamberi *et al.*, 1970*d*; 1971*b*) release.

Indoleamines. In addition, the infusion into a portal vessel of an indoleamine, serotonin or melatonin, at the rate of 2 μg/min for 30 minutes had no effect on LH (Kamberi *et al.*, 1970*b*), FSH (Kamberi *et al.*, 1970*c*) or prolactin release (Kamberi, Mical and Porter, unpublished data).

PERFUSION OF THE STALK MEDIAN EMINENCE COMPLEX

Landsmeer (1947; 1951) has shown that in the rat the peduncular artery usually supplies blood to the postpeduncular eminence and pituitary stalk, whereas the infundibular arteries supply blood to the postchiasmatic eminence. It was of interest to see if perfusion of these structures with a catecholamine could stimulate the secretion of one or more hypophysiotropic substances from the stalk median-eminence complex. When dopamine hydrochloride was infused for 30 minutes at the rate of 2 μg/min into the peduncular artery or into a ramus of an infundibular artery, no effect was seen on LH, FSH or prolactin release (Kamberi, Mical and Porter, unpublished observations).

INJECTION OF BIOGENIC AMINES INTO THE THIRD VENTRICLE

The injection of 2.5–5.0 μl of an isotonic salt solution into the third ventricle of anesthetized male rats had no effect on the release of LH, FSH or prolactin. However, the injection into the third ventricle of 2.5–5.0 μl of an isotonic salt solution containing 1.25 or 2.5 μg dopamine hydrochloride caused within 10 minutes a fourfold increase in the plasma levels of LH and FSH. During the same time, the concentration of prolactin fell to a level that was 75% that of the controls. Twenty minutes after the intraventricular injection of 1.25 or 2.5 μg dopamine, the plasma level of LH was eightfold and that of FSH was over fivefold greater than that of the controls. At the same time, the plasma level of prolactin was only one-half that of the control values. It is of interest that doses of dopamine greater than 2.5 μg caused a progressively diminished response, and a dose of 100 μg had no effect at all on the release of LH (Kamberi *et al.*, 1969*a*; 1970*b*), FSH (Kamberi *et al.*, 1970*c*; 1971*a*) or prolactin (Kamberi *et al.*, 1970*d*; 1971*b*).

Although small doses of epinephrine bitartrate or norepinephrine bitartrate (2.5–5.0 μg) had no effect on LH, FSH or prolactin release, 100 μg did cause a significant release of LH (Kamberi *et al.*, 1969*a*; 1970*b*) and FSH (Kamberi *et al.*, 1970*c*; 1970*d*) and an inhibition of release of prolactin (Kamberi *et al.*, 1970*d*; 1971).

The injection of 1, 5 or 50 μg of serotonin or melatonin suppressed the basal rate of release of LH (Kamberi *et al.*, 1970*b*) and FSH (Kamberi *et al.*, 1970*c*). The inhibitory action of these indoleamines was evident for approximately 60 minutes.

RELEASE OF HYPOPHYSIOTROPIC SUBSTANCES INTO PORTAL BLOOD

These findings support the view that the catecholamines, especially dopamine, stimulate the secretion of certain hypophysiotropic substances which, following release, diffuse into portal blood. This conclusion seems reasonable since an infusion of dopamine into the anterior pituitary has no effect on LH, FSH or prolactin release, yet small doses of dopamine injected into the third ventricle stimulate LH and FSH release while suppressing prolactin release.

To test the hypothesis that dopamine does in fact stimulate the secretion of certain hypophysiotropic substances, pituitary stalk blood and femoral artery blood were collected simultaneously from anesthetized male rats according to the procedure of Porter and Smith (1967). Blood was obtained from animals given 2.5 μg dopamine hydrochloride via the third ventricle and from rats not given dopamine. The latter were identified as untreated animals. Plasma samples from several animals were pooled and subsequently assayed for hypophysiotropic activity using *in vitro* and *in vivo* procedures.

Anterior pituitary tissue incubated in a synthetic tissue culture fluid (Difco, M-199) released LH, FSH and prolactin spontaneously. Pituitary tissue incubated in plasma from femoral artery blood from dopamine-treated or untreated donor rats released LH, FSH and prolactin at rates identical to those seen when M-199 was the incubation medium. However, pituitary tissue incubated in stalk plasma from untreated donor rats released LH, FSH and prolactin at rates that were 175, 185 and 80%, respectively, of those seen for glands incubated in femoral plasma. Glands incubated in stalk plasma from dopamine-treated animals released LH (Kamberi *et al.*, 1969*b*), FSH (Kamberi *et al.*, 1970*e*) and prolactin (Kamberi *et al.*, 1970*f*) at rates that were 450, 525 and 25%, respectively, of those observed for glands incubated in femoral plasma.

Recent results obtained by an *in vivo* procedure confirm observations made *in vitro*. When stalk plasma from dopamine-treated rats was infused via a microcannula into a portal vessel of untreated, anesthetized male rats, LH and FSH release increased and prolactin release decreased. These results show that stalk plasma from dopamine-treated rats contains luteinizing hormone-releasing activity, follicle-stimulating hormone-releasing activity and prolactin-inhibiting activity (Kamberi, *et al.,* unpublished data).

ADRENERGIC INHIBITORS

The effects of low doses of intraventricularly-administered dopamine on LH, FSH and prolactin release were completely blocked when an α-adrenergic inhibitor, phenoxybenzamine or phentolamine, was injected into the third ventricle simultaneously with dopamine. The β-adrenergic inhibitor, pronethalol, had no effect on dopamine-induced alteration of LH, FSH and prolactin release (Kamberi *et al.*, 1970*g*). These observations suggest that the effect of dopamine in the brain may be mediated by an α-adrenergic mechanism.

SUMMARY AND CONCLUSIONS

1. The techniques of cannulation of portal vessels and collection of stalk blood have been used in the investigation of the neurovascular link between the brain and the anterior pituitary.
2. By means of these procedures, it has been possible to determine the role of biogenic amines in the regulation of gonadotropin release.
3. The ventromedial region of the hypothalamus contains hypophysiotropic substances which stimulate release of LH and FSH and inhibit release of prolactin.
4. These hypophysiotropic substances are found in the portal blood of the hypothalamic-hypophysial complex.
5. Biogenic amines, particularly dopamine, induce the release of hypophysiotropic substances from neural elements of the hypothalamus.
6. These effects of dopamine may be mediated via an α-adrenergic mechanism.

REFERENCES

FRIEDGOOD, H. B. (1970): The nervous control of the anterior hypophysis. *J. Reprod. Fertil. Suppl.*, *10*, 1.

HEAPE, W. (1905): Ovulation and degeneration of ova in the rabbit. *Proc. roy. Soc. Ser, B*, *76*, 260.

HOUSSAY, B.-A., BIASOTTI, A. and SAMMARTINO, R. (1935): Modifications fonctionnelles de l'hypophyse après les lésions infundibulo-tubériennes chez le crapaud. *C. R. Soc. Biol. (Paris)*, *120*, 725.

KAMBERI, I. A., MICAL, R. and PORTER, J. C. (1969*a*): A possible role for dopamine in the stimulation of the release of the LH-releasing factor. In: *Program of the 2nd Annual Meeting of the Society for the Study of Reproduction, Davis, Calif.*, p. 4.

KAMBERI, I. A., MICAL, R. S. and PORTER, J. C. (1969*b*): Luteinizing hormone-releasing activity in hypophysial stalk blood and elevation by dopamine. *Science*, *166*, 388.

KAMBERI, I. A., MICAL, R. S. and PORTER, J. C. (1970*a*): Effect of infusion via a hypophysial portal vessel of crude hypothalamic extract on gonadotropin release in male rats. In: *Program of the 3rd Annual Meeting of the Society for the Study of Reproduction, Columbus, Ohio*, p. 14.

KAMBERI, I. A., MICAL, R. S. and PORTER, J. C. (1970*b*): Effect of anterior pituitary perfusion and intraventricular injection of catecholamines and indoleamines on LH release. *Endocrinology*, *87*, 1.

KAMBERI, I. A., MICAL, R. S. and PORTER, J. C. (1970*c*): Effect of catecholamines and indoleamines on FSH release. *Program of the 52nd Meeting of The Endocrine Society, St. Louis, Mo.*, p. 61.

KAMBERI, I. A., MICAL, R. S. and PORTER, J. C. (1970*d*): Intraventricular (V_3) injection or pituitary perfusion of catecholamines and prolactin (LtH) release. *Fed. Proc.*, *29*, 378.

KAMBERI, I. A., MICAL, R. S. and PORTER, J. C. (1970*e*): Follicle stimulating hormone releasing activity in hypophysial portal blood and elevation by dopamine. *Nature (Lond.)*, *227*, 714.

KAMBERI, I. A., MICAL, R. S. and PORTER, J. C. (1970*f*): Prolactin-inhibiting activity in hypophysial stalk blood and elevation by dopamine. *Experientia (Basel)*. In press.

KAMBERI, I. A., MICAL, R. S. and PORTER, J. C. (1970*g*): Possible role of α-adrenergic receptors in mediating the response of the hypothalamus to dopamine. *Physiologist*, *13*, 239.

KAMBERI, I. A., MICAL, R. S. and PORTER, J. C. (1971*a*): Effect of anterior pituitary perfusion and intraventricular injection of catecholamines on FSH release. *Endocrinology*. In press.

KAMBERI, I. A., MICAL, R. S. and PORTER, J. C. (1971*b*): Effect of anterior pituitary perfusion and intraventricular injection of catecholamines on prolactin release. *Endocrinology*, *88*, 1012.

LANDSMEER, J. M. F. (1947): *Het Vaatstelsel van de Hypophyse bij de Witte Rat*. Doctorate Thesis, University of Leyden.

LANDSMEER, J. M. F. (1951): Vessels of the rat's hypophysis. *Acta anat. (Basel)*, *12*, 82.

MARKEE, J. E., SAWYER, C. H. and HOLLINSHEAD, W. H. (1948): Adrenergic control of the release of luteinizing hormone from the hypophysis of the rabbit. *Rec. Progr. Hormone Res.*, *2*, 117.

POPA, G. and FIELDING, U. (1930): A portal circulation from the pituitary to the hypothalamic region. *J. Anat. (Lond.)*, *65*, 88.

POPA, G. and FIELDING, U. (1933): Hypophysio-portal vessels and their colloid accompaniment. *J. Anat. (Lond.)*, *67*, 227.

PORTER, J. C., MICAL, R. S., KAMBERI, I. A. and GRAZIA, Y. R. (1970): A procedure for the cannulation of a pituitary stalk portal vessel and perfusion of the pars distalis in the rat. *Endocrinology*, *87*, 197.

PORTER, J. C. and SMITH, K. R. (1967): Collection of hypophysial stalk blood in rats. *Endocrinology*, *81*, 1182.

WISLOCKI, G. B. (1937): The vascular supply of the hypophysis cerebri of the cat. *Anat. Rec.*, *69*, 361.

WISLOCKI, G. B. (1938): The vascular supply of the hypophysis cerebri of the rhesus monkey and man. *Ass. Res. nerv. Dis. Proc.*, *17*, 48.

WISLOCKI, G. B. and KING, L. S. (1936): The permeability of the hypophysis and hypothalamus to vital dyes, with the study of the hypophyseal vascular supply. *Amer. J. Anat.*, *58*, 421.

HYPOTHALAMIC RECEPTORS FOR FSH AND ESTROGEN*

V. D. RAMÍREZ, S. R. OJEDA and E. O. ALVAREZ

Institute of Physiology, University Austral, Valdivia, Chile

It is beyond dispute that the function of the anterior pituitary gland is mainly under the control of the hypothalamus, through the so-called hypothalamic pituitary stimulating and inhibiting hormones (McCann and Porter, 1969). The synthesis of the first releasing factor, thyrotropin releasing factor (TRF), achieved by Bowers *et al.* (1970) and Vale *et al.* (1970) represent a milestone in this research, which originated more than ten years ago.

How do the classical (long loop) and internal (short loop) feedback signals, following the nomenclature of Motta *et al.* (1969), act in the controlling system of gonadotrophins to modify the secretion of the hypothalamic hormones? This paper will discuss the interrelationships of estrogen (as an example of classical feedback loop) and FSH (as an example of short or internal feedback loop) at the hypothalamic level, particularly in the area called the medial basal hypothalamus (MBH).

It is well known that estrogen can be taken up by the MBH of rats (Eisenfeld and Axelrod, 1966; Kato and Villee, 1967; Presl *et al.*, 1970). We have confirmed these results using intact adult diestrous rats as can be seen in Figure 1. The highest counts detected in the MBH are

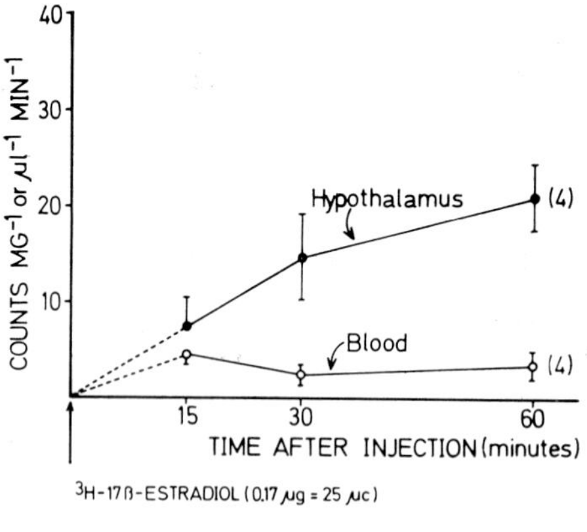

Fig. 1. Uptake of ^{3}H-estradiol by the medial basal hypothalamus (MBH) of diestrous rats. A single dose of 25 μC was injected i.p. At the times indicated 4 animals per point were bled and the MBH was dissected out. The Kato and Villee procedure slightly modified was used to extract the steroid (Kato and Villee (1967).
Mean values $\pm$ SEM are shown. Notice that at 30 minutes and 60 minutes after the injection of the radioactive steroid higher levels of radioactivity are found in the MBH than in blood.

found 60 minutes after a single i.p. injection of ^{3}H-estradiol, reaching a level 5 times higher than the blood. It is also well established that tritiated estradiol is concentrated especially in the nuclei of several hypothalamic nuclei as has been revealed by autoradiographic techniques (Stumpf, 1968*a*; *b*; Pfaff, 1968; Conwell and Greenwald, 1969).

This phenomenon may represent a real binding of estrogen to hypothalamic neurones as is clearly shown in Figure 2, redrawn from the experiment of Kato and Villee (1967). Subcutaneous injection of 17-β-estradiol 3 hours before the label pulse blocks the uptake of

* This work was supported by grant M.70.60.C from the Population Council.

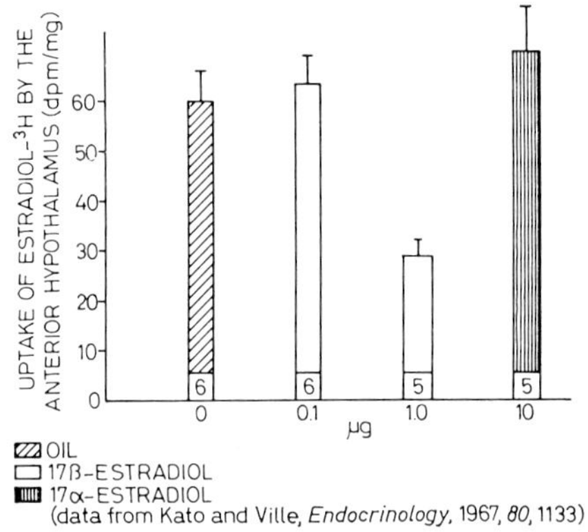

Fig. 2. Effect of unlabeled 17-β-estradiol and the 17-α isomer on ^{3}H-estradiol uptake by MBH. 0.3 μg of 6,7-^{3}H-estradiol (specific activity 42 Ci/mmol) was injected i.p. into adult ovariectomized rats 3 hours after the subcutaneous administration of 17-β- or 17-α-estradiol in 0.2 ml sesame oil. The animals were killed 1 hour after the injection of tritiated estradiol. Mean values $\pm$ SEM are shown. Number of animals in each group are inside the bars. (Redrawn from Kato and Villee (1967),

estradiol by the MBH 1 hour after i.p. injection in ovariectomized rats. The effect seems to be very specific because the 17-α isomer of estrogen in higher doses was not able to block the uptake of ^{3}H-estradiol.

There must be a physiological reason for the capacity of this area to take up and retain estrogen. This is exemplifed in Figure 3, taken from Palka *et al.* (1966). In intact adult rats, implantation of estrogen in the median eminence is capable of inducing LH secretion 4 or 5 days later, but not 18 days later. Interestingly enough, pituitary estrogen did not increase plasma LH although it was very effective in increasing pituitary weight. Another example is the well-known capacity of estrogen to release prolactin (Ramírez and McCann, 1964),

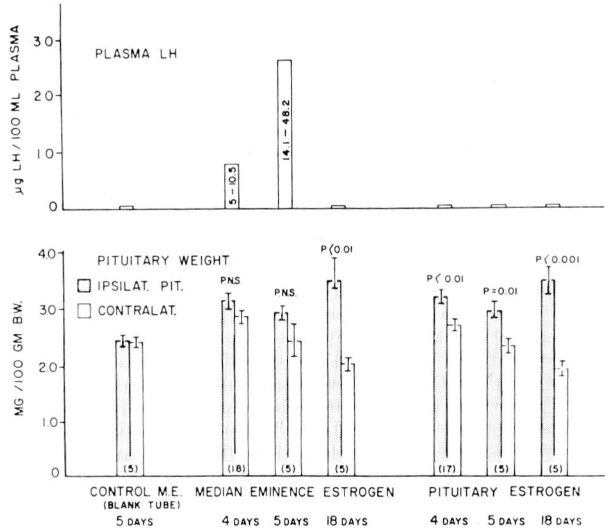

Fig. 3. Comparison of the effects on pituitary weight and plasma LH of tritiated estradiol and estradiol acetate implanted in the median eminence and pituitary. Values 5 days post-implantation were obtained with estradiol acetate; all others with estradiol. Vertical lines indicate standard error of the mean: the numbers inside the bars indicating plasma LH values refer to the 95% confidence limits. Ipsilateral and contralateral pituitary indicates the halves of the anterior pituitary on the same and opposite sides, respectively, as the implanted estrogen. Note that, while pituitary implants induced greater unilateral hypertrophy, they had no effect on the release of LH (from Palka *et al.* (1966).

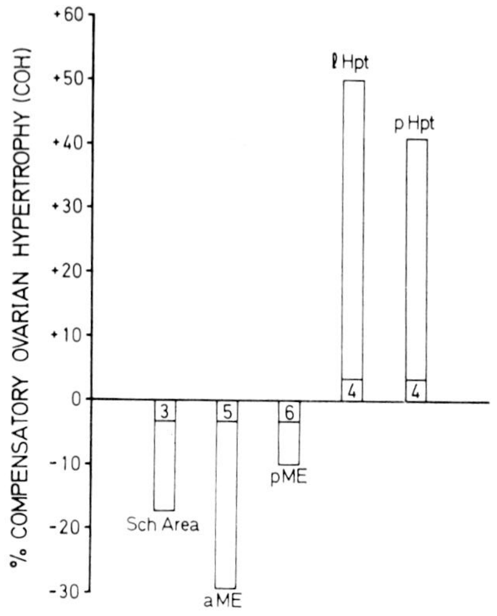

Fig. 4. Inhibition of compensatory ovarian hypertrophy (COH) by brain estrogen-implantation in hemicastrated adult rats. Notice that 14 days after hemicastration and implantation the estrogen implanted in the MBH had a strong inhibitory effect on COH. (Redrawn from Fendler and Endröczi (1965).
lHpt = lateral hypothalamus; pHpt = posterior hypothalamus; aMe = anterior median eminence; pMe = posterior median eminence; Sch area = supra-chiasmatic area.

and recently Nagasawa *et al.* (1969) have demonstrated this, using radioimmunoassay to measure blood prolactin levels. Furthermore implanted estrogen in the MBH inhibits compensatory ovarian hypertrophy (COH) as was shown by Fendler and Endröczi (1965). Figure 4, redrawn from their data, shows that 14 days after hemiovariectomy and implantation of estrogen in the MBH, the local steroid was capable of inhibiting the COH, which might suggest an inhibition of FSH release by the pituitary as was recently shown by Benson *et al.* (1969). The lateral or posterior hypothalamus were ineffective hypothalamic structures.

These actions of estrogen might be mediated through the existence of particular molecules that may be called receptors following the general ideas on the mechanism of action of estrogen (Jensen *et al.*, 1968; Soloff and Szego, 1969). The existence of a possible 'receptor' obtained from the cytoplasm of the female bovine hypothalamus and rat hypothalamus respectively has been recently shown by Kahwanago *et al.* (1969) and Eisenfeld (1969). Preliminary data from our laboratory also suggest the existence of molecules capable of binding ^{3}H-estrogen. Samples of the 75,000 *g* supernatant of female rat hypothalamus

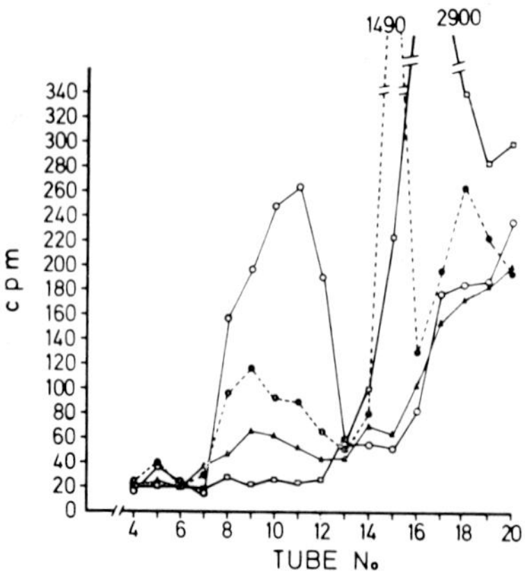

Fig. 5. Chromatographic elution pattern from small Sephadex G-25 columns (21 × 0.8 cm), loaded with 2 ml of a 75,000 *g* supernatant of different specimens. After homogenization of 15 adult female hypothalami or cortices in 0.04 M tris-C1, 0.0015 M EDTA buffer, pH 7.4 the samples were centrifuged at 75,000 *g* × 90′ in a Spinco L2-65B. Two ml of supernatant fractions (50 mg/ml) were incubated at 4°C for 3 hours with 3.4 × 10^{3} μg of ^{3}H-estradiol (0.5 μC). The ^{3}H-estradiol alcohol solution was previously evaporated. Each elution fraction was of 0.5 ml. The samples were evaporated and counted directly from the vial after adding the scintillation mixture. Counting efficiency was 35%. Note the appearance of a peak of radioactivity associated with molecules eluted in the void volume.
○——○ MBH + ^{3}H-E; ●---● cortex + ^{3}H-E;
▲——▲ MBH + cold-E (1 μg) + ^{3}H-E;
□——□ Buffer + ^{3}H-E

homogenates were incubated at 4°C with tritiated estradiol for 3 hours. Afterwards a sample was placed on a small Sephadex-G-25 column and several fractions were collected at room temperature. A representative distribution of radioactivity in the different fractions (0.5 ml per fraction) is presented in Figure 5. The ^{3}H-estradiol incubated with buffer is eluted beyond the void volume of the column and practically all the estradiol is found in the fractions corresponding to the internal volume of the column. When the supernatant from cortex tissue (50 mg/ml) is incubated with ^{3}H-estradiol some of the radioactivity is distributed in the fractions corresponding to the void volume but most of the estrogen is free estrogen. On the other hand, when the cytoplasmic fraction of the MBH is incubated with the labeled estrogen most of the radioactivity is associated with molecules eluted in the void volume. When cold estrogen is incubated with a sample of the same MBH cytoplasmic fraction together with labeled estrogen there was a competition between both estrogens, as suggested by a marked diminution of the radioactivity in the molecules eluted in the void volume. This experiment and those of Kahwanago *et al.* and Eisenfeld using different tissues and methods to separate the molecules of the supernatant fraction suggest the existence of possible receptors to estrogen, located in the MBH.

Against this background the question arises, how does FSH interact with estrogen to modulate the secretion of endogenous FSH by the pituitary? First of all we need to know if FSH really plays a role in controlling pituitary function.

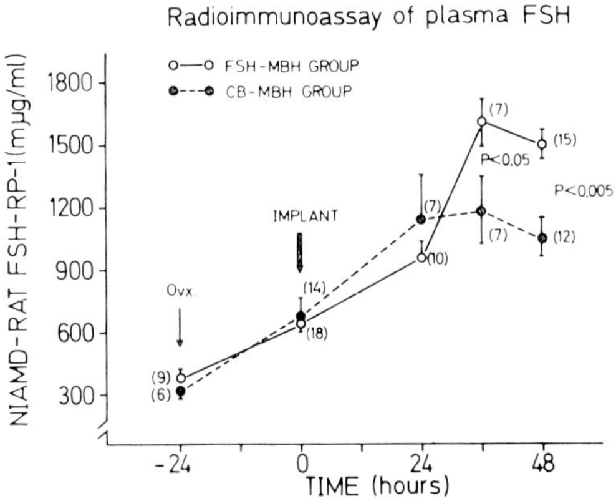

Fig. 6. Changes in plasma FSH concentration in 24-hour ovariectomized rats implanted in the MBH with local FSH or cocoa butter (CB). Number in parenthesis indicates number of animals used. Day of implantation is considered as time zero. Mean ± SEM are shown.
○——○ FSH-MBH group; ●---● CB-MBH group

Figure 6 shows that a minute amount of ovine FSH (NIH-FSH-S6) implanted in the MBH of 24-hr ovariectomized rats is capable of releasing pituitary FSH into the systemic blood as measured by radioimmunoassay. There is a latent period of about 36 hours and the effect continues for at least 12 hours more. Control animals bearing cocoa-butter-MBH implants did not present any suggestion of enhanced release of FSH. Figure 7 shows that the pituitary gland is depleted of FSH around 48 hours post-implantation of FSH in the MBH, recovering its normal level at 96 hours. The controls showed small pituitary FSH fluctuations which were not significant.

This positive feedback action of exogenous FSH to increase the release of pituitary FSH in ovariectomized adult rats is quite specific since simultaneous determination of LH in these same animals did not reveal any alteration in immunoreactive plasma LH (Fig. 8).

It is possible therefore to postulate that FSH placed in the hypothalamus can alter the

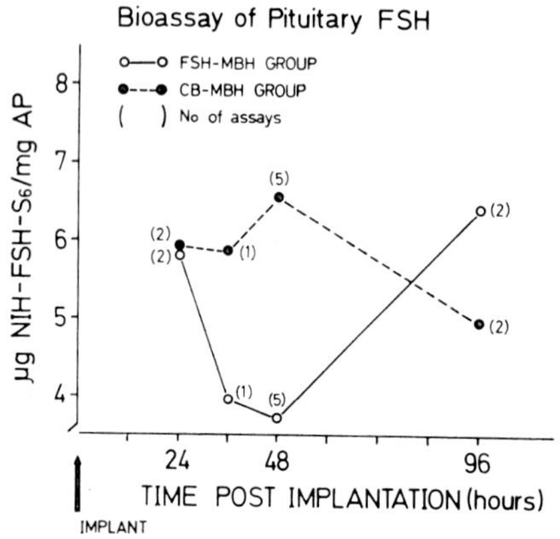

Fig. 7. Depletion of pituitary FSH following implantation of FSH in the MBH (○——○). Compare the results with the control implanted with CB in the MBH (●---●). The rats were implanted with 27-gauge needles immediately after ovariectomy. FSH was determined by the Steelmann-Pohley method injecting the equivalent of 1 pituitary per assay rat. Each point represents the mean value obtained from the total number of assays run. The points at 48 hours are significantly different ($p < 0.05$).
In each assay both the pituitary of the control and the experimental groups were run simultaneously.

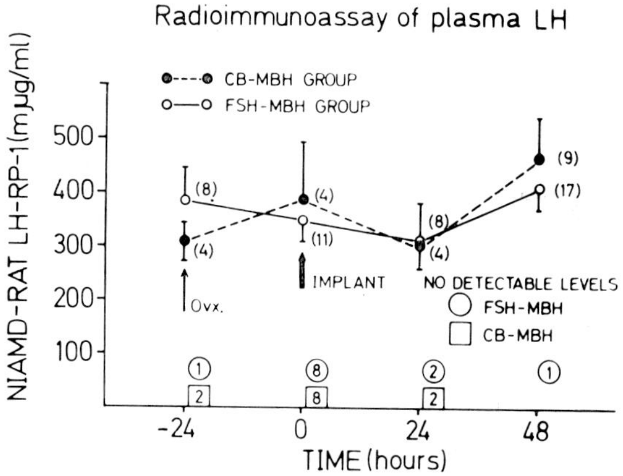

Fig. 8. Effect of FSH-MBH implants on plasma LH concentration of 24-hour ovariect omized rats Mean value ± SEM. Undetectable levels: FSH-MBH ○
CB-MBH □
The implantation was carried out 24 hours after ovariectomy. It is clear that LH concentration determined by radioimmunoassay is not changed by FSH-MBH implants.

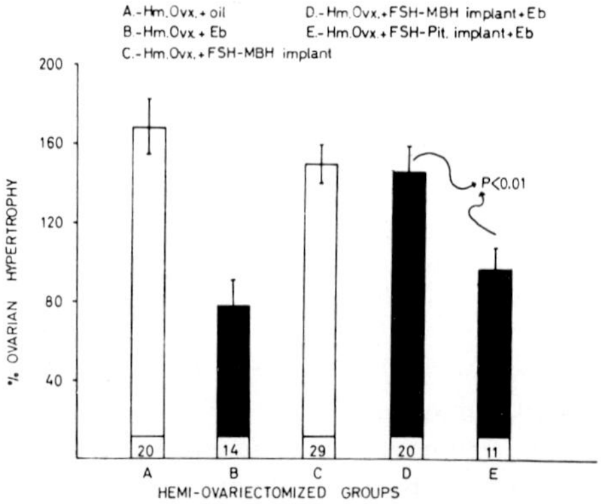

Fig. 9. Effect of estradiol benzoate (Eb) treatment on compensatory ovarian hypertrophy (COH) of hemicastrated immature rats without implants and in rats bearing MBH-FSH or adenohypophyseal implants. Groups B, D and E were treated daily with 0.1 µg Eb for 10 days after hemiovariectomy. Vertical lines indicate standard error of the mean. Number inside the bars indicate number of animals used. Hm.Ovx-hemiovariectomy; FSH-MBH implants of FSH in the medial basal hypothalamus; FSH-Pit implants of FSH in the anterior pituitary (from *Endocrinology*, *86*, 50, 1970).

release of FSH-RF which secondarily modifies the release of pituitary FSH. This has been clearly shown by the experiments of Corvin *et al.* (1970).

If one hemiovariectomizes 30–31-day-old rats and places FSH locally in the MBH there is an obvious COH 10 days later, as can be seen in Figure 9. The most interesting finding in this type of preparation was the demonstration that FSH implanted in the MBH was capable of blocking the inhibitory effect of systemic estrogen on COH. The animals received 24 hours after implantation and hemicastration 0.1 μg of estradiol benzoate daily for 10 days.

Control animals bearing an FSH implant in the pituitary or withour an implant showed the characteristic inhibition of COH. The effect of estrogen was only blocked by FSH-MBH implants since LH-MBH implants or LTH-MBH implants were not able to inhibit the effect of estrogen on COH, as shown in Figure 10.

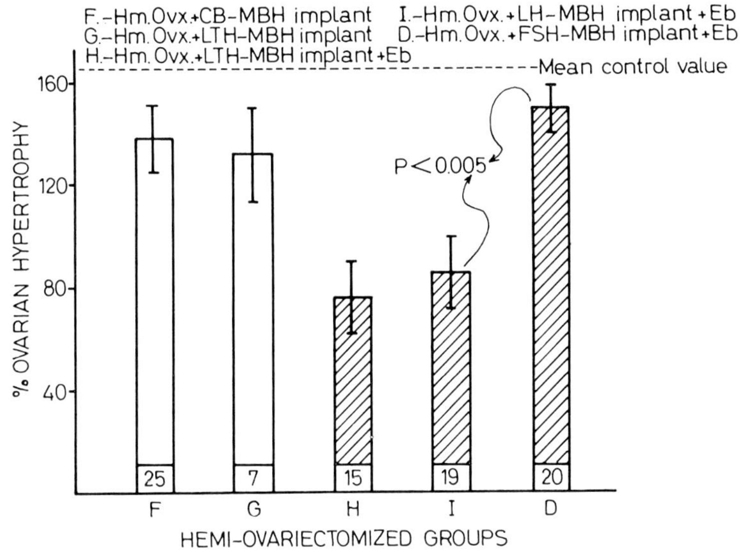

Fig. 10. COH in rats implanted with CB, LH, LTH or FSH in MBH with or without EB (0.1 μg daily × 10 days treatment). The mean control value represents the mean COH present in hemicastrated rats injected with oil. Total number of rats used inside the bars. CB-MBH implants of cocoa butter in the medial basal hypothalamus; LTH-MBH implants of prolactin; LH-MBH implants of LH (from *Endocrinology*, *86*, 50, 1970).

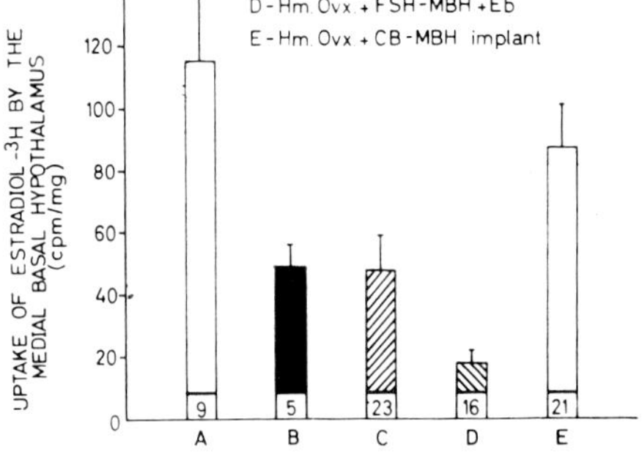

Fig. 11. Uptake of 17-β-6,7-^{3}H-estradiol by the MBH in hemiovariectomized rats with implants of FSH or CB in the MBH or without implants. Mean ± SEM are shown. Total number of rats used inside the bars. The net counts were obtained subtracting the free compartment of estrogen from the bound compartment according to the procedure described by Eisenfeld (1967). The same procedure has been carried out in all the figures where the results are expressed as cpm/mg.

In another experiment (Fig. 11) these same animals received 1 hour before being killed a single injection of 25 μC of 17-β-6, 7-^{3}H-estradiol i.p. It can be seen that the rats bearing FSH-MBH implants showed lower ^{3}H-estradiol uptake than the control animals bearing CB-MBH implants ($p < 0.01$). When the rats received cold estrogen (0.1 μg daily for 10 days) previous to the single-label estrogen pulse, the uptake was even lower.

This peculiar action of FSH-implants is not limited to immature rats but is also present in adult animals. Figure 12 presents the results in hemiovariectomized adult rats bearing different FSH implants. It also shows, close to the SE of each column, the values of pituitary FSH expressed as μg/mg (NIH-FSH-S6 equivalents). It is evident that rats treated with estrogen (2 μg daily for 10 days) and bearing FSH implants in the cortex, pituitary, or implanted with cocoa butter (CB) in the MBH or without implants, presented a marked

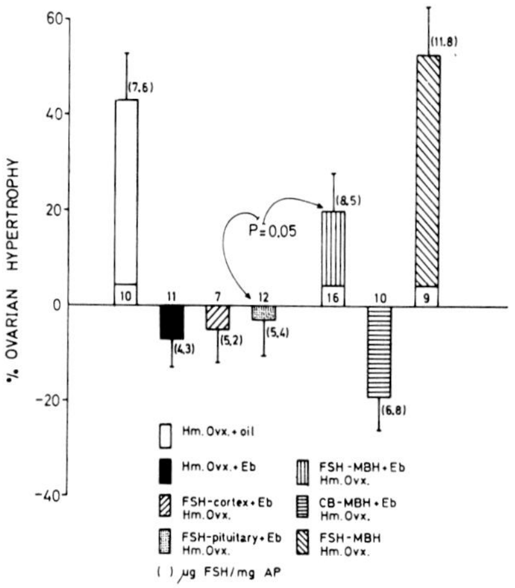

Fig. 12. COH in hemiovariectomized adult rats bearing different implants, untreated or treated with estrogen (2 μg $\times$ 10 days). Pituitary FSH determinations were made by bioassay. Number of rats employed in the differents groups is indicated on the x-axis. Mean values $\pm$ SEM are presented. Close to the vertical line of each column (SE) is shown the concentration of FSH determined in each group.

inhibition of COH. On the other hand, rats bearing FSH-MBH implants and treated with estrogen similarly to the other groups did have some degree of COH that was significantly different ($p < 0.01$). Also, the rats bearing FSH-MBH implants showed a greater ovarian hypertrophy than the controls without implants. Furthermore, the concentration of FSH in the rats bearing FSH-MBH implants and treated with estrogen was significantly higher than all the other estrogen-treated groups bearing FSH implants in other regions, or with CB-MBH implant. Interestingly enough, the concentration of FSH in the pituitary glands of rats with FSH-MBH implants and treated with estrogen was higher than in the controls without implants and estrogen treatment.

Thus, all these results tend to support the idea that FSH blocks the effect of estrogen upon certain pituitary functions that require the normal connections of the hypothalamic-pituitary unit.

In order to clarify this hypothesis we decided to study the action *in vivo* of an acute injection of exogenous FSH (kindly given to us by Dr. Parlow) upon the uptake of estradiol by the MBH of 24-hour ovariectomized rats or hypophysectomized animals. Figure 13 shows that 100 μg of FSH injected intravenously 30 minutes before a single i.p. injection of labeled estrogen were able to block, 1 hour later, the ability of the MBH area of ovariectomized animals to pick up estrogen. This was not true when the FSH was injected 15 minutes previous to the labeled estrogen, because the value found 1 hour later was similar to the one observed in rats receiving only labeled estrogen at time zero.

Since pituitary gonadotrophin secretion might alter the uptake of ^{3}H-estradiol, 8–9-day

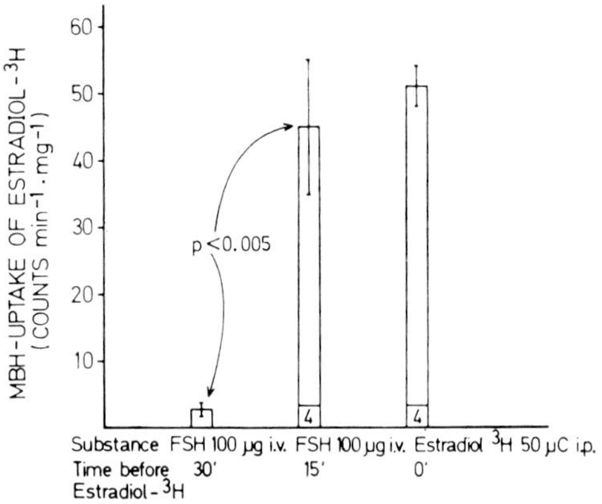

Fig. 13. Blocking action of FSH upon uptake of ^{3}H-estradiol by the MBH in 24-hour ovariectomized rats. One hundred μg of FSH was given intravenously 30 minutes and 15 minutes previous to a single i.p. injection of 50 μC of tritiated estradiol. All the animals were killed 1 hour later by bleeding under light ether anesthesia. Mean $\pm$ SEM are shown. The net counts shown were obtained subtracting the free compartment (pons tissue) of estrogen from the bound compartment according to the procedure of Eisenfeld (1967).

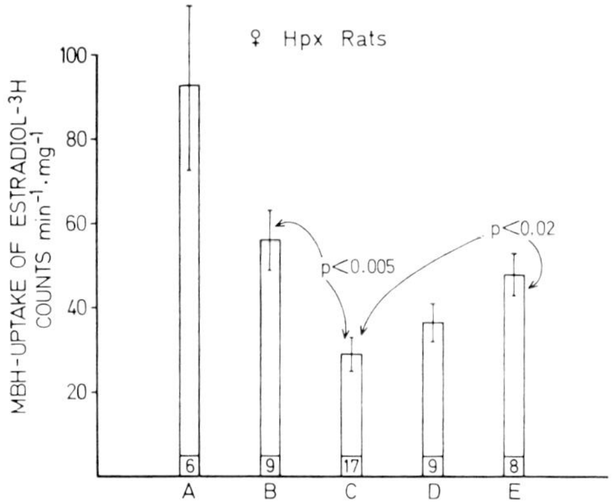

Fig. 14. Effect of different substances on the uptake of H^3-estradiol by the MBH of 8-day hypophy sectomized rats. Each female animal was injected i.v. with either saline (A, 0.1 ml), albumin (B, 100 μg), FSH (C, 100 μg), LH (D, 100 μg), or prolactin (E, 100 μg) 30′ previous to a single i.p. injection of tritiated estradiol (50 μC). Mean $\pm$ SEM are indicated.

hypophysectomized rats were prepared and injections of several substances 30 minutes previous to a single labeled estradiol pulse were given i.v. The results of this procedure can be seen in Figure 14 and their analysis shows that all the substances decrease the ability of the MBH area to concentrate the estradiol from the blood. However, the most effective substances were apparently FSH and LH (notice that LH was given in very high doses relatively to FSH). Since the blood level in each of the animals studied can be different, and was in fact, the results are expressed in Figure 15 as the ratio between radioactivity detected in the MBH (counts/mg) and the blood radioactivity (counts/μl). This particular way of expressing the results indicates that estradiol uptake is practically zero in the case of prolactin and close to unity in the case of FSH.

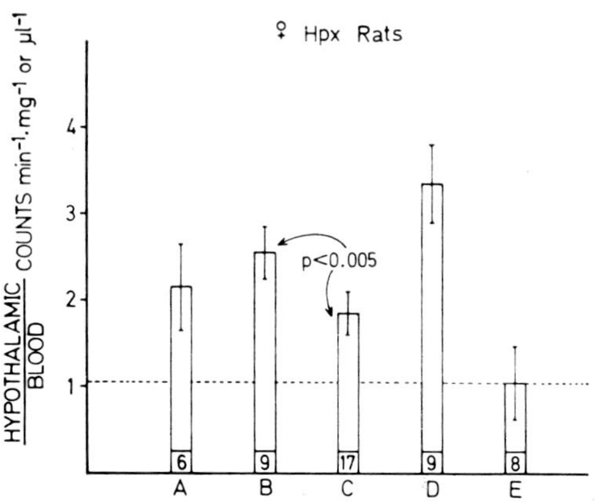

Fig. 15. Hypothalamic: blood radioactivity ratio calculated from the animals of Fig. 14. Notice that FSH and prolactin are the most effective hormones in blocking the uptake of tritiated estradiol by MBH if the results are expressed in this way. Mean $\pm$ SEM are shown.

Summing up the evidence so far presented, we may elaborate the following hypothesis: in the MBH of the diencephalon of the rat there exists a macromolecule able to bind estrogen which has been tentatively called a 'receptor'. It is possible that the first step in the chain of physiological events initiated by estrogen at hypothalamic level is the binding of estrogen to this receptor. On the other hand, we have demonstrated *in vivo*, both in acute and chronic experiments, that FSH competes with estrogen in such a way that it reduces the uptake of estrogen by the MBH area, and blocks the inhibitory effect of estrogen on compensatory ovarian hypertrophy. There are also apparently other hormones, such as prolactin or LH, that may alter the uptake of estrogen by the MBH. The physiological meaning of these findings will be revealed by future experimentation.

ACKNOWLEDGMENTS

The authors wish to thank Mr. Victor Saldivia, for his valuable help, and Mrs. Marcia González and Miss Silvia Neira for their kind assistance in preparing this manuscript.

REFERENCES

BENSON, B., SORRENTINO, S. and EVANS, J. S. (1969): Increase in serum FSH following unilateral ovariectomy in the rat. *Endocrinology*, *84*, 369.

BOWERS, C. Y., SCHALLY, A. V., ENZMANN, F. BØLER, J. and FOLKERS, K. (1970): Porcine thyrotropin releasing hormone is (Pyro) Glu-His-Pro (NH_2). *Endocrinology*, *86*, 1143.

CONWELL, H. A. and GREENWALD, G. S. (1969): Autoradiographic analysis of estradiol uptake in the brain and pituitary of the female rat. *Endocrinology*, *85*, 1160.

CORVIN, A., DANIELS, E. L. and MILMORE, J. E. (1970): An internal feedback mechanism controlling follicle stimulating hormone releasing factor. *Endocrinology*, *86*, 735.

EISENFELD, A. J. (1969): Hypothalamic oestradiol-binding macromolecules. *Nature*, *224*, 1202.

EISENFELD, A. J. and AXELROD, J. (1966): Effect of steroid hormones, ovariectomy, estrogen pretreatment, sex and immaturity on the distribution of H^3-estradiol. *Endocrinology*, *79*, 38.

FENDLER, K. and ENDRÖCZI (1965): Effects of hypothalamic steroid implants on compensatory ovarian hypertrophy of rats. *Neuroendocrinology*, *1*, 129.

ISAO KAHWANAGO, LEROY HEINRICHS, W. and HERRMANN, WALTER L. (1969): Isolation of oestradiol 'receptors' from bovine hypothalamus and anterior pituitary gland. *Nature (Lond.)*, *223*, 313.

JENSEN, E. V., SUZUKI, T., KAWASHIMA, T., STUMPF, W. E., JUNGBLUT, P. W. and DESOMBRE, E. R. (1968): A two-step mechanism for the interaction of estradiol with rat uterus. *Proc. nat. Acad. Sci. (Wash,). 59*, 632.

KATO, J. and VILLEE, C. A. (1967): Factors affecting uptake of estradiol-6,7 H^3 by the hypophysis and hypothalamus. *Endocrinology, 80*, 1133.

MCCANN, S. M. and PORTER, J. C. (1969): Hypothalamic pituitary stimulating and inhibiting hormones. *Physiol. Rev., 49*, 240.

MOTTA, M., FRASCHINI, F. and MARTINI, L. (1969): 'Short' feedback mechanism in the control of anterior pituitary function. In: *Frontiers in Neuroendocrinology*. p. 211. Editors: F. Ganong and L. Martini. Oxford University Press, London.

NAGASAWA, H., CHEN, C. L. and MEITES, J. (1969): Effects of estrogen implant in median eminence on serum and pituitary prolactin levels in the rat. *Proc. Soc. exp. Biol. (N.Y.), 132*, 859.

PALKA, Y. S., RAMIREZ, V. D. and SAWYER, C. H. (1966): Distribution and biological effects of tritiated estradiol implanted in the hypothalamo-hypophysial region of female rats. *Endocrinology, 78*, 487.

PFAFF, D. W. (1968): Uptake of H^3-estradiol by the female rat brain. An autoradiographic study. *Endocrinology, 82*, 1149, 1155.

PRESL, J., RÖHLING, S., HORSKY, J. and HERZMANN, J. (1970): Changes in uptake of H^3-estradiol by the female rat brain and pituitary from birth to sexual maturity. *Endocrinology, 86*, 899.

RAMIREZ, V. D. and MCCANN, S. M. (1964): Induction of prolactin secretion by implants of estrogen into the hypothalamo-hypophysial region of female rats. *Endocrinology, 75*, 206.

SOLOFF, M. S. and SZEGO, CLARA M. (1969): Purification of estradiol receptor from rat uterus and blockade of its estrogen binding function by specific antibody. *Biochem. biophys. Res. Commun. 34*, 141.

STUMPF, W. E. (1968*a*): Cellular and subcellular localization of H^3-estradiol in target and non-target tissues by autoradiography. In: Abstracts, *III International Congress of Endocrinology, Mexico*, 1968, p. 10. Editor: C. Gual. ICS No. 157. Excerpta Medica, Amsterdam.

STUMPF, W. E. (1968*b*): Estradiol-concentrating neurons: topography in the hypothalamus by dry-mount autoradiography. *Science, 162*, 1001.

VALE, W., BURGUS, R., DUNN, T. F. and GUILLEMIN, R. (1970): Release of TSH by oral administration of synthetic peptide derivatives with TRF activity. *J. clin. Endocr., 30*, 148.

NEONATAL HORMONAL EFFECTS AND ENVIRONMENTAL STIMULATION ON BRAIN DEVELOPMENT AND BEHAVIOR

SHAWN SCHAPIRO*

Developmental Neuroendocrinology Laboratory, Veterans Administration Hospital, San Fernando, California, and Department of Psychiatry, University of California, Los Angeles, California, U.S.A.

It is generally recognized that environmental influences during certain periods of early post-natal life have an effect upon later development and behavior. In many species this perinatal period of CNS plasticity is also characterized by behavioral and homeostatic immaturity. The primary responsibility of the neonate is to survive. It therefore seemed possible that this perinatal functional immaturity may ensure a relatively stable biochemical climate for developing neurones during periods in their ontogenesis when environmental stimuli are having an organizing influence upon the CNS. It may also aid survival of the newborn and/or optimize survival potential at later stages of the life cycle. To test this assumption, infant rats from separate litters received (1) large amounts of either thyroxine or cortisol or (2) a wide range of sensory stimuli superimposed on their normal neonatal routine. The following observations were made:

Neonatal corticoid administration

(1) impairs later immunological reactivity; (2) delays behavioral, neurophysiological and biochemical development of the brain; (3) retards the ontogeny of the cerebral cortical pyramidal cell and its fine dendritic structure; and (4) results in a consistent, non-statistically significant, improvement in performance on several learning tasks.

Neonatal thyroxine administration

(1) accelerates biochemical, behavioral and neurophysiological development of the brain; (2) advances the ontogeny of the pyramidal cell and its dendritic structure; (3) improves the learning ability of infant rats, but impairs learning ability of older animals.

Extra sensory stimulation during the pre-weaning period

(1) increases the rate of development of the cortical pyramidal cell and its fine dendritic structure; (2) increases the ontogeny of total EEG energy output; (3) increases brain acetylcholinesterase activity.

These results indicate that both sensory stimuli impinging on the growing neurone and the hormonal climate in which this is occurring may play an important role in determining the rate of functional and organizational development of the brain.

---

* Deceased.

THYROCALCITONIN

CONTENTS

SECRETION OF THYROCALCITONIN AND ITS REGULATION*

CARY W. COOPER**, T. KENNEY GRAY***,
JAMES D. HUNDLEY† and AHMED M. MAHGOUB

Department of Pharmacology, School of Medicine, University of North Carolina, Chapel Hill, N. C., U.S.A.

Since the initial development of the calcitonin concept (Copp *et al.*, 1962) and the subsequent discovery (Hirsch *et al.*, 1963) of thyrocalcitonin (TC), additional evidence has been obtained demonstrating that the secretion of this hypocalcemic, hypophosphatemic hormone from the mammalian thyroid gland is regulated by the concentration of calcium in the blood (reviewed in Hirsch and Munson, 1969).

During the last five years, several studies attempting to elucidate more fully the control of secretion of TC (Care *et al.*, 1968*a*; *b*; Lee *et al.*, 1969; Cooper *et al.*, 1971) and the possible physiological factors which signal the thyroid gland to secrete increased amounts of hormone (Gray and Munson, 1969; Munson and Gray, 1970) have been reported. In our own laboratory Care *et al.* (1968*a*; *b*), by bioassay of thyroid venous effluent blood collected from the isolated, perfused thyroid gland, were able to demonstrate that the secretion of pig TC was directly proportional to the concentration of blood calcium at levels of calcium above normocalcemia. These studies were limited by the sensitivity of the bioassay method for TC to the measurement of hormone in hypercalcemic blood. However, the subsequent recent development by Deftos *et al.* (1968) of a radioimmunoassay for porcine TC has allowed us to further explore the relationship between blood calcium levels and TC secretion using the pig.

RADIOIMMUNOASSAY OF PORCINE TC

Details of the procedures for the radioimmunoassay of porcine TC have been described previously (Lee *et al.*, 1969; Deftos *et al.*, 1968). Free and antibody-bound ^{125}I-TC were separated by a double antibody precipitation procedure (Morgan and Lazarow, 1963).The concentration of hormone in each plasma sample was calculated by comparing the displacement of antibody-bound ^{125}I-TC produced by the sample to that produced by known amounts of pure porcine TC.

Figure 1 illustrates a representative radioimmunoassay response curve and also shows the presence of TC in two thyroid venous plasma samples obtained from a pig, one taken during

* This investigation was supported by a Research Grant from the National Institute of Arthritis and Metabolic Diseases (AM-10558) and by a U.S. Public Health Service Research Support Grant (FR-5406).

** Recipient of a Merck grant for faculty development.

*** U.S.P.H.S. Special Research Fellow 1968–70.

† Present address: Division of Orthopedics, Department of Surgery, University of North Carolina School of Medicine, Chapel Hill, North Carolina 27514.

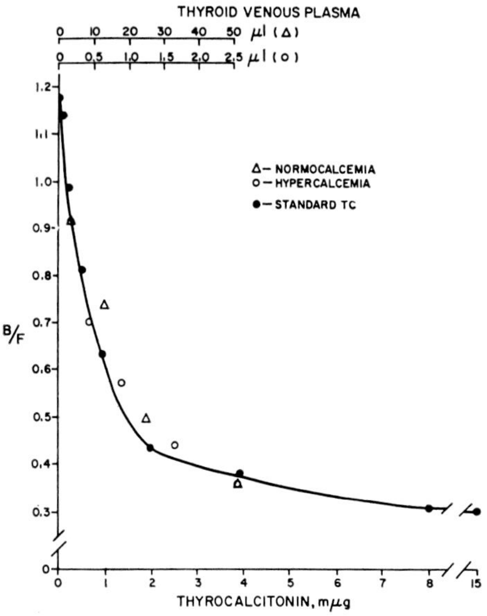

Fig. 1. Determination by radioimmunoassay of thyrocalcitonin (TC) in pig thyroid venous blood. Aliquots of 2 thyroid venous plasma samples from a pig, one (-Δ-) obtained during normocalcemia (11.2 mg Ca/100 ml) and one (-o-) taken during hypercalcemia (16.7 mg Ca/100 ml), produced a progressive displacement of antibody-bound ^{125}I-labeled TC (drop in ratio of bound to free ^{125}I-TC (B/F)) which was indistinguishable from that produced by pure porcine TC (-●-). The much smaller aliquots of hypercalcemic thyroid venous plasma required to produce a response, compared to normocalcemic plasma, illustrate the 20-fold increase in TC concentration in the thyroid effluent blood obtained during hypercalcemia. The pig was a male and weighed 17.5 kg. Final dilution of antiserum in the immunoassay was 1:100,000.

normocalcemia and one taken during hypercalcemia. Increasing aliquots of both plasma samples caused a progressive decrease in the ratio of bound to free labeled TC (B/F) which was indistinguishable from that produced by pure standard TC. Estimation of the concentration of TC in each aliquot of a given sample provides multiple estimates of the mean concentration of TC in that sample. The much smaller amounts of hypercalcemic thyroid venous plasma required to obtain a response (decrease in B/F), compared to normocalcemic plasma, demonstrates about a 20-fold increase in the TC concentration in the hypercalcemic sample.

MEASUREMENT OF SECRETION OF PIG TC BY RADIOIMMUNOASSAY

Experimental procedures involving anesthesia, surgical isolation of the *in situ* pig thyroid gland, and the continuous and complete collection of thyroid venous effluent blood from the heparinized animal have been described previously (Care *et al.*, 1968*a*).

Figure 2 shows one of our representative, earlier experiments in the pig in which large changes in plasma calcium levels were deliberately induced by systemic infusion of first calcium chloride and then EDTA. After isolation of the thyroid vein, thyroid venous effluent blood was continuously and completely collected. The thyroid gland continued to receive blood from the thyroid artery but no venous effluent blood was permitted to reenter the systemic circulation. The results shown in Figure 2 illustrate the sequential changes in concentrations of immunoreactive TC in thyroid venous plasma and peripheral (femoral arterial) plasma which occurred following experimental elevation or reduction of the blood calcium concentration. Within minutes after induction of hypercalcemia, TC concentrations in thyroid venous blood rose several hundredfold to 2000–3000 mμg/ml. A decline in blood calcium to hypocalcemic levels after EDTA was matched by an equally rapid fall in TC to essentially undetectable levels. Since the thyroid venous blood was not allowed to reenter the general circulation, peripheral (femoral arterial) hormone concentrations did not rise in response to the hypercalcemic challenge. The results of this and other similar experiments agreed with our earlier bioassay results (Care *et al.*, 1968*a*; *b*) in showing that the concentration of TC in blood leaving the thyroid gland was directly proportional to the existing concentration of

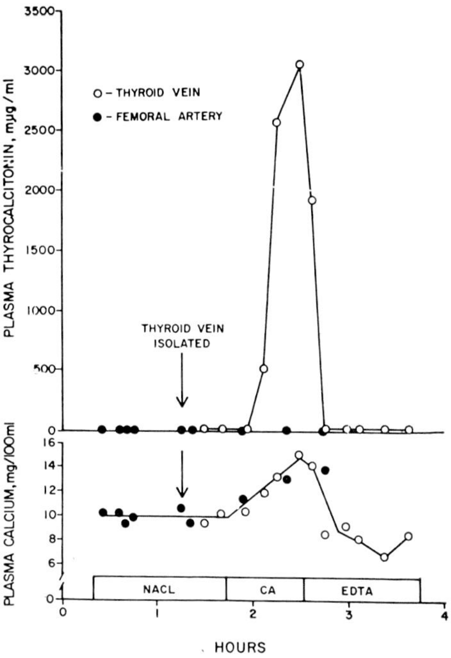

Fig. 2. Changes in the concentration of TC in thyroid venous effluent plasma of a fasted pig (♂, 26 kg) after sequential induction of systemic hyper- and hypocalcemia. Hypercalcemia was produced by i.v. infusion (femoral vein) of 0.11 M calcium chloride at rates of 3–5 ml/min; hypocalcemia by infusion of 1.25% disodium EDTA at a rate of 3 ml/min. A control period of infusion with 0.15 M NaCl preceded the infusions of Ca and EDTA. The duration of administration of these solutions is shown in blocks in the lower portion of the figure. Vertical arrows (↓) indicate the time at which the thyroid vein was isolated and complete, continuous collection of thyroid venous effluent blood was begun. Each point in the bottom graph represents the plasma calcium concentration in either a thyroid venous plasma sample (-o-) or a femoral arterial plasma sample (-●-). Each point in the top graph represents the mean concentration of TC determined by radioimmunoassay in 3-5 aliquots of each of these same plasma samples. From C. W. Cooper *et al.* (1971).

blood calcium. Since blood flow rates through the thyroid gland remained approximately constant throughout each experiment, the changes in hormone concentration represented changes in the secretion rate of TC.

We also concluded from these earlier experiments that the thyroid gland was extremely sensitive to changes in the blood calcium level and that secretion of TC could rise rapidly more than a hundredfold in response to an acute hypercalcemic challenge (Cooper *et al.*, 1971).

PROTECTION BY THYROID GLAND AGAINST HYPERCALCEMIA–NORMAL FUNCTION?

Our more recent studies in the pig have been designed to examine possible physiological conditions for stimulation of secretion of TC – namely, absorption of calcium from the gastrointestinal tract. Presumably such stimulation of TC would provide additional circulating hormone which, in turn, could act on bone to counteract hypercalcemia.

Figure 3 illustrates the results of one of several recent experiments by Munson and Gray (1970) which show that the rat thyroid gland can protect against hypercalcemia following oral administration of a calcium salt at doses ranging from 10 to 80 mg calcium/kg body weight. In this particular experiment intragastric administration of 3 or 6 mg Ca^{++} to young rats, immediately after removal of their thyroid glands (by thyroparathyroidectomy), produced significant hypercalcemia one hour later. Similarly-treated rats with intact thyroid glands (SHAM) did not exhibit hypercalcemia one hour after gavage.

This finding prompted Gray and Munson (1969; Munson and Gray, 1970) to suggest that during rapid intestinal absorption of calcium the blood calcium level rises enough to stimulate an increased release of TC which, in turn, acts on bone to rapidly restore normocalcemia. However, this hypothesis raised two important questions which required further study:

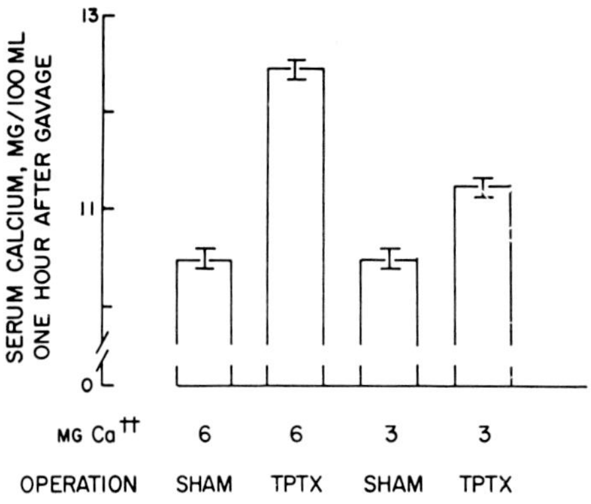

Fig. 3. Development of hypercalcemia in acutely thyroparathyroidectomized (TPTX) young rats 1 hour after intragastric administration of small amounts of calcium chloride. After being fasted for 48 hours, the rats were either TPTX or sham-operated and immediately given, via a stomach tube, a volume of 1% $CaCl_2$ sufficient to deliver either 3 or 6 mg Ca^{++}. One hour after gavage the rats were bled by cardiac puncture. The height of each bar represents the mean serum calcium concentration of a separate group of rats, and the vertical lines show the SE. From P. L. Munson and T. K. Gray (1970).

1. Does release of TC indeed increase following oral administration and subsequent intestinal absorption of calcium?
2. If the secretion of TC is increased, then what is the nature of the stimulus to the thyroid gland?

Since detectable elevation of the blood calcium level has not been observed in Ca-gavaged (Fig. 3) or parathyroid hormone-treated rats (Cooper *et al.*, 1970) when the thyroid gland was present, our working hypothesis has been that the thyroid gland is so sensitive to the concentration of calcium in the blood that it responds to increases too small to be detected by our analytical procedures for calcium (Gray and Munson, 1969; Munson and Gray, 1970; Cooper *et al.*, 1970).

STIMULATION OF PIG TC SECRETION BY INTRAGASTRIC CALCIUM

We have attempted to further explore the two questions just posed using the pig, because concentrations of TC in blood can be directly measured in this species using the radioimmunoassay. Our initial studies involved measuring the concentrations of TC in the thyroid venous plasma of young, fasted pigs following intragastric administration of calcium. The results of several experiments are shown in Figures 4–7. As in the experiment shown in Figure 2, after isolation of the thyroid vein the effluent venous blood was collected continuously.

Figure 4 shows an experiment in which a pig was administered sufficient calcium chloride via an intragastric tube to deliver a total dose of 20 mg Ca/kg body weight. Despite the fact that no detectable hypercalcemia became evident during the period following the calcium gavage, the TC concentration in thyroid venous blood rose 2- to 3-fold within about 30 minutes. Since blood flow rates through the thyroid gland remained approximately constant throughout the experiment, the increase in TC concentration represented an increase in the secretion rate of the hormone. As expected, peripheral TC levels did not rise.

Figure 5 shows a similar experiment. However, in this study calcium was administered intragastrically at 2-dose levels during the 4-hour experiment (10 mg Ca/kg and 40 mg Ca/kg). With this pig, also, no consistent elevation in plasma calcium was detected after oral calcium administration. However, even after oral administration of the lower dose of calcium (10 mg/kg), the TC concentration in thyroid venous blood approximately doubled, and a further elevation of TC was observed after the second gavage (40 mg/kg). Systemic i.v. infusion of calcium toward the end of the experiment produced hypercalcemia, and TC secretion rose markedly, indicating that the secretory capacity of the gland greatly exceeded that demanded by even the largest oral dose of calcium given.

Figure 6 shows the results of another pig experiment in which 3 doses of calcium were sequentially administered intragastrically (10, 20 and 40 mg Ca/kg). Again there was no

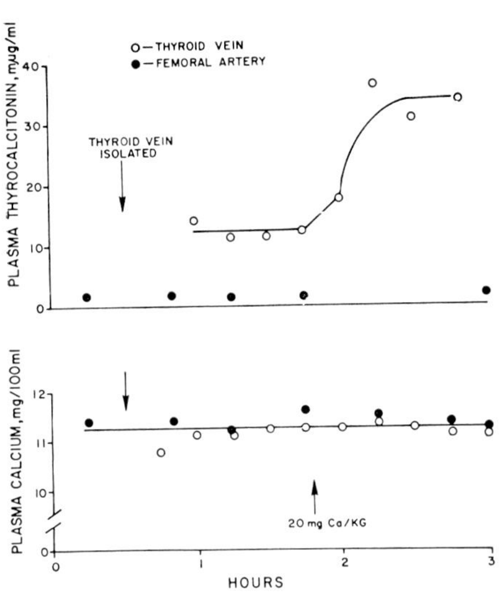

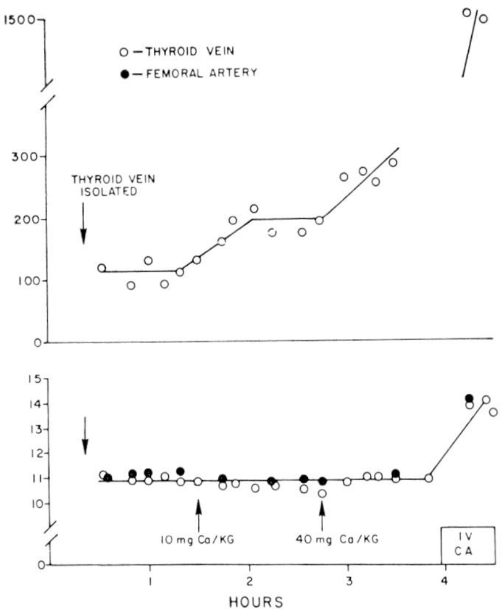

Fig. 4. Increase in the concentration of TC in the thyroid venous plasma of a fasted pig (♀, 16.5 kg) after intragastric administration of calcium. A volume of 2% calcium chloride sufficient to deliver 20 mg Ca/kg body weight was given rapidly via a feeding tube at the time indicated by the vertical arrow (↑). See Fig. 2 legend for additional explanation.

Fig. 5. Increase in the concentration of TC in the thyroid venous plasma of a fasted pig (♀, 16 kg) after intragastric administration of calcium at 2 dose levels (10 and 40 mg Ca/kg). See legends of Figs. 2 and 4 for additional explanation.

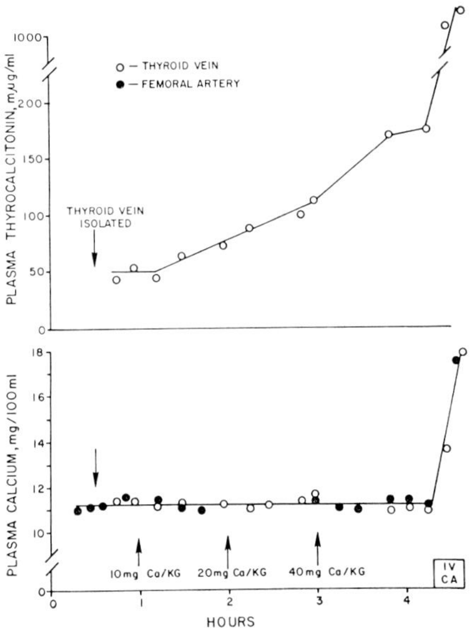

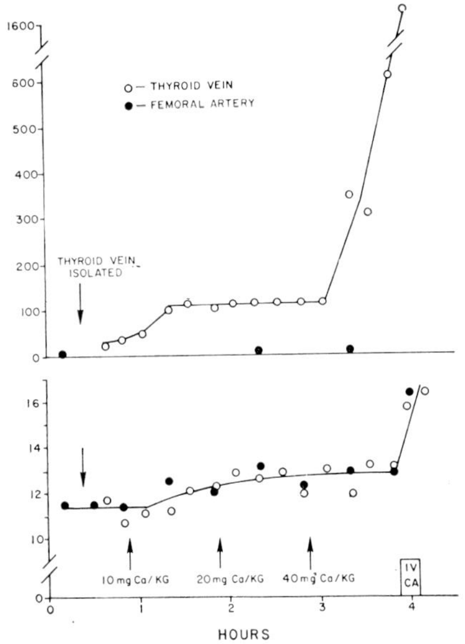

Fig. 6. Increase in the concentration of TC in the thyroid venous plasma of a fasted pig (♀, 15,2 kg) after intragastric administration of calcium sequentially at 3 dose levels (10, 20, and 40 mg Ca/kg). See legends of Figs. 2 and 4 for additional explanation.

Fig. 7. Increase in the concentration of TC in the thyroid venous plasma of a fasted pig (♀ ,22.5 kg) after intragastric administration of calcium sequentially at 3 dose levels (10, 20, and 40 mg Ca/kg). See legends of Figs. 2 and 4 for additional explanation.

obvious elevation in the plasma calcium concentration after oral calcium administration. However, the TC concentration in thyroid venous blood rose approximately 2-fold during the first few hours and reached concentrations approaching 4 times greater than basal by the period just before calcium was infused. In this experiment, sufficient calcium to produce hypercalcemia again evoked a further marked rise in TC concentration.

When this experiment was repeated in another pig (Fig. 7) some elevation of the plasma calcium concentration appeared to occur after oral administration of calcium. The concentration of TC in thyroid effluent blood (but not femoral arterial blood) rose even after the first gavage and remained at a fairly constant level after about a 4-fold increase. Within 30 minutes after the highest oral dose of calcium (40 mg/kg) was given, the concentration of hormone rose further and reached levels at least 10 times greater than those observed at the beginning of the experiment. Again marked hypercalcemia, produced by i.v. calcium, caused a further stimulation of TC secretion.

STIMULATION OF PIG TC SECRETION BY INCREASED INTESTINAL ABSORPTION OF CALCIUM

In the series of experiments just presented (Figs. 4–7), neither consistent nor dramatic changes in blood calcium were observed after intragastric administration of calcium at doses (10–40 mg/kg) corresponding to those used in rats by Munson and Gray (Fig. 2; Gray and Munson, 1969; Munson and Gray, 1970). However, since increased secretion of TC occurred, we inferred that increased intestinal absorption of calcium must somehow be involved in the signal to the thyroid gland. In order to evaluate this possibility, our most recent studies have involved *in vivo* measurement of calcium absorption across a 30-cm test segment of pig jejunum according to the method described by Wensel *et al.* (1969). A triple-lumen polyvinyl tube was used for both intraluminal perfusion of solutions and sampling of intestinal contents by aspiration. Polyethylene glycol was employed as a nonabsorbable concentration marker. The total amounts of calcium delivered into the intestinal lumen during these experiments ranged from 5 to 30 mg Ca/kg body weight, dose-levels which were similar to those administered intragastrically in the studies just presented (Figs. 4–7).

In the experiment shown in Figure 8, solutions, with or without added calcium, were perfused directly into the jejunum. Concentrations of calcium were chosen to deliver 24 or 72 mg Ca/hour, and these solutions were administered for 1½ to 2 hours. Irrespective of whether or not calcium was perfused, little change in plasma calcium levels occurred. Intestinal perfusion of 24 mg Ca/hour produced a limited increase in intestinal absorption of calcium, and thyroid venous TC concentrations did not increase. However, following introduction of the higher amount of calcium (72 mg/hour) into the intestinal lumen, a 2- to 3-fold increase in TC concentration occurred, and the pattern of this increase appeared to reflect that observed in intestinal absorption of calcium.

Figure 9 illustrates that perfusion of the pig jejunum with even higher amounts of calcium (72 and 216 mg Ca/hour) produced even higher rates of intestinal calcium absorption. Plasma calcium levels in this pig may have risen slightly following the initiation of perfusion with calcium. A rapid increase in the concentration of TC in thyroid venous blood occurred shortly after the introduction of calcium into the intestinal lumen (again, like Figure 8, at 72 mg Ca/hour), and the concentration of hormone continued to increase throughout the course of the experiment reaching levels about 4 times greater than those found initially by the time the experiment was terminated. These marked changes in the concentration of TC in thyroid effluent blood appeared to reflect the large increases in calcium absorption observed during intestinal perfusion of calcium.

Figure 10 represents an experiment similar to the previous two, except that calcium was perfused at the outset of the study and collection of thyroid venous blood was not begun until after initiation of perfusion with a calcium-free solution. At the time we began to collect

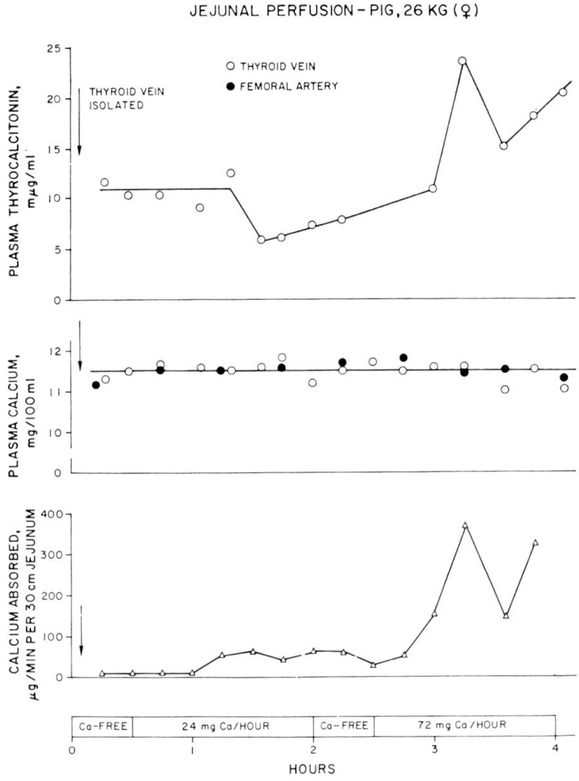

Fig. 8. Increase in the concentration of TC in the thyroid venous plasma of a fasted pig (♀, 26 kg) during increased intestinal absorption of calcium and in the absence of detectable hypercalcemia. The upper and middle graphs show the changes in plasma calcium and TC concentration as before (see Fig. 2 legend). The bottom graph shows the measured values of calcium absorption across a 30 cm test segment of jejunum during the treatments whose duration is indicated in blocks at the bottom of the figure. These blocks show the times during which a buffered isotonic saline solution containing either 2 mM Ca (24 mg Ca/hour), 6 mM Ca (72 mg Ca/hour), or no Ca (Ca-free) was perfused intraluminally at a rate of 5 ml/min. A triple-lumen polyvinyl tube was used for perfusion and sampling of intestinal contents according to the method described by Wensel *et al.* (1969). Polyethylene glycol was used as the non-absorbable dilution-concentration marker.

thyroid venous blood, TC levels appeared to be falling, reaching a baseline only after the calcium perfusion had been re-initiated. Thus the changes in hormone secretion reflected, but appeared to lag behind, the observed changes in calcium absorption, perhaps because a decrease in TC secretion from a high level (produced by increased intestinal absorption of calcium) requires a longer period of time than stimulation of secretion from a baseline level.

CONCLUSIONS

Physiological condition leading to stimulation of secretion of TC

The results of our studies involving measurement of secretion of TC in the pig by radioimmunoassay provide some answers to the two questions posed at the outset of this presentation.

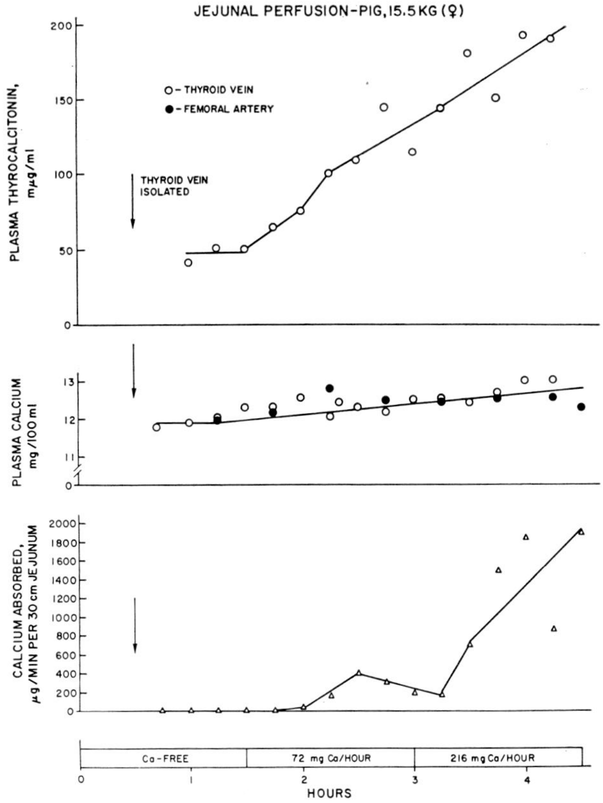

Fig. 9. Increase in the concentration of TC in the thyroid venous plasma of a fasted pig (♀, 15.5 kg) during increased intestinal absorption of calcium. The solutions perfused into the jejunum contained either 6 mM Ca (72 mg Ca/hour), 18 mM Ca (216 mg Ca/hour), or no Ca (Ca-free). See Fig. 8 legend for complete explanation.

In answer to our first question 'Does release of TC increase after oral administration of calcium?', we feel that the results of our studies directly demonstrate that the introduction of calcium into the gastrointestinal tract produces an increased absorption of calcium which is followed by an increased release of TC from the thyroid gland. This increased release of hormone occurs even when there is no detectable increase in the plasma calcium concentration.

However, because increased TC secretion does occur in the absence of detectable hypercalcemia, the answer to our second question 'What is the nature of the stimulus to the thyroid gland?' is less easily resolved.

Nature of the stimulus for increased secretion of TC following increased gastrointestinal absorption of calcium.

The results shown in Figure 11 were drawn from earlier studies in two pigs, one of which was presented in Figure 2. In Figure 11 we have plotted TC concentrations in thyroid venous plasma samples against the concentrations of plasma calcium in the same samples. The plasma calcium levels in both animals were deliberately altered markedly by i.v. administration of calcium or EDTA so that regression curves could be calculated. Although the slope

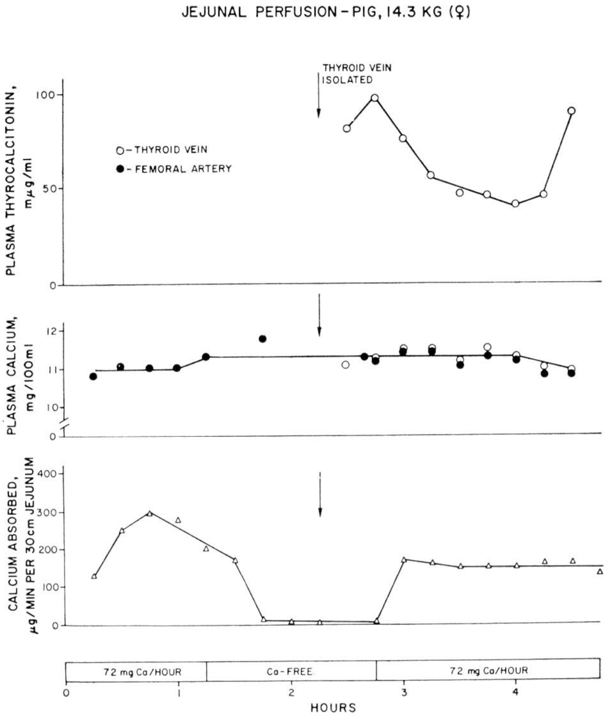

Fig. 10. Changes in the concentration of TC in the thyroid venous plasma of a fasted pig (♀, 14.3 kg) during changes in intestinal absorption of calcium. The solutions perfused into the jejunum contained either 6 mM Ca (72 mg Ca/hour) or no Ca (Ca-free). See Fig. 8 legend for complete explanation.

of the curve varies among individual animals (as previously noted: Care *et al.*, 1968*a*; Lee *et al.*, 1969), the steepness of the slopes of the two curves shown in Figure 11 is apparent. Using the slopes of these two curves, one can calculate that an increase in the concentration of TC in thyroid venous blood in the order of 2- to 4-fold from normocalcemic baseline levels of 10–50 mμg/ml would require only a minor elevation in plasma calcium – as little as 0.1 to 0.3 mg/100 ml. This calculation is in harmony with the results of our studies shown in Figures 4–10 which illustrate that such increases in TC concentration in thyroid venous blood can be detected during changes in blood calcium too small to be detected with surety by our present analytical procedures for blood calcium.

Our findings do not eliminate the possibility that factors other than absorbed calcium – perhaps gastrointestinal in origin – may be involved in the stimulation of secretion of TC. For example, Care (1970) has suggested that secretion of pancreozymin, in response to increased absorption of calcium, may stimulate secretion of TC. In our own laboratory, we have entertained the possibility that 'gut glucagon' (Unger *et al.*, 1968) or a related gastrointestinal hormone might be involved in the stimulus to the thyroid gland following oral calcium administration. This idea seemed attractive particularly in view of the fact that under certain conditions pancreatic glucagon has been shown to increase release of TC from the pig thyroid gland (Cooper *et al.*, 1971; Care *et al.*, 1970). In our early exploratory studies along this line, we have on occasion seen a TC response to infusion of intestinal extract, but our results have been inconsistent.

At present our own findings support the hypothesis (Cooper *et al.*, 1970; 1971; Gray and

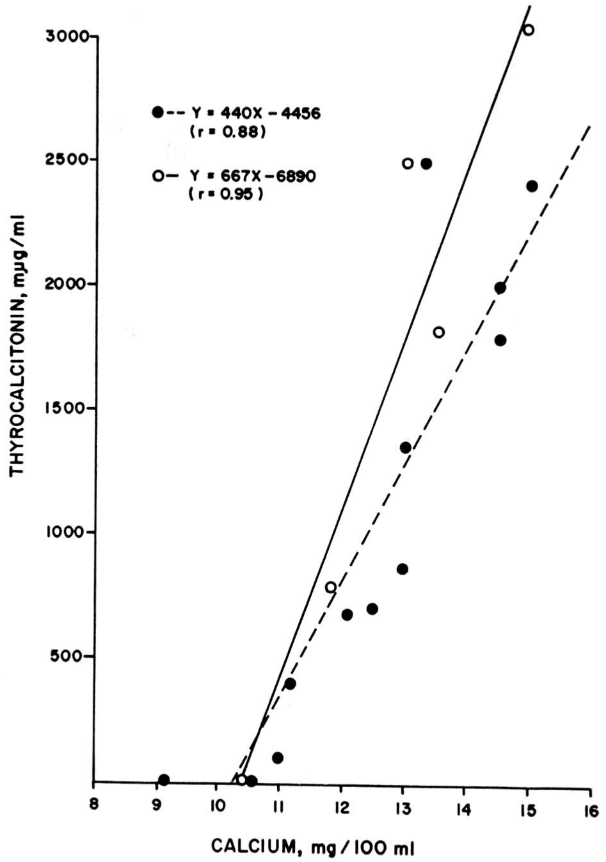

Fig. 11. Relationship between the concentrations of calcium (independent variable) and of TC (dependent variable) in the thyroid venous effluent blood of 2 pigs, one of which was shown in Fig. 2 (-o-) and one not shown (-●-). Regression equations are shown in the top left portion of the figure with the significant ($p < 0.01$) correlation coefficients (r) indicated in parentheses. From C. W. Cooper *et al.* (1971).

Munson, 1969; Munson and Gray, 1970) that the thyroid gland is extremely sensitive to small elevations in the concentration of calcium in blood and that even minor increases, occurring during absorption of calcium from the gastrointestinal tract, are sufficient to produce an increased secretion of TC which, in turn, acts to restrict hypercalcemia.

ACKNOWLEDGMENTS

We are indebted to Dr. Paul L. Munson and Dr. Philip F. Hirsch for their advice and encouragement during the course of this work and preparation of the manuscript.

REFERENCES

CARE, A. D. (1970): The effects of pancreozymin and secretin on calcitonin release. *Fed. Proc.*, *29*, 253 (abstract).

CARE, A. D., BATES, R. F. L. and GITELMAN, H. J. (1970): A possible role for the adenyl cyclase system in calcitonin release. *J. Endocr.*, *48*, 1.

CARE, A. D., COOPER, C. W., DUNCAN, T. and ORIMO, H. (1968*a*): A study of thyrocalcitonin secretion by direct measurement of *in vivo* secretion rates in pigs. *Endocrinology*, *83*, 161.

CARE, A. D., COOPER, C. W., DUNCAN, T. and ORIMO, H. (1968*b*): The direct measurement of thyrocalcitonin secretion rate *in vivo*. In: *Parathyroid Hormone and Thyrocalcitonin (Calcitonin)*, pp. 417–427. Editors: R. V. Talmage and L. F. Belanger. ICS No. 159. Excerpta Medica, Amsterdam.

COOPER, C. W., DEFTOS, L. J. and POTTS, J. T., JR. (1971): Direct measurement of *in vivo* secretion of pig thyrocalcitonin by radioimmunoassay. *Endocrinology*, *88*, 747.

COOPER, C. W., HIRSCH, P. F. and MUNSON, P. L. (1970): Importance of endogenous thyrocalcitonin for protection against hypercalcemia in the rat. *Endocrinology*, *86*, 406.

COPP, D. H., CAMERON, E. C., CHENEY, B. A., DAVIDSON, A. G. F. and HENZE, K. G. (1962): Evidence for calcitonin – a new hormone from the parathyroid that lowers blood calcium. *Endocrinology*, *70*, 638.

DEFTOS, L. J., LEE, M. R. and POTTS, J. T., JR. (1968): A radioimmunoassay for thyrocalcitonin. *Proc. Nat. Acad. Sci. (Wash.)*, *60*, 293.

GRAY, T. K. and MUNSON, P. L. (1969): Thyrocalcitonin: Evidence for physiological function. *Science*, *166*, 512.

HIRSCH, P. F., GAUTHIER, G. F. and MUNSON, P. L. (1963): Thyroid hypocalcemic principle and recurrent laryngeal nerve injury as factors affecting the response to parathyroidectomy in rats. *Endocrinology*, *73*, 244.

HIRSCH, P. F. and MUNSON, P. L. (1969): Thyrocalcitonin. *Physiol. Rev.*, *49*, 548.

LEE, M. R., DEFTOS, L. J. and POTTS, J. T., JR. (1969): Control of secretion of thyrocalcitonin in the rabbit as evaluated by radioimmunoassay. *Endocrinology*, *84*, 36.

MORGAN, C. R. and LAZAROW, A. (1963): Immunoassay of insulin: Two antibody system. *Diabetes*, *12*, 115.

MUNSON, P. L. and GRAY, T. K. (1970): Function of thyrocalcitonin in normal physiology. *Fed. Proc.*, *29*, 1206.

UNGER, R. H., OHNEDA, A., VALVERDE, I., EISENTRAUT, A. M. and EXTON, J. (1968): Characterization of the responses of circulating glucagon-like immunoreactivity to intraduodenal and intravenous administration of glucose. *J. clin. Invest.*, *47*, 48.

WENSEL, R. H., RICH, C., BROWN, A. C. and VOLWILER, W. (1969): Absorption of calcium measured by intubation and perfusion of the intact human small intestine. *J. clin. Invest.*, *48*, 1768.

CALCIUM HOMEOSTASIS, PARATHYROID HORMONE AND CALCITONIN IN HEALTH AND DISEASE*

CLAUDE D. ARNAUD,[1] E. TRAVIS LITTLEDIKE,[4] HANG SHENG TSAO,[1] ALBERT E. FOURNIER,[5] JACOB FURSZYFER,[5] WILLIAM J. JOHNSON[2] and RALPH S. GOLDSMITH[3]

[1] Department of Endocrine Research, [2] Division of Nephrology and Internal Medicine, [3] Russell M. Wilder Clinical Study Unit, Mayo Clinic and Mayo Foundation, Rochester, Minn.; [4] National Animal Disease Laboratory, Ames, Iowa; [5] Mayo Graduate School of Medicine, University of Minnesota, Rochester, Minn., U.S.A.

In this report we describe our published and recent studies of the effect of perturbations of calcium and magnesium metabolism on the secretion of parathyroid hormone and calcitonin in the young pig and some results of the use of a new radioimmunoassay for human parathyroid hormone in the study of pathologic states of human parathyroid function.

METHODS

Radioimmunoassays

New, sensitive radioimmunoassay systems have been developed for the measurement of calcitonin (CT) in porcine serum or plasma and for parathyroid hormone (PTH) in porcine (Arnaud *et al.*, 1970*a; b*), bovine, and human serum or plasma (Arnaud *et al.*, 1971). The principles described by Yalow and Berson (1964) were used. The radioimmunoassays for PTH use a guinea-pig anti-porcine-PTH antiserum which has a high affinity for porcine, bovine, and human PTH. The radioimmunoassays for CT were done with a guinea-pig anti-porcine-CT antiserum which has a high affinity for porcine CT. The details of these procedures have been published (Arnaud *et al.*, 1970*a*; *b*; 1971). In general, all of the assays can measure in the range of 50 pg of peptide per ml.

Standard preparations of hormones were all highly purified except in the case of the human PTH assay in which a standard hyperparathyroid serum was used in multiple dilutions because there was a clear immunologic difference between the PTH in serum and that extracted from parathyroid adenomata (Arnaud *et al.*, 1970*c*). Serum concentrations in immune mixtures never exceeded 40% and were considerably less most of the time. It was found that rigid control of the assays, with respect to excluding nonspecific effects of serum and replication at various dilutions of serum, was necessary to achieve results which were meaningful and precise (Arnaud *et al.*, 1971).

Other Analyses

Plasma or serum concentrations of total calcium (Ca_T) and magnesium (Mg) were determined

* This investigation was supported in part by Research Grant AM-12302 and Contract Grant 69-2168 from the National Institutes of Health, Public Health Service.

by atomic absorption spectrophotometry (Slavin, 1968); ionized calcium (Ca_I) was determined by the series 99–20 calcium activity flow-through system (Orion Research Company). Total inorganic phosphorus (Pi) was measured by the method of Taussky and Shorr (1953) or by an automated version of the Fiske and Subbarow technique (1925).

Protocols

Animal experiments: Young pigs were used. They were fed a diet providing a normal calcium intake. They had chronically implanted femoral artery and vein catheters. Parathyroidectomy and thyroidectomy procedures were done as previously reported (Littledike *et al.*,1968). Thyroidectomized pigs were given USP thyroid powder, 4 g/day, after the operation. Femoral artery catheters and heparinized syringes were used to obtain blood samples. The blood was cooled and centrifuged immediately, and the plasma was frozen (–15°C) within 15 minutes after collection. Hypocalcemia, hypercalcemia, and hypermagnesemia were induced by intravenous infusions of 0.1M EGTA (sodium ethylenebisoxyethylene nitrilotetraacetic acid), 0.1 M calcium gluconate, and 1.38 M magnesium chloride, respectively, at various rates. Pigs were conscious and restrained in cages (2 by 5 feet) during experiments. In three experiments, plasma was obtained from the thyroid veins of anesthetized pigs without touching the thyroid glands.

Human Studies: Measurements of all constituents were done in serum except that plasma was used when patients were undergoing chronic hemodialysis. The blood was allowed to clot at room temperature for 2 hours and then was centrifuged. The serum was removed, frozen, and stored at –15°C. Sera designated as normal were obtained from subjects 13 to 76 years old who were certified, by specialists in internal medicine, as not having disorders of calcium, phosphate, or magnesium metabolism. In all surgically proved cases of primary hyperparathyroidism, the pathologic diagnosis was either parathyroid adenoma or adenomatous hyperplasia of the parathyroid gland (Hoehn *et al.*, 1969). Cases suspected to be primary hyperparathyroidism were designated as such if agreement was reached on this diagnosis by four endocrinologists.

RESULTS

Animal Experiments

Plasma immunoreactive parathyroid hormone (IPTH) and calcitonin (ICT) were not detectable during control, hypocalcemic, hypercalcemic, or hypermagnesemic periods in thyroparathyroidectomized pigs; however, as reported previously in dogs by Sanderson *et al.* (1960), induced changes in plasma Ca_T were more marked and prolonged than in intact animals.

In intact pigs, IPTH was present in the peripheral plasma during the control period at levels of 300 to 700 pg/ml and, when measurable, ICT was present at levels of 150 to 600 pg/ml. In thyroid vein plasma of three normocalcemic anesthetized pigs, ICT was 7,000 to 15,000 pg/ml. In experiments in which acute hypocalcemia and then hypercalcemia were produced in sequence in five intact pigs, an inverse relationship between Ca_T and IPTH and a direct relationship between Ca_T and ICT were found (Fig. 1). Although these studies are the first in which IPTH and ICT were measured simultaneously, similar results have been obtained previously in separate studies of CT in the pig (Arnaud *et al.*, 1968; Care *et al.*, 1968; Lee *et al.*, 1969) and PTH in the cow, sheep, and goat (Sherwood *et al.*, 1966; 1968; Care *et al.*, 1966). In the present acute studies, the patterns of responses of the two hormones (Fig. 1) to their respective disturbing signals are different. Maximal IPTH levels were reached later and the levels were little more than twice control, whereas for ICT there was a rapid, early increase and maximal levels were at least eight times control values. Additionally, the

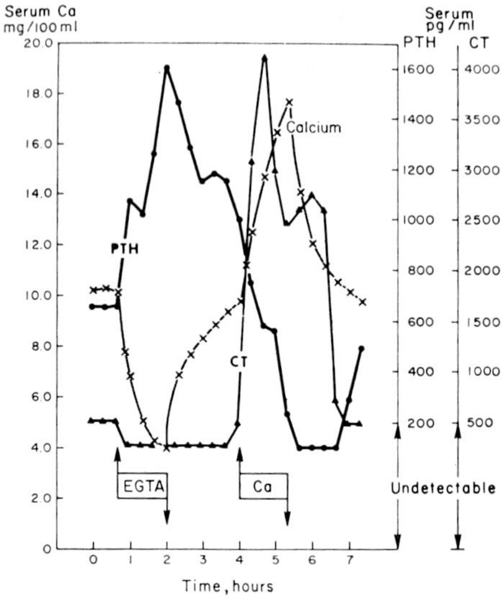

Fig. 1. Interrelationships between peripheral plasma ICT *(triangles)* and IPTH *(solid circles)* during sequential, induced changes in Ca_T *(x)*. (From Arnaud, C. D., Tsao, H. S., Littledike, T. (1970): Calcium homeostasis, parathyroid hormone, and calcitonin: preliminary report. *Mayo Clin. Proc.*, *45*, 125. By permission.)

apparent rate of disappearance of IPTH during hypercalcemic inhibition of PTH secretion was much slower than that of ICT when CT secretion was inhibited by return of CA_T to control levels. It is important to note, however, that, in separate studies of acute hypocalcemic stimulation of PTH secretion with either EGTA in pigs or CT administration in humans with Paget's disease (Arnaud *et al.*, 1971), an early-peaking IPTH response occasionally has been observed.

When secretion of CT or PTH was stimulated by slow step increases or decreases in Ca_T, respectively, a directly proportional increase in ICT and an inversely proportional increase in IPTH were observed (Fig. 2). A plot of the values for IPTH and ICT obtained in these experiments as a function of Ca_T is shown in Figure 3. The regression lines shown were obtained by the method of least squares and they have correlation coefficients near negative unity for IPTH and near positive unity for ICT. They intersect at $Ca_T = 9.3$ mg/100 ml, 0.2 mg/100 ml lower than the mean control level in the pigs studied.

The production of hypocalcemia by induced hypermagnesemia has been previously reported in dogs by Kemeny *et al.* (1961) and Knippers and Hehl (1965), in man by Kelly *et al.* (1960) and Jones and Fourman (1966), and in cats by Nielsen (1970). Figure 4 illustrates the changes in ICT, Ca_T, Ca_I, Mg, and P_i which occurred in an intact and a thyroparathyroidectomized pig during and after an 80-minute intravenous infusion of a large dose of magnesium chloride (27.6 μmol/kg/min). Plasma Mg had increased to 11.6 mEq/l at the end of the infusion period, and narcosis occurred at this concentration. Subsequently, Mg decreased gradually but was still 1 mEq/l higher than the preperfusion level 4 hours after the infusion was stopped. In the intact pig, a significant progressive decrease in Ca_T, Ca_I, and P_i occurred during the magnesium infusion—coincident with a dramatic increase in ICT. All of these indices returned toward control levels after the infusion was discontinued and Mg had decreased, except for P_i which briefly increased above control and finally decreased to control at 24 hours. In contrast, in the thyroparathyroidectomized pig, a similar magnesium infusion led to no change in ICT and an increase in Ca_T and Ca_I, with an increase in P_i after the infusion was discontinued. Similar experiments in parathyroidectomized pigs showed changes comparable to those in intact pigs.

When various doses of magnesium were given by infusion (13.8, 5.2, and 2.76 μmol/kg/min), ICT increased and Ca_I and P_i decreased in proportion to the degree of hyper-

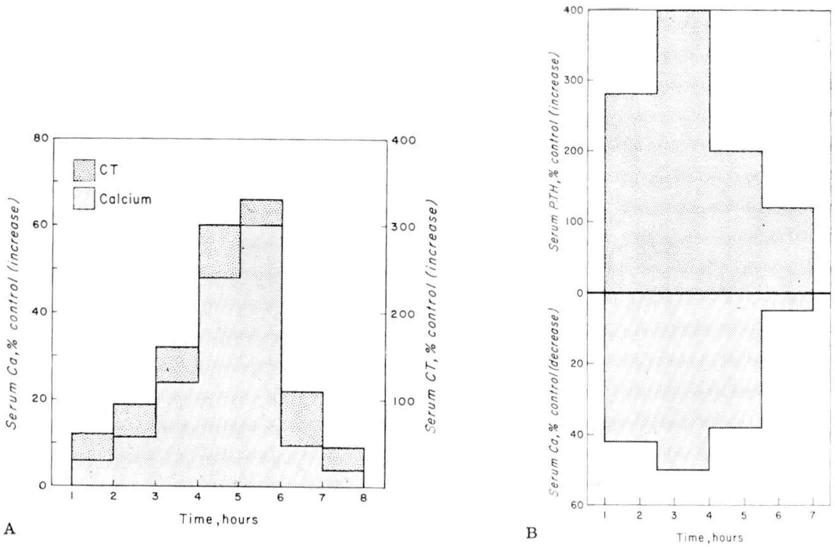

Fig. 2. A, Changes in ICT caused by step increases in Ca_T. *B*, Changes in IPTH caused by step decreases in Ca_T produced by EGTA infusion. (From Arnaud, C. D., Littledike, T., Tsao, H. S. (1970): Calcium homeostasis and the simultaneous measurement of calcitonin and parathyroid hormone in the pig. In: *Proceedings of the Second International Symposium on Calcitonin.* Heinemann, London. By permission.)

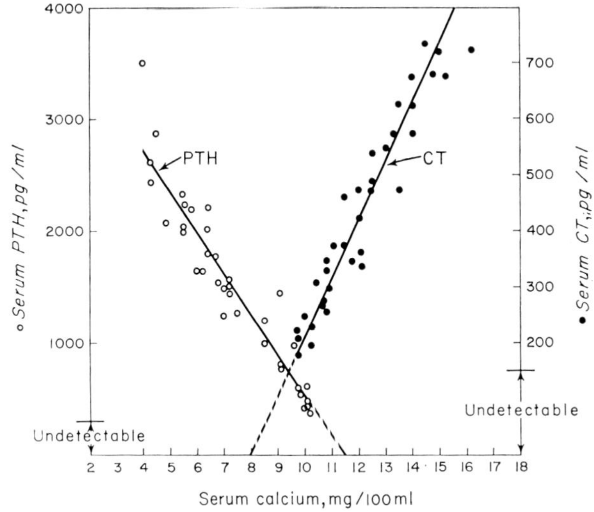

Fig. 3. Plot of ICT and IPTH values as a function of Ca_T in the same plasma samples; $r = +0.964$ for ICT and —0.942 for IPTH. *P* for both <0.001. (From Arnaud, C. D., Littledike, T., Tsao, H. S. (1969): Calcium homeostasis and the simultaneous measurement of calcitonin and parathyroid hormone in the pig. In: *Proceedings of the Second International Symposium on Calcitonin.* Heinemann, London. By permission.)

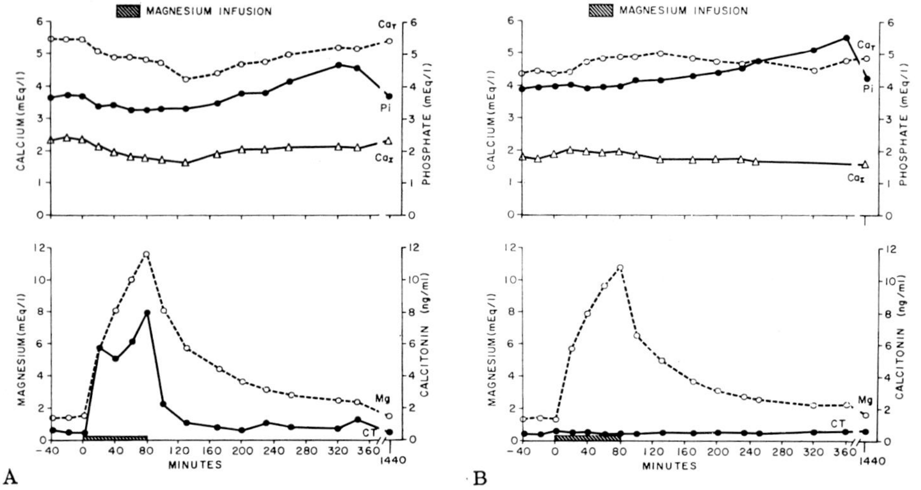

Fig. 4. Interrelationships between peripheral plasma ICT, Ca_T, Ca_I, P_i, and Mg during induced hypermagnesemia (27.6 μmol/kg/min). *A*, In intact young pig. *B*, In thyroparathyroidectomized pig.

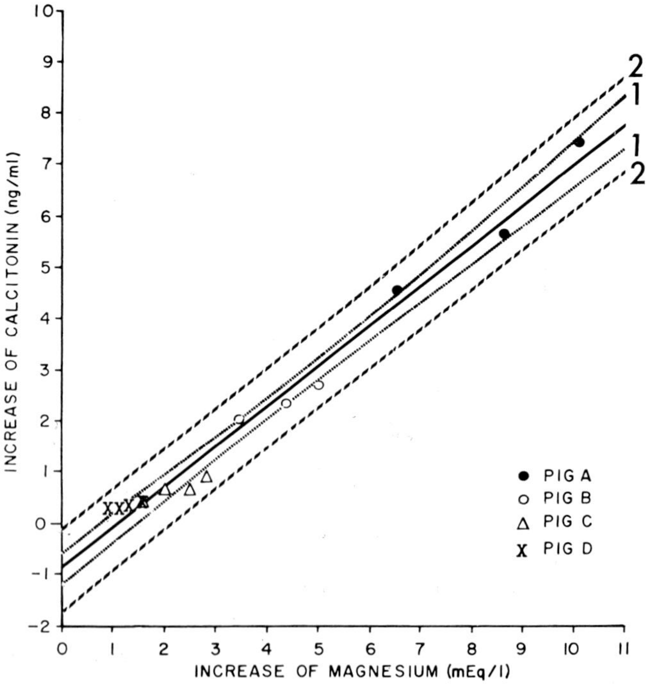

Fig. 5. Increase in ICT as a function of increase in Mg during the latter part of infusions of magnesium at various concentrations. Solid line = population line; broken lines *1* = 95% confidence interval of the population line; broken lines *2* = 95% confidence interval for the predicted CT values.

magnesemia produced. The direct, proportional relationship between Mg and ICT after the first 40 minutes of infusions of various doses of magnesium is shown in Figure 5. Changes in ICT occurring during the first 40 minutes of the infusion are complex (resembling early responses to hypercalcemia; see Figure 1); they do not appear to be directly proportional to Mg and will require further study before they can be characterized. The smallest increase in Mg which elicited a detectable, significant increase in ICT was 50%; however, a lesser increase in Mg induced by an infusion at 1.38 μmol/kg/min was associated with a significant decrease (0.2 mEq/l) in Ca_T after 100 minutes. This suggests that our failure to demonstrate changes in ICT with small increases in Mg is due to insensitivity of the ICT radioimmunoassay.

Human Studies

Typical standard curves obtained in equilibrium and non-equilibrium incubations of a 1:75,000 dilution of guinea-pig anti-porcine-PTH antiserum (G.P. 1), ^{131}I-labeled bovine PTH, and varying dilutions of a standard hyperparathyroid serum are shown in Figure 6.

Figure 7 summarizes our experience in measuring IPTH in serum from normal subjects and hypocalcemic, hypoparathyroid, and hyperparathyroid patients. Serum IPTH was undetectable in 10 patients with surgical hypoparathyroidism. In the small sample of 51 normal subjects, IPTH did not differ significantly with age or sex, was measurable in 94% of sera studied, and ranged between undetectable and 38 μl eq/ml. Serum IPTH ranged from 25 to 6,500 μl eq/ml in patients with surgically proved parathyroid adenomata, and there was a significant correlation between IPTH and the weight of the tumor. In patients suspected of having primary hyperparathyroidism, IPTH ranged from 22 to 430 μl eq/ml. Although the hormone was easily measured in all of these sera, values for IPTH were within the normal

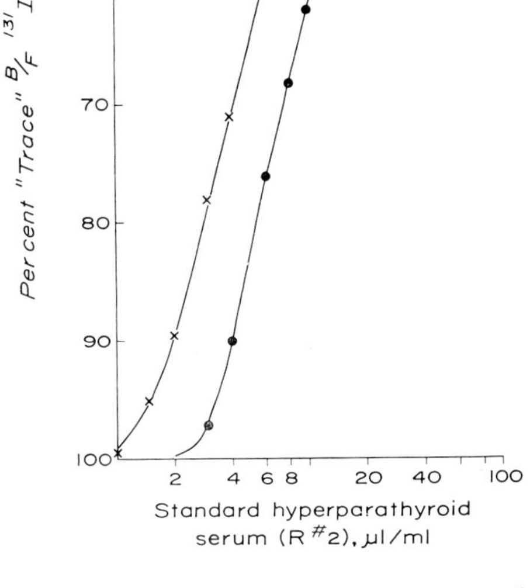

Fig. 6. Inhibition of binding of bovine PTH-^{131}I to G. P. 1 anti-porcine-PTH antiserum (1:75,000) by standard hyperparathyroid serum (R 2) in equilibrium *(circles)* and non-equilibrium *(x)* systems. (From Arnaud, C. D., Tsao, H. S., Littledike, T. (1971): Radioimmunoassay of human parathyroid hormone in serum. *J. clin. Invest., 50,* 21. By permission of the Rockefeller University Press.)

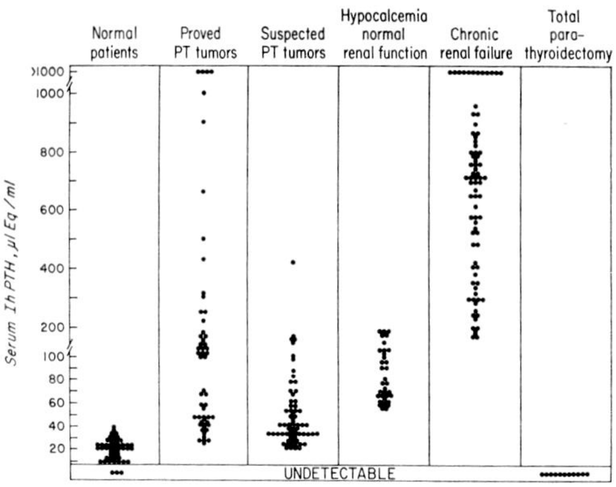

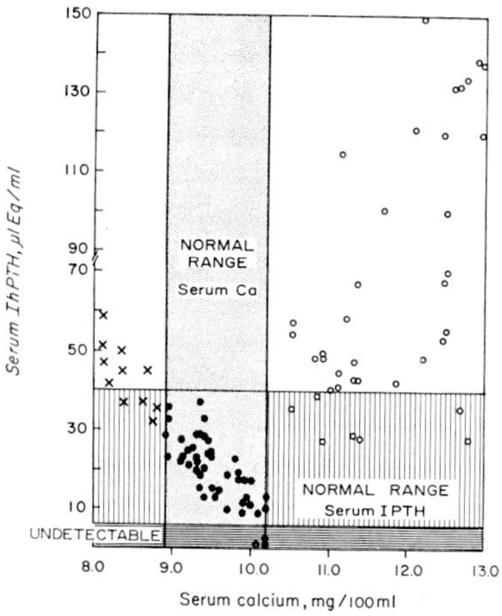

Fig. 7. Serum IPTH in normal humans and patients with various disorders of parathyroid function. (From Arnaud, C. D., Tsao, H. S., Littledike, T. (1971): Radioimmunoassay of human parathyroid hormone in serum. *J. clin. Invest., 50,* 21. By permission of the Rockefeller University Press.)

Fig. 8. Serum IPTH as a function of Ca_T in normals *(solid circles)*, hypocalcemic patients *(x)*, and patients with surgically proved primary hyperparathyroidism *(open circles)* and IPTH values less than 150 μl eq/ml (r for normals = —0.569; $P < 0.0001$). (From Arnaud, C. D., Tsao, H. S., Littledike, T. (1971): Radioimmunoassay of human parathyroid hormone in serum. *J. clin. Invest., 50,* 21. By permission of the Rockefeller University Press.)

range in 22% of patients with proved primary hyperparathyroidism and 49% of those with suspected hyperparathyroidism.

Figure 8 shows the overlap for IPTH in normal subjects and patients with IPTH values less than 150 μl eq/ml plotted as a function of the serum calcium. There is a highly significant negative correlation between serum calcium and IPTH in the normal group. IPTH is appropriately increased above the normal range in patients with hypocalcemia due to causes other than hypoparathyroidism or renal failure (that is, intestinal malabsorption or osteomalacia) (also see Figure 7). Visual inspection of this plot shows complete discrimination between normal subjects and patients with primary hyperparathyroidism. A formal discriminant analysis of these data produced the expected separation free of overlap (this is in marked contrast to the poor discrimination between these two groups obtained when only IPTH was used).

Serum IPTH is uniformly increased from 3 to 100 times normal in patients with renal failure (Fig. 7), as previously reported by Berson and Yalow (1966). In extensive studies of the etiology of hyperparathyroidism and bone disease during chronic hemodialysis (Fournier *et al.*, 1971*a*; *b*) we have been able to show a significant relationship between the dialysate concentration of calcium and the presence or absence of roentgenologic evidence of bone disease (subperiosteal resorption) but other predialysis or intradialysis factors, such as age, sex, and duration of renal failure, could not be implicated. Dialysate concentrations of calcium less than 5.7 mg/100 ml significantly favored the development of symptomatic and radiographically apparent bone disease; those patients dialyzed against a calcium concentration greater than 5.7 mg/100 ml were largely without such bone disease. We found that IPTH was significantly higher in patients with bone disease ($P < 0.01$) and that there was a significant positive correlation between the predialysis Ca_T and the predialysis IPTH. The factors which best correlated with IPTH were mean dialysate calcium (negative) and mean dialysis P_i during the entire period of dialysis (positive).

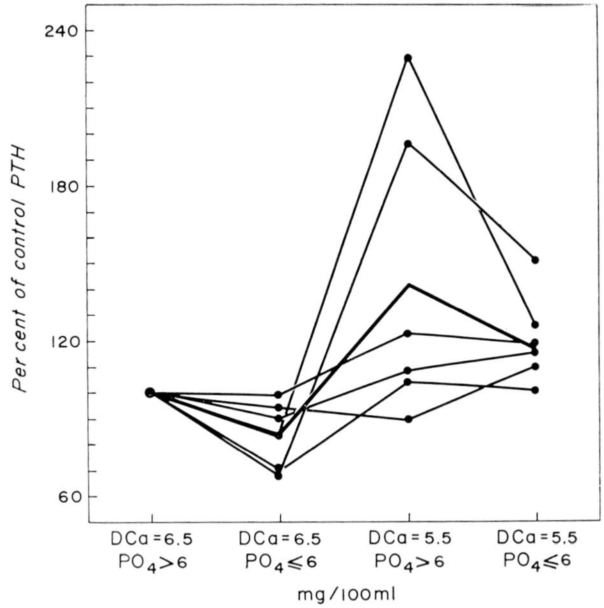

Fig. 9. Serum IPTH as a function of hemodialysis regimen in patients with chronic renal failure. DCa = dialysate calcium concentration in mg/100 ml; PO_4 = serum phosphate concentration in mg/100 ml. Heavy line represents the mean of IPTH values for six patients on each regimen.

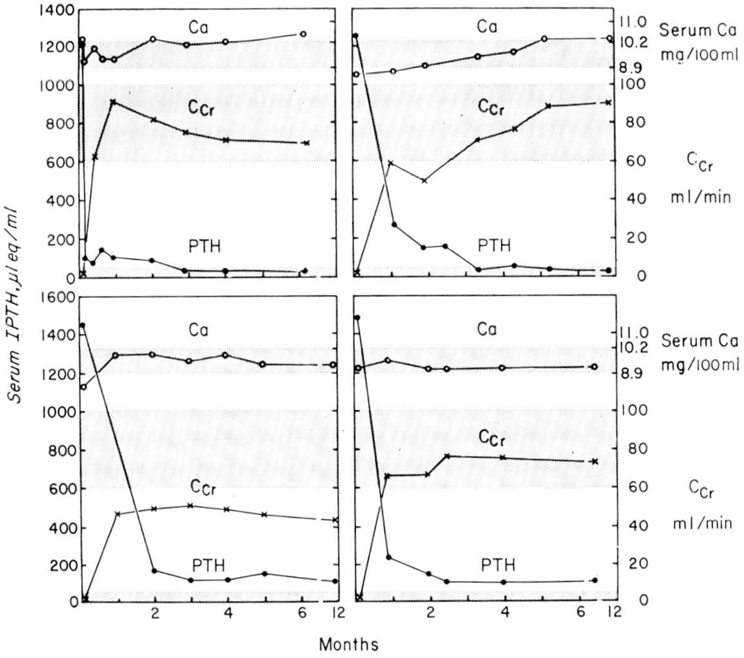

Fig. 10. Serum IPTH, serum Ca_T, and creatinine clearance in patients who have received renal transplants at time 0.

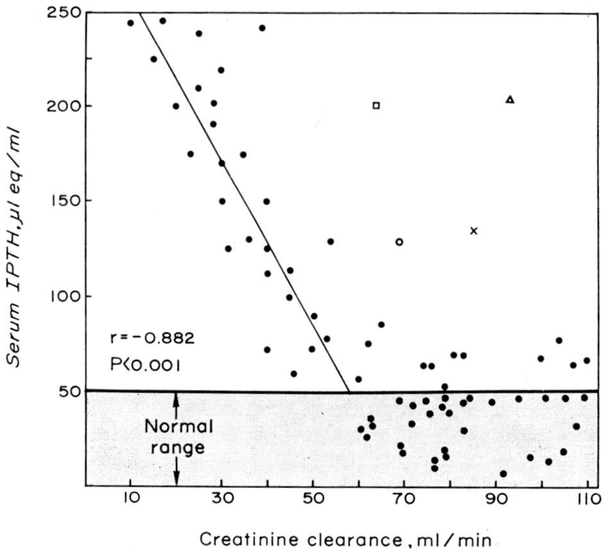

Fig. 11. Serum IPTH as a function of glomerular filtration rate in patients with renal transplants. o, x, □, and Δ represent patients who had hypercalcemia 6 to 12 months after transplantation.

Because of these relationships, we designed a 2-by-2 factorial study which permitted evaluation of the effects of high and low dialysate concentrations of calcium as well as high and low plasma phosphate concentrations. Six patients were sequentially placed on four different regimens for 2 to 3 weeks each (Fig. 9). The plasma phosphate concentration was decreased by oral administration of a phosphate binding agent ($Al(OH)_3$). IPTH was lowest with the combination of high dialysate calcium and low plasma phosphate, highest with the combination of low dialysate calcium and high plasma phosphate, and intermediate with the other two combinations. In these short-term studies, none of the therapeutic regimens decreased IPTH levels to normal; however, these principles now are being applied in chronic studies and the preliminary results appear promising.

Figure 10 shows examples of four different IPTH responses in patients who have undergone renal transplantation for chronic renal failure. In successful transplantations *(upper left* and *lower right)*, IPTH decreased from very high levels toward normal rapidly, but it remained either at the upper limit of normal or at two to three times normal in relation to the Ca_T (Fig. 8) for as long as these patients were followed. When the IPTH responses of all of the patients with glomerular filtration rates (C_{cr}) greater than 60 ml/min (Kemeny *et al.*, 1961) are considered, it appears that the degree to which IPTH is increased 6 months after transplantation is directly correlated with the IPTH prior to transplantation. In partially successful transplantations *(lower left* and *upper right)*, the decrease in IPTH was related to the glomerular filtration rate and, as shown in Figure 11, there is a significant correlation (negative) when the glomerular filtration rate is less than 60 ml/min.

DISCUSSION

The data we have presented on the plasma CT and PTH responses to induced hypercalcemia and hypocalcemia in young pigs serve to show quantitatively the dynamic interrelationships of these hormones in extracellular fluid calcium homeostasis. The differences in the patterns of their responses and the observations that CT is at least 50 to 100 times more potent on a weight basis and has a more rapid but shorter action than PTH suggest a working model of this control system. We visualize CT as a potent, rapidly acting, damping factor which suppresses oscillations of Ca_T above physiologic levels and PTH as a major controlling factor which maintains Ca_T in the physiologic range and suppresses oscillations of Ca_T below physiologic levels, by virtue of its relatively long half-life in plasma and slow, prolonged action.

The stimulation of CT secretion by induced hypermagnesemia is a new observation and probably accounts for the associated hypocalcemia and hypophosphatemia observed. Plasma CT levels were proportional to the degree of hypermagnesemia induced, as were the degree and duration of the hypocalcemia and hypophosphatemia. However, an early-peaking CT response was observed early in the course of magnesium infusion and was similar to that which occurs during calcium infusion. We have postulated that these types of responses are related to the quantity of hormone stored in the gland at the time of study and that the status of glandular storage depots may condition the character of the secretory response. However, these phenomena require intensive further study before definitive information can be obtained. The question of the physiologic importance of magnesium as a secretagogue of CT cannot be answered until this system is examined with a more sensitive radioimmunoassay for ICT, but our studies indicate that increases of Mg of 50% to 100% result in measurable increases in ICT. Mg increases of this degree are not uncommon in a number of clinically important human and animal diseases.

Several features of our radioimmunoassay for human PTH deserve discussion. Bovine ^{131}I-labeled PTH was used to compete with human PTH for binding to an antibody to porcine PTH. Although unusual, there does not appear to be any objection, theoretical or otherwise, to this practice since, in this system, unlabeled bovine PTH and human PTH appear to react similarly (Arnaud *et al.*, 1971*c*; 1970).

The antiserum to porcine PTH used in this immunoassay distinguishes between the human IPTH in hyperparathyroid sera and that extracted and purified from parathyroid adenomata. A similar antiserum (to bovine PTH) has been reported by Berson and Yalow (1968). We have concluded that this finding in our immunoassay system probably reflects a difference between the native species of the hormone which is secreted and that which is chemically extracted from the parathyroid gland (Arnaud *et al.*, 1971*c*). Because of this, we have concluded that it is imperative that the human PTH present in hyperparathyroid serum be used as the standard preparation in this assay.

The ability of our immunoassay for human PTH to measure the hormone present in 94% of normal sera tested is indicative of its great sensitivity. Unfortunately, it is not reasonable to discuss the concentrations of hormone in serum in gravimetric terms because purified human PTH is not suitable as a standard in this immunoassay.

Perhaps the most important criterion for the validity of any hormone assay is its ability to demonstrate appropriate levels of hormone concentrations in the serum under conditions known to be associated with increased or decreased secretion of the hormone. The present radioimmunoassay for human PTH in serum has good support in this regard. Values for Ca_T correlated negatively with those of IPTH over the normal Ca_T range (Fig. 8) and hypocalcemic subjects with disorders other than renal failure had appropriately increased IPTH values (Figs. 7 and 8). Serum IPTH generally was increased in patients with hyperparathyroidism (Fig. 7), and there was a positive correlation between Ca_T and IPTH values when the hyperparathyroidism was due to the presence of a parathyroid adenoma. Serum IPTH was undetectable in patients with hypoparathyroidism.

The large overlap in IPTH values in normal subjects and patients with primary hyperparathyroidism (Figs. 7 and 8) has been reported previously by Berson and Yalow (1966). However, the complete separation of normal subjects from patients with primary hyperparathyroidism by formal discriminant analysis of both variables, Ca_T and IPTH, has not been reported before and has been of practical importance to us in making the diagnosis of mild hyperparathyroidism. Whether this advantage will prove to be consistent will require further long-term studies, but it is clear that the separation of the normal from the hyperparathyroid state on this basis requires an assay system which is sufficiently sensitive to quantitate, not merely detect, low levels of IPTH in serum.

Very pertinent to our observations on parathyroid gland function in chronic renal failure are those of others (Potts *et al.*, 1969; Genuth *et al.*, 1970) indicating that suppression of PTH secretion to 'normal' can be accomplished by the brief induction of hypercalcemia by a 4-hour calcium infusion. Our experience is more in line with that of Riess *et al.* (1968) in that only minimal suppression (0 to 20%) is achieved by this manipulation. Even hypercalcemia over a period of 8 hours results only in a 40% to 60% decrease in IPTH. Furthermore, our current work using high dialysate calcium concentrations (8 mg/100 ml) and reduction of plasma phosphate to normal with aluminum hydroxide gel (oral) in patients undergoing chronic hemodialysis for chronic renal failure suggests that only after several months of this treatment do IPTH values decrease to a range between normal and two to three times normal. These discrepancies are probably related to differences in the sensitivities of the various PTH assays used. If, as our data indicate, it is not easy to render the hyperplastic parathyroid glands of chronic renal failure functionless, it will be important to carry out more precise, better designed, inductive investigations of the control mechanisms (perhaps other than Ca_I and P_i) involved in regulating PTH secretion by these glands. Also, it appears that more strenuous measures to restore calcium and phosphate homeostasis to or toward normal in these patients are mandatory if prevention or treatment of severe secondary hyperparathyroidism is to be accomplished.

Our observations concerning the greater incidence of roentgenographically apparent bone disease in chronic renal failure patients dialyzed against a dialysate calcium concentration less than 5.7 mg/100 ml strongly suggest that, in some patients, clinically evident renal osteodystrophy may be iatrogenically induced by chronic hemodialysis. The significantly higher IPTH values in these patients as a group support this notion, and the studies in which IPTH was measured when plasma phosphate and dialysate calcium were independently varied (Fig. 9) suggest simple therapeutic measures which might provide a rational prophylactic approach to this problem.

The disturbance in calcium metabolism after renal transplantation for chronic renal failure which has attracted the greatest attention and concern is hypercalcemia. This is wholly justified because of the probable adverse influence of hypercalcemia on the parenchyma of the transplanted kidney. In our experience the complication of hypercalcemia is infrequent; however, when present, it may be due to any one or a combination of factors which are operative in most transplanted patients: persistent hyperparathyroidism, phosphate depletion, restoration of vitamin D metabolism to normal, variations in glucocorticoid therapy, and possible further stimulation of hyperplastic parathyroid glands by hypomagnesemia. However, it is probable that the single most important factor is a concentration of circulating PTH which is unphysiologic for the conditions which exist in the individual patient. Our studies show that IPTH decreases dramatically, from markedly increased values, within a short time after renal transplantation (Fig. 10). Whether this phenomenon is due to altered metabolism of PTH or to an actual decrease in secretion of PTH is not yet known, but the answer to this question is important because it may provide a clue to an as yet unknown factor involved in the regulation of PTH secretion. It appears that the percentage decrease in IPTH immediately after transplantation is approximately the same in all patients, but IPTH does not decrease to the normal range in most cases for 4 to 6 months and, in some patients, IPTH is still 10 times normal at this time. Even in patients whose IPTH is in the normal range at 12 months, it is probably inappropriately increased for the level of Ca_T. We have been conservative in our approach to the problem of post-transplantation hyperparathyroidism and have subjected only 2 of 71 patients to subtotal parathyroidectomy. Although the surgical approach appears to be curative, the problem of inadvertent production of hypoparathyroidism is not inconsequential because it raises the frightening prospects of treatment with pharmacologic doses of vitamin D and the intrinsic hazard of iatrogenic production of hypercalcemia, hypercalciuria, and nephrocalcinosis in a transplanted kidney. Clearly, a systematic and broad medical approach to the treatment and prevention of hyperparathyroidism prior to renal transplantation is needed and, as described briefly in this paper, the rudiments of such a program are at hand.

SUMMARY

1. Using sensitive radioimmunoassays for porcine calcitonin and parathyroid hormone, we have demonstrated quantitatively the dynamic interrelationships of these hormones during acute perturbations of calcium homeostasis in the young pig. A working model of this contro system is proposed on the basis of these observations.

2. Induced hypermagnesemia in young pigs stimulates the release of immunoreactive calcitonin from the thyroid gland and probably accounts for associated hypocalcemia and hypophosphatemia.

3. Using a new, sensitive radioimmunoassay for human parathyroid hormone in serum, based on cross reaction with an antibody to porcine parathyroid hormone, we have studied the relationship between the concentrations of this hormone and total calcium in the serum of normal subjects, in patients with hyperparathyroidism associated with adenomatous disease of the parathyroid glands or chronic renal failure, and in patients who have undergone renal transplantation. Only representative data from extensive work with this assay are presented with the purpose of demonstrating its usefulness as a diagnostic and research tool. Perhaps the most important information obtained from these studies is that, in patients with chronic renal failure being treated by chronic hemodialysis, restoration of calcium and phosphate homeostasis toward normal results in suppression of previously overactive parathyroid glands and a diminished frequency of roentgenographic evidence of parathyroid-induced bone disease.

ACKNOWLEDGMENTS

We thank Miss Judith A. Hess, Mrs. Karen J. Laakso, Miss Juliana Bischoff, Mr. Wayne V. Blanchard, and Mrs. Janette Winge for expert technical assistance. We are indebted to numerous physicians at the Mayo Clinic for their generous cooperation, especially Drs. F. Raymond Keating, Jr.,* Don C. Purnell, Donald A. Scholz, Lynwood H. Smith, B. Lawrence Riggs, David L. Hoffman, Carl F. Anderson, and James C. Hunt.

* Deceased.

REFERENCES

ARNAUD, C. D., LITTLEDIKE, T. and TSAO, H. S. (1970*a*): Calcium homeostasis and the simultaneous measurement of calcitonin and parathyroid hormone in the pig. In: *Calcitonin 1969: Proceedings of the Second International Symposium on Calcitonin*, pp. 95–101. Editor: S. Taylor. Heinemann, London.

ARNAUD, C. D., LITTLEDIKE, T., TSAO, H. S. and KAPLAN, E. L. (1968): Radioimmunoassay of calcitonin: a preliminary report. *Mayo Clin. Proc.*, *43*, 496.

ARNAUD, C. D., TSAO, H. S. and LITTLEDIKE, T. (1970*b*): Calcium homeostasis, parathyroid hormone, and calcitonin: preliminary report. *Mayo Clin. Proc.*, *45*, 125.

ARNAUD, C. D., TSAO, H. S. and LITTLEDIKE, T. (1971): Radioimmunoassay of human parathyroid hormone in serum. *J. clin. Invest.*, *50*, 21.

ARNAUD, C. D., TSAO, H. S. and OLDHAM, S. B. (1970*c*): Native human parathyroid hormone: an immunochemical investigation. *Proc. nat. Acad. Sci. (Wash.)*, *67*, 415.

BERSON, S. A. and YALOW, R. S. (1966): Parathyroid hormone in plasma in adenomatous hyperparathyroidism, uremia, and bronchogenic carcinoma. *Science*, *154*, 907.

BERSON, S. A. and YALOW, R. S. (1968): Immunochemical heterogeneity of parathyroid hormone in plasma. *J. clin. Endocr., 28*, 1037.
CARE, A. D., COOPER, C. W., DUNCAN, T. and ORIMO, H. (1968): A study of thyrocalcitonin secretion by direct measurement of *in vivo* secretion rates in pigs. *Endocrinology, 83*, 161.
CARE, A. D., SHERWOOD, L. M., POTTS, J. T., JR. and AURBACH, G. D. (1966): Perfusion of the isolated parathyroid gland of the goat and sheep. *Nature (Lond.), 209*, 55.
FISKE, C. H. and SUBBAROW, Y. (1925): The colorimetric determination of phosphorus. *J. biol. Chem., 66*, 375.
FOURNIER, A. E., ARNAUD, C. D., JOHNSON, W. J., TAYLOR, W. F. and GOLDSMITH, R. S. (1971*a*): Etiology of hyperparathyroidism and bone disease during chronic hemodialysis. II. Factors affecting serum immunoreactive parathyroid hormone *J. clin. Invest., 50*. 599.
FOURNIER, A. E., JOHNSON, W. J., TAVES, D. R., BEABOUT, J. W., ARNAUD, C. D. and GOLDSMITH, R. S. (1971*b*): Etiology of hyperparathyroidism and bone disease during chronic hemodialysis. I. Association of bone disease with potentially etiologic factors *J. clin. Invest., 50*, 592.
GENUTH, S. M., SHERWOOD, L. M., VERTES, V. and LEONARDS, J. R. (1970): Plasma parathormone, calcium and phosphorus in patients with renal osteodystrophy undergoing chronic hemodialysis. *J. clin. Endocr., 30*, 15.
HOEHN, J. G., BEAHRS, O. H. and WOOLNER, L. B. (1969): Unusual surgical lesions of the parathyroid gland. *Amer. J. Surg., 118*, 770.
JONES, K. H. and FOURMAN, P. (1966): Effects of infusions of magnesium and of calcium in parathyroid insufficiency. *Clin. Sci., 30*, 139.
KELLY, H. G., CROSS, H. C., TURTON, M. R. and HATCHER, J. D. (1960): Renal and cardiovascular effects induced by intravenous infusion of magnesium sulphate. *Canad. med. Ass. J., 82*, 866.
KEMENY, A., BOLDIZSAR, H. and PETHES, G. (1961): The distribution of cations in plasma and cerebrospinal fluid following infusion of solutions of salts of sodium, potassium, magnesium and calcium. *J. Neurochem., 7*, 218.
KNIPPERS, R. and HEHL, U. (1965): Die renale Ausscheidung von Magnesium, Calcium und Kalium nach Erhöhung der Magnesium-Konzentration im Plasma des Hundes. *Z. ges. exp. Med., 139*, 154.
LEE, M. R., DEFTOS, L. J. and POTTS, J. T., JR. (1969): Control of secretion of thyrocalcitonin in the rabbit as evaluated by radioimmunoassay. *Endocrinology, 84*, 36.
LITTLEDIKE, E. T., ST. CLAIR, L. E. and NOTZOLD, R. A. (1968): Effects of parathyroidectomy of the pig. *Amer. J. vet. Res., 29*, 635.
NIELSEN, S. P. (1970): Abolition of magnesium-induced hypocalcaemia by acute thyro-parathyroidectomy in the cat. *Acta endocr. (Kbh.), 64*, 150.
POTTS, J. T., JR., REITZ, R. E., DEFTOS, L. J., KAYE, M. B., RICHARDSON, J. A., BUCKLE, R. M. and AURBACH, G. D. (1969): Secondary hyperparathyroidism in chronic renal disease. *Arch. intern. Med., 124*, 408.
RIESS, E., CANTERBURY, J. M. and EGDAHL, R. H. (1968): Experience with a radioimmunoassay of parathyroid hormone in human sera. *Trans. Ass. Amer. Phycn., 81*, 104.
SANDERSON, P. H., MARSHALL, F. and WILSON, R. E. (1960): Calcium and phosphorus homeostasis in the parathyroidectomized dog: evaluation by means of ethylenediamine tetraacetate and calcium tolerance tests. *J. clin. Invest., 39*, 62.
SHERWOOD, L. M., MAYER, G. P., RAMBERG, C. F., JR., KRONFELD, D. S., AURBACH, G. D. and POTTS, J. T., JR. (1968): Regulation of parathyroid hormone secretion: proportional control by calcium, lack of effect of phosphate. *Endocrinology, 83*, 1043.
SHERWOOD, L. M., POTTS, J. T., JR., CARE, A. D., MAYER, G. P. and AURBACH, G. D. (1966): Evaluation by radioimmunoassay of factors controlling the secretion of parathyroid hormone: intravenous infusions of calcium and ethylenediamine tetraacetic acid in the cow and goat. *Nature (Lond.), 209*, 52.
SLAVIN, W. (1968): *Atomic Absorption Spectroscopy*, pp. 78–188. Interscience Publishers, New York.
TAUSSKY, H. H. and SHORR, E. (1953): A microcolorimetric method for the determination of inorganic phosphorus. *J. biol. Chem., 202*, 675.
YALOW, R. S. and BERSON, S. A. (1964): Immunoassay of plasma insulin. In: *Methods of Biochemical Analysis, Vol. 12*, pp. 69–96. Editor D. Glick. Interscience Publishers, New York.

GROWTH HORMONE

CONTENTS

RELATIONSHIP BETWEEN CHEMICAL STRUCTURE AND BIOLOGICAL ACTIVITY OF HUMAN GROWTH HORMONE*

JORGE BROVETTO-CRUZ, THOMAS A. BEWLEY, LIN MA and CHOH HAO LI

The Hormone Research Laboratory, University of California,
San Francisco, California, U.S.A.
Cathedra of Medicine and Service of Obstetrical Physiology,
University of Uruguay, Uruguay

INTRODUCTION

The search for the unique features, the special molecular characteristics that differentiate a protein with hormonal properties from thousands of other proteins, is one of the most provocative challenges for molecular biologists as well as for endocrinologists.

Since the interaction of a protein hormone with its receptor must be of great stereochemical precision, a detailed knowledge of the primary, secondary and tertiary structure of the molecule, and the relationship of its structural characteristics with its biological properies must be the basis for the understanding of the molecular mechanism of protein hormone action.

The conformation of a protein is a consequence not only of the amino-acid sequence but also of other covalent linkages like the disulfide bonds, which exert restrictions in the conformations which a protein can possess. Moreover, it is now accepted that nonconvalent intramolecular forces, arising from the amino-acid side-chains, play a prime role in the determination of the native three-dimensional configuration.

In the last years, extensive studies performed on human growth hormone (HGH), which was first isolated from the pituitary gland by Li and Papkoff in 1956, have provided abundant information on the chemical, physical and biological properties of the hormone, and have permitted the disclosure of the complete primary structure (amino-acid sequence) of the protein (Li *et al.*, 1969).

We summarize here our investigations oriented to evaluate the specific function of certain selected amino-acid residues in the maintenance of the molecular conformation and in the manifestation of the growth-promoting and lactogenic activities of the hormone.

SPECIFIC CHEMICAL MODIFICATIONS

One of the procedures employed for these structure-biological activity relationship studies was the chemical modification of certain functional groups in the molecule by specific reagents in mild reaction conditions. This approach can have great significance only if the

* This work is supported in part by the American Cancer Society, the Geffen Foundation and the Allen Foundation.

native conformation is not altered by the modification and by the procedure used. Therefore a detailed biological, chemical and biophysical characterization of the derivative molecules, obtained by the modification reactions, was performed before drawing any difinitive conclusion.

Disulfide bonds

The role of the nonpeptidic covalent bonds, introduced by the disulfide bridges, in achieving or stabilizing the protein conformation, or both, and the question of whether some of these disulfide bonds may be intrinsically involved in the active site(s) of the hormone, have been the subject of our early investigations.

It was shown by Dixon and Li (1966) that the reductive cleavage of the disulfide bonds of HGH followed by alkylation with iodoacetamide, produce a reduced carbamidomethylated derivative that possesses growth-promoting and lactogenic potencies comparable with those of the native hormone. It is remarkable that even though quite drastic conditions were used (reduction with mercaptoethanol in 8 M urea solutions), an active derivative was obtained. These results were further confirmed by Bewley *et al.* (1968). They reported the preparation in high yield of a biologically active reduced-tetra-S-carbamidomethylated (RCAM)-HGH by a procedure developed by Bewley and Li (1969), which involves no denaturants. However, it was also found (Bewley, 1968) that when iodoacetic acid was used as the alkylating agent instead of iodoacetamide, the reduced-tetra-S-carboxymethylated (RCOM)-HGH obtained retained considerable lactogenic activity but was essentally devoid of growth-promoting activity (Tables I and II). The measurements (Bewley *et al.*, 1969) of the chemical composition, molecular weight by osmotic pressure determinations, viscosity, spectrophotometric titrations of tyrosyl groups, and circular dichroism have shown that the secondary and tertiary structure of HGH is only very little, if at all, perturbed by reduction and alkylation of the disulfide bonds. Moreover, it was not possible to demonstrate any significant difference between the two derivatives, RCAM and RCOM.

Figure 1 shows the rates of tryptic hydrolysis of native, RCAM, RCOM and performic acid oxidized HGH. A considerable difference in their relative rates of proteolysis can be clearly seen. An average of 8 bonds of the RCOM and the performic acid oxidized hormone are digested in 30 minutes while the RCAM is digested much more slowly (5 bonds in

TABLE I

Growth-promoting activity of HGH and reduced-alkylated derivatives as measured by the rat tibia test

	Tibia width (μ)* for total dose (μg)			
Preparation	0	20 μg	60 μg	80 μg
Saline	168 ± 2 (12)	—	—	—
Native HGH	—	211 ± 4 (12)	269 ± 5 (11)	—
RCAM-HGH	—	197 ± 6 (12)	257 ± 4 (12)	
RCOM-HGH	—	—	194 ± 14 (5)	199 ± 22 (4)

* Expressed as the mean plus and minus standard error of the mean followed by the number of test animals in parentheses.

TABLE II

Lactogenic activity of HGH and reduced-alkylated derivatives as measured by the pigeon local crop-sac assay

Protein	Dry mucosal wt. (mg)* for dose (μg)	
	2 μg	8 μg
Native HGH	13.5 ± 3.1 (6)	18.2 ± 4.7 (5)
RCAM-HGH	12.6 ± 1.8 (5)	20.1 ± 5.8 (5)
RCOM-HGH	11.9 ± 2.8 (6)	15.1 ± 3.9 (4)

* Uninjected controls give mucosal weights of 8–9 mg expressed as in Table I.

30 minutes). The native hormone is even slower, less than 3 bonds being digested on average in the same period of time. This rapid proteolysis of RCAM and RCOM proteins must indicate a difference in the rigidity of the secondary and tertiary structures of these molecules relative to the native HGH, perhaps due to a very small conformational difference which escapes detection by other criteria. The higher rigidity of the native protein may be of considerable importance for the molecule to be able to survive within the organism in an active form from the time it is synthetized in the pituitary until it performs its intended function at the receptor site. It is very likely that the loss of growth-promoting activity by the RCOM-HGH, is due to destruction, probably by enzymatic degradation, during the passage from the site of injection to the receptor site. In the rat tibia bioassay used, the preparation to be tested must reach the receptor through the circulatory system, where it does come in contact with proteolytic enzymes. Under these conditions, the RCOM derivative may never reach the target, due to faster enzymatic degradation. On the other hand, the lactogenic activity is estimated by the local pigeon crop-sac bioassay, in which the substance tested is injected directly into the tissue which contains the lactogenic receptor.

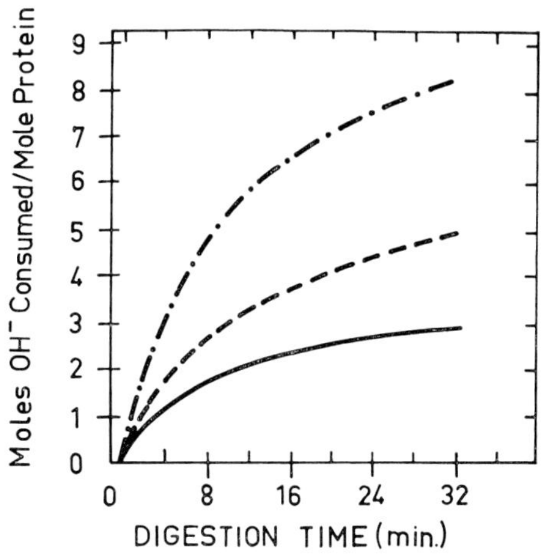

Fig. 1. Rates of tryptic hydrolysis of native (————), RCAM, (— — — — —), RCOM, and performic acid oxidized HGH (—.—.—.). The RCOM and performic acid oxidized proteins were digested at the same rate and are shown as a single curve (Bewley *et al.*, 1969).

From all these studies we conclude that the disulfide bonds in the HGH molecule are not necessary for the manifestation of biological activity, nor are they required for the maintenance of the secondary and tertiary structure. The presence of these bonds does serve, however, to stabilize the molecular architecture against perturbing forces.

Tryptophan residue

The fact that the disulfide bridges are neither essential for the biological activities nor for the three-dimensional structure, suggests that the conformation of the HGH molecule must be mainly a consequence of noncovalent forces.

Since tryptophan residues are known to play an important role in stabilizing the structure of proteins by hydrophobic interactions with other nonpolar residues (Kauzmann, 1959) it was of interest to determine the importance of this amino-acid residue for the maintenance of the biological property and structure of HGH.

These investigations (Brovetto-Cruz and Li, 1969) have been carried out using two specific tryptophan reagents: 2-nitophenyl-sulfenyl chloride (NPS-Cl) reported by Scoffone *et al.* (1968) and 2-hydroxy-5-nitrobenzyl bromide (HNB-Br) introduced by Koshland *et al.* (1964).

Different reaction conditions were used. When 50% acetic acid was used as reaction medium, quantitative alkylation of the tryptophan residue by NPS-Cl was obtained. As may be seen in Table III, full growth-promoting activity is retained in the HGH-NPS

TABLE III

Growth-promoting activity of the NPS derivative of HGH and control preparations, assayed by the rat tibia test

Preparation	Mean responses (μ) $\pm$ S.D. for total doses (μg) of: 40	100	Potency	Statistical evaluation: Fiducial limits for P = 0.05
HGH (untreated)	253 $\pm$ 6 (10)*	271 $\pm$ 15 (10)		
HGH (50% AcOH treated)	259 $\pm$ 5 (6)	271 $\pm$ 20 (6)		
HGH-NPS	250 $\pm$ 7 (5)	282 $\pm$ 24 (6)	0.98	0.49 – 1.83

* Number of experimental test animals in parentheses.

TABLE IV

Lactogenic activity of the NPS derivative of HGH and control preparations, assayed by the pigeon crop-sac test

Preparation	Total dose (μg)	Response: Visual (a)	Mean wt. (b) $\pm$ S.E.
HGH (untreated)	2	2.3	17.2 $\pm$ 2.9
	16	3.4	30.0 $\pm$ 8.9
HGH (50% AcOH treated)	2	2.2	17.5 $\pm$ 6.3
	16	3.5	28.0 $\pm$ 8.0
HGH-NPS	5	0	9.7 $\pm$ 2.8
	40	1.6	12.4 $\pm$ 3.4

(a) Subjectively evaluated using the scale: 0, no stimulation; 1, minimal stimulation; 2, moderate stimulation; 3, marked stimulation; 4, maximum stimulation. Values shown are the means of 10 observations.
(b) Dry weight of crop-sac mucosal epithelium in mg.

derivative as well as in a 50% acetic acid treated preparation used as control. Conversely, in the pigeon crop-sac (Table IV) only this control preparation was as active as the native hormone, while the HGH-NPS derivative was almost devoid of lactogenic activity.

It must be pointed out that it was not possible to uncover any significant difference between this derivative, the control preparation, and the native hormone, by studies on the chemical composition, chromatographic behavior on gel filtration, spectrophotometric titrations of the tyrosyl residues, and tryptic digestions. This indicates that no gross irreversible changes in the conformation of the HGH molecule occur as a consequence of the 50% acid treatment, or by the alkylation of the tryptophan residue.

It may therefore be concluded that the Trp_{25} residue in the human growth hormone molecule is not essential for the growth-promoting activity, but, on the other hand, it seems to play an important role in the lactogenic activity of the hormone. This would mean that two different 'active sites' exist in the HGH molecule: one for the growth-promoting activity and the other for the lactogenic activity.

When the reaction was performed in diluted acetic acid media (0.2 M) only partial conversion occurred. Since total alkylation of tryptophan by NPS-Cl can be effected in this 0.2 M acetic acid solution, as is shown by an experiment performed with a model heptadecapeptide (α^{1-17}-ACTH) (Brovetto-Cruz and Li, 1969), some reversible conformational changes in the HGH molecule, sufficient to expose a masked tryptophan residue, must occur in 50% acetic acid.

Studies performed with the other tryptophan derivatives obtained by reaction of HGH with HNB-Br (Brovetto-Cruz and Li, 1969) further support the assumption that the Trp_{25} residue of HGH is located in the interior of the molecule, and is reversibly exposed in 50% acetic acid.

Tyrosyl residues

The HGH molecule contains 8 tyrosyl residues (Li *et al.*, 1966) that appear to be quite evenly distributed along the polypeptide chain. The environmental sensitivity of the ionization of this amino-acid phenolic group was used to obtain information concerning their environment in the molecule. The spectrophotometric titration technique was employed. On the basis of these studies (Bewley *et al.*, 1969), the 8 tyrosines can be separated, according to their location in the HGH molecule, in 2 groups: (1) 6 exposed or semi-exposed residues, and (2) 2 deeply buried within the protein molecule.

Using the same technique, Fønss-Bech and Schmidt (1969) have arrived at the same conclusion that some of the tyrosyl residues in the native hormone are shielded from the solvent by being buried in the molecule.

Further investigations by specific nitration of the tyrosyl residues (Ma *et al.*, 1970*a*) using

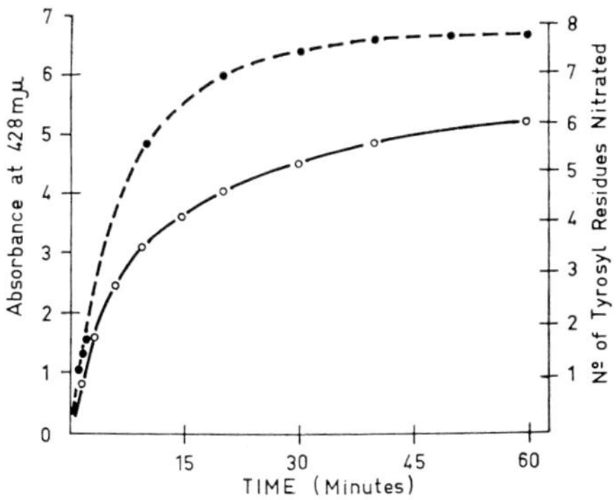

Fig. 2. Rates of nitration of HGH in pH 8.0 tris buffer (○ ——— ○) and in the same tris buffer containing 5 M guanidine hydrochloride (● — — — — ●). (Ma *et al.*, 1970*b*.)

TABLE V

Lactogenic activity of nitrated HGH as assayed by the pigeon crop-sac test

Preparation	Total dose (μg)	Response	
		Mean weight* $\pm$ S.D.	Potency
Native HGH	1	10 $\pm$ 2 (6)	
	4	18 $\pm$ 4 (6)	
HGH-$_6NO_2$	1	12 $\pm$ 2 (6)	
	4	17 $\pm$ 4 (6)	99.6%

* Mean dry weight of crop-sac epithelium in mg.

TABLE VI

Growth-promoting activity of nitrated HGH as assayed by the rat tibia test

Preparation	Mean response (μ) $\pm$ S.D. for total doses (μg) of:				Potency
	20	40	100	200	
Native HGH	233 $\pm$ 16	—	284 $\pm$ 12	—	
HGH-$_6NO_2$	—	236 $\pm$ 16	—	295 $\pm$ 14	59%

tetranitromethane (Sokolovsky *et al.*, 1966) have confirmed these results. Figure 2 shows the kinetics of the nitration reaction. It can be seen that in the presence of a potent denaturant agent (5 M guanidine hydrochloride) that completely unfolds the protein molecule, all 8 tyrosyl residues were nitrated in 1 hour, whereas in the absence of guanidine only 6 were nitrated. Moreover, these studies showed that the derivative obtained by nitration of the 6 exposed tyrosines (HGH-$_6NO_2$) retains full lactogenic potency (Table V). Therefore, it can be concluded that the 6 'exposed' tyrosyl residues are not involved in the lactogenic activity of the hormone. It is interesting to point out that, as was described by us for ovine prolactin (Ma *et al.*, 1970), despite the significant conformational changes produced by the nitration, no appreciable alteration of the activity was found.

As is shown in Table VI, the growth-promoting potency of this derivative was only 59% of the potency of the native hormone. Since the derivative has a faster enzymatic degradation rate it can be partially hydrolyzed by proteolytic enzymes present in the circulatory system of the rat used for the bioassay. For this reason it is more difficult to evaluate the role played by the 6 'exposed' tyrosyl residues on the growth-promoting activity of the hormone.

PARTIAL ENZYMATIC HYDROLYSIS

Investigations carried out in the last few years have shown that hormonal activities do not depend upon the integrity of the whole molecule. Li and Samuelsson (1965) have reported that growth-promoting activity as well as lactogenic activity are retained after tryptic digestion of as much as 25% of the bonds of HGH susceptible to hydrolysis by trypsin. Recently, we have reinvestigated the tryptic hydrolysis of the hormone using insoluble polymer-supported enzyme as well as soluble trypsin (Brovetto-Cruz *et al.*, 1970). After an average of 4 bonds were cleaved, a fraction of lower molecular weight, as judged by gel filtration chromatography in different experimental conditions, was obtained. New additional C- and N-terminal amino-acids were found in this smaller complex fraction that almost completely retains both growth-promoting and lactogenic activities.

On the basis of these studies, it is certain that the whole molecule of HGH is not necessary for its hormonal potency.

CONCLUSIONS

Human growth hormone is a very stable molecule that firmly retains its biological properties: (1) it can withstand, without diminution of its hormonal activities, the cleavage of the 2 disulfide bridges; (2) it is not irreversibly damaged by such extreme conditions as dilution in 50% acetic acid, or in aqueous solution at pH 13.4; (3) significant conformational changes can be produced in the molecule without important alterations of the hormonal properties, as is demonstrated by the partially nitrated derivative HGH-$_6NO_2$.

The two biological activities studies (growth-promoting and lactogenic) seem to be located in two different sites in the hormone molecule, and derivatives possessing only one of these activities can be obtained.

Moreover, it looks possible to isolate, after partial enzymatic hydrolysis, a polypeptide smaller than the native molecule, which retains biological activity. The identification of such a fragment will greatly diminish the work involved in the synthesis of compounds with HGH activity.

REFERENCES

Bewley, T. A. (1968): Physico-chemical studies of human hypophyseal growth hormone. Ph. D. Dissertation, University of California, San Francisco, Calif.

Bewley, T. A., Brovetto-Cruz, J. and Li, C. H. (1969): Human pituitary growth hormone. Physico-chemical investigations of the native and reduced-alkylated protein. *Biochemistry*, *8*, 4701.

Bewley, T. A., Dixon, J. S. and Li, C. H. (1968): Human pituitary growth hormone. XVI. Reduction with Di thiothreitol in the absence of urea. *Biochim. biophys. Acta (Amst.)*, *154*, 420.

Bewley, T. A. and Li, C. H. (1969): The reduction of protein disulfide bonds in the absence of denaturants. *Int. J. Protein Res.*, *1*, 117.

Brovetto-Cruz, J. and Li, C. H. (1969): Human pituitary growth hormone. Studies of the tryptophan residue. *Biochemistry*, *8*, 4695.

Brovetto-Cruz, J., Martin, M. and Li, C. H. (1970): Unpublished results.

Dixon, J. S. and Li, C. H. (1966): Retention of the biological potency of human pituitary growth hormone after reduction and carbamidomethylation. *Science*, *154*, 785.

Fønss-Bech, P. and Schmidt, K. D. (1969): Studies on human somatotropin. Preparation and some physico-chemical properties. *Int. J. Protein Res.*, *1*, 85.

Kauzmann, W. (1959): Some factors in the interpretation of protein denaturation. *Advanc. Protein Chem.*, *14*, 1.

Koshland, D. E., Jr., Karkhanis, Y. D. and Latham, H. G. (1964): An environmentally-sensitive reagent with selectivity for the tryptophan residue in proteins. *J. Amer. chem. Soc.*, *86*, 1448.

Li, C. H., Dixon, J. S. and Liu, W. K. (1969): Human pituitary growth hormone. XIX. The primary structure of the hormone. *Arch. Biochem. Biophys.*, *133*, 70.

Li, C. H., Liu, W. K. and Dixon, J. S. (1966): Human pituitary growth hormone. XII. The amino acid sequence of the hormone. *J. Amer. chem. Soc.*, *88*, 2010.

Li, C. H. and Papkoff, H. (1956): Preparation and properties of growth hormone from human and monkey pituitary gland. *Science*, *124*, 1293.

Li, C. H. and Samuelsson, G. (1965): Human pituitary growth hormone. XI. Rate of hydrolysis by trypsin, chymotrypsin and pepsin. Effect of trypsin on the biological activity. *Molec. Pharmacol.*, *1*, 47.

MA, L., BROVETTO-CRUZ, J. and LI, C. H. (1970*a*): Pituitary lactogenic hormone. The reaction of tetranitromethane with the ovine hormone. *Biochemistry*, *9*, 2302.
MA, L., BROVETTO-CRUZ, J. and LI, C. H. (1970*b*): Human pituitary growth hormone. XXVII. Reaction with tetranitromethane. *Biochim. biophys. Acta (Amst.)*, in press.
SCOFFONE, E., FONTANA, A. and ROCCHI, R. (1968): Sulfenyl halides as modifying reagent for polypeptides and proteins. I. Modification of tryptophan residues. *Biochemistry*, *7*, 971.
SOKOLOWSKY, M., RIORDAN, J. F. and VALLEE, B. L. (1966): Tetranitromethane. A reagent for the nitration of tyrosyl residues in proteins. *Biochemistry*, *5*, 3582.

PLASMA GROWTH HORMONE-LIKE ACTIVITY*

R. M. BALA, K. A. FERGUSON** and J. C. BECK

The McGill University Clinic, Royal Victoria Hospital, Montreal 112, Canada

INTRODUCTION

Human growth hormone (HGH) extracted from pituitary glands has been studied extensiveiy and the amino acid sequence reported by Li (1968). Human plasma contains pituitary-dependent substance(s) with antigenic similarity to extracted pituitary HGH (ep-HGH). Berson and Yalow (1966) and Boucher (1968) have presented evidence suggesting that immunoreactive HGH (IR-HGH) in plasma exists in an unassociated monomeric form which resembles ep-HGH, whereas others have presented direct and indirect evidence suggesting that IR-HGH in plasma may occur in different molecular sizes or may be associated with other proteins (Ferguson *et al.*, 1967; Hadden and Prout, 1964; 1965; MacMillan *et al.*, 1967; Irie and Barrett, 1962; Collip *et al.*, 1964).

Many investigators have demonstrated that physiological amounts of ep-HGH lack biological activity *in vitro* (Rigal, 1964; Daughaday and Kipnes, 1966; Daughaday and Mariz, 1962; Daughaday and Reeder, 1966; Salmon and Daughaday, 1957; Kostyo and Knobil, 1959; Wettenhall *et al.*, 1969), and that there is a time lag in the expression of certain biological activities when HGH is administered *in vivo*. Plasma contains a biologically active substance(s) as measured *in vitro* by stimulation of incorporation of radioactive sulfate (Daughaday and Kipnis, 1966; Salmon and Daughaday, 1958; Daughaday *et al.*, 1959; Kogut *et al.*, 1963; Almqvist, 1961), thymidine (Daughaday and Reeder, 1966) and proline (Daughaday and Mariz, 1962) into chondroitin sulfate, DNA and hydroxyproline, respectively, by cartilage from hypophysectomized rats. This activity, usually referred to a sulfation factor (SF), is pituitary-dependent and in general reflects the plasma levels of IR-HGH. Figure 1 summarizes some of the arguments which raise the question as to whether plasma and pituitary growth hormone are identical. On the one hand biologic and IR-HGH in plasma are increased in acromegaly and decreased in dwarfism, Sheehan's syndrome, and after hypophysectomy. In the latter group of disorders, the levels of activity can be restored to normal by treatment with HGH extracted from pituitaries. These observations are strong arguments in favor of plasma- and pituitary-HGH being identical. On the other hand, the discrepancy between clinical evidence of biological activity and IR-HGH levels measured in conditions such as the dwarfism described by Laron *et al.* (1966), Daughaday *et al.* (1969) and Rimoin *et al.* (1967), and in cerebral gigantism, partial hypopituitarism with gigantism and paradoxical growth after removal of craniopharyngiomas suggests non-identity. This series of observations suggests that pituitary-HGH is converted to biologically active form(s) before or after entering plasma, or that it induces the synthesis of biologically active substance(s) in

* Supported by the Medical Research Council of Canada, grant MT-631.

** Visiting Scientist C.S.I.R.O. Paramatta, New South Wales, Australia.

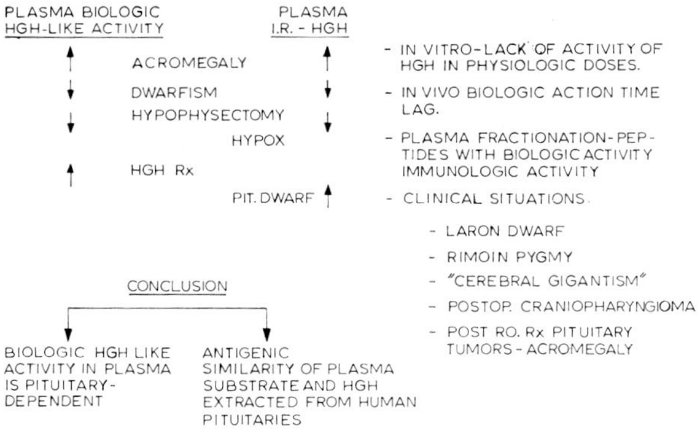

Fig. 1

plasma or in a tissue from which it is secreted into the circulation. Alternatively, plasma HGH may be associated with a larger protein playing a transport-storage role.

We have attempted to study the distribution and correlation of biologic and IR-HGH-like activity in plasma after fractionation of large volumes of plasma by gel filtration on Sephadex, producing a series of fractions of progressively smaller molecular weight. The molecular weight has been estimated from the distribution coefficient (Kd) (Andrews, 1964; 1966; Laurent and Killander, 1964) where:

$$Kd = \frac{Ve - Vo}{Vi},$$

Ve, Vo, and Vi represent the elution volume for the protein, the gel column void volume, and the gel imbibed volume, respectively (Flodin).

MATERIALS AND METHODS

Blood samples from 3 normal (Boucher, 1968) and 15 acromegalic patients were collected in anticoagulant ACD solution and centrifuged at 4°C, yielding plasma samples varying from 80 to 350 ml. The plasma samples were kept at 4°C and were used within 24 hours of venipuncture ('fresh' samples). One plasma sample was stored at 4°C for one month after the addition of 0.02% sodium azide ('non-fresh' sample). The lyophilized plasma samples were processed shortly after collection, stored at 4°C and reconstituted immediately prior to use. The plasma samples were fractionated by gel filtration utilizing large closed-end columns, 10 × 100 cm, with a minimum gel bed volume (Vi) of 7000 ml, containing Sephadex G-75 superfine (Pharmacia). Elution was carried out at 4°C in a reverse flow manner with 0.15 M NH_4HCO_3, at pH 8.1, which contained 0.02% sodium azide as a bactericidal agent. On the column, albumin was eluted with a Kd value of 0.05 and ep-HGH at 0.30. The absorbance (OD) of the eluate at 280 mμ was continuously monitored and the eluate was divided into successive fractions; these were concentrated by ultrafiltration, at 4°C, through Diaflo UM-2 membranes (Amicon Corp.) specified to retain proteins of greater than 1000 molecular weight. The total amount and concentration of protein was rechecked after ultrafiltration.

The amount of IR-HGH in the concentrated fraction was determined by a modified solid phase tube method (Bala *et al.*, 1969), consistently sensitive to less than 0.05 ng HGH and often to values of 0.025 ng HGH. Similarly fractionated bovine plasma was used as a control for non-specific protein effects on the radioimmunoassay.

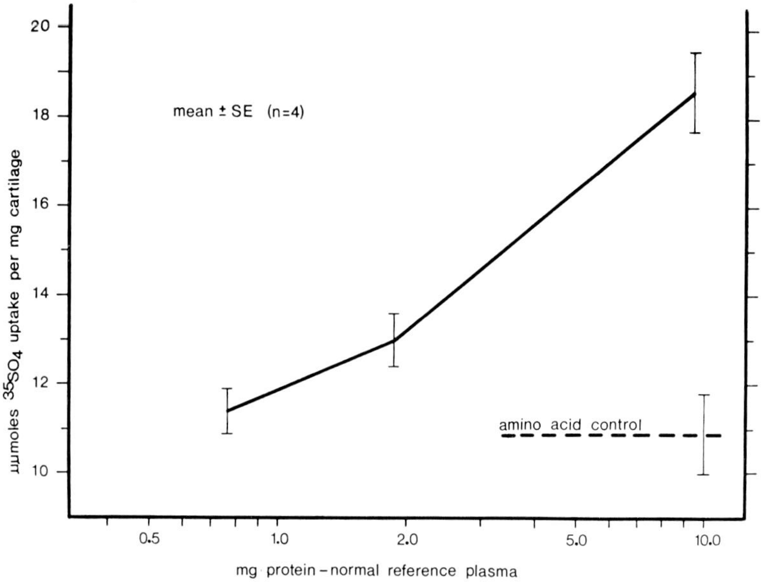

Fig. 2. In vitro sulfation factor assay standard curve. Uptake of $^{35}SO_4$ of 4 groups of 4 cartilage segments from a randomized pool of hypophysectomized rat costal cartilages. Expressed as mean ± SE mµ moles of $^{35}SO_4$ incorporated per mg dry weight cartilage versus the amount of plasma protein added in the form of normal reference plasma.

Sulfation factor assays of the concentrated samples were carried out as described by Daughaday *et al.* (1959), using the modifications of Kogut *et al.* (1963) with further modifications. The amino acid medium was prepared as described except that serine was added to result in a final concentration of 0.11 mM (Daughaday and Reeder, 1966). At least two dose levels were assayed and pooled normal human plasma was used as a reference standard. A standard curve, Figure 2, shows the mean ±S.E. uptake of $^{35}SO_4$ per mg of cartilage versus mg of protein in the normal pooled plasma which was added. A unit of SF activity was arbitrarily defined as the activity of 10 mg protein in the normal pooled reference plasma.

RESULTS

Fractionations of three representative plasma samples are shown in Figures 3–5. The protein concentration of the eluate is plotted at the mid-sample Kd. The magnified scale reveals minor secondary peaks at a Kd greater than 1.0, implying adsorption by Sephadex of material with significant absorbance at 280 mµ. This could represent aromatic amino acids alone or in small peptides. The height of the hatched bars represents the total nanograms (ng) of IR-HGH eluted in the fractions, and the elution volumes are represented by the width of the bars along the Kd scale. The potency of the eluted proteins is shown by the height of the solid bars in ng of IR-HGH per mg of protein in these fractions. In all of these examples, more than 50% of the total IR-HGH recovered was eluted in the Kd area less than 0.25, that is in a molecular size range greater than ep-HGH. The maximum potency occurred in the Kd interval corresponding to the molecular size of ep-HGH in all the plasmas. It is noted that some fractions of the normal plasma (Fig. 3) do not have detectable levels of IR-HGH. The acromegalic plasmas (Figs. 4 and 5), fresh and lyophilized respectively, have a greater relative proportion of the total IR-HGH in the ep-HGH molecular size range in comparison with the

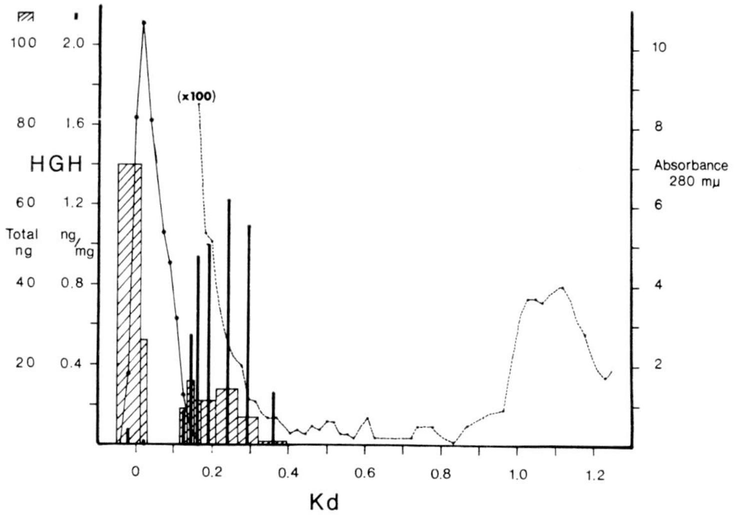

Fig. 3. Fractionation of 115 ml of fresh normal plasma by gel filtration with Sephadex G75. Protein concentration of the eluate (280 mμ OD) plotted at mid fraction Kd ●———● and magnified 100 × ●-----------●. The height of the hatched bars represents the total ng of IR-HGH in the fractions, while the width of the hatched bars represents the volume of elution corresponding to the Kd area covered. The heights of the solid bars represent the potency of the fractions in ng IR-HGH per mg of protein. Original plasma IR-HGH 1.9 ng per ml; 0.047 ng per mg protein.

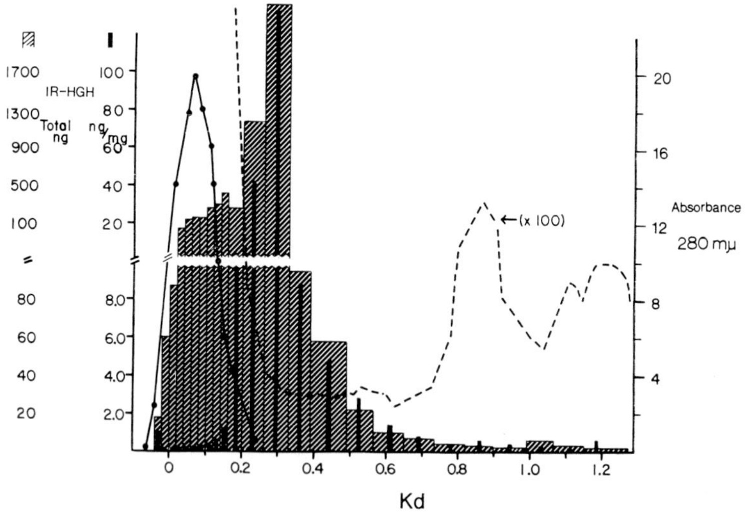

Fig. 4. Fractionation of 272 ml of fresh acromegalic patient plasma. Plotted similarly to Fig. 2. Original plasma IR-HGH 27.8 ng per ml; 0.623 ng per mg protein.

normal plasma. The lyophilized acromegalic plasma (Fig. 5) reveals material of high IR-HGH potency eluted after Kd 1.0 compared with fresh acromegalic plasma.

To allow interexperimental comparison of the plasma fractions, 0.10 Kd intervals were selected semi-arbitrarily. The total amount of protein eluted in each Kd interval for each experiment was expressed as a percentage of the total protein recovered in that experiment,

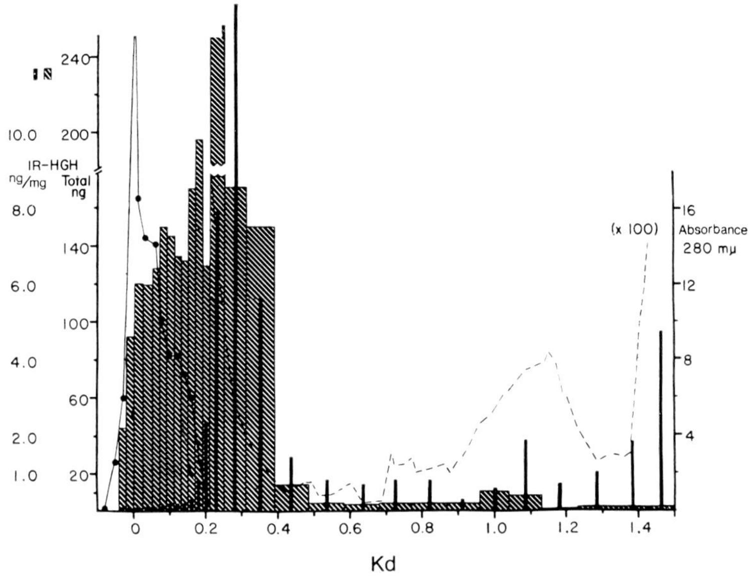

Fig. 5. Fractionation of 200 ml of lyophilized acromegalic patient plasma. Similarly plotted to Fig. 2. Original plasma IR-HGH 11.6 ng per ml, 0.159 ng per mg protein.

TABLE I

Mean percent of the total protein recovered per Kd interval after gel filtration of plasma*

Plasma	Kd interval										
	.05	.05-.15	.15-.25	.25-.35	.35-.45	.45-.55	.55-.65	.65-.75	.75-.85	.85-.95	.95
Normal** (3)	64.4 ±1.7	33.7 ±1.4	1.0 ± .3	.22 ±.05	.13 ±.02	.09 ±.01	.07 ±.01	.07 ±.01	.05 ±.01	.05 ±.01	.20 ±.03
Acromegalic (4) (Fresh)	62.9 ±4.1	33.9 ±3.1	1.7 ± .8	.34 ±.07	.19 ±.07	.16 ±.08	.12 ±.05	.09 ±.04	.11 ±.01	.13 ±.03	.27 ±.07
Acromegalic (11) (Lyophilized)	62.4 ±3.6	32.1 ±2.5	3.4 ±1.2	.81 ±.35	.32 ±.16	.16 ±.05	.14 ±.04	.12 ±.04	.12 ±.05	.19 ±.09	.55 ±.31

The number of experiments with each type of plasma is shown in brackets.
* Mean percentages ± SE. ** Includes 1 normal non-fresh plasma.

and the mean percentages ±SE of the various plasmas are shown in Table I. The mean final recovery of proteins in the experiments was 89% (range 83–129). The number of experiments with each type of plasma is shown in brackets. The lyophilized plasmas from acromegalic patients revealed greater relative secondary retarded peaks after Kd 0.95, implying that lyophilization resulted in increased amounts of small-sized molecular material with a high aromatic molecular structure component. The relatively similar proportions of protein eluted in the other Kd intervals indicate consistency in column behaviour between experiments.

The mean per cent ±SE of the total IR-HGH recovered is similarly shown for each Kd interval in Figure 6. Pooling of the data broadens the zone of activity compared with the

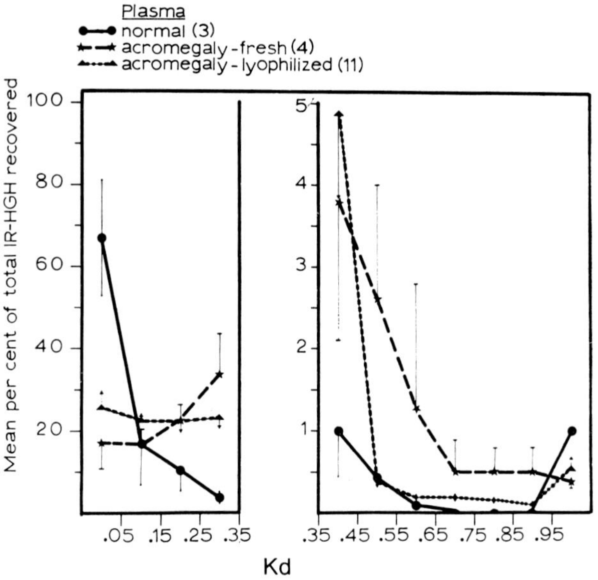

Fig. 6. The total amount of IR-HGH in each Kd interval calculated as a percent of the total IR-HGH recovered in each experiment, the mean percent ±SE is shown for the different types of plasmas. The increased value in the Kd interval greater than 0.95 was mainly due to the 1 non-fresh normal plasma.

individual experiments shown in Figures 2–4. The mean final recovery of IR-HGH in all experiments was 108% (range 60–137). The mean levels of IR-HGH in the normal, fresh and lyophilized acromegalic plasma were 1.7, 27.1, 37.7 ng/ml, respectively. The normal plasmas have a greater proportion of the total IR-HGH eluted before Kd 0.25 areas compared to plasmas from acromegalics. The latter show a higher percentage of the total IR-HGH in the Kd area corresponding to the molecular size of ep-HGH compared with the normal plasmas. This suggests that, in acromegaly, the IR-HGH molecules are of different size or exhibit less aggregation or perhaps less association with other plasma proteins concomitant with the higher levels of initial plasma IR-HGH. A relatively greater proportion of the total IR-HGH occurs in the larger molecular size area in lyophilized compared with fresh acromegalic plasma, indicating aggregation of IR-HGH molecules or association with other protein molecules due to lyophilization. Significant individual variation occurred in the percentages of the total IR-HGH eluted per Kd interval; however, in all plasmas more than 50% of the total IR-HGH was eluted before Kd 0.25.

The mean potency of the various plasma fractions in ng IR-HGH per mg of protein for each Kd interval is shown in Figure 7. The mean potencies of the original plasmas were 0.028, 0.496, and 0.501 ng IR-HGH per mg of protein for the normal, fresh, and lyophilized acromegalic plasmas, respectively. The highest IR-HGH potency of eluted proteins in all the plasmas was found in the Kd interval 0.25–0.45 and in most plasmas in the 0.25–0.35 Kd interval which corresponds to the molecular size interval of ep-HGH. The fractions of acromegalic plasma showed higher potencies than normal plasma fractions throughout. Even in the Kd area corresponding to very large and small molecular sizes the potency of the acromegalic fractions approximated the peak potency of the normal plasmas in the Kd interval of ep-HGH.

Plasma fractions from Kd 0.15 to 0.85 were assayed for SF activity. To allow interexperimental comparison, the total SF activity in each Kd interval for each plasma was expressed

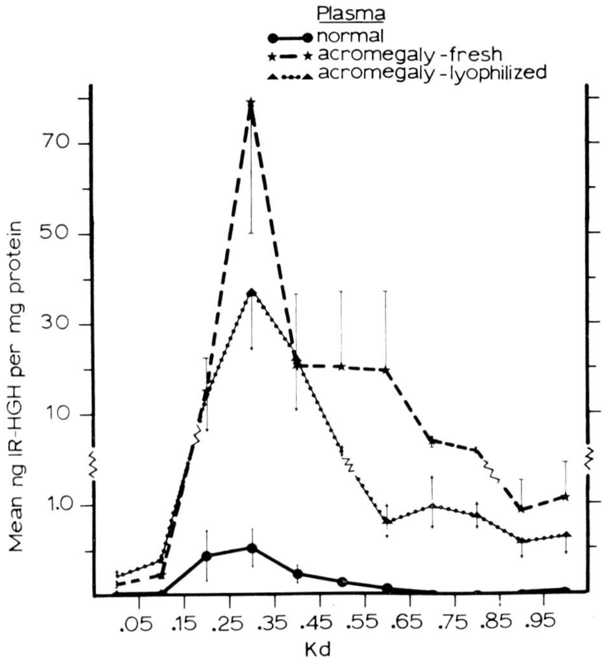

Fig. 7. The potencies of the eluted proteins in each Kd interval for each experiment calculated in ng IR-HGH per mg of protein. The mean ±SE potencies are plotted for the different types of plasmas.

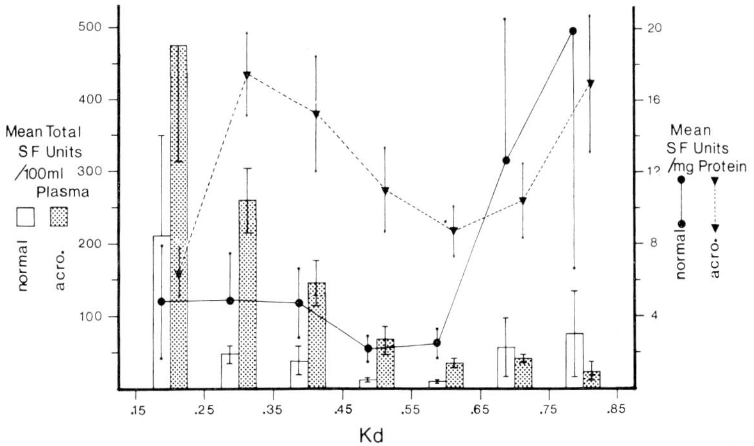

Fig. 8. The total SF units of activity in each Kd interval of each experiment was calculated per 100 ml of original plasma found. The potency in SF units per mg of protein in each Kd interval for each experiment was calculated. The mean ±SE total SF activities and potencies are plotted for acromegalic and normal plasma.

per 100 ml of original plasma. The mean ±SE totals per Kd interval for normal and acromegalic patient plasma are shown in Figure 8. Considerable variation in the SF activity by the various plasmas occurred when expressed per 0.1 Kd intervals. The maximum total SF activity occurred in the 0.15–0.25 Kd interval in all plasmas, except in three lyophilized acromegalic plasmas in which the maximal total activity occurred in the 0.25–0.35 Kd area.

In the Kd area less than 0.65, the potency in SF units per mg of eluted protein was greatest in the 0.25–0.35 Kd interval area in most plasmas. The potency of all but two acromegalic plasmas was higher than the normal plasmas in the Kd intervals before 0.65 Kd. This suggests that acromegalic plasma contains a greater amount of a more potent SF activity stimulating substance than does normal plasma. In the Kd area greater than 0.65 the elution of an increased amount of more potent SF activity-stimulating substance suggests a substance of a different nature or a dissociated form.

Added ep-HGH in amounts up to 0.1 mg/ml of the amino acid medium or of plasma had no direct SF-stimulating activity. SF activity in acromegalic and normal plasma was not reduced by addition of HGH antiserum.

DISCUSSION

We have attempted to investigate the nature of endogenous IR-HGH in plasma. Large volumes of plasma were fractionated by gel filtration, and the eluate fractions subsequently concentrated by ultrafiltration. We feel that this approach has allowed detection of IR-HGH activity in plasma fractions which might otherwise not have been apparent. Since electrophoresis might have disruptive effects on protein associations (Ferguson, 1964; Franglen and Gosselin, 1958; Reithel, 1963), we have avoided this technique as an initial separative method. Our results showed that more than 50% of the IR-HGH activity in acromegalic and normal plasma was present in a molecular size area greater than that of ep-HGH after fractionation of the plasmas by gel filtration. It is possible that ep-HGH is an altered form or subunit structure of endogenous pituitary HGH and is therefore different from part of the total plasma IR-HGH (Leaver, 1966; Roos *et al.*, 1963; Rhode and Dörner, 1969). If endogenous pituitary HGH is identical to ep-HGH then either these IR-HGH molecules in plasma are aggregated forms or they are associated with other plasma proteins, and these complexes are not disrupted by gel filtration. There is convincing evidence that ep-HGH does aggregate under appropriate conditions (Andrews, 1966; Leaver, 1966; Sluyser, 1964; Hunter, 1963; 1965; Saxena and Henneman, 1966; Squire and Pedersen, 1961; Hanson *et al.*, 1966; Lewis *et al.*, 1969; Cheever and Lewis, 1969; Li, 1964); however, convincing evidence with respect to endogenous plasma IR-HGH is lacking.

Our results showing an increased proportion of the total IR-HGH of lyophilized acromegalic plasma in a larger molecular size Kd area may support the findings of others (Squire *et al.*, 1963) that lyophilization does favour aggregation of proteins, but this does not explain our findings with fresh plasmas. Similarly fractionated lyophilized ep-HGH resulted in more than 95% of the IR-HGH being eluted in the same Kd area on refractionation. These results are similar to the findings of others using different buffer systems (Hunter, 1963; 1965; Saxena and Henneman, 1966). This suggests that the conditions in which our plasmas were fractionated did not result in the apparent larger molecular size units for IR-HGH by favouring aggregation of IR-HGH.

The finding that the relative proportions of IR-HGH with a Kd similar to ep-HGH were increased in acromegalic plasma compared to normal plasma, supports the possibility of the association of IR-HGH with plasma proteins (Hadden and Prout, 1964; 1965; MacMillan *et al.*, 1967; Irie and Barrett, 1962; Collipp *et al.*, 1964), with saturation occurring at higher levels of plasma IR-HGH analogous to the distribution of cortisol in states of hypercortisolism. Preliminary studies of mixtures of rechromatographed ep-HGH added to plasma or to solutions of various plasma proteins and similarly fractionated by gel filtration, suggest that some degree of IR-HGH association with plasma proteins is occurring. Further studies including attempts to dissociate the IR-HGH proteins from plasma proteins are required. The ratio of the total plasma protein to IR-HGH protein in plasma is high, and it is recognized that part of this IR-HGH in the molecular size area larger than ep-HGH may be due to molecular size zone spreading on gel filtration in spite of the conditions chosen to minimize this effect.

The elution of IR-HGH peptides with Kd values corresponding to molecular sizes smaller than ep-HGH suggests a metabolically changed endogenous plasma HGH, or that low molecular weight IR-HGH is produced during storage of the plasma or during gel filtration. One similarly fractionated plasma after prolonged storage in a frozen state (not included) revealed six distinct peaks of IR-HGH which were maximal in the small molecular size range. Others have shown that degradation of ep-HGH may occur during extraction, storage, freezing, or lyophilization (Berson and Yalow, 1966; Leaver, 1966; Rhode and Dörner, 1969; Hunter, 1965; Lewis *et al.*, 1969; Cheever and Lewis, 1969) and this conversion may be prevented to some extent by enzyme inhibitors (Ellis *et al.*, 1968; Lewis and Cheever, 1965). In general, however, our data show that the plasmas with the highest initial IR-HGH levels were associated with increased relative amounts of IR-HGH in the small molecular size area, suggesting that part of this IR-HGH may reflect increased levels of metabolically changed IR-HGH in plasma. Since we did not add enzyme inhibitors to our plasmas, this is only speculative. Our findings, however, do imply that molecules much smaller than ep-HGH can be immunoreactive with it. It is possible that part of the high molecular weight IR-HGH may be due to binding of small IR-HGH molecules with plasma proteins. Preliminary fractionation studies (unpublished) of plasma from hypopituitary patients after treatment with ep-HGH revealed a similar distribution of IR-HGH to that found in normal plasma, with the relative proportions of IR-HGH with smaller and larger molecular size than ep-HGH increasing with the time from treatment to withdrawal of plasma.

Similarly fractionated plasmas from hypophysectomized patients revealed that all the fractions were devoid of IR-HGH activity; this study was carried out by one of us (K.A.F.) using slightly different conditions from the present study and consequently has not been included.

We have attempted to use the sulfation factor assay as an *in vitro* assay for pituitary HGH-dependent biological activity in plasma. It is established that SF in plasma is, to a large degree, dependent upon pituitary HGH. This plasma SF is not due to pituitary HGH directly, as is shown by absence of SF activity in physiological amounts of ep-HGH tested *in vitro*, and by the time lag of restoration of SF activity in the plasma of hypophysectomized rats or humans after administration of ep-HGH *in vivo*, as well as the subsequent persistence of the SF in plasma for much longer than IR-HGH (Daughaday and Kipnis, 1966). The greatest total amount of SF in all the plasma fractions assayed over the 0.15–0.85 Kd interval corresponded to a molecular size range larger than that of ep-HGH. In all the Kd areas less than 0.65, all but two acromegalic plasmas contained a greater amount of more potent SF activity than normal plasma. The peak mean potencies in the Kd interval corresponding to ep-HGH molecular size suggest that the most potent SF activity-stimulating material has a molecular size similar to ep-HGH. The approximate parallelism, in general, of SF activity and IR-HGH in these plasmas is interesting. Since ep-HGH is biologically inactive *in vitro* in physiological amounts, this could represent an altered pituitary HGH molecule in plasma that has both IR-HGH and *in vitro* biological activity. Alternatively it may be an *in vitro* biologically active substance(s) in plasma, which is pituitary HGH-dependent, that is distinct from IR-HGH but is similar in size. The increase in SF activity after Kd 0.65 suggests an SF of a different nature. Preliminary assays of immunoreactive insulin (IRI) and insulin-like activity (ILA) of these fractions show peak activity at Kd 0.65, but the amount of insulin would not fully account for the level of SF activity found according to our studies (unpublished) and from published similar observations (Salmon and Daughaday, 1957; Salmon *et al.*, 1968; Esanu *et al.*, 1969) on *in vitro* SF activity stimulation by insulin. However, insulin could account for part of the activity. Since insufficient amounts of samples were available to repeat the assays with addition of specific antisera to ep-HGH and insulin, our SF activity data are inconclusive at this time. We believe that the further isolation and characterization of the *in vitro* biologically active substances in plasma, which are pituitary HGH-dependent, would be of great experimental and clinical value.

SUMMARY

1. The amounts of protein, IR-HGH and SF activity of plasma fractions from normals and acromegalic patients obtained by gel filtration and concentrated by ultrafiltration were determined and expressed per 0.1 distribution coefficient (Kd) intervals.
2. In excess of 50% of the total IR-HGH in these plasma samples was eluted in a molecular size range greater than ep-HGH, indicating plasma IR-HGH activity in a molecular size larger than ep-HGH or in association with other plasma proteins.
3. IR-HGH activity was also found in the Kd areas corresponding to a molecular size smaller than ep-HGH.
4. The plasma from acromegalic patients showed a relatively greater amount of IR-HGH in the ep-HGH molecular size area compared to normal plasma.
5. The maximal total SF activity occurred in a molecular size greater than ep-HGH but the maximum SF potency of the eluted proteins occurred in the ep-HGH molecular size area, and plasma from acromegalic patients contained a greater amount of more potent SF activity.
6. The general parallelism between SF and IR-HGH activity in the plasma fractions suggests that the SF is similar in size to ep-HGH but they cannot be identical. It is possible that ep-HGH is different from plasma HGH and from endogenous pituitary HGH. The possible mechanisms by which this may be brought about are discussed.

REFERENCES

Almqvist, S. (1961): Studies on sulfation factor (SF) activity of human serum. *Acta endocr. (Kbh.)*, *36*, 31.

Andrews, P. (1964): Estimation of the molecular weights of proteins by Sephadex gel-filtration. *Biochem. J.*, *91*, 222.

Andrews, P. (1966): Molecular weights of prolactins and pituitary growth hormones estimated by gel filtration. *Nature*, 209, 155.

Bala, R. M., Ferguson, K. A. and Beck, J. C. (1969): Modified solid-phase (tube) radioimmunoassay of human growth hormone. *Canad. J. Physiol.*, *47*, 803.

Berson, S. A. and Yalow, R. S. (1966): State of human growth hormone in plasma and changes in stored solutions of pituitary growth hormone. *J. biol. Chem.*, *241*, 5745.

Boucher, B. J. (1968): The molecular weight of radioimmunoassayable growth hormone in human serum. *J. Endocr.*, *42*, 153.

Cheever, E. V. and Lewis, U. J. (1969): Estimation of the molecular weights of the multiple components of growth hormone and prolactin. *Endocrinology*, *85*, 465.

Collipp, P. J., Kaplan, S. A., Boyle, D. C. and Shimizu, C. S. N. (1964): Protein bound human growth hormone. *Metabolism*, *13*, 532.

Daughaday, W. H. and Kipnis, D. M. (1966): The growth promoting and anti-insulin action of somatotropin. *Recent Progr. Hormone Res.*, *22*, 49.

Daughaday, W. H., Laron, Z. and Heins, J. N. (1969): Defective sulfation factor generation: a possible etiological link in dwarfism. *Clin. Res.*, *17*, 472 (Abstract).

Daughaday, W. H. and Mariz, I. K. (1962): Conversion of proline-U-C^{14} to labeled hydroxyproline by rat cartilage *in vitro*. Effects of hypophysectomy, growth hormone, and cortisol. *J. Lab. clin. Med.*, *59*, 741.

Daughaday, W. H. and Reeder, C. (1966): Synchronous activation of DNA synthesis in hypophysectomized rat cartilage by growth hormone. *J. Lab. clin. Med.*, *68*, 357.

Daughaday, W. H., Salmon, W. D. and Alexander, F. (1959): Sulfation factor activity of sera from patients with pituitary disorders. *J. clin. Endocr.*, *19*, 743.

ELLIS, S., MENKE, J. M. and GRINDELAND, K. E. (1968): Identity between growth hormone degrading activity of the pituitary gland and plasmin. *Endocrinology*, *83*, 1029.
ESANU, C., MURAKAWA, S., BRAY, G. A. and RABEN, M. S. (1969): DNA synthesis in human adipose tissue in vitro. I. Effect of serum and hormones. *J. clin. Endocr.*, *29*, 1027.
FERGUSON, K. A. (1964): Starch-gel electrophoresis – application to the classification of pituitary proteins and polypeptides. *Metabolism*, *13*, 985.
FERGUSON, K. A., LAZARUS, L., VANDOOREN, P. and YOUNG, J. D. (1967): The nature of the growth-promoting substances in human plasma. *Acta endocr. (Kbh.)*, *Supp. 119,* 238 (Abstract).
FLODIN, P.: In: *Dextral Gels and their Application in Gel Filtration.* Pharmacia, Uppsala, Sweden.
FRANGLEN, G. and GOSSELIN, C. (1958): Separation of metastable polymers by starch gel electrophoresis. *Nature (Lond.)*, *181*, 1152.
HADDEN, D. R. and PROUT, T. E. (1964): A growth hormone binding protein in normal human serum. *Nature (Lond.)*, *202*, 1342.
HADDEN, D. R. and PROUT, T. E. (1965): Studies on human growth hormone. II. The effect of human serum on growth hormone labelled with radioactive iodine. *Bull. Johns Hopk. Hosp.*, *116*, 1965.
HANSON, L. A., ROOS, P. and RYMO, L. (1966): Heterogeneity of human growth hormone preparations by immuno-gel filtration and gel filtration electrophoresis. *Nature (Lond.)*, *212*, 948.
HUNTER, W. M. (1963): Proceedings of the Society of Analytical Chemistry. 87th Ordinary Meeting of the Physical Methods Group. *Analyst, 88*, 251.
HUNTER, W. M. (1965): Homogeneity studies on human growth hormone. *Biochem. J.*, *97*, 199.
IRIE, M. and BARRETT, R. J. (1962): Immunologic studies of human growth hormone. *Endocrinology*, *71*, 277.
KOGUT, M. D., KAPLAN, S. A. and SCHIMIZU, C. S. N. (1963): Growth retardation; use of sulfation factor as a bioassay for growth hormone. *Pediatrics*, *31*, 538.
KOSTYO, J. L. and KNOBIL, E. (1959): The stimulation of leucine-Z4-C^{14} incorporation with the protein of isolated rat diaphragm by simian growth hormone added *in vitro*. *Endocrinology*, *65*, 525.
LARON, Z., PERTZELAN, A. and MANNHEIMER, S. (1966): Genetic pituitary dwarfism with high serum concentration of growth hormone. A new inborn error of metabolism. *Israel J. med. Sc.*, *2*, 152.
LAURENT, J. C. and KILLANDER, J. (1964): A theory of gel filtration and its experimental verification. *J. Chromat.*, *14*, 317.
LEAVER, F. W. (1966): Evidence for the existence of human growth hormone-ribonucleic acid complex in the pituitary. *Proc. Soc. exp. Biol. Med. (N.Y.)*, *122*, 188.
LEWIS, U. J. and CHEEVER, E. V. (1965): Evidence for two types of conversion reactions for prolactin and growth hormone. *J. biol. Chem.*, *240*, 247.
LEWIS, U. J., PARKER, D. C., OKERLUND, M. D., BOYER, R. M., LITTERIA, M. and VANDERLAAN, W. P. (1969): Aggregate-free human growth hormone. II. Physicochemical and biological properties. *Endocrinology*, *84*, 332.
LI, C. H. (1968): The chemistry of human pituitary hormone; review 1956–1966. In: *Growth Hormone, Proceedings of the First International Symposium, Milan*, pp. 3–28. Editors: A. Pecile and E. E. Müller. ICS No. 158. Excerpta Medica, Amsterdam.
LI, C. H., TANAKA, A. and PICKERING, B. T. (1964): Human pituitary hormone. VII. *In vitro* lipolytic activity. *Acta endocr. (Kbh.)*, *45*, *Sypp. 90*, 155.
MACMILLAN, D. R., SCHMID, J. M., EASH, S. A. and READ, C. H. (1967): Studies on the heterogeneity and serum binding of human growth hormone. *J. clin. Endocr.*, *27*, 1090.
REITHEL, F. J. (1963): The dissociation and association of protein structures. *Advanc. Protein Chem.*, *18*, 123.
RIGAL, W. M. (1964): Site of action of growth hormone in cartilage. *Proc. Soc. exp. Biol. Med. (N.Y.)*, *117*, 794.
RIMOIN, D. L., MERIMEE, T. J., RABINOWITZ, D., CAVALLI-SFORZA, L. L. and MCKUSICK, V. (1968): Genetic aspects of isolated growth hormone deficiency. In: *Growth Hormone, Proceedings of the First International Symposium, Milan,* pp. 418–432. Editors: A. Pecile and E. E. Müller. ICS No. 158. Excerpta Medica, Amsterdam.
ROHDE, W. and DORNER, G. (1969): Immunochemical studies on the heterogeneity of human growth hormone (HGH). *Acta endocr. (Kbh.)*, *60*, 101.
ROOS, P., FEVOLD, H. R. and GEMZELL, C. A. (1963): Preparation of human growth hormone by gel filtration. *Biochim. biophys. Acta (Amst.)*, *74*, 525.
SALMON, W. D. and DAUGHADAY, W. H. (1957): A hormonally-controlled serum factor which stimulates sulfate incorporation by cartilage *in vitro*. *J. Lab. clin. Med.*, *49*, 825.

Salmon, W. D. and Daughaday, W. H. (1958): The importance of amino acids as dialyzable components of rat serum which promotes sulfate uptake by cartilage from hypophysectomized rats *in vitro*. *J. Lab. clin. Med.*, *51*, 167.

Salmon, W. D., DuVall, R. M. and Thompson, E. Y. (1968): Stimulation by insulin *in vitro* of incorporation of (^{35}S) sulfate and (^{14}C) leucine into protein-polysaccharide complexes, (^{3}H) uridine into RNA, and (^{3}H) thymidine into DNA of costal cartilage from hypophysectomized rats. *Endocrinology*, *82*, 493.

Saxena, B. B. and Henneman, P. H. (1966): Isolation and properties of the electrophoretic components of human growth hormone by Sephadex-gel filtration and preparative polyacrylamide-gel electrophoresis. *Biochem. J.*, *100*, 711.

Sluyser, M. (1964): Possible causes of electrophoretic and chromatographic heterogeneity of pituitary hormones. *Nature (Lond.)*, *204*, 574.

Squire, P. G. and Pedersen, K. O. (1961): Sedimentation behavior of human pituitary growth hormone. *J. Amer. chem. Soc.*, *83*, 476.

Squire, P. G., Starman, B. and Li, C. H. (1963): Studies of pituitary lactogenic hormone. XII. Analysis of the state of aggregation of the ovine hormone by ultracentrifugation and exclusion chromatography. *J. biol. Chem.*, *238*, 1389.

Wettenhall, R. E. H., Schwartz, P. L. and Bornstein, J. (1969): Actions of insulin and growth hormone on collagen and chondroitin sulfate synthesis in bone organ cultures. *Diabetes*, *18*, 280.

STIMULATION TESTS OF GROWTH HORMONE SECRETION*

THEODORE W. AvRUSKIN,** JOHN F. CRIGLER, JR.,†
PETER H. SONKSEN° and J. STUART SOELDNER

Department of Medicine (Endocrine Division), The Children's Hospital Medical Center; The Elliott P. Joslin Research Laboratory, The Peter Bent Brigham Hospital; and the Departments of Pediatrics and Medicine, Harvard Medical School, Boston, Mass.; and The Department of Pediatrics, Division of Pediatric Endocrinology, The Brookdale Hospital Center; and Department of Pediatrics, New York University School of Medicine, New York, U.S.A.

The secretion of growth hormone (GH) has been extensively studied in man and primates in recent years. Radioimmunoassay of GH (Hunter and Greenwood, 1962; Glick *et al.*, 1963*a*) employing the principles of insulin immunoassay (Yalow and Berson, 1960) has made possible the accurate measurement in plasma and serum of extremely small concentrations of this polypeptide hormone.

Since the demonstration of insulin-induced hypoglycemia as a stimulus of growth hormone secretion (Roth *et al.*, 1963*a*), the administration of many different substances has been found to be associated with significantly increased serum growth hormone concentrations. Despite these studies, however, the role of growth hormone, especially in adults, has not been clarified completely. This fact results, in part, from the multitude of tasks assigned to growth hormone and from the wide range of factors which influence its release. Plasma concentrations vary considerably in normal subjects, being influenced by age, sex, activity, sleep, body weight, period of fasting, stress in recognized and in occult forms, and many metabolic factors. In the newborn period, GH levels may be quite high, even though this hormone does not seem to be required for fetal or neonatal growth. In normal adults, baseline concentrations vary from 0 to 5 ng/ml in males whereas in females a much broader range is seen with occasional values above 25 ng/ml. Transient peaks occur commonly during the day after stress, exercise, protein meals, and during sleep. The magnitude of increases seems to be greater in females, especially midway through the menstrual cycle, and is influenced by estrogen administration. For example, GH responses are more marked in females than in males following exercise or arginine (Catt, 1970) and are accentuated in males following arginine stimulation with estrogen pretreatment (Merimee *et al.*, 1969).

This paper briefly reviews some of the factors influencing GH secretion as they relate to tests for evaluating its production and presents data on serum growth hormone levels fol-

* Supported in part by U.S. Public Health Service Research Grants AM-09748, 5TO1-HD-0056, RR-00128, and the John A. Hartford Foundation, Inc., and The Joslin Diabetes Foundation, Inc., Boston, Mass.

** Present address: The Brookdale Hospital Center, Division of Pediatric Endocrinology and Metabolism. Linden Blvd. at Brookdale Plaza, Brooklyn, New York.

† Requests for reprints should be addressed to John F. Crigler, Jr., M.D., The Children's Hospital Medical Center, 300 Longwood Avenue, Boston, Mass. U.S.A. 02115

° Recipient of a Harkness Fellowship of the Commonwealth Fund of New York City, New York.

lowing the administration of glucagon to normal children and adolescents and to patients in the same age range with genetic variations in stature or alterations in growth and development due to hypopituitarism.

FACTORS INFLUENCING GROWTH HORMONE SECRETION

It can be seen that a host of non-specific stimuli (Table I) including stress, exercise, fasting, sleep and age are associated with GH secretion and, therefore, must be taken into account when considering tests for evaluating GH production which employ specific substances. Release of ACTH and catechol amines may be part of the sequence of events leading to GH release in response to stressful stimuli. Meyer and Knobil (1967) have shown that 'stress' precipitates the release of GH and ACTH, and Muller (1966) has noted that the reduction of pituitary GH content in rats induced by insulin hypoglycemia is blocked by a variety of drugs known to suppress ACTH release in response to noxious stimuli. In addition, Franz and Rabkin (1964) demonstrated that cortisol inhibits the growth hormone release associated with insulin hypoglycemia. The existence of a hypothalamic growth releasing factor (GRF) also seems amply confirmed since GH release with insulin-induced hypoglycemia may be inhibited by stalk-section (Roth *et al.*, 1963*b*), by tumors compressing hypothalamus and portal system (Landon *et al.*, 1966) and by micro-infusion of glucose into the hypothalamus (Blanco *et al.*, 1966). Stress control is mediated by the hypothalamus (Bayliss *et al.*, 1967) and, since many such stimuli result in GH secretion, it is reasonable to infer that GRF is controlled by neural impulses from a variety of CNS sites.

Specific stimuli for growth hormone secretion are listed in Table I. Hypoglycemia, induced by insulin (Roth *et al.*, 1963*a*), tolbutamide, post-glucose infusion, fructose, ethanol, or by decreasing the peripheral uptake of glucose using 2-deoxy-glucose (Roth *et al.*, 1963*b*), results in GH secretion. In general, significant elevations in serum GH levels have occurred 30–60

TABLE I

Factors influencing growth hormone release

I. Increases growth hormone
  A. Non-specific stimuli
    1. Stress (heat, cold, pH change, noise, pyrogen administration, surgery, etc.)
    2. Exercise
    3. Prolonged fasting
    4. Sleep
    5. Age
  B. Specific stimuli
    1. Induced hypoglycemia (insulin, tolbutamide, post-glucose, fructose, ethanol, 2-deoxyglucose, etc.)
    2. Amino acids (arginine, histidine, lysine, phenylalanine, leucine, valine, methionine, isoleucine, threonine)
    3. Glucagon
    4. Lysine vasopressin
    5. Estrogens (augment responses to other stimuli)
    6. Propranolol (augments response to insulin-induced hypoglycemia)

II. Decreases growth hormone
  A. Hyperglycemia
  B. Adrenocortical hormones
  C. Phentolamine (suppresses response to insulin-induced hypoglycemia)

minutes after the lowest blood glucose concentration. Amino acids produce release of GH from the pituitary, without inducing hypoglycemia. Indeed, arginine, a glucogenic amino acid widely used to study GH secretion, produces increased GH levels at a time when blood sugar is rising. Growth hormone responses after arginine may be influenced by prior sex hormone administration (Merimee *et al.*, 1969). Others have found higher GH levels after arginine in pre-adolescent females than in males (Parker *et al.*, 1967), and that prior testosterone augments GH response to arginine in males with hypogonadism (Martin *et al.*, 1966). Arginine, on the other hand, may have also a non-specific effect on GH release (Best *et al.*, 1968). Other amino acids have had a varying effect on GH release (Knopf *et al.*, 1969). Lysine vasopressin administration (Hillman and Colle, 1969) also is associated with increased serum GH concentrations, and estrogens and propranolol have been found to augment GH responses to other stimuli.

Growth hormone secretion is suppressed by hyperglycemia, adrenocortical hormones and phentolamine, an alpha-adrenergic blocking agent (Blackard and Heidingsfelder, 1968) (Table I).

In 1968, we reported that intramuscular glucagon administration was associated with a rise in serum GH concentrations in normal children and adolescents, whose responses were compared to responses in patients with a variety of endocrine disorders (AvRuskin *et al.*, 1968). Subsequently others (Mitchell *et al.*, 1969; 1970; Cain *et al.*, 1970) have reported similar findings, although Danforth and Rosenfeld (1970) found no change in GH levels after rapid i.v. glucagon. This paper provides additional data on growth hormone secretion after various routes of glucagon administration given either two hours after intravenous tolbutamide or after an overnight fast.

MATERIAL AND METHODS

Sixty-two tests were carried out in 48 subjects. The subjects studied included 10 normal males (age 10.6 ± 0.8 yr*) and 9 normal females (age 10.3 ± 0.5 yr) within 2 standard deviations of height and weight for age (Reed and Stuart, 1959; Bayer and Bailey, 1959), the females being sexually more mature than males (stage 2.6 ± 0.3 *vs* 1.9 ± 0.3; Tanner, 1962; Johannson *et al.*, 1969); 15 genetically short males (age 8.6 ± 0.8 yr, heights outside of minus 2 SD for age, weights average for height, stage sexual maturation 1.4 ± 0.1); 7 genetically tall females (age 11.6 ± 0.6 yr, height outside plus 2 SD for age, weight average for height, stage sexual maturation 2.6 ± 0.2); and 7 hypopituitary females (age 10.0 ± 1.1 yr, heights outside minus 2 SD for age, weights average for height, stage sexual maturation 1.1 ± 0.1), 3 with idiopathic hypopituitarism and 4 with pituitary deficiencies resulting from surgery for craniopharyngioma. The latter were receiving pitressin tannate-in-oil when indicated but no other therapies. All genetically short and tall subjects had normal pituitary-thyroid-adrenal axes as determined by standard thyroid and adrenal functional test. All subjects had an overnight fast (not more than 12 hr) and were kept supine from 30 to 60 minutes before and throughout the test period. Glucagon (0.03 mg/kg; maximum 1 mg) was administered either i.m. or i.v. after the overnight fast or 2 hours after tolbutamide. Serial samples for blood sugars (BS) and serum immunoreactive growth hormone (IRGH) were obtained and measurements made by previously described methods (Boden and Soeldner, 1967).

RESULTS

Changes in mean fasting and post-glucagon BS, and serum IRGH responses for all groups are shown in Table II. These tests were performed 2 hours after tolbutamide administration.

In normal males and females, BS rose significantly with higher mean values in females

* All data expressed as mean ± standard error of mean.

TABLE II

Blood sugar (BS mg/100 ml), and serum immunoreactive growth hormone (IRGH ng/ml) levels after i.m. gluca

Group	No.		0′ BS	0′ IRGH	0″ BS	0″ IRGH	15′ BS	15′ IRGH	30′ BS	30′ IRGH
Normal males	10	M	76	2.2	68	5.1	90	4.7	114	5.5
		SE	2.5	0.7	2.2	1.0	4.6	0.8	6.6	1.6
Normal females	9	M	77	4.1	67	1.9	100	2.1	133	1.3
		SE	1.3	1.4	1.7	0.7	2.6	0.4	1.2	0.3
		P	NS	NS	NS	<0.02	NS	<0.01	<0.02	<0.0
Short males	15	M	71	3.8	60	3.2	90	2.4	115	5.9
		SE	1.7	1.1	2.4	0.8	4.1	0.4	5.6	2.2
		P	NS	NS	<0.02	NS	NS	<0.02	NS	NS
Tall females	7	M	75	2.2	67	5.7	100	4.4	120	3.1
		SE	1.1	0.4	1.8	1.1	3.8	0.9	1.5	0.5
		P	NS	NS	NS	<0.02	NS	<0.05	<0.002	<0.0
Hypopit. females	7	M	70	1.1	56	0.7	87	0.5	115	0.7
		SE	2.8	0.2	2.3	0.4	7.2	0.2	11.7	0.1
		P	<0.05	<0.05	<0.002	NS	NS	<0.001	NS	NS

Group	No.		45′ BS	45′ IRGH	60′ BS	60′ IRGH	90′ BS	90′ IRGH	120′ BS	120′ IRGH
Normal males	10	M	115	7.1	100	8.9	75	10	67	12.4
		SE	7.5	3.1	6.4	3.9	3.0	3.7	2.5	2.1
Normal females	9	M	143	1.3	134	2.4	107	8.1	76	11.8
		SE	2.4	0.5	5.8	1.5	5.1	2.5	3.1	4.2
		P	<0.002	NS	<0.002	NS	<0.001	NS	<0.05	NS
Short males	15	M	117	4.3	106	4.7	75	7.5	62	15.9
		SE	6.5	1.2	5.8	1.6	4.4	2.0	2.4	4.6
		P	NS	NS	NS	NS	NS	NS	NS	NS
Tall females	7	M	122	2.5	117	6.1	87	10.4	71	27.9
		SE	5.1	0.2	7.3	2.4	6.2	4.3	3.4	7.6
		P	<0.01	<0.05	NS	NS	<0.05	NS	NS	NS
Hypopit. females	7	M	132	0.6	127	0.6	99	0.8	68	0.8
		SE	13.4	0.2	12.5	0.2	11.5	0.3	7.9	0.3
		P	NS	NS	NS	NS	NS	<0.02	NS	<.002

0′ : Zero time before i.v. tolbutamide administration.
0″: Zero time before i.m. glucagon administration (2 hours after tolbutamide).
P=: Comparison of significance using Student's 't' test between groups of similar sex, except when normal males a females are compared.

from 30–120 minutes ($P < 0.001$–0.05). Peak BS levels in both groups, however, occurred 45 minutes after glucagon. Maximum serum IRGH levels for normal males and females of 12.4 ± 2.1 ng/ml and 11.8 ± 4.2 ng/ml, respectively, were observed at 120 minutes.

BS and serum IRGH responses after i.m. glucagon in short males were similar to normal males, significant differences being evident only in the fasting post-tolbutamide levels and in the IRGH concentrations 15 minutes after glucagon ($P < 0.02$). The greatest mean serum IRGH concentration in short males was 15.9 ± 4.6 ng/ml and occurred 120 minutes after glucagon.

Tall-statured girls had significantly lower BS levels, 30, 45 and 90 minutes after i.m. glucagon compared to normal females ($P < 0.002$–0.05). In contrast, IRGH concentrations were greater prior to and 15, 30 and 45 minutes after glucagon administration in the tall females

TABLE III

Blood sugar (BS mg/100 ml) and serum immunoreactive growth hormone (IRGH ng/ml) levels of males after glucagon with and without prior tolbutamide administration

Group	No.		0′		15′		30′		45′		60′		90′		120′	
			BS	IRGH	BS	IRGH	BS	IRGH	BS	IRGH	BS	IRGH	BS	IRGH	BS	IRGH
Prior		M	57	3.3	76	2.6	94	2.1	94	2.6	94	4.4	69	6.5	58	23.4
tolbutamide	7	SE	2.4	0.6	5.6	0.4	9.1	0.4	15.1	0.9	10.2	2.5	6.1	3.3	3.3	8.6
No prior		M	74	5.9	108	3.1	129	2.3	122	1.6	97	2.0	78	1.7	68	15.2
tolbutamide	7	SE	4.1	2.0	7.2	0.8	7.9	0.5	8.5	0.2	8.4	0.6	5.1	0.3	3.7	3.4
		P	<0.01	NS	<0.01	NS	<0.02	NS	NS	NS	NS	NS	NS	NS	NS	NS

($P < 0.01$–0.05). Although the peak response of mean serum IRGH level in tall females occurred at 120 minutes and was 27.9 ± 7.6 ng/ml, the value was not significantly different from the normal females.

The hypopituitary females had lower fasting and post-tolbutamide BS concentrations than normal females ($P < 0.002$–0.05) but BS values after glucagon were not significantly different. The significantly lower mean fasting serum IRGH level in the hypopituitary females compared to the normal females was not increased after glucagon, the mean value 15, 90 and 120 minutes being significantly lower ($P < 0.001$–0.02).

In order to exclude any effect of prior tolbutamide on subsequent glucagon-mediated GH response, i.m. glucagon tests were carried out with and without prior tolbutamide administration in 7 male subjects (4 normal, 3 short males) (Table III). Blood sugar concentrations were lower ($P < 0.01$–0.02) before and 15 and 30 minutes after glucagon in tests done after tolbutamide than in tests without prior tolbutamide. In spite of these differences, mean serum IRGH levels before and after glucagon were not significantly different under the two conditions of testing. Therefore, prior tolbutamide does not appear to influence glucagon-mediated GH secretion.

Glucagon was given i.v. to the same 7 male subjects after an overnight fast to determine whether this route of administration would affect the serum IRGH response (Table IV). Blood sugar levels after both routes of administration peaked at 30 minutes, but from 45 through 90 minutes values were significantly higher ($P < 0.2$–0.05) after i.m. glucagon. Zero time IRGH concentrations of 5.9 ± 2.0 ng/ml and 3.4 ± 1.4 ng/ml in i.m. and i.v. tests, respectively, increased to maximum values of 23.4 ± 7.8 ng/ml 150 minutes after i.m. glucagon and 9.9 ± 1.9 ng/ml 120 minutes after i.v. glucagon. Nevertheless, mean IRGH values after both routes of administration were not significantly different at any time.

The mean of the maximum IRGH levels for each subject after i.m. glucagon and the mean time of individual maximum IRGH increase for all groups are given in Table V. Significant IRGH responses were seen in all except the hypopituitary group. Maximum growth hormone responses and mean times of this response were not different in the groups showing significant increases in serum IRGH concentrations after i.m. glucagon administration.

TABLE IV

Blood sugar (BS mg/100 ml) and serum immunoreactive growth hormone (IRGH ng/ml) levels of males after i.m. and glucagon administration

			-60′		-30′		0′		3′		5′		15′		30′	
Group	No.		BS	IRGH	BS	IRGH	BS	IRGH	BS	IRGH	BS	IRGH	BS	IRGH	BS	IRG
I.m.	7	M	81	6.1	74	6.8	74	5.9	74	4.6	69	3.8	108	3.1	129	2.3
glucagon		SE	5.4	2.3	3.4	2.8	4.1	2.0	4.3	1.4	12.7	1.2	7.2	0.8	7.9	0.5
I.v.	7	M	75	6.0	72	7.3	71	3.4	81	3.4	87	3.5	102	4.9	111	5.9
glucagon		SE	1.6	1.3	1.5	2.1	1.0	1.4	2.2	1.1	2.1	1.1	3.4	1.1	5.7	2.6
		P	NS	NS	NS	NS	NS	NS	NS	NS	NS	NS	NS	NS	NS	NS

			45′		60′		90′		120′		150′		180′	
Group	No.		BS	IRGH	BS	IRGH	BS	IRGH	BS	IRGH	BS	IRGH	BS	IRG
I.m.	7	M	122	1.6	97	2.0	78	1.7	68	15.2	66	23.4	69	8.4
glucagon		SE	8.5	0.2	8.4	0.6	5.1	0.3	3.7	3.4	5.4	7.8	4.5	2.0
I.v.	7	M	91	4.0	76	2.9	63	5.1	66	9.9	66	8.6	65	7.3
glucagon		SE	5.3	1.5	3.6	0.6	1.2	1.8	1.3	1.9	1.1	1.7	2.0	1.3
		P	<0.02	NS	<0.05	NS	<0.02	NS	NS	NS	NS	NS	NS	NS

TABLE V

*Mean maximum IRGH responses after i.m. glucagon**

Group	No.	Control IRGH (ng/ml)	Max. IRGH (ng/ml)	P†	Time max. response (min)
Normal males	10	5.1 ±1.0	17.1 ±3.2	<0.01	97 ±8.7
Normal females	9	1.9 ±0.7	14.3 ±3.9	<0.01	113 ±4.4
Short males	15	3.2 ±0.8	19.5 ±6.8	<0.02	98 ±6.8
Tall females	7	5.7 ±1.1	27.4 ±6.6	<0.01	103 ±8.9
Hypopit. females	7	0.7 ±0.4	1.1 ±0.2	NS	69 ±16

* Data expressed as mean ± standard error.
† Comparison of significance using Student's 't' test between control and maximum IRGH.

DISCUSSION AND CONCLUSIONS

There is a consistent increase in serum GH levels following glucagon administration to normal children and adolescents which reaches its maximum between 60 and 150 minutes. This reproducible rise in GH was found to be of comparable magnitude to normal subjects in genetically short males and tall females of similar age and development but absent in females with hypopituitarism. The increase in serum GH occurred regardless of the route of glucagon administration although it appeared more marked after i.m. than after i.v. administration at the dosages used. The GH response to glucagon was not significantly influenced by prior administration of tolbutamide. The increase in serum GH levels occurs 45–75 minutes after peak rises in BS but is not positively correlated with the rate of BS decrease which precedes its rise. The mechanism by which glucagon induces GH secretion is being further investigated.

REFERENCES

AvRuskin, T. W., Crigler, J. F., Jr. and Sonksen, P. (1968): Growth hormone secretion after i.m. glucagon administration to normal children and adolescents and to patients with endocrine disorders. *Clin. Res.*, *16*, 520.

Bayer, L. and Bayley, N. (1959): *Growth Diagnosis.* University of Chicago Press.

Bayliss, M., Greenwood, F. C., James, V. H. T., Jenkins, J., Landon, J., Marks, V. and Samols, E. (1967): An examination of the control mechanisms postulated to control growth hormone secretion in man. In: *Proceedings, 1st International Symposium on Growth Hormone, Milan,* pp. 89–104. Editors: A. Pecile and E. Müller. ICS No 158. Excerpta Medica, Amsterdam.

Best, J., Catt, K. J. and Burger, H. G. (1968): The specificity of arginine infusion as a test for growth hormone secretion. *Lancet*, *2*, 125.

Blackard, W. G. and Heidingsfelder, S. A. (1968): Adrenergic receptor control mechanism for growth hormone secretion. *J. clin. Invest.*, *47*, 1407.

Blanco, S., Schalch, D. S. and Reichlin, S. (1966): Control of growth hormone secretion by glucoreceptors in the hypothalamic pituitary unit. *Fed. Proc.*, *25*, 91.

Boden, G. and Soeldner, J. S. (1967): A sensitive double antibody radioimmunoassay for human growth hormone (HGH): levels of serum HGH following rapid tolbutamide infusion. *Diabetologia*, *3*, 43.

Cain, J. P., Williams, G. H. and Dluhy, R. G. (1970). Glucagon stimulation of immunoreactive human growth hormone. In: *Abstracts, Program of the Fifty-second Meeting of the Endocrine Society,* p. 149.

Catt, K. J. (1970): ABC of endocrinology. III. Growth hormone. *Lancet*, *1*, 933.

Danforth, E., Jr. and Rosenfeld, P. S. (1970): Effect of intravenous glucagon on circulating levels of growth hormone and 17-hydroxycorticosteroids *J. clin. Endocr.*, *30*, 117.

FRANZ, A. G. and RABKIN, M. T. (1964): Human growth hormone. Clinical measurement response to hypoglycemia, and suppression by corticosteroids. *New Engl. J. Med.*, *271*, 1375.

GLICK, S. M., ROTH, J., YALOW, R. S. and BERSON, S. A. (1963*a*): Immunoassay of human growth hormone in plasma. *Nature (London)*, *199*, 784.

HILLMAN, D. A. and COLLE, E. (1969): Plasma growth hormone and insulin responses in short children. *Amer. J. Dis. Child.*, *117*, 636.

HUNTER, W. N. and GREENWOOD, F. C. (1962): Radioimmuno-electrophoretic assay for human growth hormone. *Acta endocr. (Kbh.)*, *Suppl.*, *67*, 60.

JOHANNSON, A. J., GUDYA, H., LIGHT, C., MIGEON, C. J. and BLIZZARD, R. M. (1969): Serum luteinizing hormone by radioimmunoassay in normal children. *J. Pediat.*, *74*, 416.

KNOPF, R. F., CONN, J. W., FAJANS, S. S., FLOYD, J. S., JR. and PEK, S. (1969): Metabolic stimuli to growth hormone release (protein). In: *Progress in Endocrinology, Proceedings, III International Congress of Endocrinology, Mexico, 1968*, pp. 610–618. Editor: C. Gual. ICS No 184. Excerpta Medica, Amsterdam.

LANDON, J., GREENWOOD, F. C., STAMP, T. C. B. and WYNN, V. (1966): The plasma sugar, free fatty acid, cortisol and growth hormone response to insulin and the comparison of this procedure with other tests of pituitary and adrenal function. II. In patients with hypothalamic or pituitary dysfunction or anorexia nervosa *J. clin. Invest.*, 45, 437.

MARTIN, L. G., CLARK, J. W. and CONNOR, T. B. (1966): Effect of androgen on plasma growth hormone response to hypoglycemia and arginine infusion. *Clin. Res.*, *14*, 477.

MERIMEE, T. J., RABINOWITZ, D. and FINEBERG, S. E. (1969): Arginine-initiated release of human growth hormone. Factors modifying the response in normal man. *New Eng. J. Med.*, *280*, 1434.

MEYER, V. and KNOBIL, E. (1967): Growth hormone secretion in the unanesthetized rhesus monkey in response to noxious stimuli. *Endocrinology*, *80*, 163.

MITCHELL, M. L., BYRNE, M. J., SANCHEZ, Y. and SAWIN, C. T. (1970): Detection of growth hormone deficiency. The glucagon stimulation test. *New Engl. J. Med.*, *282*, 539.

MITCHELL, M. L., BYRNE, M. J. and SILVER, J. (1969): Growth hormone release by glucagon. *Lancet*, *1*, 289.

MULLER, E. E., SAITO, T., KASTIN, A. J. and PECILE, A. (1966): In: *Abstracts, Program of the 48th Meeting of the Endocrine Society, June*, p. 28.

PARKER, M. L., HAMMOND, J. M. and DAUGHADAY, W. H. (1967): Arginine provocative test; aid in diagnosis of hyposomatotropism. *J. clin. Endocr.*, *27*, 1129.

REED, R. B. and STUART, H. G. (1959): Patterns of growth in height and weight from birth to eighteen years of age. *J. Pediat.*, *24*, 904.

ROTH, J., GLICK, S. M., YALOW, R. S. and BERSON, S. A. (1963*a*): Hypoglycemia, a potent stimulus to secretion of growth hormone. *Science*, *140*, 987.

ROTH, J., GLICK, S. M., YALOW, R. S. and BERSON, S. A. (1963*b*): Secretion of human growth hormone: physiologic and experimental modification. *Metabolism*, *12*, 577.

TANNER, J. M. (1962): *Growth at Adolescence.* Blackwell, Oxford.

YALOW, R. S. and BERSON, S. A. (1960): Immunoassay of endogenous plasma insulin in man. *J. clin. Invest.*, *39*, 1157.

INFLUENCE OF ADRENERGIC NERVOUS SYSTEM ON SECRETION OF GROWTH HORMONE*

ADALBERTO PARRA,** ROBERT B. SCHULTZ, THOMAS P. FOLEY and ROBERT M. BLIZZARD

Department of Pediatrics, The Johns Hopkins University School of Medicine, The Johns Hopkins Hospital, Baltimore, Maryland, U.S.A.

INTRODUCTION

This study is based on two observations: Aarskog *et al.* (1965) demonstrated that a majority of patients with idiopathic hypopituitarism reveal an abnormal response to metapirone stimulation, but have a normal response to piromen stimulation. A similar experience was reported by Landon *et al.* (1966) when the adrenal glands were stimulated with metapirone and hypoglycemia. The dichotomy of these responses suggested a defect in ACTH release rather than an inability to produce ACTH in these patients.

On the other hand, it is well known that several stimuli for growth hormone (GH) release, both in humans and in animals, are catecholamine-mediated (Schalih, 1967; Luft *et al.*, 1966; Meyer and Knobil, 1966) and there is increased evidence to support, in human adults, a definitive participation of the adrenergic nervous system in the release of GH, the α-receptors having a stimulatory role and the β-receptors an inhibitory one (Blackard and Heidingsfelder, 1968).

The present study was undertaken to determine whether the plasma GH levels obtained in children, in response to hypoglycemia and arginine stimulation, could be elevated with a simultaneous infusion of epinephrine and propranolol, a β-adrenergic receptor-blocking agent.

MATERIAL AND METHODS

The patients and their controls were admitted to the Pediatric Clinical Research Unit, The Johns Hopkins Hospital, one day prior to testing and kept at rest and fasting after midnight. The diagnostic criteria for hypopituitarism and psychosocial dwarfism have been previously reported (Brasel *et al.*, 1965; Powell *et al.*, 1967*a*; *b*). The general data regarding the subjects are presented in Table I. Four controls and four hypopituitary subjects underwent a combined insulin-arginine tolerance test (I-ATT) on day 1. After a control period of 30 minutes, crystalline insulin (0.1 U/kg) was given i.v. (time 0) and l-arginine (0.5 g/kg) was infused from

* This work was supported by Grant HD 01852, U.S.P.H.S.
Dr. Adalberto Parra was supported by an International Postdoctoral Research Fellowship (1F05 TW 1400-01), U.S.N.I.H.; Dr. T. P. Foley by Traineeship Grant TI AM 5219-09.; Dr. R. M. Blizzard is Eudowood Professor of Pediatrics.
** Current address: División de Nutrición, Departamento de Investigación Científica, Centro Médico Nacional, Instituto Mexicano del Seguro Social, México City.

TABLE I

Group	Sex		Age (yr)	Height (cm)	Weight (kg)	Endocrine function			
						HGH	TSH	ACTH	FSH-L
Control	3F + 7M	Mean Range	10.7 (5.6-16.7)	123.4 (100.2-157.8)	27.5 (11.1-65.5)	N	N	N	N
Mild GH deficiency	1M		11.0	126.8	26.8	±	N	N	NT
Hipopituitary dwarfs	2F + 4M	Mean Range	16.0 (12.4-22.0)	131.4 (111.7-152.5)	25.3 (21.7-60.0)	A (6/6)	A (2/6)	A (2/6)	A (2/6) (4
Psychosocial dwarfs	2M		3.2 7.1	80.5 105.5	11.7 18.4	A A	N N	N N	NT NT

N = normal; A = abnormal; ± subnormal; NT = not tested.

time 60 to 90 minutes. The test was ended at 120 minutes. On the second day, the I-ATT was similarly performed with a simultaneous constant infusion of epinephrine and propranolol at 0.1 μg/kg/min and 80 μg/min respectively, from time 0 to 120 minutes.

Six controls, one patient with a mild GH deficiency and two psychosocial dwarfs underwent a combined arginine-insulin tolerance test (A-ITT) on day 1. The second day, the A-ITT was similarly performed with a simultaneous constant infusion of epinephrine and propranolol at the rates already mentioned, from time 0 to 120 minutes. The two subjects with isolated growth hormone deficiency (D.S. and K.D.) were differently studied. On day 1 they were given an insulin tolerance test (ITT). After a control period of 30 minutes, crystalline insulin (0.1 U/kg) was given i.v. at time 0. Simultaneously, a propranolol constant infusion (80 μg/min) was given from 0 to 90 minutes; the test ended at 120 minutes. On the second day, they were given an arginine tolerance test (ATT) (0.5 g/kg) along with a constant infusion of epinephrine and propranolol (0.1 μg/kg/min and 80 μg/min, respectively), from time 0 to 90 minutes. The test ended at 120 minutes.

All subjects had blood samples drawn every 15 minutes. The plasma was immediately separated, kept frozen at –20°C and later analyzed in duplicate for GH, using the radioimmunoassay technique of Schalch and Parker (1964) and for glucose, using a glucose oxidase method (McCann and Jude, 1958).

RESULTS

The results obtained in the controls who underwent the I-ATT are shown in Figure 1. Three out of four of them showed a two-peak GH response during the control test, the first during the hypoglycemic phase and the second during the arginine stimulation. Both peaks were greater than 6 mμg/ml (our criteria for normal response). On the next day, all subjects also had a distinct two-peak GH response and the values were consistently higher than the day before, including one patient who had an initial basal GH level of 10 mμg/ml. When the plasma GH and glucose changes from basal level were analyzed by means of pair test analysis (Table II), the plasma GH differences were significantly so at all times, except at 15/ and 105 minutes. All subjects achieved a comparable degree of hypoglycemia on both days, except at 15/and 120 minutes, when there was a greater hypoglycemia on day 1 than on day 2.

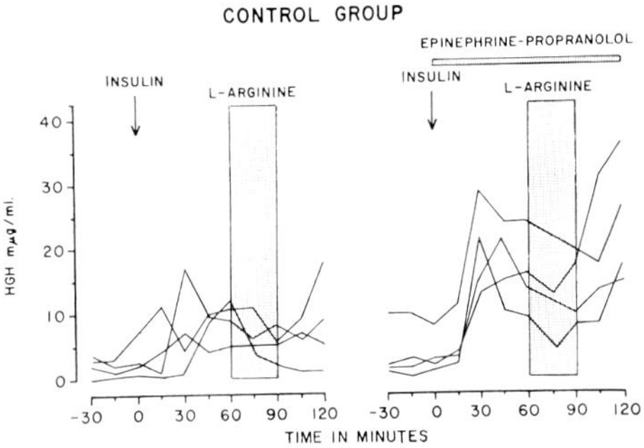

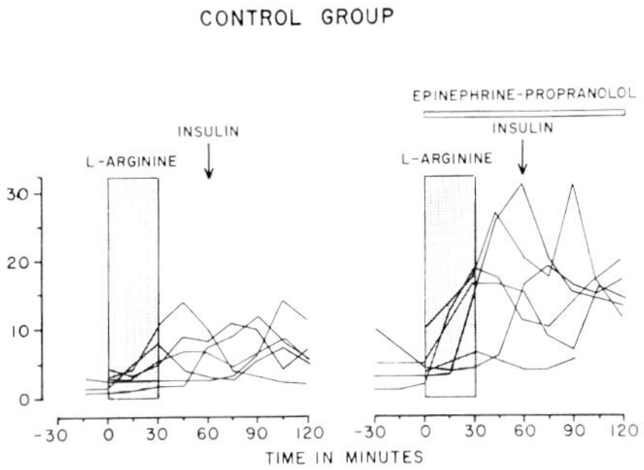

Fig. 1. Plasma GH values in 4 control subjects during the I-ATT alone and during the I-ATT together with a simultaneous infusion of epinephrine and propranolol.

Fig. 2. Plasma GH values in six control subjects during the A-ITT alone and during the A-ITT together with a simultaneous infusion of epinephrine and propranolol.

Figure 2 shows the results in the controls who underwent the A-ITT. Three out of six had a two-peak GH response and all six had values above 6 mμg/ml. On the second day, all subjects but one had a marked elevation in the plasma GH levels in response to the epinephrine-propranolol infusion. One subject, who had had a basal GH level of 10 mμg/ml even showed a significant rise. Pair-test analysis is shown in Table III. On the second day, the GH values were significantly greater than on day 1, at 45, 60, 75, 105 and 120 minutes.

Figure 3 illustrates the results in one patient in whom a moderate form of GH deficiency was suspected. Again, the increases in plasma GH levels were significantly greater during the epinephrine-propranolol infusion than during the control A-ITT.

Figure 4 shows that none of the four hypopituitary subjects had a significant rise in plasma GH levels in response to either I-ATT alone or in combination with epinephrine and propranolol. All hypopituitary dwarfs achieved a comparable degree of hypoglycemia on both days

TABLE II

Pair-test analysis of the plasma growth hormone and glucose changes from basal levels during the insulin-arginine tolerance test in the control group, before and during the epinephrine-propranolol infusion ('P' values)

	Time in minutes							
	15	30	45	60	75	90	105	120
Growth hormone	NS	< .01	< .02	< .05	< .05	< .05	NS	< .05
Plasma glucose	< .01	NS	NS	NS	NS	NS	0.5	< .05

TABLE III

Pair-test analysis of the plasma growth hormone changes from basal level during the arginine-insulin tolerance test in the control group, before and during the epinephrine-propranolol infusion ('P' values)

	Time in minutes							
	15	30	45	60	75	90	105	120
Growth hormone	NS	NS	< .05	.04	< .05	NS	< .01	.03

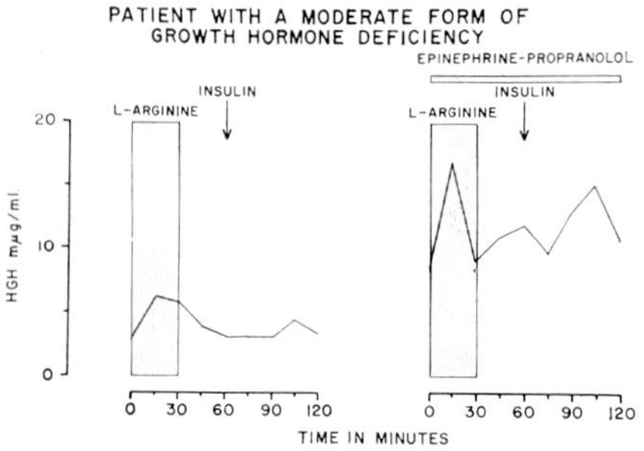

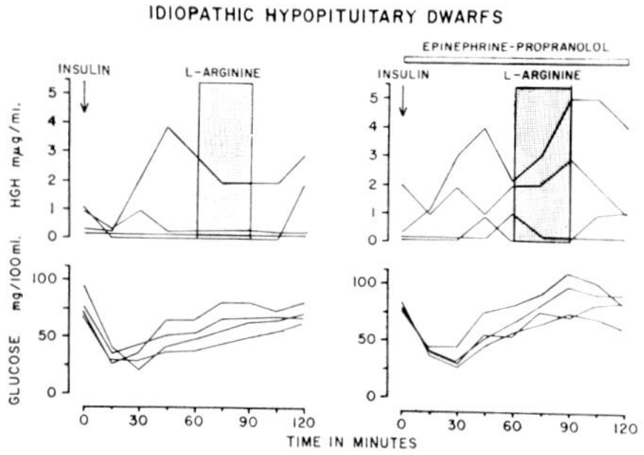

Fig. 3. Changes in plasma GH values during the A-ITT alone and during the A-ITT combined with a simultaneous infusion of epinephrine and propranolol.

Fig. 4. Plasma GH and glucose concentrations during the I-ATT alone and during the I-ATT together with a simultaneous infusion of epinephrine and propranolol.

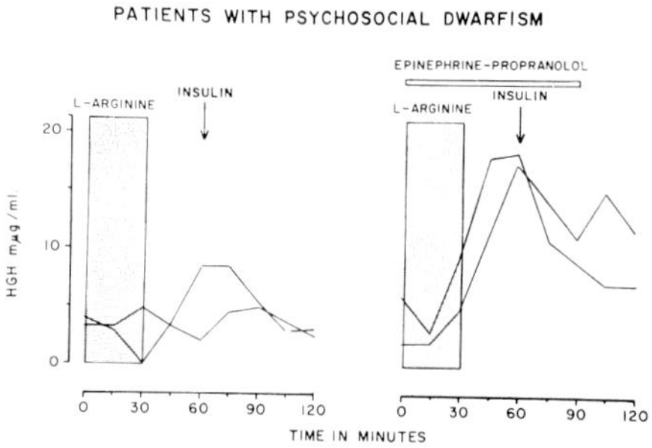

Fig. 5. Plasma GH levels during the A-ITT alone and combined with a simultaneous infusion of epinephrine-propranolol.

and the recovery of the glucose level was slightly better, if any, on the second day.

The results obtained in two subjects with isolated growth hormone deficiency are shown in Table IV. There were no measurable levels of GH on either day. The abnormally high plasma glucose levels are partially related to the epinephrine infusion that was simultaneously given with the arginine.

Figure 5 shows that both psychosocial dwarfs had an augmented GH response when the

TABLE IV

Isolated growth hormone deficiency

			Growth hormone (mμg/ml)								Glucose (mg/100 ml)						
			Minutes								Minutes						
Name	Test*	Drug infused	0	15	30	45	60	75	90	120	0	15	30	45	60	75	90
D.S.	ITT	propranolol	1	2	2	1	0	1	1	1	68	37	18	48	32	53	61
	ATT	epinephrine/+ propranolol	0	0	0	0	0	0	1	1	81	122	161	201	193	191	197
K.D.	ITT	propranolol	1	1	0	1	1	1	1	1	79	63	34	25	40	57	69
	ATT	epinephrine/+ propranolol	1	1	1	2	1	1	1	1	69	130	143	144	139	129	110

* ITT = insulin tolerance test
ATT = arginine tolerance test

A-ITT stimuli were combined with a simultaneous infusion of epinephrine and propranolol.

During the control I-ATT and A-ITT, both controls and hypopituitary patients developed symptoms of hypoglycemia. However, during the simultaneous infusion of epinephrine and propranolol none of the subjects had such symptoms. The cardiovascular response to epinephrine was completely abolished by propranolol and the subjects had bradycardia but no rise in the systolic blood pressure. No other side effects were recorded.

DISCUSSION

The present study has shown that the simultaneous infusion of epinephrine and propranolol markedly enhances the plasma GH response to hypoglycemia and arginine stimulation in 10 control subjects and in 2 children with psychosocial dwarfism. No attempt was made to distinguish between the stimulatory effects upon GH release of epinephrine vs. propranolol.

Our observations are in agreement with the existence of an adrenergic receptor mechanism controlling the release of GH in normal children as well as in adults. The present data support the hypothesis that β-adrenergic receptors in the hypothalamic-pituitary unit exert an inhibitory effect on the release of GH in normal (Blackard and Heidingsfelder, 1968) as well as in non-hypopituitary patients.

None of the 6 idiopathic hypopituitary dwarfs had a significant elevation in plasma GH levels, during the I-ATT combined with a simultaneous infusion of epinephrine and propranolol. This observation does not support the concept that idiopathic hypopituitarism is a defect in the releasing mechanism of GH, rather than in the synthesis of the hormone. However, more studies are necessary before a definitive statement can be made.

ACKNOWLEDGEMENTS

We gratefully acknowledge the assistance of Professor Arturo Almaraz Ugalde for statistical analysis and to Miss Luz María Luna for secretarial work.

REFERENCES

AARSKOG, D., BLIZZARD, R. M. and MIGEON, C. J. (1965): Response to methopyrapone (Su-4885) and pyrogen test in idiopathic hypopituitary dwarfism. *J. clin. Endocr.*, *25*, 439.

BLACKARD, W. C. and HEIDINGSFELDER, S. A. (1968): Adrenergic receptor control mechanism for growth hormone secretion. *J. clin. Invest.*, *47*, 1407.

BRASEL, J. A., WRIGHT, J. C., WILKINS, L. and BLIZZARD, R. M. (1965): An evaluation of seventy-five patients with hypopituitarism beginning in childhood. *Amer. J. Med.*, *38*, 484.

LANDON, J., GREENWOOD, F. C., STAMP, T. C. B. and WYNN, V. (1966): The plasma sugar, free fatty acid, cortisol and growth hormone response to insulin and the comparison of this procedure with other tests of pituitary and adrenal function. II. In patients with hypothalamic or pituitary dysfunction or anorexia nervosa. *J. clin. Invest.*, *45*, 437.

LUFT, R., CERASI, E., MADISON, L., von EULER, V. S., DELLA CASA, L. and ROOVETE, A. (1966): Effect of a small decrease in blood glucose on plasma growth hormone and urinary excretion of catecholamines in man. *Lancet*, *2*, 254.

MCCANN, W. P. and JUDE, J. R. (1958): The synthesis of glucose by the kidney. *Bull. Johns Hopkins Hosp.*, *103*, 77.

MEYER, V. and KNOBIL, E. (1966): Stimulation of growth hormone secretion by vasopressin in the rhesus monkey. *Endocrinology*, *79*, 1016.

POWELL, G. F., BRASEL, J. A. and BLIZZARD, R. M. (1967*a*): Emotional deprivation and growth retardation simulating idiopathic hypopituitarism. I. Evaluation of the syndrome. *New Engl. J. Med.*, *276*, 1271.
POWELL, G. F., BRASEL, J. A., RAITI, S. and BLIZZARD, R. M. (1967*b*): Emotional deprivation and growth retardation simulating idiopathic hypopituitarism. II. Endocrinologic evaluation of the syndrome. *New. Engl. J. Med.*, *276*, 1279.
SCHALCH, D. A. and PARKER, M. L. (1964): A sensitive double antibody immunoassay for human growth hormone in plasma. *Nature (Lond.)*, *203*, 1141.
SCHALCH, D. S. (1967): The influence of physical stress and exercise on growth hormone and insulin secretion in man. *J. Lab. clin. Med.*, *69*, 256.

EFFECTS OF GROWTH HORMONE IN DWARFISM*

M. S. RABEN**

New England Medical Center Hospitals and the Department of Medicine, Tufts University School of Medicine, Boston, Mass., U.S.A.

Although it is widely known that human growth hormone promotes growth in hypopituitary dwarfs, rather few endocrinologists have had the opportunity to actually treat patients with growth hormone or even to observe such patients. I should therefore like to present several examples of successful treatment with growth hormone. At their best, the results are truly remarkable and thrilling to observe. Such is the case in my first example, an 18-year-old hypopituitary female with the height of a 9-year-old child (133.7 cm). Three years of treatment with HGH added 24.8 cm to her height and brought her close to the mean adult height (within 0.5 SD) (Fig. 1). This girl was uncommon among hypopituitary patients in exhibiting an extreme degree of retardation of dental development. When thyroid was added to her treatment after a year of growth hormone, rapid dental maturation ensued. Despite this evidence of thyroid deficiency, as well as a low serum thyroxine iodine (1.6 $\mu g\%$), there was an excellent response to HGH even before thyroid was prescribed.

The inverse result in regard to thyroid medication is that some hypopituitary patients temporarily grow faster with this treatment alone. It is therefore not always helpful in differentiating hypothyroidism and hypopituitarism to test the effect of thyroid on the growth rate. N.S., Jr., was 119 cm tall at age $12^{4}/_{12}$, 21.6 cm below the 3rd percentile, 34.3 cm below

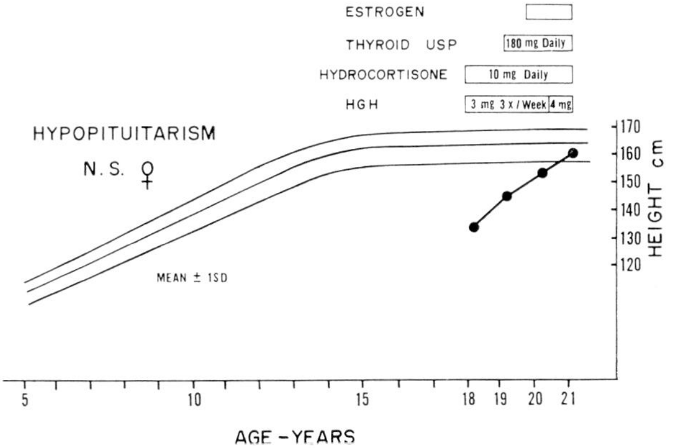

Fig. 1. Treatment of an 18-year-old hypopituitary dwarf for 3 years with HGH.

* This study was supported by USPHS grant AM01567.
** Recipient of a Research Career Award from the U.S. Public Health Service.

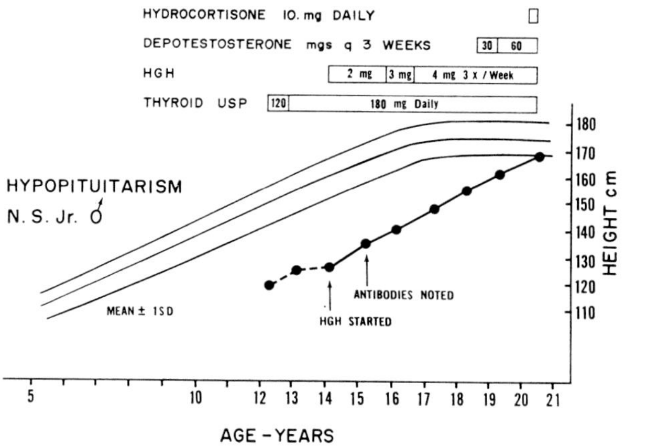

Fig. 2. Temporary stimulation of growth in a hypopituitary dwarf by thyroid alone. When the effect waned, the patient was treated for $6^5/_{12}$ years with HGH.

the 50th percentile (Fig. 2). On thyroid alone, he grew 5 cm in 10 months, but then only 2.3 cm in the subsequent year. On HGH, he then grew 40.1 cm in $6^5/_{12}$ years (6.1 cm/yr), reaching the 16th percentile of adult heights. Antibodies to HGH were noted after one year of treatment but, as is almost always the case, the antibodies did not seem to decrease his responsiveness to HGH. The dose of HGH was increased during the course of therapy from 2 mg to a maximum of 4 mg three times a week, but this increase was in fact proportionately less than his weight increase during the period of treatment. Neither in this patient nor in others have we seen any spurt in growth when testosterone was added to the treatment. We have used sex hormones, both androgen and estrogen, only for maturation, not for growth, and have added sex hormone only when the usual pubertal height has been attained.

F.H., a 17-year-old male hypopituitary dwarf, grew 38.1 cm in $6^1/_2$ years, from 130.8 cm to 168.9 cm. In this case, treatment with thyroid for eight months before starting HGH produced no stimulation of growth.

In general, the more clearly hypopituitary a patient is, the more likely is he to respond well to HGH. However, C.R. was studied at the age of five, in 1962, and no endocrine abnormality was found. Current evaluation would probably reveal him as having an isolated GH deficiency in view of the extreme short stature of his father (140 cm) and his dramatic response to HGH. Treated with HGH from age $5^{11}/_{12}$ to age $12^{10}/_{12}$, $6^{11}/_{12}$ years, he grew an average of 7.6 cm/year, moving up on the growth chart from 11 cm below the 3rd percentile to about the 40th percentile in height (Fig. 3). The dose of HGH increased from 1 mg to 3 mg three times a week, but his weight increased more than three times during that period.

Despite the concern of some investigators that even rather small doses of corticosteroids may inhibit the growth response to HGH, we have usually given with impunity 10–15 mg of hydrocortisone or cortisone per day to hypopituitary patients who weighed 25 kg or more. Large doses will of course inhibit growth, and our recent studies have shown how completely cortisone can prevent the stimulation by GH of DNA synthesis and thymidine kinase activity in the rat (Epstein *et al.*, 1969).

The diabetogenicity of growth hormone has not been a problem despite prolonged treatment. Perhaps the infrequent injections (three times a week) as well as the small dose needed for growth help minimize the diabetogenicity. It should be remembered nonetheless that 12 hours after a single injection of 10 mg HGH in a normal adult there is diminished glucose tolerance even in the face of increased insulin response to the administered glucose (Mitchell *et al.*, 1970).

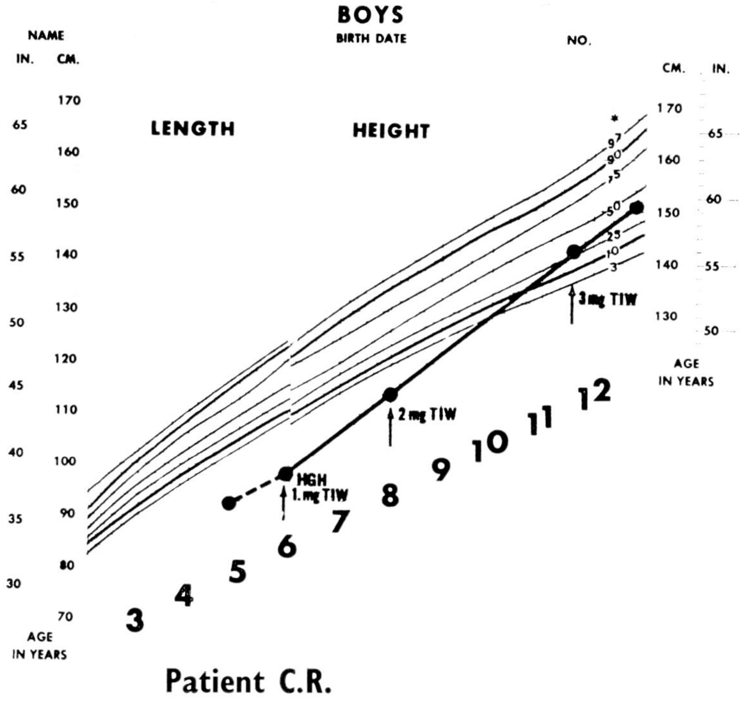

Fig. 3. Treatment of a patient with presumptive diagnosis of isolated growth hormone deficiency with HGH for $6^{11}/_{12}$ years.

To obtain HGH in substantial amounts, pituitaries obtained at autopsy must be assiduously collected and properly stored either in reagent-grade acetone or frozen. Dr. Fukashi Matsuzaki and I have been preparing large batches of HGH once a year, and these batches have been a major source of HGH for investigators around the world as well as for the National Pituitary Agency, which organizes the collection of pituitaries and distribution of hormone in the United States. Our method (Raben, 1957) lends itself to large-scale preparation, and as many as 40,000 pituitaries have been extracted in one annual batch. A collection of 23,000 human pituitaries is shown in Figure 4. If recovery of gonadotropins and thyrotropin is desired, the procedure can be preceded by a pre-extraction for these substances, as has been done by Hartree for the British national collection (Hartree, 1966).

For the moment, there is no substitute for HGH. Primate GH would be a small source and has not been tested in long-term use. Human placental lactogen cannot replace HGH. Synthetic HGH or an active portion of the molecule is not yet available. Hypothalamic GH-releasing factor (GRF), if a preparation active in man became available, might be useful in cases of pituitary deficiency secondary to hypothalamic damage. If there are intermediary effector substances in growth hormone's action, such as 'sulfation factor', perhaps they could be put to therapeutic use. Speculative thoughts about other possibilities are encouraged by the remarkable recent observation of Mueller that infestation with the larvae of the cat tapeworm, *Spirometra mansonoides*, causes growth in hypophysectomized rats (Mueller, 1968). Worms provided by Dr. Mueller are shown in Figure 5. The worms may be injected through a #18 needle, either intraperitoneally or subcutaneously. In Figure 6 is shown the growth stimulation following worm injection in animals hypophysectomized more than six months earlier. Serum from worm-infested rats is also growth-promoting and appears to have a longer period of action than growth hormone. Resistance, presumably due to antibodies,

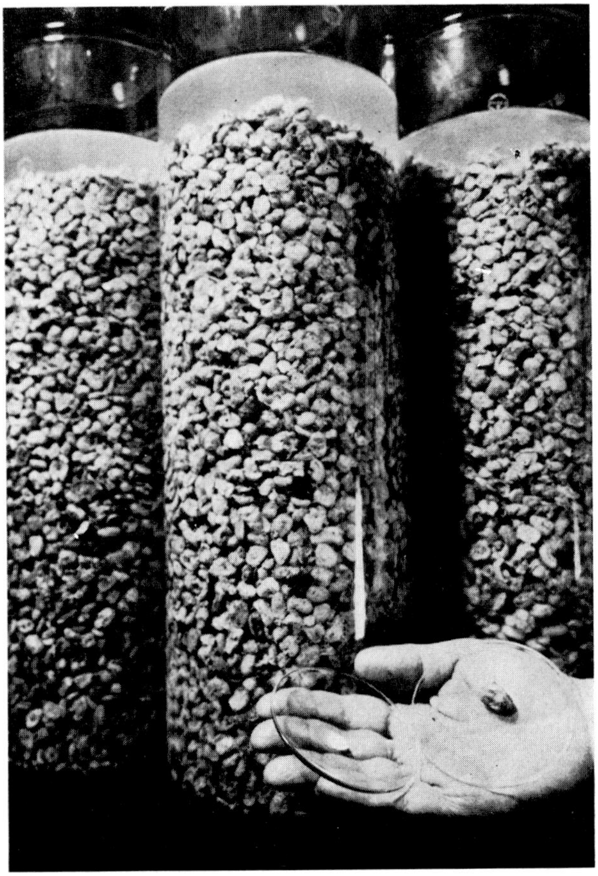

Fig. 4. Approximately 23,000 human pituitaries stored in reagent-grade acetone.

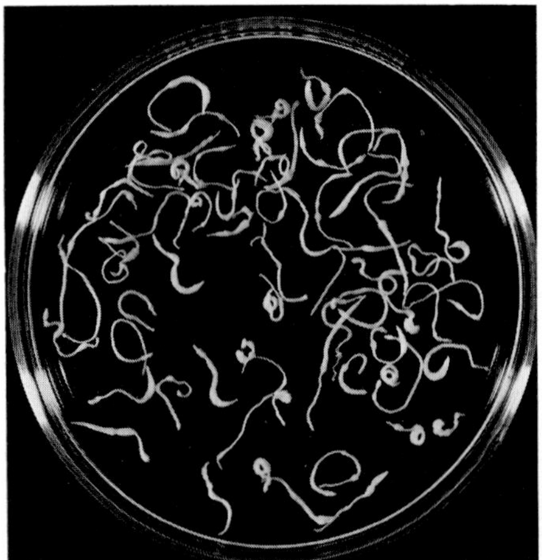

Fig. 5. Larvae of the cat tapeworm, *Spirometra mansonoides*.

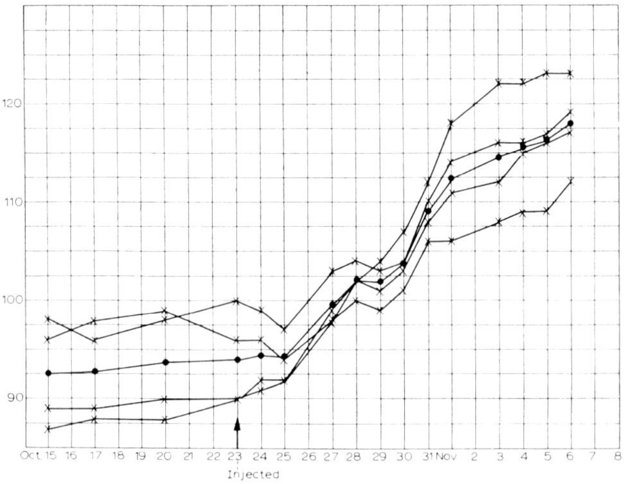

Fig. 6. Stimulation of growth by larvae of *Spirometra mansonoides*. Hypophysectomized rats were injected with 10 worms each intraperitoneally on the day indicated by the arrow.

develops after a few weeks. These unusual findings serve as a reminder that the solution to some human growth problems may yet come from equally unexpected sources.

REFERENCES

EPSTEIN, S., ESANU, C. and RABEN, M. S. (1969): The effect of growth hormone and of cortisone on thymidine kinase activity in rat adipose tissue. *Biochim. biophys. Acta (Amst.)*, *186*, 280.

HARTREE, A. S. (1966): Separation and partial purification of the protein hormones from human pituitary glands. *Biochem. J.*, *100*, 754.

MITCHELL, M. L., RABEN, M. S. and ERNESTI, M. (1970): The use of growth hormone as a diabetic stimulus in man. *Diabetes*, *19*, 196.

MUELLER, J. F. (1968): Growth stimulating effect of experimental sparganosis on thyroidectomized and hypophysectomized rats, and comparative activity of different species of *Spirometra*. *J. Parasit.*, *54*, 795.

RABEN, M. S. (1957): Preparation of growth hormone from pituitaries of man and monkey. *Science*, *125*, 883.

INSULIN SECRETION – DIABETES MELLITUS

CONTENTS

INSULIN, PROINSULIN AND THE COMPONENTS OF PLASMA INSULIN IMMUNOREACTIVITY

JESSE ROTH, PHILLIP GORDEN, BARRY SHERMAN and PIERRE FREYCHET

National Institute of Arthritis and Metabolic Diseases, National Institutes of Health, Bethesda, Md., U.S.A.

PROINSULIN

Proinsulin, the single chain intrapancreatic precursor of insulin, consists of the insulin molecule in which the C-terminus of the insulin B-chain is linked by a connecting segment to the N-terminus of the A-chain (Steiner *et al.*, 1969). The connecting segment consists of a pair of basic amino acids, the C-peptide, and another pair of basic amino acids. Proinsulin, which constitutes only a few percent of total pancreatic insulin, is converted within the β-cell into insulin and C-peptide. The β-cell granules contain equimolar amounts of insulin and C-peptide, and insulin release is accompanied by release of equimolar quantities of C-peptide (Melani *et al.*, 1970*a*). Some proinsulin is also released. Proinsulin is not converted to insulin in plasma, nor, so far as it is known, in any other site in the body outside of the β-cell. *In vitro*, trypsin at low concentrations produces a similar but not identical transformation of proinsulin and yields dealanated insulin and C-peptide (Steiner *et al.*, 1969).

A variety of intermediates between proinsulin and insulin have been described but which of these are actually present *in vivo* is not certain. Proinsulin has essentially all of the biological properties of insulin but its potency is only a few percent of that of insulin (Steiner *et al.*, 1969; Chance, 1971, in press). The bioactivity of the intermediates is between that of proinsulin and insulin; increased degree of conversion produces increased bioactivity (Steiner *et al.*, 1969; Chance, 1971, in press).

Proinsulin and its intermediates react with anti-insulin antibodies almost as well as does insulin (Steiner *et al.*, 1969; Chance, 1971, in press; Steiner *et al.*, 1968). Thus their immunoreactivity is often relatively greater than their bioactivity. Anti-proinsulin antisera contain populations of antibodies that react with insulin and antibodies that are specific for the C-peptide portion of the proinsulin molecule and therefore react with proinsulin, proinsulin intermediates and free C-peptide (Melani *et al.*, 1970*a*). Since the amino acid sequences of the C-peptides vary widely among different species, antibodies react strongly only with the C-peptide of that species used in the immunization. Heterologous C-peptides react weakly or not at all (Melani *et al.*, 1970*a*). By way of contrast, anti-insulin antibodies cross react strongly with heterologous insulins; in general the mammalian insulins differ much less in structure from one another than do the C-peptides.

CIRCULATING IMMUNOREACTIVITY

When plasma is filtered on G-50 Sephadex, the insulin immunoreactivity is recovered in two peaks (Roth *et al.*, 1968). The first peak, which nearly always constitutes a minority of the total immunoreactivity, is proinsulin-like; for convenience the immunoreactive components recovered from plasma in the region of proinsulin following gel filtration are called 'big' insulin because they are presumed to be of higher molecular weight. Most of the plasma insulin immunoreactivity is recovered after gel filtration in the same region as insulin and is referred to as 'little' insulin (Roth *et al.*, 1968).

CHARACTERIZATION OF PLASMA INSULINS

Because the plasma insulins are too low in concentration to be isolated in pure form for direct chemical characterization, a series of experiments were performed to compare the properties of 'big' insulin with the properties of purified proinsulin and other proinsulin-like materials that had been isolated from the pancreas (Sherman *et al.*, 1971). 'Big' insulin, like proinsulin, is stable in plasma and is not transformed with time. When purified proinsulin or insulin were added to plasma, they were recovered entirely as increments in the 'big' and 'little' insulin peaks, respectively (Roth *et al.*, 1968). When a tracer of ^{125}I-proinsulin was mixed with whole plasma or with 'big' insulin that was isolated from plasma and filtered on G-50 Sephadex, the immunoreactivity and radioactivity eluted coincidentally (Sherman *et al.*, 1971). Analogous results were obtained when 'little' insulin was filtered with a tracer of ^{125}I-insulin. When a mixture of the isolated 'big' insulin and a tracer of ^{125}I-proinsulin were treated with trypsin the extent of transformation of both immunoreactivity and radioactivity were identical over a wide range of enzyme concentrations. The decreases in 'big' insulin were accounted for completely by increases in 'little' insulin; recoveries of total immunoreactivity were 80–120% (Sherman *et al.*, 1971).

With a guinea-pig anti-porcine insulin serum and ^{131}I-porcine insulin, 'big' insulin and 'little' insulin gave curves of reactivity of identical shape over a wide range of concentrations (Sherman *et al.*, 1971). In addition, since trypsin-treatment caused decrements of 'big' insulin equal to increments of 'little' insulin, we concluded that the antibody reacted quantitatively equally with both components. We also tested these components with a guinea pig anti-porcine proinsulin serum that contained insulin-specific as well as proinsulin-specific antibodies. When this serum was reacted with ^{131}I-proinsulin in the presence of an excess of unlabeled insulin to block the insulin-specific sites, porcine proinsulin and 'big' insulin produced substantial displacement in the assay, though the latter was less potent than the former; porcine insulin and 'little' insulin were completely unreactive (Sherman *et al.*, 1971). Thus we concluded that 'big' insulin has the immunological properties of a proinsulin-like material and that its reduced reactivity with the anti-porcine proinsulin serum, relative to porcine proinsulin, is what would be reasonably expected for a heterologous proinsulin.

To study the biological potencies of the plasma components, the 'big' and 'little' insulins were re-filtered to reduce their contamination with plasma proteins and to free each insulin component from the other. With isolated fat cells, 'little' insulin stimulated glucose oxidation as much as did pure porcine insulin, while 'big' insulin had activity that was quantitatively indistinguishable from that of proinsulin (Sherman *et al.*, 1971). Based on our other studies, the bioassay data have led us to conclude that 'big' insulin is probably proinsulin or a proinsulin in which only a single peptide bond in the connecting segment has been broken. We presume, based on data of others (Chance, 1971, in press), that if the 'big' insulin represented a proinsulin intermediate that was at a further stage of conversion to insulin, its bioactivity would be substantially higher than that observed. We also concluded that the circulating form of insulin was indistinguishable from insulin purified from the pancreas.

FLUCTUATIONS IN THE CONCENTRATIONS OF 'BIG' AND 'LITTLE' INSULIN

Patients with islet cell tumors, hypokalemia, and diabetes mellitus with severe hypoinsulinemia are the only three groups of patients in whom abnormalities in the relative or absolute amounts of 'big' insulin have been observed; they will be discussed below. Set forth here are the characteristics observed in thin, obese, and acromegalic subjects; the fluctuations occurred irrespective of the body weight, glucose tolerance, or the total plasma insulin or growth hormone concentrations. 'Big' insulin constitutes 10–30% of the insulin immunoreactivity in plasma obtained at rest after an overnight fast (Gorden *et al.*, 1971*b*). Glucose, administered orally, causes a prompt release of insulin so that by 15 minutes the total plasma insulin concentration is increased many times. All of this increase is accounted for by a rise in the 'little' insulin concentration; the concentration of 'big' insulin is unchanged (Gorden *et al.*, 1971*b*; Gorden and Roth, 1969). Thus the fraction of total insulin that is 'big' insulin at 15 min is reduced, with the degree of reduction dependent on the total plasma insulin concentration in the fasting state and the increase in 'little' insulin release. By 2 hr after oral glucose, irrespective of the total plasma insulin concentration, the 'big' insulin concentration increases significantly. The fraction of total insulin that is 'big' insulin is about equal to that observed in the fasting state (Gorden *et al.*, 1971*b*). In a few cases, when tolbutamide was used as the stimulating agent, results were qualitatively quite similar (Gorden *et al.*, 1969).

Hypokalemia frequently produces impaired glucose tolerance associated with hypoinsulinism. In patients with hypokalemia from a variety of causes the fraction of total insulin that is 'big' insulin at each time point (0, 15, and 120 min) is higher than normal, usually due to decreases in the concentration of 'little' insulin. The general pattern of response is qualitatively normal, *i.e.*, the concentration of 'big' insulin is unchanged at 15 min after oral glucose but is increased by 120 min (Gordon *et al.*, 1970). Patients with severe idiopathic glucose intolerance associated with hypoinsulinism show results quite similar to those observed in patients with hypokalemia (Gorden and Roth, unpublished observations).

In patients with islet cell tumors, the fraction of total insulin that is 'big' insulin ranges from the upper range of normal to as high as 80% (Gorden *et al.*, 1971*b*; Lazarus *et al.*, 1970; Goldsmith *et al.*, 1969; Melani *et al.*, 1970*b*) usually due to an absolute increase in the concentration of 'big' insulin. Following stimulation of insulin release by glucose, tolbutamide, or leucine results are qualitatively the same as those described following oral glucose in normal subjects (Gorden *et al.*, 1971*b*). The finding of a marked increase in the fraction of total insulin that is 'big' insulin in the fasting state is suggestive of but not diagnostic of islet cell tumors – we have observed one severely obese patient with chloride-losing diarrhea and hypokalemia in whom 'big' insulin often is the majority of the circulating insulin (Gorden *et al.*, unpublished observations). Another abnormality detected in plasma of patients with islet cell tumors are immunoreactive components that elute from G-50 Sephadex in positions different from those of proinsulin and insulin (Gutman *et al.*, 1970; Gorden *et al.*, 1971*a*).

CONCLUSION

Because the concentration of proinsulin in plasma is normally low, its reduced biological activity relative to its immunologic potency does not significantly alter the interpretations of results obtained by many laboratories in which total insulin immunoactivity was measured; the pathophysiology of blood glucose and plasma insulin changes of diabetes and obesity are unexplained by studies of plasma proinsulin. Only in patients with islet cell tumors, hypokalemia and possibly diabetes with severe insulinopenia are the levels of proinsulin-like substances sufficiently high to have possible clinical significance. This presumes, from current data, that proinsulin has reduced biological potency but that it does not interfere with the normal action of insulin; if the latter should obtain, its role in disorders of glucose tolerance might be increased.

REFERENCES

CHANCE, R. E. (1971): Chemical, physical, biological and immunological studies on porcine proinsulin and related polypeptides. In: *Proceedings, VII Congress of the International Diabetes Federation, Buenos Aires 1970*, p. 292-305. ICS No. 231. Excerpta Medica, Amsterdam.

GOLDSMITH, S. J., YALOW, R. S. and BERSON, S. A. (1969): Significance of human plasma insulin Sephadex fractions. *Diabetes, 18*, 834.

GORDEN, P., FREYCHET, P. and NANKIN, H. (1971*a*): New form of circulating insulin in islet cell carcinoma. *Clin. Res., 19*, 560.

GORDEN, P. and ROTH, J. (1969): Plasma insulin: fluctuations in the 'big' insulin component in man after glucose and other stimuli. *J. clin. Invest., 48*, 2225.

GORDEN, P. and ROTH, J., unpublished observations.

GORDEN, P., SHERMAN, B. and ROTH, J. (1971*b*): Proinsulin-like component of circulating insulin in the basal state and in patients and hamsters with islet cell tumors. *J. clin. Invest.*, in press.

GORDEN, P., SHERMAN, B., ROTH, J. and SIMOPOULOS, A. P. (1970): 'Big' insulin secretion: Increased with hypokalemia. In: *Program of the 52nd Meeting of the Endocrine Society, St. Louis,*

GUTMAN, R. A., LAZARUS, N. R., PENHOS, J. C., RECANT, L. and FAJANS, S. S. (1970): Proinsulin (PI) and proinsulin-like material (PI-LM) in serum of patients with islet cell tumors. *Diabetes, 19*, 360.

LAZARUS, N. R., TANESE, T., GUTMAN, R. A. and RECANT, L. (1970): Synthesis and release of proinsulin and insulin by human insulinoma tissue. *J. clin. Endocr., 30*, 273.

MELANI, F., RUBENSTEIN, A. H., OYER, P. E. and STEINER, D. F. (1970*a*): Identification of proinsulin and C-peptide in human serum by a specific immunoassay. *Proc. nat. Acad. Sci. (Wash.), 67*, 148.

MELANI, F., RYAN, W. G., RUBENSTEIN, A. H. and STEINER, D. F. (1970*b*): Proinsulin secretion by a pancreatic beta-cell adenoma. *New Engl. J. Med., 283*, 713.

ROTH, J., GORDEN, P. and PASTAN, I. (1968): 'Big insulin': a new component of plasma insulin detected by immunoassay. *Proc. nat. Acad. Sci. (Wash.), 61*, 138.

SHERMAN, B., GORDEN, P., ROTH, J. and FREYCHET, P. (1971): Circulating insulin: the proinsulin-like properties of 'big' insulin in patients without islet cell tumors. *J. clin. Invest., 50*, 849.

STEINER, D. F., CLARK, J. L., NOLAN, C., REUBENSTEIN, A. H., MARGOLIASH, E., ATEN, B. and OYER, P. E. (1969): Proinsulin and the biosynthesis of insulin. *Recent Progr. Hormone Res., 25*, 207.

STEINER, D. F., HALLUND, O., RUBENSTEIN, A., CHO, S. and BAYLISS, C. (1968): Isolation and properties of proinsulin intermediate forms, and other minor components from crystalline bovine insulin. *Diabetes, 18*, 725.

VARIABLE SENSITIVITY OF THE PERFUSED RAT PANCREAS TO GLUCOSE*

GEROLD M. GRODSKY, V. LICKO and H. LANDAHL

Metabolic Research Unit, Department of Biochemistry and Biophysics and Department of Pathology, University of California, San Francisco, California, U.S.A.

INTRODUCTION

Previous experiments performed *in vitro* (Grodsky *et al.*, 1967*a*; Curry *et al.*, 1968) and *in vivo* (Porte and Pupo, 1969; Cerasi and Luft, 1967) have shown that the pancreas responds to constant stimulation with a multiphasic pattern of insulin release. This presentation summarizes our studies, indicating that each phase reflects different pancreatic phenomena which can vary in both magnitude and time sequence of their contribution to release. The mathematical two-compartmental model, previously suggested (Grodsky *et al.*, 1969; Grodsky *et al.*, 1970), was modified to reproduce typical insulin responses caused by glucose presented in a variety of stimulation patterns. The modified model also reproduced the typical insulin secretion patterns occurring during glucose stimulation of the mild diabetic subject.

MATERIALS AND METHODS

Specific details for the *in vitro* perfusion technique of the rat pancreas and the radioimmunoassay for rat insulin have been described in our earlier publications (Curry *et al.*, 1968; Grodsky *et al.*, 1967*b*). In brief, the pancreas with the adjacent stomach, spleen, and part of the duodenum was removed from fasted rats and placed on the perfusion apparatus. Perfusion media, consisting of 4% albumin (Cutter Laboratory, Berkeley, Calif.) and phosphate-bicarbonate buffer, was introduced into the celiac artery. The complete effluent was collected from the portal vein at 30–60-second intervals after a single passage through the pancreas. Thus, with this dynamic system it was possible to measure rapid changes of insulin secretion during a variety of experimental conditions.

RESULTS AND DISCUSSION

Figure 1 shows the results when different concentrations of glucose were continuously perfused through the isolated pancreas for one hour. As previously noted (Grodsky *et al.*, 1967*a*), insulin release was not detectable at glucose concentrations below 50 mg/100 ml. At 100 mg/100 ml, a small early phase occurred; however, release in the second phase was below the level of sensitivity of our radioimmunoassay for rat insulin (1–1.5 mμg/ml). With increased glucose concentration, both the initial and secondary phases were observed; insulin secretion

* This project was supported in part by U.S. Public Health Service Grant 01410.

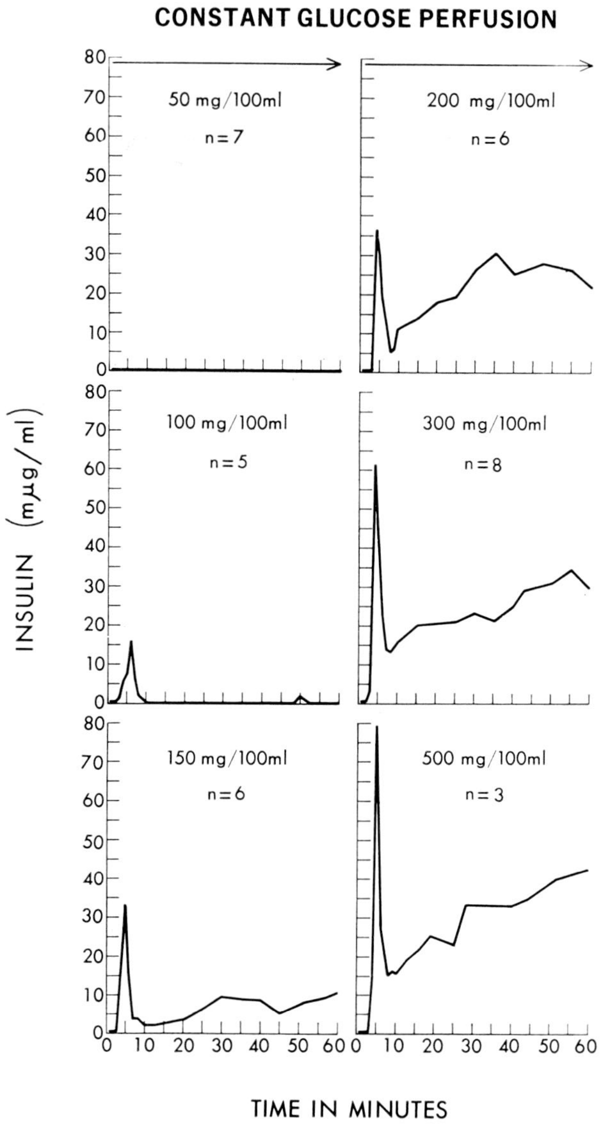

Fig. 1. Effect of constant concentrations of glucose on insulin secretion. Perfusion period was 1 hour.

in both phases increased as glucose concentrations were raised, approaching a maximum at around 500 mg glucose per ml.

The total insulin secreted during one hour at each glucose concentration is summarized in Figure 2. Insulin release, when plotted against glucose concentration, followed a sigmoidal pattern almost identical with that previously seen by Malaisse *et al.* (1967) using a static pancreatic system. It was also similar to the effect of glucose concentration on glucose oxidation in rat islet tissue (Ashcroft and Randle, 1968). Though the existence of a sigmoidal pattern for insulin release has not yet been evaluated in man or the intact animal, this type of curve permits several considerations: (1). As shown in Figure 2, the curve can be mathemati-

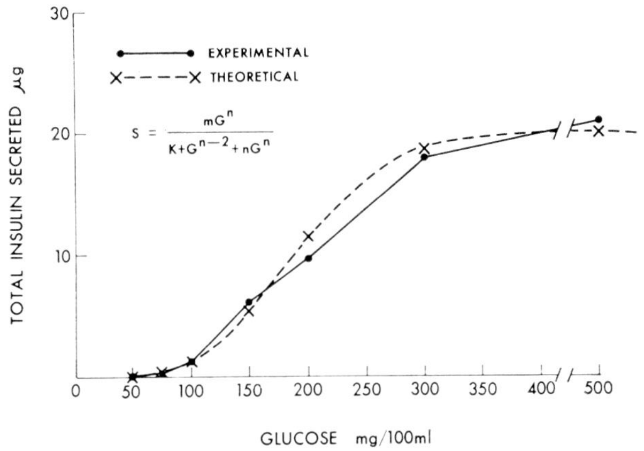

Fig. 2. Total insulin secreted during 1 hour of perfusion with various constant concentrations of glucose. Dashed line is a mathematical approximation using the formulation shown.

cally approximated if insulin release is assumed a power function of glucose concentration. Therefore, attempts in man to relate insulin responses to glucose levels in a linear fashion may be inaccurate, particularly at basal and very high blood-sugar levels. (2). Glucose is comparatively ineffective on insulin secretion at concentrations corresponding to those found in the fasting basal state. Thus, basal secretion of insulin may be regulated to a proportionately greater extent by amino acids, lipids, and hormones. (3). Small increments in glucose concentration above basal level may produce comparatively large changes in the rate of insulin secretion; *e.g.*, in Figure 2, an increase in glucose from 100 to 110 mg/100 ml results in more than a two-fold increase in insulin release. This characteristic may be particularly relevant in the intact animal when evaluating the effects of various substances on insulin release which are associated with 'only minor' glucose elevations. (4). Finally 'enhancement', 'synergism', or 'potentiation', often defined as an effect of a mixture of two agents which exceeds the sum of their individual actions, may be a simple additive effect in the non-linear sigmoidal system. This is illustrated in Table I in which for purposes of illustration, glucose is hypothetically

TABLE I

Non-linear 'potentiation'

Data was taken from Fig. 2. The predicted insulin release based on the arithmetical sum of effects of 2 glucose concentrations were compared to that observed.

	Glucose mg/100 ml	Insulin μg	Glucose mg/100 ml	Insulin μg	Glucose mg/100 ml	Insulin μg
	50	0	100	2	200	9.5
	100	2	200	9.5	300	18
Arithmetic sum	150	2	300	11.5	500	27.5
Observed	150	6.5	300	17.5	500	21
'Potentiation' observed ÷ arithmetic sum × 100		320%		150%		64%*

* Apparent inhibition of 36%

TABLE II

Characteristics of multiphasic response

Characteristic	Early phase	Late phase
Pancreatic insulin	1–2%	20%
Puromycin	No effect	Partial inhibition
Oligomycin	Minor inhibition	Complete inhibition
Visual (E.M.)	Granule secretion only	New granules in Golgi
Proinsulin	1–2%	15%
Calcium	Dependent	Dependent

taken as both the agents. Though obviously both agents are identical, the calculations indicate how an assumed linearity of a sigmoidal response can result in different levels of 'potentiation' and even 'inhibition', depending on the concentrations chosen.

Table II summarizes observations indicating that the characteristic early and late phases seen during stimulation with a high concentration of glucose reflect different, though possibly related, phenomena. The second phase is more sensitive to inhibitors of protein synthesis (Curry *et al.*, 1968) and is completely blocked when electron transport is inhibited by oligomycin (unpublished observations). The electron microscopic appearance of the beta cells in the early and late phases are in sharp contrast (Lee *et al.*, 1970). At the peak of the early phase, insulin-like granules were observed in the extracellular fluid similar to those previously noted by others (Orci, 1970; Lacy, 1964). At one hour, however, there was evidence of provision of additional insulin to the secretory mechanism characterized by new granules in the Golgi apparatus.

We previously suggested that the insulin releasing system may involve a small labile compartment of easily releasable hormone as well as the main compartment of storage granules (Curry *et al.*, 1968). A mathematical model of the two-compartmental system, including a provisionary aspect, was devised (Grodsky *et al.*, 1969; Grodsky *et al.*, 1970) which permitted simulation of curves closely approximating those seen during typical square-wave stimulations by glucose. The mathematical expression for the sigmoidal character of glucose effectiveness for both the early and late phases has now been incorporated into current calculations. This automatically produces the necessary thresholds and maximum activities previously made empirically (Grodsky *et al.*, 1968).

In recent experiments, glucose was presented to the pancreas in a staircase series of continuous steps of increasing concentration; results suggested that the basic two-compartmental model was not sufficient. As shown in Figure 3, 50 mg/100 ml glucose produced no detectable insulin release. When the concentration was increased to 100 mg/100 ml, there was a prompt rise followed by a rapid fall in secretion rate. According to the basic model, the 80% decrease in secretion rate would have represented an 80% depletion of the labile compartment; however, when the concentration was increased to 150 mg/100 ml, large amounts of insulin were still available for release. One feature of the model was therefore modified (Fig. 4); the contents of the small compartment were no longer assumed to be non-physiologically homogeneous but to consist of granule components whose threshold sensitivity to glucose fits a gaussian distribution curve. Thus, some components respond to lower concentrations of glucose, most are sensitive to mid-range concentrations, and a small number have high thresholds. Introduction of the concept of a gaussian distribution did not alter the effectiveness of the model to duplicate the previous square-wave experiments performed at high glucose concentration (Grodsky *et al.*, 1969; Grodsky *et al.*, 1970) and, in addition, permitted approximation of those results observed with the single steps shown in Figure 5. During the 20 minutes of this experiment, the provisionary factor, P (Fig. 4) slowly increased

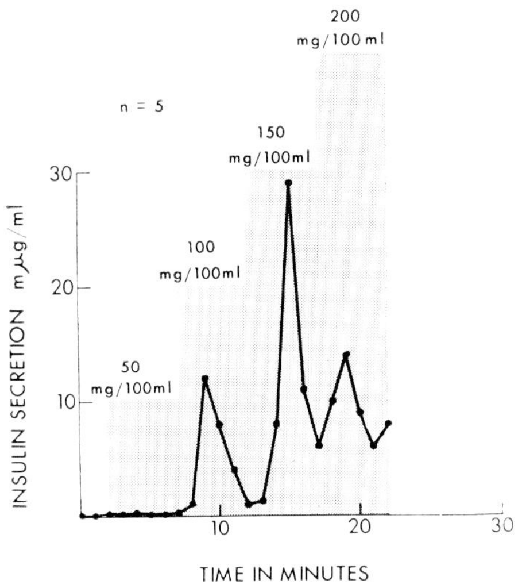

Fig. 3. Effect of staircase increments of glucose on insulin release.

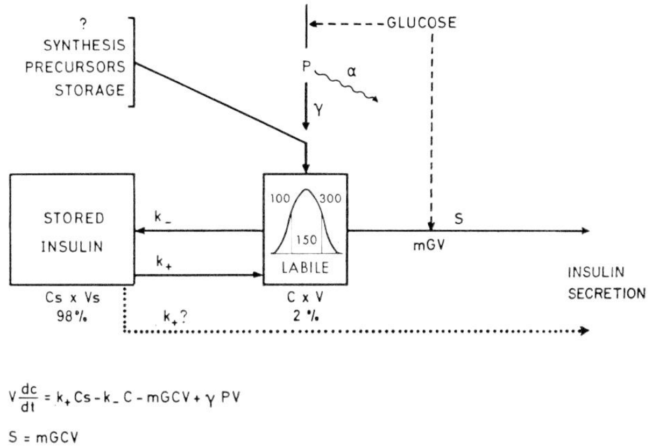

$$V\frac{dc}{dt} = k_+ Cs - k_- C - mGCV + \gamma PV$$

$$S = mGCV$$

Fig. 4. Two-compartmental model for insulin secretion modified to incorporate a gaussian distribution of components with varying thresholds to glucose in the small compartment.

as a function of glucose concentration so that insulin secretion rates fell during each square-wave but to progressively higher values. A similar pattern for insulin release in man during stepwise continuous perfusion has been noted in studies performed with Dr. John Karam in this laboratory.

Concurrently, the existence of granule components in the beta cell, which differ in their threshold sensitivity to glucose, has been suggested by Matthews and Dean (1970), who found an increasing percentage of cells to initiate action-potential discharges as glucose levels were increased.

Figure 6 shows both the experimental and theoretical results obtained when glucose was presented to the pancreas as continuous increasing gradients instead of instantaneous square waves. Though the data in Figure 6 were originally published in 1967 (Grodsky *et al.*, 1967*a*), the current two-compartmental model closely approximated the older experimental results. In these experiments, the diphasic response still occurred when glucose concentration was increased to high levels during a five-minute period. When one hour was used to increase

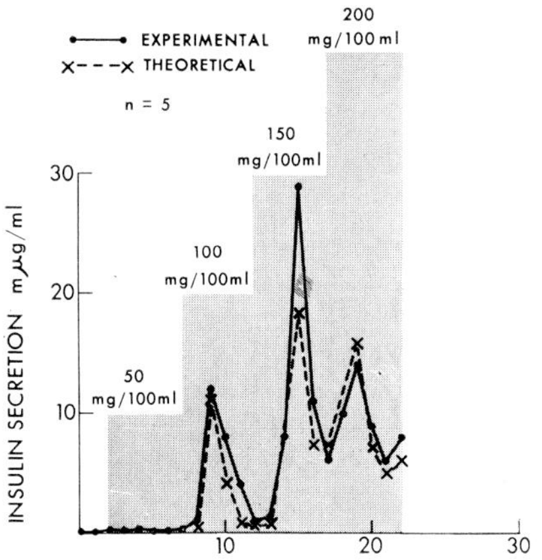

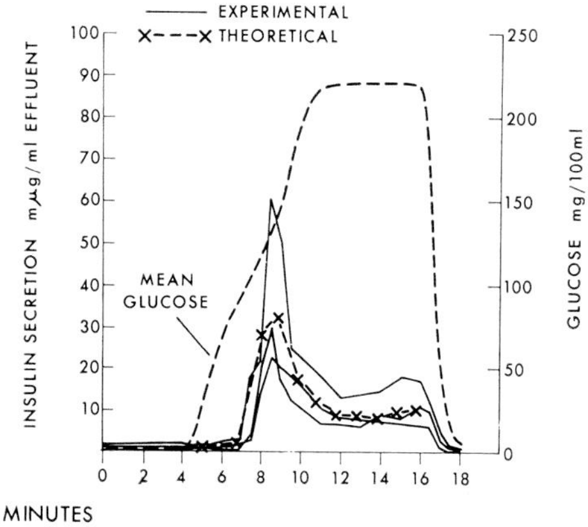

Fig. 5. Effect of staircase increments of glucose on insulin release. Data taken from Fig. 3. Theoretical curve was obtained from the modified model in Fig. 4.

Fig. 6. Effect of brisk, gradient increase of glucose on insulin release.

glucose from 50 to 250 mg/100 ml (Fig. 7), secretion increased at a smoothly accelerating rate, without detectable evidence of phasic responses. These results were also consistent with the theoretical prediction that depletion of the components in the small compartment was too slow to produce the typical 'dumping' seen during square-wave stimulations. In both types of experiments (Figs. 6 and 7), the threshold for secretion at glucose levels of 80–100 mg/100 ml was approximated by the sigmoidal characteristics for glucose activity, mathematically incorporated into the model.

It is anticipated that the two-compartmental model may prove useful to interpret the patterns of insulin release seen in man and particularly in the diabetic subject. Although clinical observations vary, most studies suggest that insulin secretion in the mild diabetic is characterized by an early impaired release, sometimes followed by hyperinsulinism (Fig. 8, taken from Hales *et al.*, 1968). In the simulation shown in Figures 9 and 10, we used the

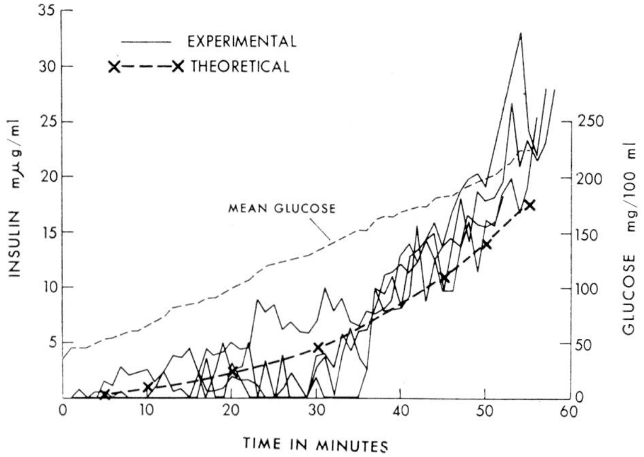

Fig. 7. Effect of slow, gradient increase of glucose on insulin release.

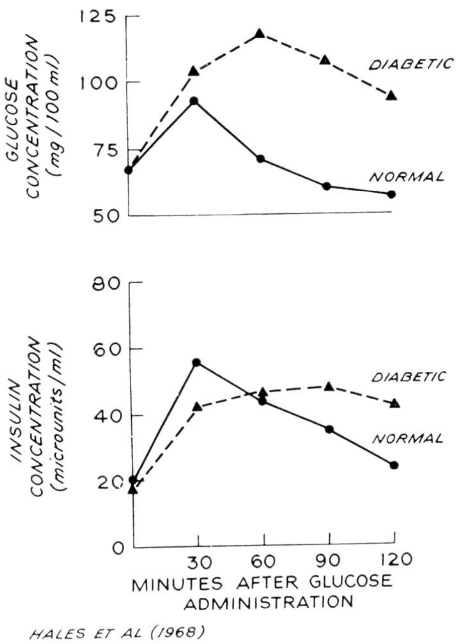

Fig. 8. Response to oral glucose (50 g) of subjects with mild abnormality of glucose metabolism (taken from Hales *et al.*, 1968).

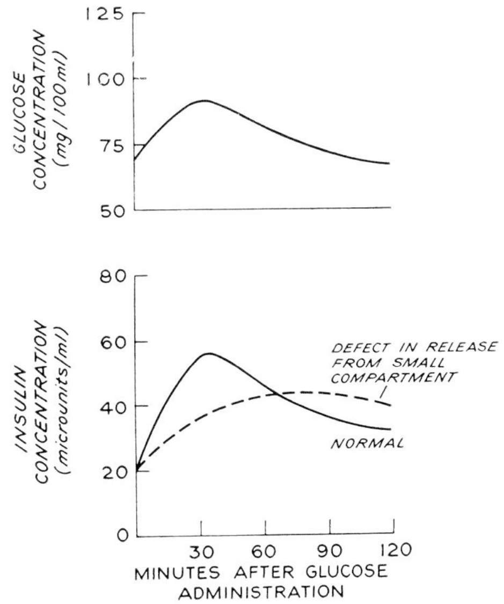

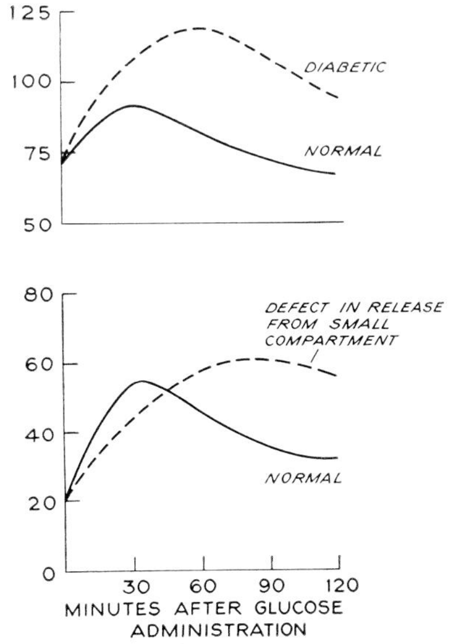

Figs. 9 and 10. Mathematical simulation of insulin secretion curves by the 2-compartmental model. For the dashed line, a defect in release from the small compartment was assumed but normal glucose levels were used to generate the curve.

mathematical constants developed with the perfused rat pancreas, which at best represent only a crude approximation for man. Nevertheless, using normal oral glucose tolerance values, an insulin release pattern was generated similar to that observed (Fig. 9). It is possible to introduce into the mathematical model a defect in release from the small compartment, while maintaining a normal action of glucose on the provisionary phase. In this case, insulin release is impaired but in time the provisionary action causes an overfilling of the small compartment and a delayed hyperinsulin response. Despite the fact that normal glucose levels were used to generate the theoretical curves in Figure 9, the introduction of a single constant defect in release produced secretion patterns showing both the early impairment and later hypersensitivity. When the abnormal glucose levels of the mild diabetic were used to generate the theoretical insulin response from this defective system, an even closer approximation to the clinical response was seen (Fig. 10). Thus, a shift from a hypo- to a hyperinsulin response during glucose stimulation in the diabetic subject can be a mathematically required resultant of a constant impairment in release from a small compartment of labile insulin. The model can generate a family of curves, in which release becomes smaller and hyperinsulinism disappears as the severity of the defect in the release step is increased. Though such a defect in release from a small compartment is consistent with general observations that early release is impaired in the mild diabetic (Cerasi and Luft, 1967; Simpson *et al.*, 1966), it is probable that other defects in the synthetic or provisionary machinery of the beta cell occur with increased severity of the diabetic state. In addition, the wide variation in response of diabetics (Cerasi and Luft, 1967) indicates underlying causes of the disease may differ. The two-compartmental model, however, may permit qualitative analysis of insulin secretion patterns and thereby provide insight into the state of various beta cell phenomena regulating insulin release.

SUMMARY

The multiphasic pattern of insulin release seen during constant stimulation of the perfused rat pancreas was further investigated. Based on inhibition studies with puromycin and oligomycin and electronmicroscopic examination of the tissues at various times during stimulation, the early transient release and the later prolonged secretion of insulin seemed to reflect related, but different, pancreatic phenomena. The effectiveness of glucose, for both release and provision of insulin to the release system, followed a sigmoidal pattern approximated mathematically by assuming that insulin release is a power function of glucose concentration. This formulation automatically produces the typical thresholds and maximum responses. The significance of the sigmoidal response in terms of basal glucose effectiveness and apparent potentiations were discussed.

The mathematical two-compartmental scheme for insulin release which we previously described was modified to include (1) the sigmoidal aspect of glucose effectiveness and (2) the existence, within the small compartment, of a gaussian distribution of components with different thresholds of glucose sensitivity. Substrate-induced feedback inhibition (Bennett and Grodsky, 1969) and inhibition of insulin secretion by insulin can eventually be included in the model; however, in its present form and using a single set of constants, it can simulate a large variety of glucose stimulations including constant square-waves, step-square-waves and gradually increasing gradients. The model also provides at least one explanation for the impaired early release followed by hyperinsulinism observed in some mild maturity-onset diabetic subjects.

REFERENCES

Aschroft, S. J. H. and Randle, P. J. (1968): Glucose metabolism and insulin release by pancreatic islets. *Lancet*, *1*, 278.

BENNETT, L. L. and GRODSKY, G. M. (1969): Multiphasic aspects of insulin release. In: *Diabetes: Proceedings, VI Congress International Diabetes Federation, Stockholm, 1967*, p. 462. Editors: J. Östman and R. D. G. Milner. ICS No. 179 Excerpta Medica, Amsterdam.

CERASI, E. and LUFT, R. (1967): The plasma insulin response to glucose infusion in healthy subjects and in diabetes mellitus. *Acta endocr. (Kbh.)*, *55*, 278.

CURRY, D. L., BENNETT, L. L. and GRODSKY, G. M. (1968): Dynamics of insulin secretion by the perfused rat pancreas. *Endocrinology*, *83*, 572.

GRODSKY, G. M., BENNETT, L. L., SMITH, D., and NEMECHECK, K. (1967*a*): The effect of tolbutamide and glucose on the timed release of insulin from the isolated perfused pancreas. In: *Tolbutamide . . . after Ten Years*, p. 11. Editors: W. J. H. Butterfield and W. van Westering. ICS No. 149 Excerpta Medica, Amsterdam.

GRODSKY, G. M., BENNETT, L. L., SMITH, D. F. and SCHMID, F. G. (1967*b*): Effect of pulse administration of glucose or glucagon on insulin secretion *in vitro*. *Metabolism*, *16*, 222.

GRODSKY, G. M., CURRY, D. L., BENNETT, L. L. and RODRIGO, V. V. (1968): Factors influencing different rates of insulin release *in vitro*. In: *Mechanism and Regulation of Insulin Secretion*, p. 140. Editors: L. Levine and E. F. Pfeiffer. Casa Editrice IL Ponte, Milan.

GRODSKY, G. M., CURRY, D. L., LANDAHL, H. and BENNETT, L. L. (1969): Further studies on the dynamic aspects of insulin release *in vitro* with evidence for a two-compartmental storage system. *Acta diabet. lat. 6, Suppl.* 1, 554.

GRODSKY, G. M., LANDAHL, H., CURRY, D. L. and BENNETT, L. L. (1970): A two-compartmental model for insulin secretion. In: *Early Diabetes. First International Symposium on Early Diabetes, Marbella, Spain, 1968*, p. 45. Editors: R. A. Camerini-Davalos and H. S. Cole. Academic Press, New York.

HALES, C. N., GREENWOOD, F. C., MITCHELL, F. L. and STRAUSS, E. T. (1968): Blood-glucose, plasma-insulin and growth hormone concentrations of individuals with minor abnormalities of glucose tolerance. *Diabetologia*, *4*, 73.

LACY, P. E. (1964): Pancreatic beta cell. In: *Ciba Foundation Colloquia on Endocrinology, Vol. 15, Etiology of Diabetes Mellitus and its Complications*, p. 75. Churchill, London.

LEE, J. C., GRODSKY, G. M., BENNETT, L. L., SMITH, D. and CRAW, L. (1970): Ultrastructure of β cells during the dynamic response to glucose and tolbutamide *in vitro*. *Diabetologia*, *6*, 542.

MALAISSE, W., MALAISSE-LAGAE, F. and WRIGHT, P. H. (1967): A new method for the measurement *in vitro* of pancreatic insulin secretion. *Endocrinology*, 80, 99.

MATTHEWS, E. K. and DEAN, P. M. (1970): Electrical activity in islet cells. In: *The Structure and Metabolism of the Pancreatic Islets*, p. 305. Editors: S. Falkmer, B. Hellman and I.-B. Täljedal. Pergamon Press, Oxford.

ORCI, L. (1970): Personal communication.

PORTE, D. and PUPO, A. A. (1969): Insulin responses to glucose: evidence for a two pool system in man. *J. clin. Invest.*, *48*, 2309.

SIMPSON, R. G., BENEDETTI, A., GRODSKY, G. M. KARAM, J. H. and FORSHAM, P. H. (1966): Stimulation of insulin release by glucagon in non-insulin-dependent diabetics. *Metabolism*, *15*, 1046.

A MULTICOMPARTMENTAL SYSTEM FOR THE REGULATION OF INSULIN SECRETION *IN VIVO*

DANIEL PORTE, JR., ARMANDO A. PUPO and ROGER L. LERNER

Veterans Administration Hospital, 4435 Beacon Avenue South, Seattle, Washington, U.S.A.

It has become apparent in recent years that insulin secretion is regulated by a variety of hormone and substrates in addition to glucose (Porte and Bagdade, 1970). The purpose of this paper is to indicate that even the insulin response to glucose is a highly complex non-linear process. Thus in man (Porte and Pupo, 1969), as in the isolated perfused pancreas (Curry *et al.*, 1968), there is no straight line relationship between the glucose presented to the islet, and the insulin secreted by the islet. A precise model which will always predict insulin levels from known glucose concentrations is not available as yet. However the data that I will present today indicate that there are at least two functional pools for insulin secretion with markedly different response characteristics to glucose stimulation. This model is depicted in Figure 1. The use of this model in pathologic states of insulin secretion has been extremely

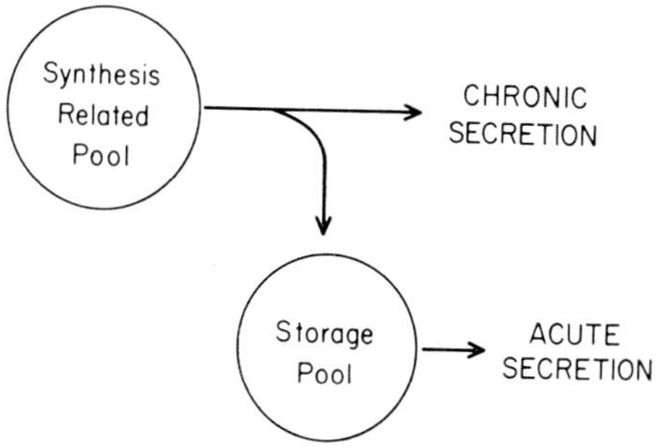

Fig. 1. The proposed model for insulin secretion in man.

useful in our attempt to relate the amount of insulin secreted during a carbohydrate tolerance test to the glucose load, since the insulin output from the two functional pools can be identified during appropriate measures of insulin secretion. In this model, one compartment is a small storage pool available for immediate release. It responds to sudden changes in glucose concentration and its output is evident within 3–5 minutes after an intravenous glucose challenge. Supply from this pool is from a second probably synthesis-related pool, which is stimulated by prolonged glucose administration and whose output is proportional to glucose concentration over time. Its output is represented in the basal insulin secretion and in steady state insulin levels during prolonged glucose infusions. The major experimental evidence for this hypothesis has been developed from the complex experiment shown in Figure 2 (Porte and Pupo, 1969). Normal subjects were given 4 small, 5 g glucose pulses rapidly i.v. One was given one hour prior to a 300 mg/min glucose infusion, another one hour after stopping the infusion, and two pulses were given during the infusion, one after 45 minutes, the other after

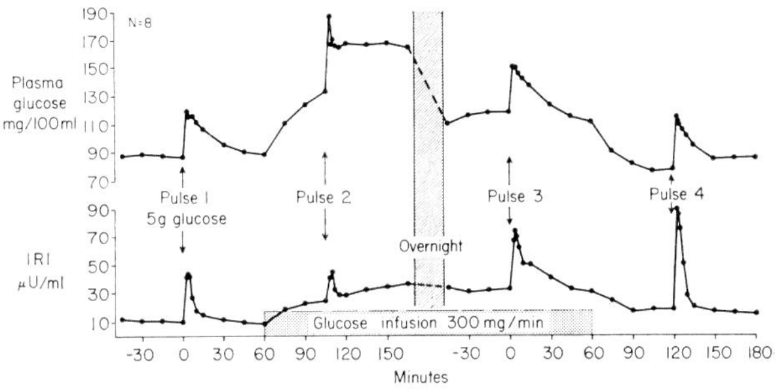

Fig. 2. Insulin responses to glucose pulses (rapid intravenous injections) and glucose infusions in 8 normal subjects. Note the variable rapid insulin response to 5 g of glucose. (Porte, D., Jr. and Pupo, A. A. (1969), *J. clin. Invest.*, *48*, 2309.)

20 hours. Between the second and third glucose pulse the glucose infusion was continued, but the subjects were allowed to eat meals in their usual fashion. The first glucose pulse was followed by a rapid rise in glucose with a plateau between 3–5 minutes followed by its characteristic curvilinear return to basal level. This curvilinear decline can be represented as a first order removal constant and/or glucose disposal rate (Kg) which correlates well with glucose tolerance. Associated with these glucose changes is an immediate peak insulin output within 3–5 min with a rapid return between 30–45 min to the original basal level. Note that after 45 minutes of glucose infusion the acute insulin response to the second glucose challenge is reduced by approximately 60%. Thus at the apparent new steady state after a short glucose infusion the acute response is diminished, and this is associated with a marked decrease in glucose disappearance rate (Kg) which is almost zero for the next hour. Continuation of the glucose infusion for 20 hours produces elevated steady-state insulin levels, with a paradoxical decline in steady-state glucose concentrations. At this new steady state acute insulin responses are restored and glucose disappearance rate (Kg) is almost identical to that observed during the first glucose pulse. Therefore a short glucose infusion produces drastically different effects upon acute insulin responses and the Kg for glucose from that of a prolonged glucose infusion. Of even further interest are the insulin and glucose responses one hour after stopping the overnight glucose infusion. Despite the return to basal glucose and insulin values that were present prior to beginning the experiment, a fourth identical 5 g glucose pulse results in a doubling of the acute insulin response, and acceleration of glucose Kg. In this experiment the same 5 g glucose challenge which produces the same sudden change in glucose concentration is followed by three different insulin responses, *i.e.*, a decrease from control, no change from control, and an increase from control. The simplest model that we have been able to devise to explain these results is available as Figure 1. This model was derived in the following way. We would suggest that the initiation of a glucose infusion is similar to multiple small glucose pulses and that the function of this short infusion is to deplete the pool of glucose available for immediate release. Continuation of the glucose infusion for 20 hours stimulates output from the chronic or basal pool which in turn refills the acute pool available for immediate release, restoring the acute insulin response to pulse # 3. Stopping the glucose infusion is associated with an immediate decrease in insulin output, but the stimulation to synthesis which was delayed in its onset is also delayed in its termination. Since glucose levels are falling, little of this additional insulin is released; it is stored in the acute releasable pool and enlarges it. When the last 5 g stimulus is administered, twice as much insulin is released for the same challenge. Thus this simple model is able to explain qualitatively the complex type of insulin secretion pattern observed. The observation that there is a good correlation between the acute insulin response and the glucose disappearance rate or Kg, suggests that

glucose tolerance may be an important function of output from this small pool. The other studies to be presented describing findings in other normal and diabetic subjects also support this relationship. First, the studies performed in thin, adult diabetic subjects with varying degrees of carbohydrate intolerance (Lerner and Porte, 1970). Thin subjects were chosen to eliminate the confusing effects of obesity on basal insulin and glucose responses that we have discussed previously (Bagdade *et al.*, 1967; Porte *et al.*, 1970). In those diabetic subjects with a fasting plasma glucose less than 115 mg/100 ml (mild diabetes), there was a modest reduction in the acute insulin response to 5 g of glucose which was further reduced after 45 minutes of glucose infusion (Fig. 3). There was considerable variability in these responses and in this

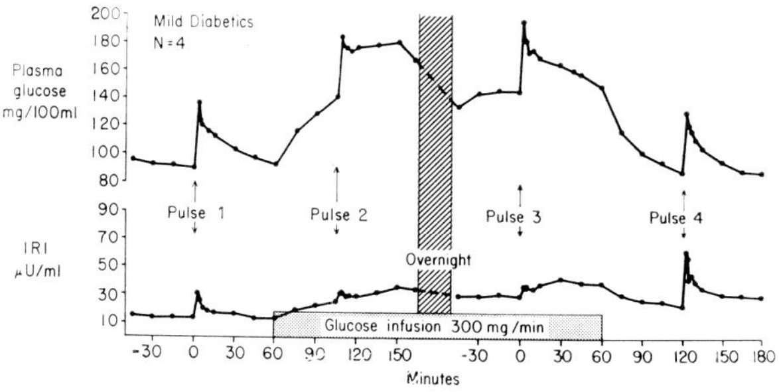

Fig. 3. The same 4-pulse study in 4 mildly diabetic subjects (fasting plasma glucose < 115 mg/100 ml). Note the poor response in pulse 3.

small group of subjects they were not statistically significantly different from the normal group. After 20 hours of glucose infusion, insulin levels were now two-fold increased over their original basal levels and the same as the normal group. But in sharp contrast, the insulin responses from the acute pool during continued glucose administration were almost non-existent or markedly reduced compared to the controls.

In Figure 4 this same pattern was observed in the more severely diabetic subjects with fasting plasma glucose of greater than 115 mg/100 ml. In this group there was essentially no acute insulin response to pulse 1, and a small negative response to pulse 2. Despite this

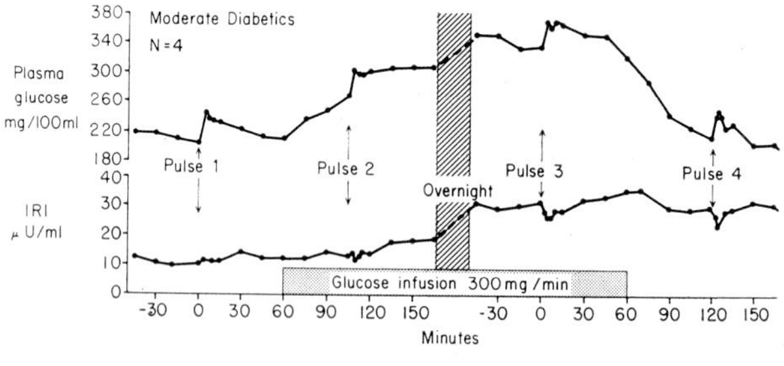

Fig. 4. The same 4-pulse study in 4 moderately diabetic subjects (fasting plasma glucose > 115 mg/100 ml). Note the negative acute responses to pulses 2, 3, and 4.

defective acute insulin response, insulin levels after 20 hours of glucose infusion were comparable to the normal and mildly diabetic group. These minor decreases in acute insulin response to glucose in pulse 2 were exaggerated in both pulses 3 and 4 in which all subjects tested showed a definite *fall* in insulin responses to a sudden *rise* in glucose concentration.

Thus acute insulin responses appeared to be defective in these diabetic patients and most defective in those that are most severely diabetic. In contrast, as summarized in Figure 5,

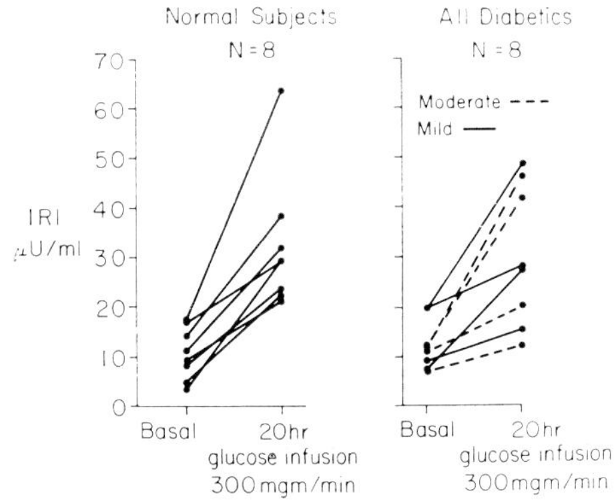

Fig. 5. The effect of a 20-hour 300 mg/min glucose infusion on steady state insulin levels in normal and diabetic subjects.

the effect of a 20-hour glucose infusion results in the same steady-state insulin levels in both the diabetic groups when compared with the normal subjects. We would conclude from this study that carbohydrate intolerance appears to be associated with a defect in the acutely releasable insulin from the small storage pool, but that output in the basal state and during prolonged glucose infusions appears to be unaffected. This correlation between a deterioration of glucose tolerance with defective acute insulin release is another piece of evidence that it is output from this pool which is primarily responsible for determining intravenous glucose tolerance.

To investigate this question further, a series of studies was performed in a group of normal subjects who were given various acute glucose injections from 0.5 to 40 g (Lerner and Porte, 1969). As shown in Figure 6, there is a progressive linear rise in the hyperglycemia induced from 0.5 to 40 g of glucose. This is associated with a progressive curvilinear rise in acute insulin response, which plateaus beyond 10 g. Thus the height of the initial insulin response appears to be unaffected by larger glucose loads. The glucose stimulus in this case could either be expressed as the grams of glucose given, the absolute plasma glucose levels achieved, or the change in glucose concentration between 0 and the first 3–5 minutes, since all of these parameters show extremely high linear intercorrelations ($r = .98$; $p < .001$). As shown in Figure 7, any of these parameters can be used to indicate the magnitude of the glucose challenge. Thus from any point of view the glucose stimulus was linearly increased

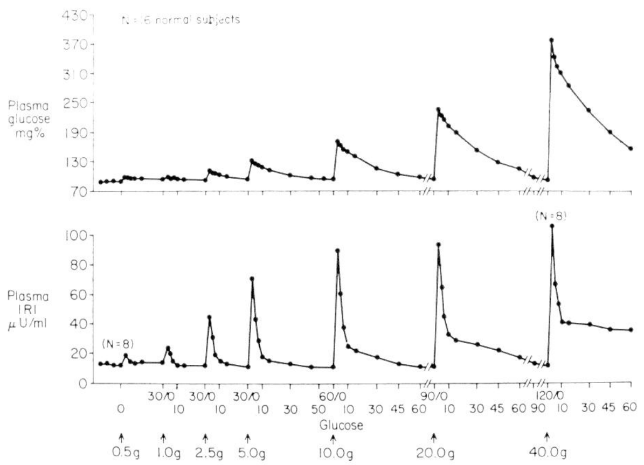

Fig. 6. The glucose and insulin responses of normal subjects to glucose pulses from 0.5 to 40 g.

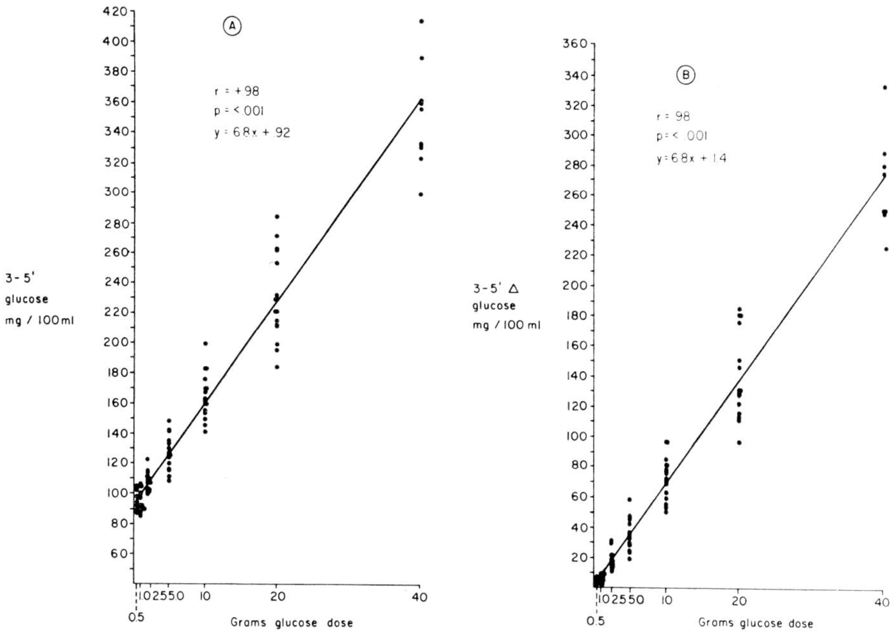

Fig. 7. The relation between the size of a glucose pulse and (A) the plasma glucose levels achieved between 3 and 5 minutes, and (B) the change in plasma glucose levels between 3 and 5 minutes. Same subjects.

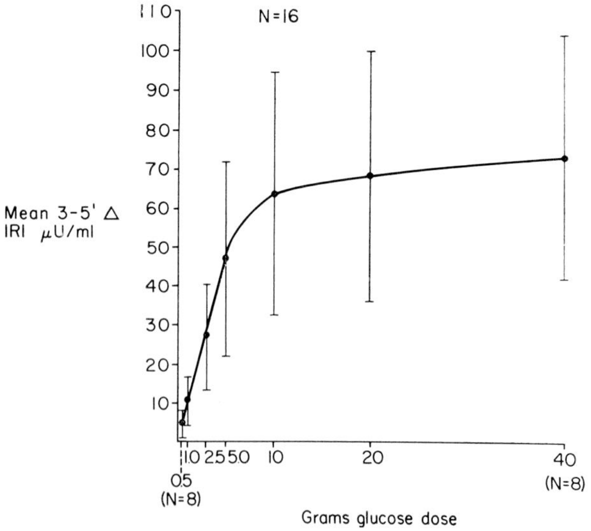

Fig. 8. The mean ± S.D. acute insulin response (Δ3–5 IRI) related to glucose dose. Same subjects.

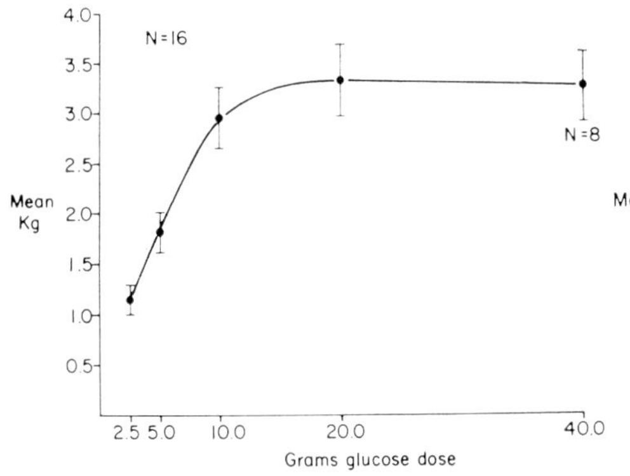

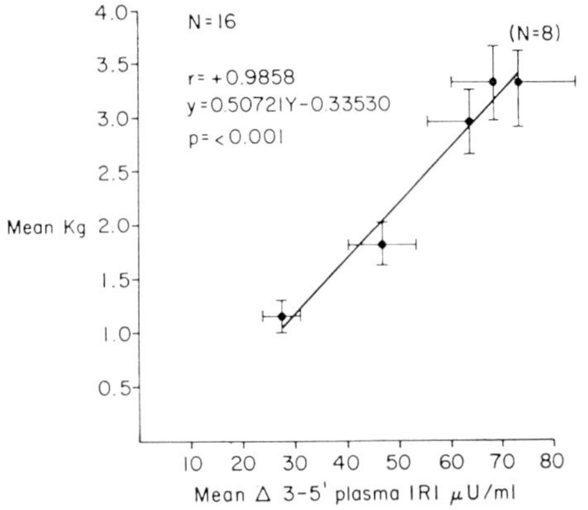

Fig. 9. The mean ± SEM glucose disappearance rate (Kg 10–30) related to glucose dose. Same subjects.

Fig. 10. The mean ± SEM acute insulin response, related to glucose disappearance rate (Kg 10–30). Same subjects.

from 0.5 to 40 g, but as shown in Figure 8 there is a curvilinear acute insulin response which is not significantly increased beyond 10 g. Because the glucose changes are so small after 0.5 and 1.0 g of glucose it is not possible to calculate a glucose disappearance rate, but it is quite evident from Figure 9 that glucose disappearance rate (Kg) from 2.5–40 g is also a curvilinear function of the glucose dose. Since both the acute insulin response and the glucose disappearance rate are curvilinear functions of the glucose dose, it is not surprising that they show a good straight-line relationship with high correlation as indicated in Figure 10. Thus, although the size of the glucose dose administered is a linear function of the total insulin secreted after this challenge ($r = +.85$; $p < 0.01$), both the acute insulin response and the glucose disappearance rates are curvilinear functions of this glucose stimulus, and in this group of normal subjects showed no further increase beyond 10 g of glucose given rapidly intravenously. This relationship supplements the observations made during the 4-pulse study in normal subjects and in the diabetic subjects and further supports the concept that glucose disappearance (Kg) and glucose tolerance are largely determined by the acute insulin response from a small finite pool of immediately available insulin.

SUMMARY AND CONCLUSIONS

Studies of insulin responses to small glucose pulses and prolonged glucose infusions indicate a multicompartmental system for insulin secretion in man. Insulin release occurs from both compartments and both are sensitive to glucose. Release from the small storage pool appears to be dependent upon a sudden change in glucose concentration and its output is a curvilinear function of glucose dose. It appears to be primarily responsible for glucose disappearance and its output is defective in diabetes mellitus. Output from the basal insulin pool is a complex function of glucose metabolism. Time plays an important role in its response to glucose, and therefore output from this pool is probably coupled closely to insulin synthesis. It is responsible for refilling the storage pool and maintaining steady insulin output in the basal state and after prolonged glucose administration. Output from this pool appears to be unaffected by the diabetic state.

REFERENCES

BAGDADE, J. D., BIERMAN, E. L. and PORTE, D., JR. 1967): The significance of basal insulin levels in the evaluation of the insulin response to glucose in diabetic and nondiabetic subjects. *J. clin. Invest.*, *46*, 1549.

CURRY, D. L., BENNETT, L. L. and GRODSKY, G. M. (1968): Dynamics of insulin secretion by the perfused rat pancreas. *Endocrinology*, *83*, 572.

LERNER, R. L. and PORTE, D., JR. (1969): A two-pool mechanism for insulin secretion in man. *Clin. Res.*, *17*, 388.

LERNER, R. L. and PORTE, D., JR. (1970): The acute insulin response to intravenous glucose: a non-linear relationship. *Clin. Res.*, *18*, 186.

PORTE, D., JR. and Bagdade, J. D. (1970): Human insulin secretion: an integrated approach. *Ann. Rev. Med.*, *21*, 219.

PORTE, D., JR., BAGDADE, J. D. and BIERMAN, E. L. (1970): The critical role of obesity in the interpretation of serum insulin levels. In: *Early Diabetes*, pp. 191–198. Editors: R. A. Camerini-Davalos and H. S. Cole. Academic Press, New York.

PORTE, D., JR. and PUPO, A. A. (1969): Insulin responses to glucose: evidence for a two pool system in man. *J. clin. Invest.*, *48*, 2309.

THE ROLE OF INTESTINAL FACTORS IN SECRETION OF INSULIN AND GLUCAGON – CLINICAL AND PHYSIOLOGICAL IMPLICATIONS*

ROGER H. UNGER

Department of Internal Medicine, University of Texas Southwestern Medical School at Dallas and Veterans Administration Hospital, Dallas, Texas, U.S.A.

INTRODUCTION

The idea of an 'enteroinsular axis', a system of hormonal messages from the small bowel to the islets of Langerhans, transmitting qualitative and quantitative information about ingested food, is almost as old as endocrinology itself. Bayliss and Starling's discovery of the first hormone, secretin, in 1903, quickly led to the idea that it might affect the secretory activity, not only of the exocrine pancreas, but of the endocrine pancreas as well. Over the ensuing seven decades considerable evidence for its existence has emerged, but absolute proof is still lacking.

The present communication will review the more recent evidence favoring a secretin and pancreozymin-cholecystokinin mediated enteroinsular axis.

THE ALPHA-BETA CELL 'ORGAN'

There is reason to view the anatomically juxtaposed α- and β-cells as a single bihormonal functional unit, which, through the diametrically opposed actions of glucagon and insulin on their common target tissues, serves to control the movement of nutrients *into* cellular storage sites in time of feasting, and *out of* these sites in time of fasting (Unger, 1970). When exogenous glucose is absorbed, prompt and quantitatively sufficient secretion of insulin, coupled with a similarly prompt and sufficient reduction in glucagon secretion, is associated with an optimal rate of glucose storage in liver and adipose tissue (Müller *et al.*, 1970). When this occurs, the glucose level in extracellular fluid stays within the relatively narrow range of 'normal', despite the huge variation in carbohydrate intake. Wasteful urinary losses of glucose after heavy meals are, thereby, avoided. On the other hand, when exogenous amino acids are absorbed after a protein meal, insulin release is coupled with a parallel secretion of glucagon (Ohneda *et al.*, 1968). This aminogenic glucagon secretion is thought to increase hepatic glucose production, thereby replacing glucose entering tissues under the impact of aminogenic insulin secretion (Unger *et al.*, 1969). Wool and Krahl (1959) have suggested that glucose may be required under certain circumstances for optimal incorporation of amino

* Supported by NIH Grant AM 02700-10, Hoechst Pharmaceutical Company, Cincinnati, Ohio, The Upjohn Company, Kalamazoo, Michigan, Eli Lilly and Company, Indianapolis, Ind., Pfizer Laboratories, N.Y. N.Y. Bristol Myers Company, N.Y. N.Y. and Dallas Diabetes Association, Dallas, Texas.

acids into protein. If glucose is ingested with the amino acids, aminogenic secretion of glucagon does not occur, presumably because endogenous glucose is not then needed (Unger *et al.*, 1969).

The insulin response to ingested glucose is greater than can be accounted for by the hyperglycemia, suggesting enhancement by a message arising from the gastrointestinal tract. In addition, very large glucose loads provoke a much greater insulin response without provoking a proportionally greater hyperglycemic peak, suggesting an anticipatory signal to the beta cells to make ready for the greater glucose load; such an arrangement would prevent a greater degree of hyperglycemia which would occur if hyperglycemia alone were the determinant of the beta cell response (Unger and Eisentraut, 1969). In other words, there is evidence for both premonitory and augmenting influence upon the beta cell response to glucose. In addition, it appears that the reduction of glucagon secretion after a carbohydrate meal occurs at a lower plasma glucose level than after a glucose infusion, raising the question of a potentiator of hyperglycemic suppression of glucagon secretion.

Amino acids have also been reported to elicit a greater response of both insulin and glucagon secretion when administered enterically than when given by intravenous infusion despite comparable hyperaminoacidemia (Ohneda *et al.*, 1968; Dupré *et al.*, 1969). An anticipatory response of insulin and glucagon preceding the rise in amino nitrogen level, is said to occur (Unger and Eisentraut, 1969).

These findings are suggestive of enteric modulation of islet-cell hormone secretion, either neural or humoral. If humoral, the hormone(s) involved would have the following properties: (1) They would be released promptly at the start of nutrient absorption; (2) They would enhance the stimulatory (or suppressive) effect of the nutrient on islet-cell hormone secretion; and (3) Their stimulatory (or suppressive) action would be instant and would be qualitatively similar to that of the particular nutrient.

EVIDENCE THAT SECRETIN INFLUENCES ISLET CELL RESPONSE TO GLUCOSE

Secretin has the three required properties and is well qualified to serve as a mediator of the anticipatory and an augmentor of the β-cell response to ingested glucose: (1) Chisholm and associates (1969) report a prompt rise in immunoassayable secretin after the ingestion of glucose. (2) Endoportal administration of secretin to dogs elicits an immediate release of insulin which reaches a peak within a minute and then returns rapidly to normal (Fig. 1) (Unger *et al.*, 1967). (3) Secretin augments the insulin response to infused glucose for as long as 25 minutes after its injection, a time at which it has disappeared from the circulation (Kraegen *et al.*, 1970). If these three observations are correct, secretin has the necessary properties to serve as an afferent limb of an enteroinsular axis for glucose.

EVIDENCE THAT PANCREOZYMIN-CHOLECYSTOKININ INFLUENCES THE ISLET CELL RESPONSE TO PROTEIN

Pancreozymin-cholecystokinin also appears to possess the three characteristics required to serve as the afferent arc of a protein-stimulated enteroinsular circuit. (1) Protein ingestion is a most powerful stimulus to pancreozymin release (Wang and Grossman, 1951). (2) The endoportal administration of pancreozymin elicits the instant release of *both* insulin *and* glucagon, a bihormonal response otherwise produced only by hyperaminoacidemia (Unger *et al.*, 1967). Figure 2 shows the prompt response of insulin and glucagon to a peak, respectively, one minute and three minutes later. The hormone levels return to the baseline level within 20 minutes. During an infusion of pancreozymin, a striking rise in both hormones again occurs

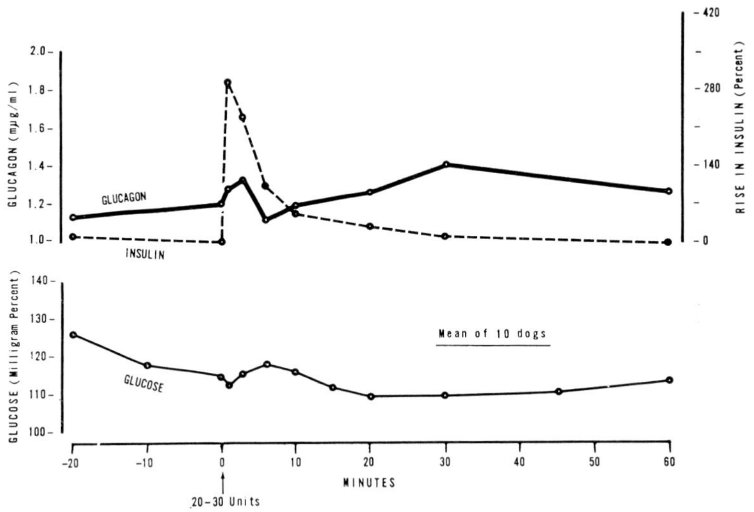

Fig 1. Effect of the rapid endoportal injection of secretin on pancreaticoduodenal venous plasma insulin and glucagon levels and arterial plasma glucose concentration.

(Reproduced with permission of the *Journal of Clinical Investigation*)

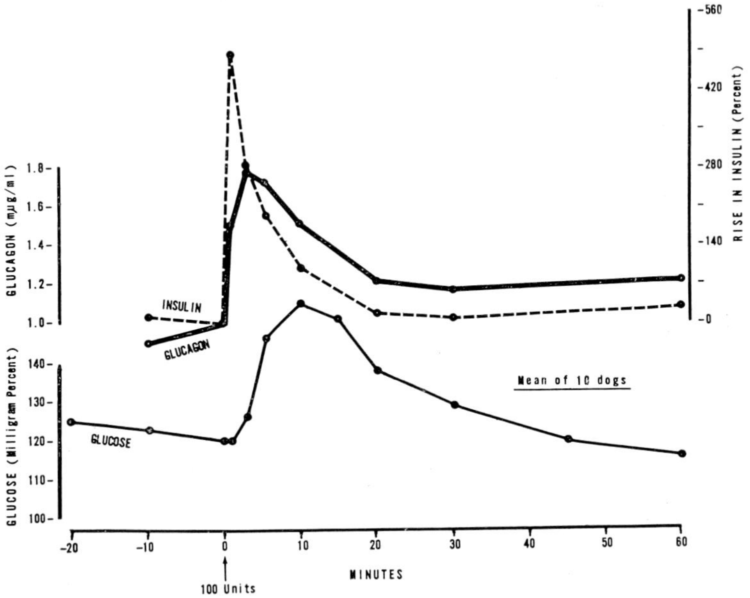

Fig. 2. Effect of the rapid endoportal injection of pancreozymin on pancreaticoduodenal venous plasma levels of insulin and glucagon and arterial plasma glucose concentration.

(Reproduced with permission of the *Journal of Clinical Investigation*)

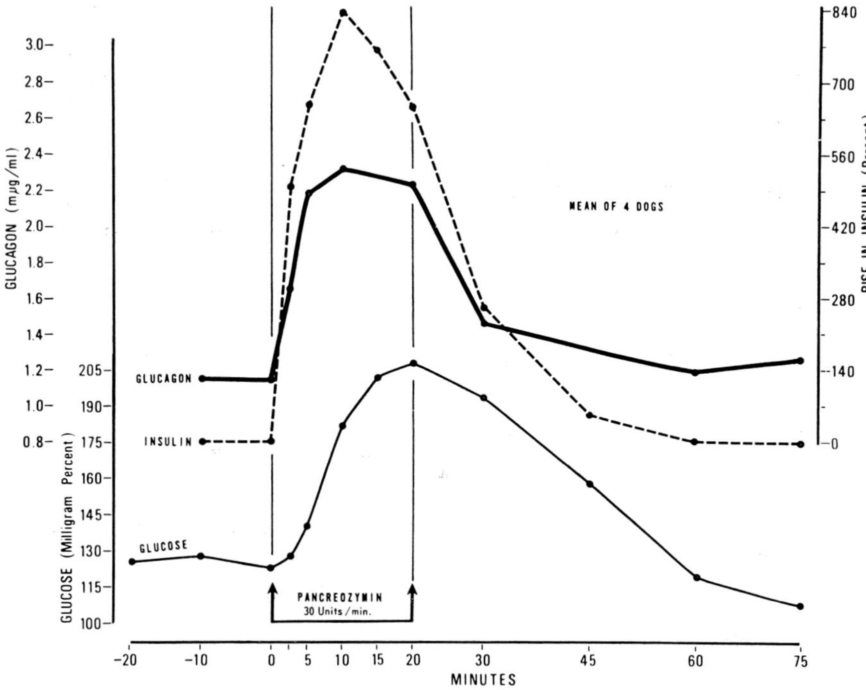

Fig. 3. Effect of endoportal infusion of pancreozymin upon pancreaticoduodenal venous plasma levels of insulin and glucagon and arterial plasma levels of glucose.

(Reproduced with permission of the *Journal of Clinical Investigation*)

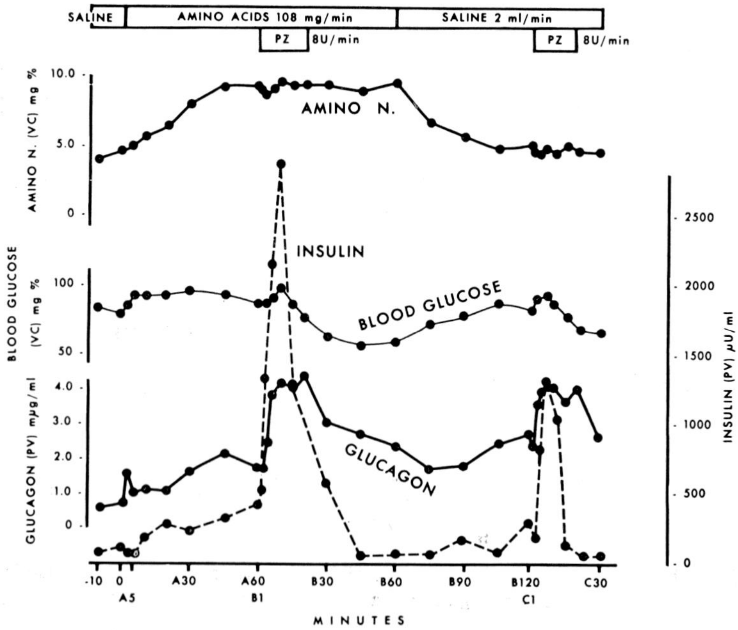

Fig. 4. The effect of pancreozymin infusion (PZ) upon the levels of pancreaticoduodenal vein insulin and glucagon during hyperaminoacidemia.

(Reproduced with permission of the *Journal of Clinical Investigation*) promptly and persists throughout the infusion (Fig. 3). (3) Pancreozymin causes a remarkable enhancement of the insulin and glucagon response to hyperaminoacidemia (Fig. 4) (Ohneda *et al.*, 1968).

SUMMARY

The evidence in favor of enterohumoral control of the secretory response of the islet cells to ingested carbohydrate and protein has been reviewed, and the qualifications of secretin and pancreozymin-cholecystokinin, respectively, to modulate the timing and the magnitude of these responses have been cited. It was concluded that the evidence supports, but does not definitively prove, the postulated roles for these hormones as the afferent limbs of entero-insular axes for carbohydrate and protein.

REFERENCES

Chisholm, D. J., Young, J. D. and Lazarus, R. (1969): The gastrointestinal stimulus to insulin release. I. Secretin. *J. clin. Invest.*, *48*, 1453.

Dupré, J., Curtis, J. D., Unger, R. H., Waddell, R. W. and Beck, J. C. (1969): Effects of secretin, pancreozymin, or gastrin on the response of the endocrine pancreas to administration of glucose or arginine in man. *J. clin. Invest.*, *48*, 745.

Kraegen, E. W., Chisholm, D. J., Young, J. D. and Lazarus, L. (1970): The gastrointestinal stimulus to insulin release. II. A dual action of secretin. *J. clin. Invest.*, *49*, 524.

Müller, W. A., Faloona, G. R., Aguilar-Parada, E. and Unger, R. H. (1970): Abnormal alpha cell function in diabetes: Response to carbohydrate and protein ingestion. *New Engl. J. Med.*, *283*, 109.

Ohneda, A., Aguilar-Parada, E., Eisentraut, A. M. and Unger, R. H. (1968): Characterization of response of circulating glucagon to intraduodenal and intravenous administration of amino acids. *J. clin. Invest.*, *47*, 2305.

Unger, R. H. (1970): The organ of Langerhans in new perspective. *Amer. J. med. Sci.*, *260*, 79.

Unger, R. H. and Eisentraut, A. M. (1969): Entero-insular axis. *Arch. intern. Med.*, *123*, 261.

Unger, R. H., Ketterer, H., Dupré, J. and Eisentraut A. M. (1967): The effects of secretin, pancreozymin and gastrin upon insulin and glucagon secretion in anesthetized dogs. *J. clin. Invest.*, *46*, 630.

Unger, R. H., Ohneda, A., Valverde, I., Eisentraut, A. M. and Exton, J. (1968): Characterization of the responses of circulating glucagon-like immunoreactivity to intraduodenal and intravenous administration of glucose. *J. clin. Invest.*, *47*, 48.

Wang, C. C. and Grossman, M. I. (1951): Physiological determination of release of secretin and pancreozymin from intestine of dogs with transplanted pancreas. *Amer. J. Physiol.*, *164*, 527.

Wool, I. G. and Krahl, M. E. (1959): Incorporation of C_{14} histidine into protein of isolated diaphragm. Interaction of fasting, glucose, and insulin. *Amer. J. Physiol.*, *197*, 367.

INSULIN RESPONSE TO NORMAL DIET

J. A. RULL, M. GARCIA-VIVEROS, F. GOMEZ-PEREZ, V. VALLES and O. LOZANO-CASTAÑEDA

Clinica de Diabetes, Instituto Nacional de la Nutricion, Mexico, D.F., Mexico

It is generally accepted that glucose is the major stimulus to insulin secretion (Metz, 1960; Yalow *et al.*, 1960; Grodsky *et al.*, 1963; Coore and Randle, 1964; Mayhew *et al.*, 1969). Furthermore, it is tacitly assumed that ingestion and absorption of glucose are necessary steps preceding post-alimentary, glucose-induced insulin release. Thus, although it has been shown that amino-acids (Floyd *et al.*, 1966*b*), proteins (Floyd *et al.*, 1966*a*; Rabinowitz *et al.*, 1966), fats (Horino *et al.*, 1968), and mixed foodstuffs (Cohn *et al.*, 1968) can produce increases in peripheral insulin levels, these have been usually considered secondary stimuli. Nevertheless, it is becoming increasingly apparent that, in the intact animal, insulin response to carbohydrates, or for that matter to any other foodstuff, is modified by a number of gastrointestinal (Elrick *et al.*, 1964; McIntyre *et al.*, 1965; Unger *et al.*, 1967) and neural (Frohman *et al.*, 1967; Daniel and Henderson, 1967; Kaneto *et al.*, 1968) factors related to the actual ingestion of food. Some of these have been extensively studied, but seldom under physiological conditions. Thus, available information on insulin response to normal feeding is practically limited to marginal observations realized during studies on circadian variations of plasma insulin (Lambert and Hoet, 1965; Malherbe *et al.*, 1969), or on insulin response to meals during treatment with hypoglycemic sulfonamides (Chu *et al.*, 1968; Quabbe and Kliems, 1969).

Initially, Lambert and Hoet (1965) suggested the existence of a circadian rhythm in plasma insulin fluctuations with the surprising finding that 'a higher insulin concentration was observed during the night, when there is no stimulation brought about by food ingestion, than during the day when normal feeding occurred'. Later this conclusion was attributed to certain deficiencies in subject sampling by Malherbe *et al.* (1969), but they insisted on the existence of a circadian periodicity in the regulation of insulin secretion characterized by a higher insulin release after breakfast, even when three identical meals were given. Results obtained by Quabbe and Kliems (1969) in 7 normal subjects do not support the previous findings, but the sampling intervals were different and the diet distribution was not indicated. Moreover, Cohn *et al.* (1968) have reported that plasma insulin response to a given meal is a function of the magnitude of the calorie load, but their results are difficult to evaluate because their study was made over a short morning period. From this brief review it becomes apparent that the physiological pattern of food-induced insulin response is yet to be established.

The studies on insulin response to normal diet now to be presented include some previously reported observations in 5 normal subjects (Lozano-Castañeda *et al.*, 1969) and the results obtained in 13 additional cases with a slight change in the experimental protocol.

MATERIAL AND METHODS

All subjects included as normals had a negative family history of diabetes mellitus and normal fasting blood glucose. Their mean age was 24.9 years (range 22 to 27) and actual weight was within 5% of the ideal weight in every case. Three days prior to testing their usual diet was established from their free choice and distribution of food.

The experimental diet (Table I) was calculated by a dietitian on this basis. The mean total caloric content, composition and distribution were found to be in close accordance with the usual Mexican diet in their social group. As can be seen, lunch was the biggest meal with 39.6% of the daily caloric intake, followed closely by dinner with 36%, while only 24.4% of the total calories were consumed at breakfast. Nevertheless, the proportional distribution of carbohydrates, proteins and fats was similar in each one of the three feedings. All meals were composed of mixed and complex foodstuffs and no special instructions were given for cooking.

On the day of testing, an indwelling teflon catheter was placed in one of the antecubital veins and left throughout the day. The subjects were all medical residents and normal activity was permitted and encouraged whenever necessary. The first sample was obtained at 7.55 a.m. after a 12-hour fast and meals were given at 8 a.m., 12.15 and 5.30 p.m. A period of 15 minutes was allowed to finish each meal.

In the first 5 subjects, samples were drawn 5, 10, 15, 30, 60, 90, 120 and 180 minutes after breakfast, 5 minutes before and 5, 10, 15, 30, 60, 90, 120, 180 and 240 minutes after lunch, and 5 minutes before and 5, 10, 15, 30, 60 and 90 minutes after dinner. The second group, 13 cases, was studied with the same protocol, but additional samples were obtained at 5, 10 and 15 minutes during each transprandial period.

Blood glucose was measured with a modification of the Hoffman method for the Autoanalyzer and serum insulin with a modification of the Morgan and Lazarow double antibody radioimmunoassay technique.

RESULTS

In the first 5 subjects (Fig. 1), the mean glucose curve shows a clear-cut rise which starts with the first sample, 5 minutes, and peaks from 15 to 30 minutes after the end of each meal;

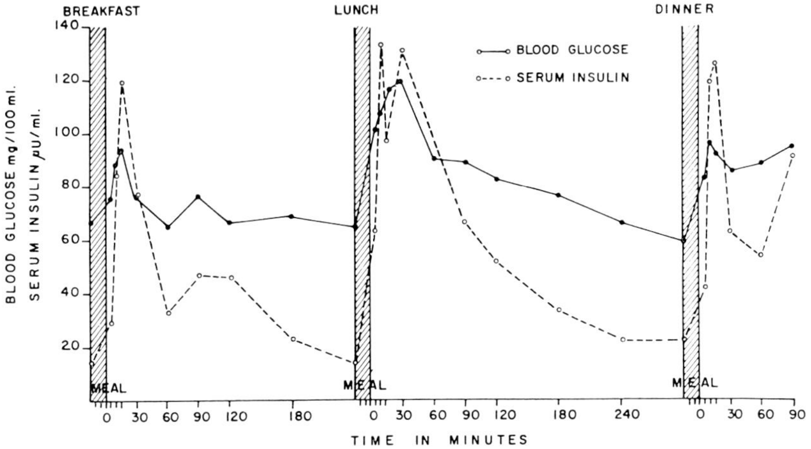

Fig. 1. Mean changes in blood glucose and serum insulin in response to the 3 daily meals in 5 normal subjects.

it then decreases sharply to reach the fasting level before the following period of ingestion. In this group, the total 90-minute glucose increment was higher at lunch than at either breakfast or dinner ($p < 0.01$). Mean insulin levels follow a similar rapid rise with peaks 15, 10 and 15 minutes after each one of the feedings and a gradual decrease thereafter, but the difference between the mean insulin increments was not statistically significant.

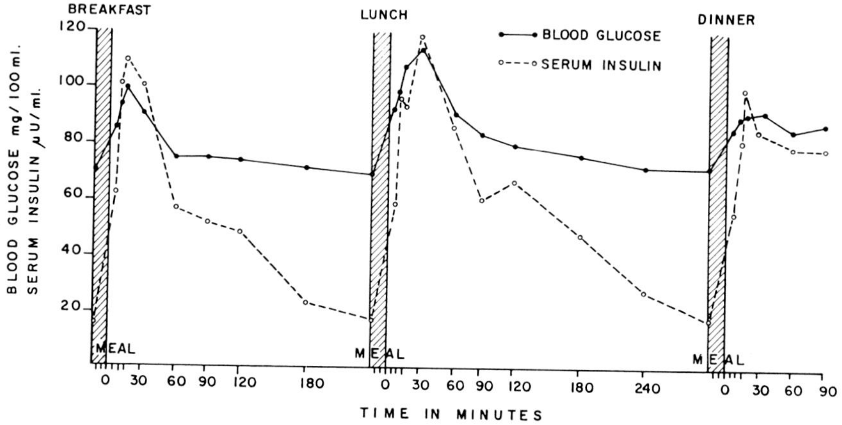

Fig. 2. Mean changes in blood glucose and serum insulin in response to the 3 daily meals in 18 normal subjects. Comparison with the results observed in 5 subjects (Fig. 1) shows a smoothing of the curves and leveling of insulin values 5 minutes after the end of each meal.

When these results are pooled with the 13 additional cases (Fig. 2), the mean glucose and insulin curves become smoother but the rapid rise, fast peaking and sharp decrease are similar. The higher glucose increment after lunch tends to decrease but it does not disappear.

In the 13 additional subjects, the mean blood glucose, serum insulin and insulin/glucose ratio values (Table II) reveal that glucose-insulin response to food starts during the transprandial period; in fact the first changes are already apparent 5 minutes after the beginning of the meal.

This transprandial rise in blood glucose and peripheral serum insulin levels can be fully appreciated in Figure 3. The general glucose-insulin profiles during the rest of the day are similar to those previously seen in the 5 subjects studied initially, including the higher absolute glucose increment at lunch.

On a different scale (Fig. 4), emphasizing the transprandial and early postprandial periods (60 minutes), the early insulin rise appears to follow a straight line with a very sharp angle.

TABLE I

Total caloric content, composition and distribution of the experimental diet

Meal	Caloric content		Carbohydrates		Proteins		Fats	
	Calories	%	g	%	g	%	g	%
Breakfast	537	24.4*	60	44.6**	22	16.3**	23.2	39.1**
Lunch	871	39.6	114.4	51	40.6	18.6	29.3	30.4
Dinner	791	36	87.6	44	40.4	20	31	36
Total	2199	100	259	47	103	19	83.5	34

* Per cent of total calories. ** Per cent of calories in each meal.

TABLE II

Mean blood glucose and serum insulin levels in 13 normal subjects

		Fasting or 5 min before meal	Transprandial			Postprandial								
			5	10	15	5	10	15	30	60	90	120	180	240
Breakfast														
Glucose		71	75	78	83	91	98	102	96	75	73	77	72	—
	±*	7	8	8	10	13	14	19	20	19	10	13	7	—
Insulin		15	26	31	64	76	107	108	105	65	54	50	24	—
	±	15	19	28	64	60	77	76	56	43	40	34	19	—
I/G ratio		.21	.34	.26	.77	.83	1.09	1.05	1.09	.86	.73	.64	.33	—
Lunch														
Glucose		71	71	74	79	90	97	105	113	91	83	79	83	73
	±	6	6	8	13	21	24	22	17	11	9	10	29	7
Insulin		19	33	29	48	55	86	93	114	82	58	74	48	39
	±	16	27	26	43	45	77	76	80	43	30	76	32	16
I/G ratio		.26	.46	.39	.60	.61	.86	.88	1.00	.90	.69	.93	.57	.53
Dinner														
Glucose		72	73	75	80	86	96	99	102	85	86	—	—	—
	±	4	4	7	12	12	21	20	17	12	9	—	—	—
Insulin		17	24	33	49	62	83	103	94	86	73	—	—	—
	±	14	12	20	50	71	83	77	56	55	50	—	—	—
I/G ratio		.23	.32	.44	.61	.72	.86	1.04	.92	1.01	.84	—	—	—

* Standard deviation.

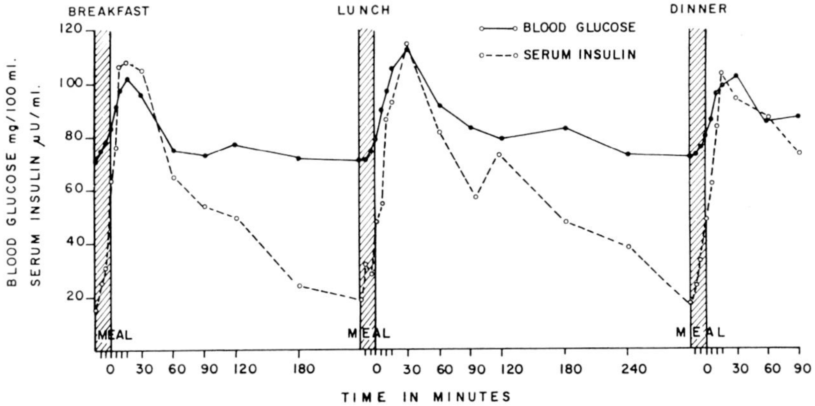

Fig. 3. Mean changes in blood glucose and serum insulin in response to the 3 daily meals with transprandial sampling in 13 normal subjects.

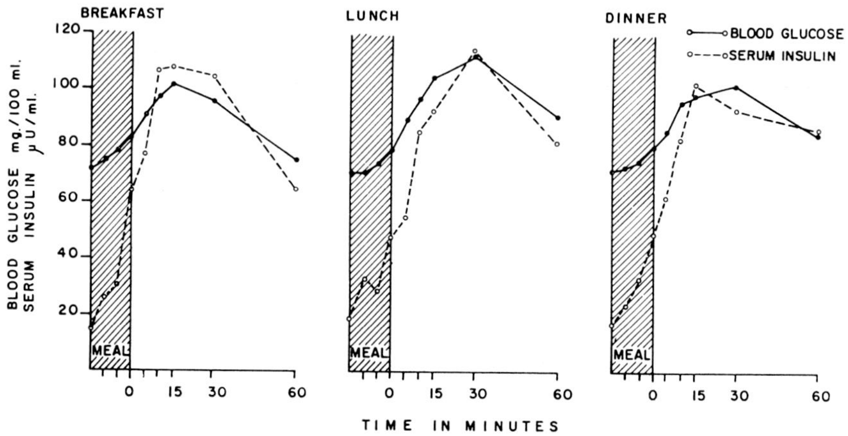

Fig. 4. Mean changes in blood sugar and serum insulin during the transprandial and early postprandial periods (13 subjects).

The pattern is similar for each one of the three meals but the curve is somewhat steeper after breakfast.

As might be expected, the insulin/glucose ratios (Fig. 5) reflect this early insulin release and they show a proportionally higher insulin than glucose increment. At the same time, it seems that the peak is reached earlier at breakfast, but that the increase in the ratio is more sustained after lunch.

Statistical comparison of the mean sum of blood glucose and serum insulin during the transprandial periods (Table III) did not reveal any significant differences between the total glucose or insulin increases after each meal, although the actual glucose value is higher at lunch. Nevertheless, separate comparison of the trans- and postprandial periods of the three meals (Table IV) shows a higher transprandial glucose increment at breakfast than at lunch or dinner, while the postprandial glucose increment is higher at lunch and dinner. As can be seen, these differences are statistically significant but they are not associated with significant differences in insulin increments during the same periods.

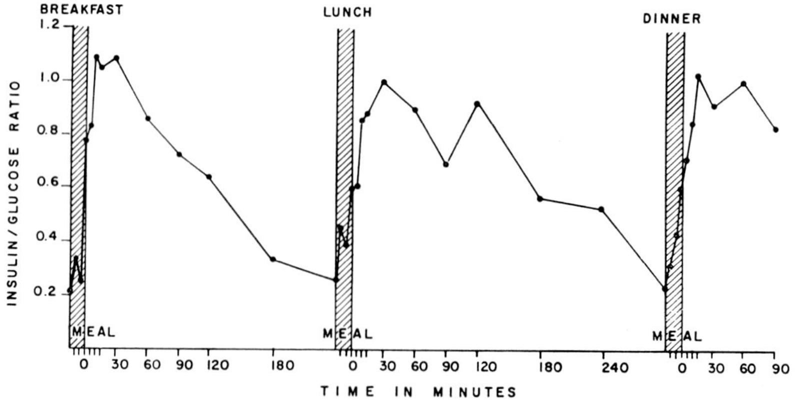

Fig. 5. Mean serum insulin/blood glucose ratios during the day in 13 normal subjects.

TABLE III

Statistical comparison of the sum of the mean increments of blood glucose and serum insulin (13 subjects)

Meal	Period	Glucose increment mg	Sum		Insulin increment μU	Sum	
	5-10-15*	7.1			25.5		
Breakfast	5-10-15**	25.2	43.1		81	164.7	
	30-60-90	10.8			59.2		
				N.S.			N.S.
	5-10-15	3.9			18.1		
Lunch	5-10-15	26.4	N.S. 55.0		59.4	N.S. 136.1	
	30-60-90	24.7			68.6		
				N.S.			N.S.
	5-10-15	3.8			18.8		
Dinner	5-10-15	20.8	43.1		53.6	137.5	
	30-60-90	18.5			65.1		

* Transprandial. ** Postprandial. N.S. Non-significant.

TABLE IV

Statistical comparison between the sum of mean glucose and insulin increments of the different periods of each meal

Period		Breakfast-Lunch	Lunch-Dinner	Breakfast-Dinner
Transprandial 5-15 minutes	Glucose	$p < 0.05$ (B)*	$p > 0.9$	$p < 0.05$ (B)*
	Insulin	$p > 0.4$	$p > 0.9$	$p > 0.4$
Postprandial 5-15 minutes	Glucose	$p < 0.05$ (L)*	$p < 0.01$ (L)*	$p > 0.3$
	Insulin	$p > 0.03$	$p > 0.7$	$p > 0.2$
Postprandial 30-90 minutes	Glucose	$p < 0.001$ (L)*	$p < 0.01$ (L)*	$p < 0.001$ (D)*
	Insulin	$p > 0.05$	$p > 0.1$	$p > 0.5$

* Higher at indicated meal.

DISCUSSION

From these results it becomes apparent that blood glucose and serum insulin levels begin to rise within 5 minutes, or at the very most 10 minutes, after the beginning of a meal consisting of mixed complex foodstuffs. Furthermore, the similarity of the slopes in the glucose and insulin increases and the lack of significant differences between the early total increments after each meal bespeak of a set and fixed postprandial response independent of the caloric content or composition of ingested food. The differences in glucose increments between the transprandial and postprandial periods of the different meals are difficult to reconcile with such an interpretation but they could be due either to the small number of cases or to some additional factors, *i.e.* the existence of a circadian rhythm (Malherbe *et al.*, 1969) capable of influencing slightly the basic pattern of response. Similarly, these secondary influences could, through a changing importance at different times of the day, modify the insulin output to each meal, thus obliterating the quantitative relationship to caloric content which has been reported by other authors (Cohn *et al.*, 1968). A final conclusion on this matter is impossible at this time although our observations seem to indicate a stronger participation of the 'preset' pattern of response, at least during the transprandial and early postprandial phases.

Since the half-time of gastric emptying is known to be approximately 50 minutes, with a range of 39–100 minutes (Harvey *et al.*, 1970), and the meals utilized in this study did not contain any readily absorbable substrates, the presence in the intestine or the absorption of even small amounts of glucose, amino-acids or free fatty acids cannot be implicated in the early glucose-insulin response which was observed. Thus, although the glucogenic-insulinogenic effect of intestinal secretagogues like secretin, pancreozymin and intestinal glucagon has been well established under experimental conditions, it is difficult to assess their role during the physiological hormonal response to feeding. Nevertheless, it has recently been shown that mechanical distension of the stomach produces gastrin release with an immediate liberation of insulinogenic intestinal factors: secretin and pancreozymin (Vague and Grossman, 1969; Kaneto *et al.*, 1970). Thus, a mechanism involving a sequential release of gastrointestinal hormones triggered by the arrival of food to the stomach could be invoked to explain the early postprandial glucose-insulin rise.

At the same time, there is ample direct and indirect evidence to support the participation of a number of neurological factors. It has been reported that the ingestion of non-caloric beverages, the tasting or even the sight of food can produce a fall in the plasma content of free fatty acids, which has to be explained through insulin release mediated by the central nervous system (Penick *et al.*, 1966). Others have failed to show any insulin changes after the intake of non-caloric beverages, but they have induced significant insulin rises during simulated food ingestion under hypnosis (Goldfine *et al.*, 1969; 1970). Moreover, the influence of the vagus nerve upon insulin secretion has been well established (Frohman *et al.*, 1967; Daniel and Henderson, 1967; Kaneto *et al.*, 1968). These observations are in accordance with the participation of a number of neurological factors in the physiological glucose-insulin response to food intake, including conditioned reflexes, and sensorial and mechanical stimuli probably mediated by the vagus nerve.

SUMMARY AND CONCLUSIONS

In summary, it can be concluded that the glucose-insulin response to the three usual meals of a normal mixed diet is part of a complex physiological phenomenon which appears to comprise a multiplicity of phases with different mechanisms. The rapid transprandial glucose-insulin rise could be triggered by several neurological stimuli and sustained by the almost immediate sequential liberation of gastro-intestinal hormones which could also be involved in the early postprandial response. During this phase the response is probably 'set' and grossly independent of the caloric content and composition of the meal. It is conceivable, however, that the actual absorption of substrates plays a role in the late postprandial phase, although this is not clearly apparent from our data. The possibility of participation of additional factors, like the existence of a circadian rhythm, which might obliterate a quantitative insulin-caloric content relationship, is not disproved by this study.

REFERENCES

Chu, P. C., Conway, M. J., Krouse, H. and Goodner, C. J. (1968): The pattern of response of plasma insulin and glucose to meals and fasting during chlorpropamide therapy. *Ann. intern. Med.*, *68*, 757.

Cohn, C., Berger, S. and Norton, M. (1968): Relationship between meal size and frequency and plasma insulin response in man. *Diabetes*, *17*, 72.

COORE, H. G. and RANDLE, P. J. (1964): Regulation of insulin secretion studied with pieces of rabbit pancreas incubated *in vitro*. *Biochem. J.*, *93*, 66.

DANIEL, P. M. and HENDERSON, J. R. (1967): Effect of vagal stimulation on plasma insulin and glucose levels in the baboon. *J. Physiol.*, *192*, 317.

ELRICK, H., STIMMLER, L., HEAD, J. C., JR. and ARAI, Y. (1964): Plasma insulin response to oral and intravenous glucose administration. *J. clin. Endocr.*, *24*, 1076.

FLOYD, J. C., JR., FAJANS, S. S., CONN, J. W., KNOPF, R. F. and RULL, J. (1966*a*): Insulin secretion in response to protein ingestion. *J. clin. Invest.*, *45*, 1479.

FLOYD, J. C. JR., FAJANS, S. S., CONN, J. W., KNOPF, R. F. and RULL, J. (1966*b*): Stimulation of insulin secretion by aminoacids. *J. clin. Invest.*, *45*, 1487.

FROHMAN, L. A., EZDINHE, E. Z. and JAIRD, R. (1967): Effect of vagotomy and vagal stimulation on insulin secretion. *Diabetes*, *16*, 443.

GOLDFINE, J. D., RYON, W. G. and SCHWARTZ, T. B. (1969): The effect of glucola, diet cola and water ingestion on blood glucose and plasma insulin. *Proc. Soc. exp. Biol. Med. (N.Y.)*, *131*, 329.

GOLDFINE, J. D., ABRAIRA, C., GRUENEWALD, D. and GOLDSTEIN, M. S. (1970): Plasma insulin levels during imaginary food ingestion under hypnosis. *Proc. Soc. exp. Biol. Med. (N.Y.)*, *133*, 274.

GRODSKY, G. M., BATTS, A. A., BENNETT, L. L., VCELLA, C., MCWILLIAMS, N. B. and SMITH, D. F. (1963): Effects of carbohydrates on secretion of insulin from isolated rat pancreas. *Amer. J. Physiol.*, *205*, 638.

HARVEY, R. F., MACKIE, D. B., BROWN, N. J. G. and KEELING, D. A. (1970): Measurement of gastric emptying time with a gamma camera. *Lancet*, *1*, 16.

HORINO, M., MACHLIN, L. J., HERTELENDY, F. and KIPNIS, D. M. (1968): Effect of short-chain fatty acids on plasma insulin in ruminant and non-ruminant species. *Endocrinology*, *83*, 118.

KANETO, A., LOSAKA, K. and NAKAO, K. (1968): Effect of stimulation of the vagus nerve on insulin secretion. *Endocrinology*, *80*, 530.

KANETO, A., MIZUNO, V., TOSAKA, Y. and KOSAKA, K. (1970): Stimulation of glucagon secretion by tetragastrin. *Endocrinology*, *86*, 1175.

LAMBERT, A. E. and HOET, J. J. (1965): Diurnal pattern of plasma insulin concentration in the human. *Diabetologia*, *2*, 69.

LOZANO-CASTEÑEDA, O., RULL, J. A., GARCIA-VIVEROS, M., GOMEZ-PEREZ, F. J., VALLES, V. and ZUBIRAN, S. (1969): Respuesta de insulina a la alimentación habitual en individuos normales. Paper presented at: IX Reunion Anual de la Sociedad Mexicana de Nutrición y Endocrinologia, San José Purua, 1969.

MALHERBE, C., DE GASPARO, M., DE HERTOGH, R. and HOET, J. J. (1969): Circadian variations of blood sugar and plasma insulin levels in man. *Diabetologia*, 5, 397.

MAYHEW, D. A., WRIGHT, P. H. and ASHMORE, J. (1969): Regulation of insulin secretion. *Pharmacol. Rev.*, *21*, 183.

MCINTYRE, N., TURNER, D. S. and HOLDSWORTH, C. D. (1965): Intestinal factors and insulin secretion. *Diabetologia*, *1*, 73.

METZ, R. (1960): The effect of blood glucose concentration on insulin output. *Diabetes*, *9*, 89.

PENICK, S. B., PRINCE, H. and HINKLE, L. F. JR. (1966): Fall in plasma content of free fatty acids associated with sight of food. *New Engl. J. Med.*, *275*, 416.

QUABBE, H. J. and KLIEMS, G. (1969): Glycémie et insuline plasmatique sous l'influence du tolbutamide et du HB-419 chez des sujets normaux et diabétiques. *Journées Ann. Diabét.*, *Hotel-Dieu*, p. 301.

RABINOWITZ, D., MERIMEE, T. J., MAFFEZZOL, R. and BURGESS, J. A. (1966): Patterns of hormonal release after glucose, protein and glucose plus protein. *Lancet*, *2*, 454.

UNGER, R. H., KETTERER, H., DUPRÉ, J. and EISENTRAUT, A. M. (1967): The effects of secretin, pancreozymin and gastrin on insulin and glucagon secretion in anesthetized dogs. *J. clin. Invest.*, *46*, 630.

VAGUE, M. and GROSSMAN, M. J. (1969): Gastrin and pancreatic secretion in response to gastric distention in dogs. *Gastroenterology*, *57*, 300.

YALOW, R. S., BLACK, H., VILLAZON, M. and BERSON, S. A. (1960): Comparison of the plasma insulin levels following administration of tolbutamide and glucose. *Diabetes*, *9*, 356.

INSULIN RESPONSE TO NORMAL DIET IN PREDIABETIC SUBJECTS

O. LOZANO-CASTAÑEDA, M. GARCIA-VIVEROS, F. GOMEZ-PEREZ, V. VALLES and J. A. RULL

Diabetes Clinic, Instituto Nacional de la Nutricion, Mexico, D.F., Mexico

We have previously reported (Lozano-Castañeda *et al.*, 1970) the results of certain simple metabolic studies realized in 139 offspring of double-diabetic marriages, followed longitudinally since 1963. In this unselected group of genetically potential prediabetic subjects, the first glucose tolerance test revealed a high prevalence of unknown asymptomatic diabetics and a large number of non-diagnostic abnormalities including hypoglycemia or isolated peaks of hyperglycemia or both. Only 32.4% of the subjects studied had a completely normal glucose tolerance test and could thus be considered truly pre-diabetic. In this last group, free fatty acids changes after glucose and serial blood lipid determinations were found useless for clinical diagnostic purposes.

Earlier at this meeting (Rull *et al.*, 1970), we have presented studies on the physiological insulin response to the three daily meals in normal subjects. It was shown that the insulin-glucose response to the meals of a normal diet appears to be a complex physiological phenomenon which probably constitutes an integrated response resulting from the interaction of several stimulant factors. Thus, the transprandial and early postprandial (60 minutes) phases are characterized by an almost immediate rise of glucose and insulin peripheral levels, which seem to be independent of the absorption of substrates and which probably represent a set, prefixed pattern of response to food ingestion triggered by multiple neurological stimuli and sustained by a rapid sequential release of gastro-intestinal hormonal factors.

Since it has been reported that in genetic potential prediabetes there is a diminished insulin response both to intravenous (Cerasi and Luft, 1967; Soeldner *et al.*, 1968) and oral glucose (Rull *et al.*, 1970), it was thought of interest to study the physiological insulin response to food in prediabetic subjects and to compare it to that previously observed in normal subjects.

MATERIAL AND METHODS

All subjects included as prediabetic were offspring of 2 diabetic parents with a completely normal oral glucose tolerance test, and they were matched for age and weight to the group of normal subjects previously studied (Rull *et al.*, this volume). The mean age of the 7 prediabetic subjects was 23.8 years (range: 19 to 31) and their actual weight was within 5% of the ideal in every case.

Three days prior to testing, their usual diet was established from their free choice and distribution of food. The experimental diet was calculated by a dietician on this basis. The mean total caloric content was similar to that observed in normal subjects but it was found that the meal composition and distribution was slightly different. In the prediabetic group, the main meal was also lunch with 41.6% of the total calories but it was followed by breakfast instead of dinner. Furthermore, carbohydrates contributed a higher percentage, roughly

55%, to the total amount of calories, while the percentage of fats decreased from 34 to 26%. All meals were composed of mixed and complex foodstuffs and no special instructions were given for their cooking.

On the day of testing, an indwelling teflon catheter was placed in one of the antecubital veins and left throughout the day. An amount of exercise, walking, equivalent to their usual activity was performed.

The first sample was obtained at 7.55 a.m. after a 12-hour fast, and meals were given at 8.00 a.m., 12.15 and 5.30 p.m., allowing a period of 15 minutes, which was considered the transprandial period, to finish each feeding. Samples were obtained 5 minutes before each meal, at 5-minute intervals during the transprandial period and 5, 10, 15, 30, 60 and 90 minutes after each meal. An additional 120-minute sample was drawn after breakfast and others at 120, 180 and 240 minutes after lunch.

Blood glucose was measured by a modification of the Hoffman method for the Auto-analyzer and serum insulin with a modification of the Morgan and Lazarow double antibody radioimmunoassay technique.

RESULTS

The mean blood glucose, serum insulin levels and insulin:glucose ratios appear in Table I.

The mean glucose and insulin curves in the prediabetic subjects (Fig. 1) show a daily profile similar to that previously seen in normal subjects. There is an almost immediate rise of blood glucose and insulin serum levels with early peaks and sharp decreases after each meal.

When a larger time scale is utilized to emphasize the transprandial and early postprandial periods (Fig. 2), the very fast rise of blood glucose and serum insulin, starting 5 minutes after the beginning of each meal, can be fully appreciated.

It is also of interest to observe that from the fasting level to the peak, insulin levels follow a very steep slope.

Statistical comparison of the sum of the mean increments of blood glucose and serum insulin during the different phases of each meal (Table II), shows a higher glucose increment at lunch, but the difference was only significant between lunch and breakfast. With regard to insulin, the total increment after lunch was significantly higher than those obtained after either breakfast or dinner.

The comparison of the mean glucose curves between the prediabetic and normal subjects

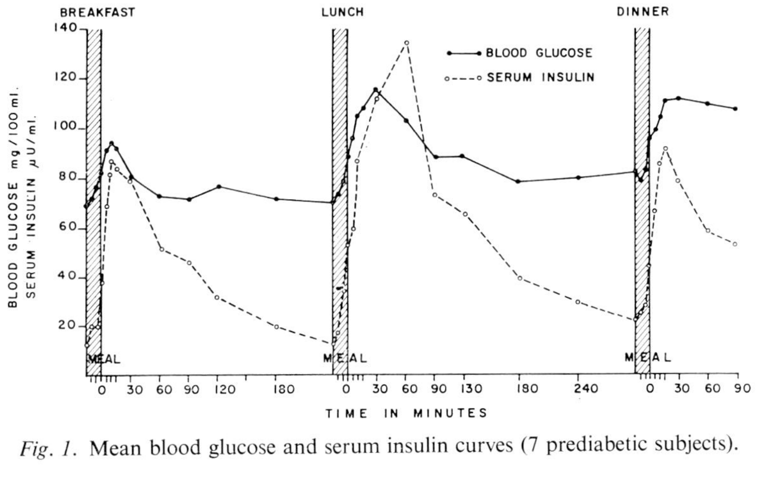

Fig. 1. Mean blood glucose and serum insulin curves (7 prediabetic subjects).

TABLE I

Mean blood glucose and serum insulin levels in 7 prediabetic subjects

		Fasting or 5 min. before meal	Transprandial 5	10	15	Postprandial 5	10	15	30	60	90	120	180	240
Breakfast														
Glucose		68	71	76	82	91	94	92	80	72	71	76	71	—
	±*	1	4	7	18	19	18	14	16	13	11	15	11	—
Insulin		12	20	20	38	68	87	83	79	51	46	31	20	—
	±	7	19	10	22	38	64	37	25	40	26	14	15	—
I/G ratio		.17	.28	.26	.46	.74	.92	.90	.98	.70	.64	.40	.28	—
Lunch														
Glucose		70	73	78	88	95	105	107	115	103	88	88	78	80
	±	7	6	7	10	15	18	20	23	23	16	17	12	10
Insulin		13	17	34	52	59	86	112	119	134	73	65	39	29
	±	9	7	16	17	20	20	33	38	94	52	48	19	12
I/G ratio		.18	.23	.43	.59	.62	.81	1.04	1.03	1.30	.82	.73	.50	.36
Dinner														
Glucose		82	79	82	95	99	104	111	112	110	108	—	—	—
	±	12	12	9	20	20	18	24	30	37	36	—	—	—
Insulin		22	25	28	44	66	85	91	78	58	53	—	—	—
	±	15	15	14	21	34	80	35	21	25	31	—	—	—
I/G ratio		.26	.31	.34	.46	.66	.81	.81	.69	.52	.49	—	—	—

* Standard deviation.

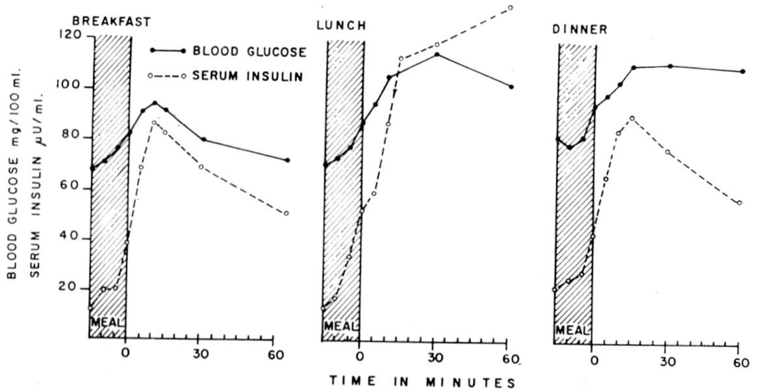

Fig. 2. Mean blood glucose and serum insulin curves, transprandial and early postprandial phase (7 prediabetic subjects).

TABLE II

Statistical comparison of the sum of the mean increments of blood glucose and serum insulin (7 prediabetic subjects)

Meal	Period	Glucose increment mg	Sum	Insulin increment μU	Sum
	5-10-15*	7.9		14.2	
Breakfast	5-10-15**	23.5	38.6	59.3	119.7
	30-60-90	7.2		46.2	
			S. (38.6 vs 70.5)		S. (119.7 vs 184.4)
	5-10-15*	9.1		21.2	
Lunch	5-10-15**	31.8	N.S. (38.6 vs 54.3) 70.5	67.6	N.S. (119.7 vs 109.9) 184.4
	30-60-90	29.6		95.6	
			N.S. (70.5 vs 54.3)		S. (184.4 vs 109.9)
	5-10-15*	3.7		9.0	
Dinner	5-10-15**	22.5	54.3	60.9	109.9
	30-60-90	28.1		40.0	

* Transprandial. ** Postprandial. S. Significant. N.S. Non Significant.

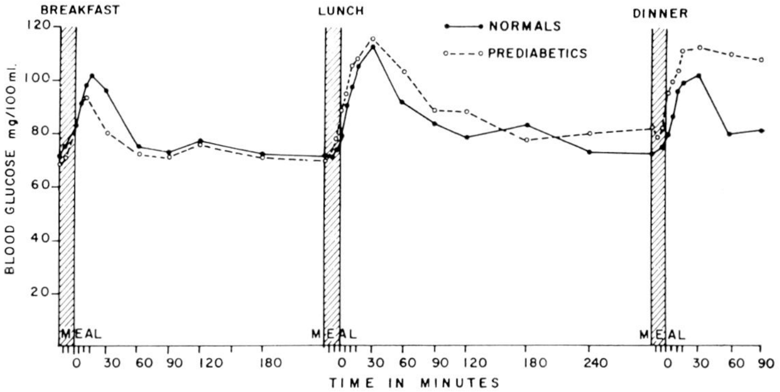

Fig. 3. Mean blood glucose curves – 13 normal and 7 prediabetic subjects.

(Fig. 3) reveals a similar pattern of response after each meal and throughout the day in both groups. Nevertheless, there seems to be a tendency to slightly higher absolute values after lunch and dinner in the prediabetic subjects, although the differences were not found to be statistically significant.

Comparison of the mean insulin curves (Fig. 4) gives a similar picture. The profile during the day, characterized by the rapid rise, early peak and gradual decrease after each meal, is the same in the two groups. Once again, some absolute quantitative differences can be observed between the two groups, but on statistical analysis they revealed themselves to be non-significant.

When the transprandial and early postprandial periods (60 minutes) are compared (Fig. 5) on a larger time scale, the same small quantitative differences in the absolute values of serum insulin can be observed, but the general insulin increment from fasting to peak follows a line with a similar slope in the two groups. Moreover, the quantitative differences are not constant and serum insulin is slightly higher at breakfast and dinner in the normals, but lower at lunch. In fact, no significant differences were found when statistical comparison of glucose and insulin increments was carried out between the two groups.

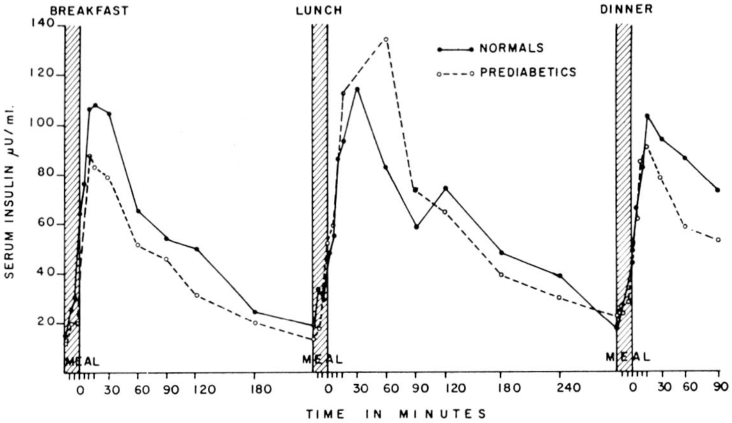

Fig. 4. Mean serum insulin curves – 13 normal and 7 prediabetic subjects.

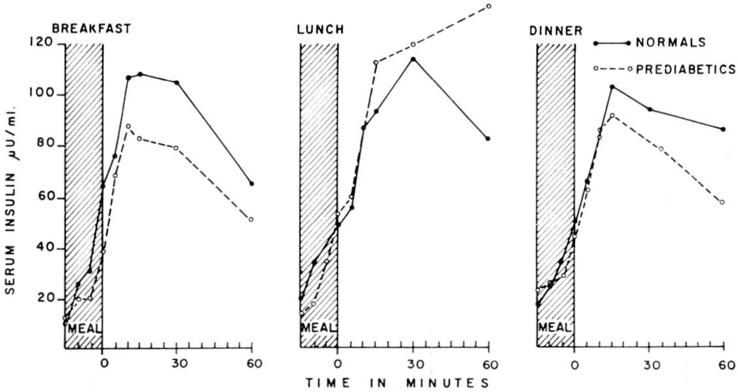

Fig. 5. Mean serum insulin curves, transprandial and early postprandial phase – 13 normal and 7 prediabetic subjects.

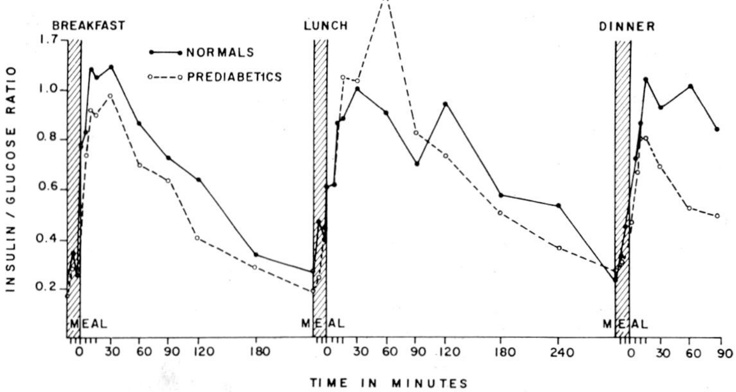

Fig. 6. Mean serum insulin-blood glucose ratios – 13 normal and 7 prediabetic subjects.

As might be expected, the insulin to glucose ratios (Fig. 6) are also similar in the two groups. The curves follow a parallel pattern throughout the day with only the slight quantitative differences previously described.

DISCUSSION

Basically, the pattern of glucose and insulin response to the three daily meals of the usual diet was the same in this group of prediabetic subjects as in the normal subjects studied previously. The peripheral levels of glucose and insulin start to rise 5 minutes after the beginning of food ingestion and they reach their peaks within a short period, 30 minutes thereafter, with the exception of lunch, where it was observed at 60 minutes after the end of the meal. However, in contrast with what was seen in normal subjects the statistical comparison of the sum of the mean increments of blood glucose and serum insulin after each meal did reveal significant differences. Thus, the glucose increment was higher after lunch than after breakfast and the insulin increment was also higher after lunch than after either breakfast or dinner in the prediabetic group. Since the usual diet in this group was found to be different from that in the normal subjects, this might explain these findings. Actually, the higher total carbohydrate content with a proportionally heavier lunch could be responsible for the higher glucose-insulin increments observed after this meal. This interpretation would be in line with the quantitative relationship between insulin levels and caloric content reported by Cohn *et al.* (1968). Nevertheless, we feel that the small numbers of cases in the two series could be an alternative explanation for these apparently contradictory findings.

Should the differences between the total glucose and insulin increments observed in the prediabetic subjects be real, it would probably not invalidate our basic explanation of the mechanisms involved in the early glucose-insulin response to food.

Thus, as was concluded for the normal group, it can be stated that in the prediabetic subjects the early glucose-insulin rise seen after a mixed meal composed of complex foodstuffs is probably a set or prefixed response mediated through multiple neurological and gastrointestinal hormonal stimuli. This hypothesis, however, does not discard the possibility of the participation of a number of additional factors that could explain the differences between the total increments after the three meals observed in prediabetic subjects. Furthermore, the similarity of the mean curves and of the slope of the rise in the early phases and the lack of statistically significant differences between the responses in the prediabetic and normal subjects lends additional support to the existence of such mechanisms. Apparently, the insulin response to food does not appear to be altered in the prediabetic state, unless the delay in reaching the insulin peak after lunch can be considered meaningful.

REFERENCES

CERASI, E. and LUFT, R. (1967): 'What is inherited, what is added' hypothesis for the pathogenesis of diabetes mellitus. *Diabetes, 16*, 615.

COHN, C., BERGER, S. and NORTON, M. (1968): Relationship between meal size and frequency and plasma insulin response in man. *Diabetes, 17*, 72.

LOZANO-CASTAÑEDA, O., QUIBRERA, R., GARCIA-VIVEROS, M., and RULL, J. A. (1970): Metabolic studies in prediabetic subjects. In: *Early Diabetes*, pp. 315–320. Editors: R. Camerini-Davalos and H. S. Cole. Academic Press, New York.

RULL, J. A., CONN, J. W., FLOYD, J. C., JR. and FAJANS, S. A. (1970): Levels of plasma insulin during cortisone glucose-tolerance test in 'nondiabetic' relatives of diabetic patients. *Diabetes, 19*, 1.

RULL, J. A., GARCIA-VIVEROS, M., GOMEZ-PEREZ, F. VALLES, V. and LOZANO-CASTAÑEDA, O.: *This Volume*, p. 442.

SOELDNER, J. S., GLEASON, R. E., WILLIAMS, R. F., GARCIA, M. J., BEARDWOOD, D. M. and MARBLE, A. (1968): Diminished serum insulin response to glucose in genetic prediabetic males with normal glucose tolerance. *Diabetes, 17*, 17.

STUDIES ON THE NATURAL HISTORY OF ASYMPTOMATIC DIABETES IN YOUNG PEOPLE*

STEFAN S. FAJANS, JOHN C. FLOYD, JR., SUMER PEK and JEROME W. CONN

Department of Internal Medicine (Division of Endocrinology and Metabolism and the Metabolic Research Unit), The University of Michigan, Ann Arbor, Mich., U.S.A.

It is the purpose of this communication to review and to bring up to date a study dealing with the natural history of asymptomatic or latent diabetes of children, adolescents and young adults. The course of diabetes in such individuals can be ascertained only by the use of prospective studies in groups of such patients. Although asymptomatic diabetes is being recognized in young people with increasing frequency, no other long-term observations of the natural history of this stage of the disease in young people have been reported.

TABLE I

Natural history of diabetes mellitus

	Prediabetes	→ ←	Subclinical diabetes	→ ←	Latent diabetes	→ ←	Overt diabetes
FBS	Normal		Normal		Normal or ↑		↑
GTT	Normal		Normal Abnormal during pregnancy, stress		Abnormal		Not necessary for diagnosis
Cortisone-GTT	Normal		Abnormal		Not necessary		——
Delayed and/or decreased insulin response to clucose	+		++		+++		++++
Vascular changes	+		+		++		++++

Before proceeding with a discussion of our findings, we need to review some definitions for purposes of identification and to put the stage of 'latent diabetes' into the perspective of the entire natural history of the disease. Table I presents a scheme depicting the natural history of diabetes as divided into four stages (Fajans and Conn, 1965). Frank or overt diabetes is the most advanced of these stages. Classical symptoms may be present; there is fasting hyper-

* Supported in part by U.S. Public Health Service Grants AM-00888, AM-02244, and T1-AM05001, National Institute of Arthritis and Metabolic Diseases, and by grants from the Upjohn Company, Kalamazoo, Michigan, Chas. Pfizer & Co., Inc., New York, and the Research Foundation of the American Diabetes Association.

glycemia and glycosuria; a glucose tolerance test is not necessary for diagnosis. Others have subdivided the stage of overt diabetes into the non-ketotic and ketotic forms of the disease.

The preceding stage is latent but clinically detectable diabetes. A latent diabetic is an individual who has no symptoms referable to the disease but in whom a definite diagnosis of diabetes can be established by presently accepted laboratory procedures such as by an elevated fasting blood sugar level or by a definitely abnormal standard glucose tolerance test. This stage has also been termed 'chemical diabetes' by some.

An earlier stage is subclinical diabetes (Conn and Fajans, 1961). Here, not only the fasting blood-sugar level but also the glucose tolerance test is normal under usual circumstances. However, diabetes may be suspected because of evidence of insufficient functional reserve of the islet cells. An example would be a woman who has a normal glucose tolerance test but who has a history of abnormality of standard glucose tolerance during pregnancy. The latter has been termed pregnancy or gestational diabetes. A high proportion of such women develop latent or overt diabetes in the years which follow. Another example of subclinical diabetes may be an individual with a normal standard glucose tolerance test but an abnormal cortisone-glucose tolerance test in the non-pregnant state.

The earliest stage is prediabetes (Conn and Fajans, 1961). The prediabetic state exists prior to the onset of identifiable diabetes mellitus, whether it be overt, latent or subclinical. It identifies the interval of time from conception until the demonstration of impaired glucose tolerance in an individual predisposed to diabetes on genetic grounds. Prediabetes can be suspected to be present on genetic grounds in the non-diabetic identical twin of a diabetic patient and in the offspring of two diabetic parents. During the prediabetic period, glucose tolerance and cortisone-glucose tolerance tests are normal. A number of findings indicate that groups of prediabetic subjects can be differentiated from groups of normal control subjects although reliable diagnostic tests are not available for detection of prediabetes in the individual. A delayed and/or decreased increase in plasma insulin in response to the stimulus of glucose has been demonstrated in groups of genetically prediabetic individuals (Cerasi and Luft, 1967; Pyke and Taylor, 1967; Colwell *et al.*, 1967; Rojas *et al.*, 1969) and in other non-diabetic relatives of diabetic patients (Fajans *et al.*, 1969*a*; Floyd *et al.*, 1968; Rull *et al.*, 1970) by a number of investigators. This defect is similar to that demonstrated in patients with overt, latent and subclinical diabetes. Vascular changes, reflected by thickening of the capillary basement membrane of muscle obtained by biopsy, have been found by Siperstein *et al.* (1968) in 52% of a group of 'prediabetic' individuals.

In the natural history of diabetes, progession or regression from one stage to the next stage (*a*) may never occur, (*b*) may occur very slowly over many years, or (*c*) may be rapid or even explosive (Fajans and Conn, 1965). The concept, supported by appropriate findings, that there may be fluctuations in the expression of the carbohydrate aspects of the disease in either direction is an important one. Such fluctuations are particularly common when carbohydrate intolerance is mild (O'Sullivan and Hurwitz, 1966; Kahn *et al.*, 1969). However, even the overt stage of the disease may regress. Extreme examples such as regression from overt ketotic diabetes to prediabetes have been reported in individuals who have been in diabetic coma and who subsequently exhibited normal standard and normal cortisone-glucose tolerance tests (Peck *et al.*, 1958). On the other hand rapid progression from prediabetes to overt or symptomatic diabetes without recognition of the intermediary stage of latent diabetes can be documented, as is illustrated by the following example. K.G. is a 16-year-old prediabetic boy who is the offspring of two asymptomatic diabetic parents and the sibling of two ketotic-type diabetics, one of whom has died of diabetic nephropathy. K.G. had normal glucose tolerance and normal cortisone-glucose tolerance tests in December, 1954, followed by symptomatic diabetes 10 months later.

It is well recognized that the carbohydrate intolerance of latent diabetes in middle age may show little or no progression in severity over many years. On the other hand, it has generally been assumed that diabetes in children and adolescents can rarely be recognized at an early stage, since the first symptoms of overt diabetes are frequently of sudden and explosive onset (White, 1956). It has also been assumed by some that the course of diabetes in the young is characterized by a rapid and progressive decrease in insulin reserves (Murthy *et al.*, 1968). Since 1960, we have reported that asymptomatic, latent or 'chemical' diabetes can be recognized in children and young adults by the finding of abnormal carbohydrate tolerance and that such patients may exhibit the nonprogressive course of the carbohydrate intolerance of 'maturity onset-type' of diabetes (Fajans and Conn, 1960, 1962, 1965; Fajans *et al.*, 1969*b*, 1970). Since 1966 at least 8 other reports have appeared which also indicate that asymptomatic diabetes can be discovered in young people by the use of the glucose tolerance test (Kahn *et al.*, 1969; Lister, 1966; Burkeholder *et al.*, 1967; Johansen and Lundbaek, 1967; Paulsen *et al.*, 1968; Sisk, 1968; Chiumello *et al.*, 1969; Rosenbloom, 1970).

We wish to report levels of blood glucose (venous whole blood) and plasma insulin obtained during glucose tolerance tests on 45 children, adolescents and young adults in whom a diagnosis of latent diabetes was made. Follow-up observations over periods of 1–16 years have been made in 35 of these individuals. These results extend observations reported previously (Fajans *et al.*, 1969*b*, 1970).

Arbitrarily these 45 patients have been divided into two groups, one consisting of 21 patients aged 9–17, and the other of 24 patients of ages 18–25 years (Table II). All have had one

TABLE II

Mild diabetes of young people

	Patients Age 9–17	Patients Age 18–25	Control subjects Age 18–25
Number of subjects	21	24	48
Mean age	12.9	22.1	21.6
FBS<99 mg%	13*	16***	35
FBS 100–120 mg%	5**	5	0
FBS>120 mg%	3	3	0
Blood glucose – Sum of increments mg/100 ml	619±53	521±38	130±10
Plasma insulin – Sum of increments μU/ml (non-obese subjects)	167±31 (14)	214±34 (13) 1175⁻ (1)	467±47
Obese	3	5	0
Years of follow-up	1–15.8 (17 patients)	1–13 (18 patients)	
Mean	7.6	6.3	
Progression to insulin dependent diabetes	4	0	0
Age at diagnosis	11 yr, 14 yr, 11 yr, 17 yr,		
Initial FBS	125 mg%, 99 mg%, 106 mg%, 77 mg%.		
Time interval from initial diagnosis	3 mth., 4½ mth. 2 yr, 2 yr.		

* Transient fasting hyperglycemia (>120 mg/100 ml) subsequently in 4 patients, FBS 100–120 mg/100 ml in one additional patient.

** Transient fasting hyperglycemia (> 120 mg/100 ml) subsequently in 1 patient.

*** Transient fasting hyperglycemia (>120 mg/100 ml) subsequently in 2 patients.

or more abnormal glucose tolerance tests by our criteria (Fajans and Conn, 1965) and all but two by the USPHS criteria (Remein and Wilkerson, 1961). Thirteen of the 45 patients have had fasting hyperglycemia (FBS > 120 mg/100 ml) at least intermittently and another 11 had fasting blood-sugar levels between 100–120 mg/100 ml (Table II). The mean sums of increments in blood glucose over control levels for all six intervals of the glucose tolerance tests for the two groups were 619 ± 53 and 521 ± 38 mg/100 ml, respectively (Table II). In 48 healthy control subjects, ages 18–25 years, the corresponding mean sum of blood glucose increments was 130 ± 10 mg/100 ml, which is significantly less than those of the two groups of patients ($p < .001$). In non-obese patients the sums of increments in plasma insulin over control levels for all 6 intervals of the glucose tolerance tests were 167 ± 31 μU/ml for the 14 younger patients, 214 ± 34 μU/ml for 13 of the older patients, both significantly less ($p < .002$ and $< .02$, respectively) than the 467 ± 47 μU/ml for the control subjects who also were non-obese (Table II). One non-obese, 19-year-old patient had an insulin response of 1175 μU/ml. His sum of increments in blood glucose was 558 mg/100 ml. Obesity was present in 3 of the younger and 5 of the older patients. A strong family history of diabetes was present in 20 of the younger and 22 of the older group of patients.

Patients in the two groups have had follow-up tests performed during periods of up to 16 and 13 years, respectively (Table II). Four patients in the younger group have progressed to insulin-dependent diabetes. The ages at diagnosis were 11, 14, 11 and 17 years, and the initial fasting blood-sugar levels were 125, 99, 106 and 77 mg/100 ml, respectively. The initial glucose tolerance tests of these 4 patients did not differ significantly from the mean of the whole group. The time interval between the diagnosis of asymptomatic diabetes and progression to insulin-dependent diabetes was 3 months, 4½ months, 2 years, and 2 years, respectively. The 35 patients who have had more than one year of follow-up have been treated either with diet alone or with a sulfonylurea in addition. It is not the purpose of this report to evaluate the effectiveness of therapy.

In the diabetic patients aged 9–17 years, both the fasting and the post-glucose blood sugar levels during the initial diagnostic glucose tolerance tests were significantly higher than in the control subjects aged 18–25 years (Fig. 1).

Plasma levels of insulin for 14 of the non-obese patients of this group are shown in Figure 1. The plasma levels of insulin in the fasting state were not different from the control group.

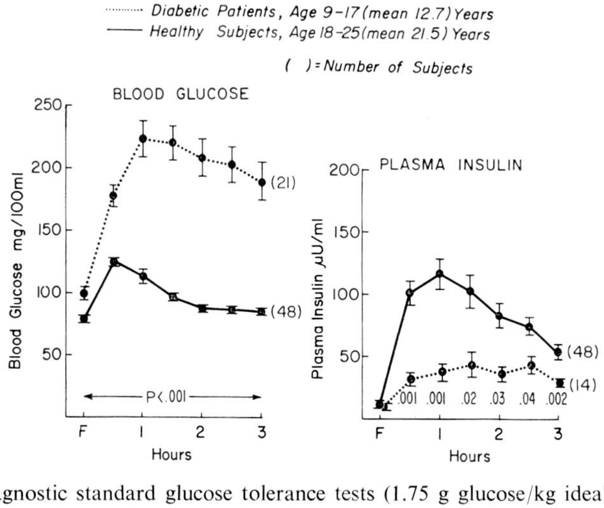

Fig. 1. Initial diagnostic standard glucose tolerance tests (1.75 g glucose/kg ideal body weight) in mildly diabetic patients ages 9–17 at diagnosis, and glucose tolerance tests in healthy control subjects.

After the administration of glucose, the diabetic group exhibited a significantly delayed and subnormal increase in plasma insulin. These results reflect determinations of plasma insulin assayed on glucose tolerance tests performed after 1961, when an immunoassay for insulin was available to us. In 5 of the 14 patients, plasma levels of insulin were not determined on the earlier glucose tolerance tests (prior to 1962) included in the mean blood glucose results of Figure 1. However, mean levels of blood glucose during the 14 glucose tolerance tests on which these initial measurements of plasma insulin were made were almost identical to those of the levels of the whole group shown in Figure 1.

The mean results of the initial diagnostic glucose tolerance tests performed in the patients aged 18–25 years are shown in Figure 2. Maximal increases in blood glucose were similar to those of the younger patients, but the subsequent decreases in blood glucose occurred somewhat faster. In 13 non-obese patients, there was a delayed and subnormal increase in plasma insulin after administration of glucose similar to that of the younger patients. In 3 of these patients, these determinations were not made on the earlier glucose tolerance tests included in the mean blood glucose results of Figure 2. One non-obese patient showed a response which, although delayed in reaching its peak, showed no delay at one half hour and was quantitatively greater than the responses of all but one of the control subjects (Fig. 2). These

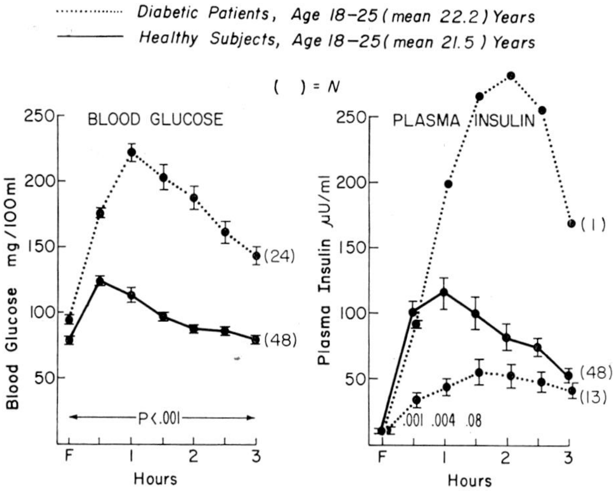

Fig. 2. Initial diagnostic standard glucose tolerance tests (1.75 g glucose/kg ideal body weight) in mildly diabetic patients ages 18–25 at diagnosis, and glucose tolerance tests in healthy control subjects.

excessive levels of plasma insulin as measured by total immunoreactive insulin in peripheral blood were shown by Dr. Donald Steiner not to be due to proinsulin or due to connecting peptide. The patient has normal sensitivity to exogenous insulin as determined by a standard insulin tolerance test. These data do not provide an explanation for the abnormal carbohydrate tolerance manifested by this patient.

In 4 of the 21 patients aged 9–17 years at diagnosis, carbohydrate tolerance deteriorated to insulin-dependent diabetes. The other 17 patients have had follow-up tests for periods of 1–15.8 years. Although the abnormality in glucose tolerance has definitely progressed in 2 of these patients, the mean glucose tolerance of this group shows no evidence of decompensation but does show significant improvement (Fig. 3). The mean plasma insulin response during glucose tolerance tests performed 1–8.4 years after the one on which the initial insulin determinations were made are subnormal and have shown no evidence of deterioration (Fig. 3).

Similar follow-up results were obtained for the older patients who have been retested at

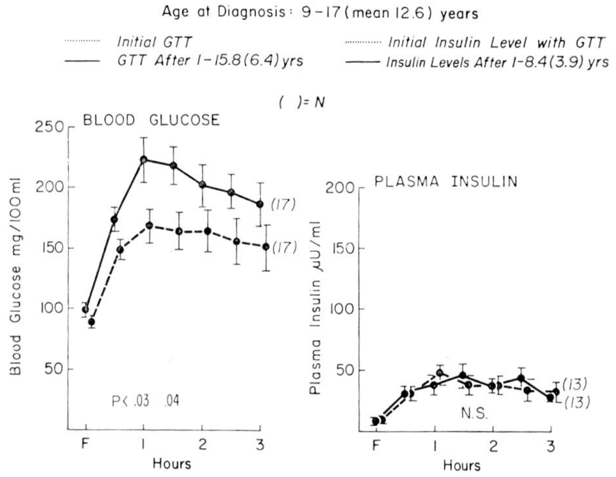

Fig. 3. Initial and last follow-up glucose tolerance tests in mildly diabetic patients, ages 9–17 years at diagnosis.

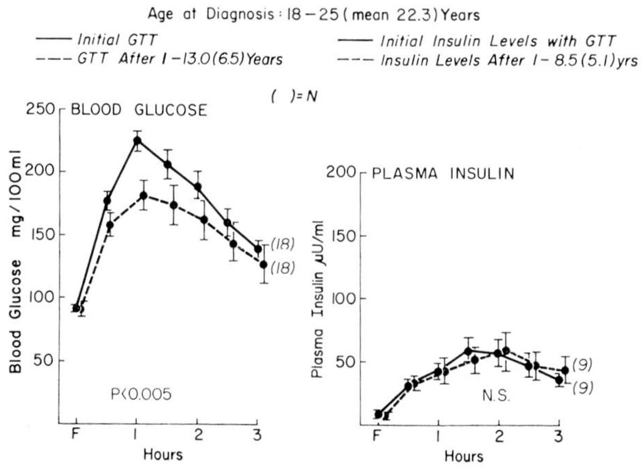

Fig. 4. Initial and last follow-up glucose tolerance tests in mildly diabetic patients, ages 18 25 years at diagnosis.

intervals for periods of 1–13 years (Fig. 4). The mean results indicate that no significant change in glucose tolerance has occurred. There is no evidence of significant change in the subnormal insulin response to glucose after intervals of 1–8½ years.

Considerable fluctuation in glucose tolerance may occur in some patients when the test is repeated at intervals of days, months or years, whether such patients are untreated or treated with diet or tolbutamide. Similar fluctuations may occur in the insulin response to glucose. Although for *groups* of diabetic patients the magnitude of the mean insulin response to glucose is inversely related to the degree of glucose intolerance, on repetitive tests in the same patient there may be no consistent relationship between glucose tolerance and the accompanying plasma insulin response as measured by levels of insulin in peripheral blood by conventional radioimmunoassay (Fajans *et al.*, 1969*b*; Fajans *et al.*, 1970). On repeated tests, there may be (*a*) the expected relationship between changes in glucose tolerance and the associated insulin response, or (*b*) glucose tolerance may vary while the insulin response is unchanged, or (*c*) the insulin response may vary while glucose tolerance remains constant. Some representative examples of these findings have been reported previously (Fajans *et al.*, 1969*b*; Fajans *et al.*, 1970). Two further illustrations of these findings are shown in Figures 5 and 6.

Patient S. N., age 11, is a sibling of a girl who has ketotic-type diabetes and the offspring of a father with latent diabetes which had been discovered by performance of a routine glucose tolerance test. The boy had an abnormal cortisone-glucose tolerance test in June, 1969, but a normal standard glucose tolerance test in July, 1969, associated with subnormal levels of plasma insulin (Fig. 5). At that time he would have been classified as being a subclinical

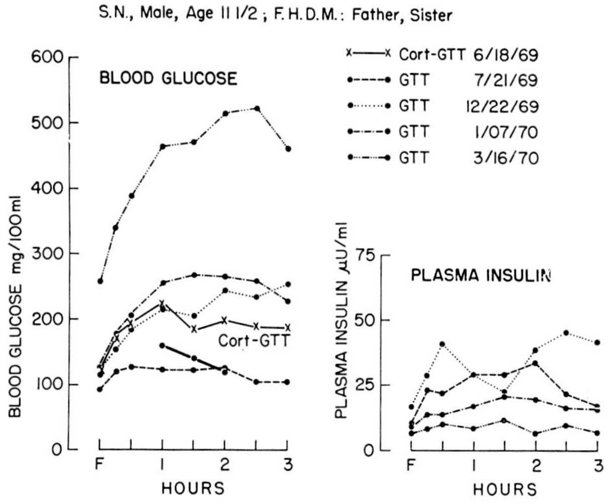

Fig. 5. Glucose tolerance tests in patient S. N.

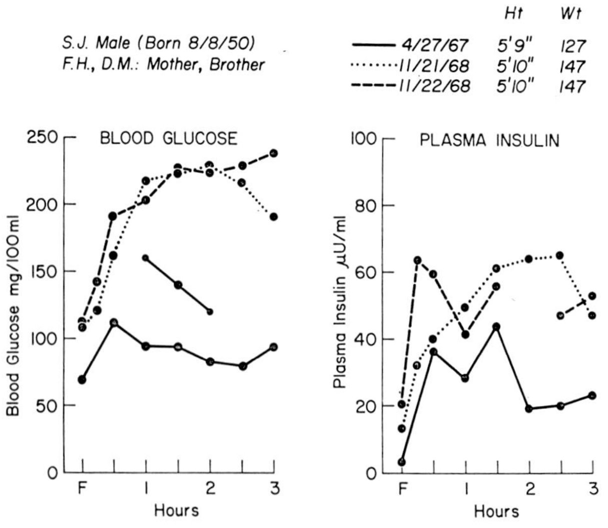

Fig. 6. Glucose tolerance tests in patient S. J.

diabetic. In December, 1969, and January, 1970, asymptomatic or latent diabetes was apparent with mild fasting hyperglycemia of 125 mg/100 ml. The abnormal glucose tolerance test in December, 1969, was associated with as rapid and somewhat greater increases in plasma insulin than when his glucose tolerance test was normal. However, in January, 1970, greater glucose intolerance was associated with a delayed and lower insulin response (Fig. 5). Diet and tolbutamide therapy were then initiated. In February, 1970, a 2-hour post-breakfast blood-sugar level was 116 mg/100 ml. In March, 1970, overt diabetes was present with a fasting blood-sugar level of 259 mg/100 ml and a history of polydipsia and nocturia during the last 5 days. At this time there was only a negligible increment in plasma insulin in response to the administration of glucose (Fig. 5).

Patient S. J. had normal glucose tolerance in April, 1967, when he was 17 years of age (Fig. 6). One and one-half years later two grossly abnormal glucose tolerance tests were associated with a more rapid insulin response on one occasion and a delayed one on another occasion. However plasma levels of insulin were higher at each time period during these two tests than one and one-half years earlier when he maintained normal glucose tolerance (Fig. 6). These levels of plasma insulin are lower than those of the mean of the control subjects.

In summary the results of these studies have led us to the following conclusions:

1. Although asymptomatic diabetes may progress to overt diabetes in some children, adolescents and young adults, in the majority of such individuals studied glucose intolerance does not increase in severity over periods of up to 16 years.

2. In the majority of these patients the mean insulin responses to glucose are delayed and subnormal, but the insulin response may not deteriorate over periods of up to 8 years.

3. In individual patients there may be no consistent relationship between glucose tolerance and the insulin response to glucose as measured by plasma levels of insulin in peripheral blood by conventional radioimmunoassay. With the assumptions that (*a*) the fractional removal rate of insulin from plasma or (*b*) the concentrations of proinsulin or connecting peptide in plasma during glucose tolerance tests do not differ from one test to another in any one individual, our findings suggest that factors in addition to the abnormal pancreatic insulin response to glucose may determine normality or abnormality of glucose tolerance. A normal glucose tolerance test may occur in some diabetic patients in the presence of a greatly delayed and subnormal insulin response. This may occur either before or after the initial recognition of the disease. Similar findings have been reported also in prediabetic subjects (Cerasi and Luft, 1967; Pyke and Taylor, 1967; Colwell and Lein, 1967; Rojas *et al.*, 1969) and in other nondiabetic relatives of diabetic patients (Fajans *et al.*, 1969*a*; Floyd *et al.*, 1968; Rull *et al.*, 1970).

4. Since a large majority of the patients in this study have shown no significant progression of the disease, validation of diagnostic criteria for the interpretation of the glucose tolerance test need not depend on a high rate of progression to more severe hyperglycemia.

5. The slow progression of latent diabetes in many children and adolescents suggests that with early detection, time may be available for the institution of prophylactic procedures which have the potentiality of being effective.

REFERENCES

BURKEHOLDER, J. M., PICKENS, J. M., and WOMACK, W. N. (1967): Oral glucose tolerance test in siblings of children with diabetes mellitus. *Diabetes, 16*, 156.

CERASI, E. and LUFT, R. (1967): Insulin response to glucose infusion in diabetic and non-diabetic monozygotic twin pairs. Genetic control of insulin response? *Acta. endocr. (Kbh.), 55*, 330.

CHIUMELLO, G., DEL GUERCIO, M. J., CARNELUTTI, M. and BIDONE, G. (1969): Relationship between obesity, chemical diabetes and beta pancreatic function in children. *Diabetes, 18*, 238.

COLWELL, J. A. and LEIN, A. (1967): Diminished insulin responses to hyperglycemia in prediabetes and diabetes. *Diabetes, 16*, 560.

CONN, J. W. and FAJANS, S. S. (1961): The prediabetic state. A concept of dynamic resistance to a genetic diabetogenic influence. *Amer. J. Med.*, *31*, 839.

FAJANS, S. S. and CONN, J. W. (1960): Tolbutamide-induced improvement in carbohydrate tolerance of young people with mild diabetes mellitus. *Diabetes*, *9*, 83.

FAJANS, S. S. and CONN, J. W. (1962): The use of tolbutamide in the treatment of young people with mild diabetes mellitus – a progress report. *Diabetes (Suppl.)*, *11*, 123.

FAJANS, S. S. and CONN, J. W. (1965): Prediabetes, subclinical diabetes and latent clinical diabetes: interpretation, diagnosis and treatment. In: *On the Nature and Treatment of Diabetes*, pp. 641–656. Editors: B. S. Leibel and G. S. Wrenshall. ICS No. 84. Excerpta Medica, Amsterdam.

FAJANS, S. S., FLOYD, J. C., JR., CONN, J. W. and PEK, S. (1970): The course of asymptomatic diabetes of children, adolescents, and young adults. In: *Early Diabetes*. p. 377. Editors: R. A. Camerini-Davalos and H. S. Cole, *Advances in Metabolic Disorders, Suppl. 1*. Academic Press, New York.

FAJANS, S. S., FLOYD, J. C., JR., CONN, J. W., PEK, S., RULL, J. and KNOPF, R. F. (1969*a*): Plasma insulin responses to ingested glucose and to infused amino acids in subclinical diabetes and prediabetes. In: *Diabetes, Proceedings VI Congress of International Diabetes Federation, Stockholm 1969*, pp. 515–521. Editor: J. Östman. ICS No. 172. Excerpta Medica, Amsterdam.

FAJANS, S. S., FLOYD, J. C., JR., PEK, S. and CONN, J. W. (1969*b*): The course of asymptomatic diabetes in young people, as determined by levels of blood glucose and plasma insulin. *Trans. Assoc. Amer. Phys.*, *82*, 211.

FLOYD, J. C., JR., FAJANS, S. S., CONN, J. W., THIFFAULT, C., KNOPF, R. F. and GUNTSCHE, E. (1968): Secretion of insulin induced by amino acids and glucose in diabetes mellitus. *J. clin. Endocr.*, *28*, 266.

JOHANSEN, K. and LUNDBAEK, K. (1967): Plasma-insulin in mild juvenile diabetes. *Lancet*, *1*, 1257.

KAHN, C. B., SOELDNER, J. S., GLEASON, R. E., ROJAS, L., CAMERINI-DAVALOS, R. A. and MARBLE, A. (1969): Clinical and chemical diabetes in offspring of diabetic couples. *New Engl. J. Med.*, *281*, 343.

LISTER, J. (1966): The clinical spectrum of juvenile diabetes. *Lancet*, *1*, 386.

MURTHY, D. Y. N., GUTHRIE, R. A. and WOMACK, W. N. (1968): Progressive decrease in insulin reserve in children with chemical diabetes. *J. Pediat.*, *72*, 567.

O'SULLIVAN, J. B. and HURWITZ, D. (1966): Spontaneous remissions in early diabetes mellitus. *Arch. intern. Med.*, *117*, 769.

PAULSEN, E. P., RICHENDERFER, L. and GINSBERG-FELLNER, F. (1968): Plasma glucose, free fatty acids, and immunoreactive insulin in 66 obese children. *Diabetes*, *17*, 261.

PECK, F. B., JR., KIRTLEY, W. R. and PECK, F. B., SR. (1958): Complete remission of severe diabetes. *Diabetes*, *7*, 93.

PYKE, D. A. and TAYLOR, K. W. (1967): Glucose tolerance and serum insulin in unaffected identical twins of diabetics. *Brit. med. J.*, *4*, 21.

REMEIN, Q. R. and WILKERSON, H. L. C. (1961): The efficiency of screening tests for diabetes. *J. chron. Dis.*, *13*, 6.

ROJAS, L., SOELDNER, J. S., GLEASON, R. E., KAHN, C. B. and MARBLE, A. (1969): Offspring of two diabetic parents: differential serum insulin responses to intravenous glucose and tolbutamide. *J. clin. Endocr.*, *29*, 1569.

ROSENBLOOM, A. L. (1970): Insulin responses of children with chemical diabetes mellitus. *New Engl. J. Med.*, *282*, 1228.

RULL, J. A., CONN, J. W., FLOYD, J. C., JR. and FAJANS, S. S. (1970): Levels of plasma insulin during cortisone glucose tolerance tests in 'nondiabetic' relatives of diabetic patients. Implications of diminished insulin secretory reserve in subclinical diabetes. *Diabetes*, *19*, 1.

SIPERSTEIN, M. D., UNGER, R. H. and MADISON, L. L. (1968): Studies of muscle capillary basement membranes in normal subjects, diabetic, and prediabetic patients. *J. clin. Invest.*, *47*, 1973.

SISK, CH. W. (1968): Application of a one-hour glucose tolerance test to genetic studies of diabetes in children. *Lancet*, *1*, 262.

WHITE, P. (1956); Natural course and prognosis of juvenile diabetes. *Diabetes*, *5*, 445.

THE EFFECT OF OBESITY IN DIABETES

J. D. BAGDADE

Department of Medicine, University of Washington School of Medicine, and the Seattle Veterans Administration Hospital, Seattle, Wash., U.S.A.

It has been known for many years that weight gain complicates the management of both insulin-requiring and adult-onset diabetic patients. Until recently, the cause for the almost invariable deterioration of diabetic control and glucose tolerance associated with weight gain has been unexplained. Recent studies, however, employing precise methods for quantitating the cellularity of human adipose tissue have provided a basis for understanding how adiposity influences glucose tolerance.

Hirsch, Salans and their co-workers at the Rockefeller University have made the important basic observation that adipose tissue cells are increased in both size and number in patients with long-standing obesity (Salans *et al.*, 1968). This group has shown that adipocytes from these patients are relatively insensitive to the metabolic actions of insulin. Furthermore, these investigators demonstrated that weight reduction is associated with an improvement in glucose tolerance, restoration of insulin sensitivity, and no alteration in adipocyte number. Simm's observation that adipose tissue cell number also remained constant in non-obese volunteers in whom obesity was induced by overfeeding (Simms *et al.*, 1968) has established conclusively that the number of adipocytes is predetermined and maintained in the adult in states of both caloric excess and deprivation. In addition, and of particular interest to the diabetologist, Simms noted a slight but uniform deterioration of glucose tolerance following weight gain in these subjects. It thus appears that the enlarged adipocyte is a morphologic feature of the obese state and with this increased cell size there is an associated resistance to insulin action.

Since obesity seems to be associated with insulin resistance, β-cell hyperfunction and compensatory hypersecretion of insulin might be anticipated. Indeed, not only have β-cell hypertrophy and hyperplasia been demonstrated (Ogilvie, 1933) but probably as a reflection of this increased secretory activity, immunoreactive insulin levels (IRI) after an overnight fast have been shown to be increased in the obese (Fig. 1). The lack of any demonstrable correlation between basal IRI and glucose tolerance (Bagdade *et al.*, 1967), along with other studies (Porte and Bagdade, 1970) indicate that basal IRI secretion is intact in diabetes. In both diabetic and nondiabetic subjects the basal IRI level and obesity correlate so closely that it has been suggested that basal IRI may be the simplest accurate index of adiposity and the coexisting level of tissue insulin antagonism in man (Bierman *et al.*, 1968).

Our recent demonstration that the close association between weight and basal IRI is preserved after weight reduction in obese patients indicates that basal hyperinsulinism is a reversible consequence of obesity (Fig. 2). The decline observed in basal IRI following weight loss is consistent with an *in vivo* reduction in tissue insulin resistance, as Salans has shown *in vitro* in adipocytes from obese subjects (Salans *et al.*, 1968).

The elevation of IRI levels which also have been observed in the obese after a variety of insulinogenic stimuli indicate that β-cell secretion is exaggerated in the stimulated as well as

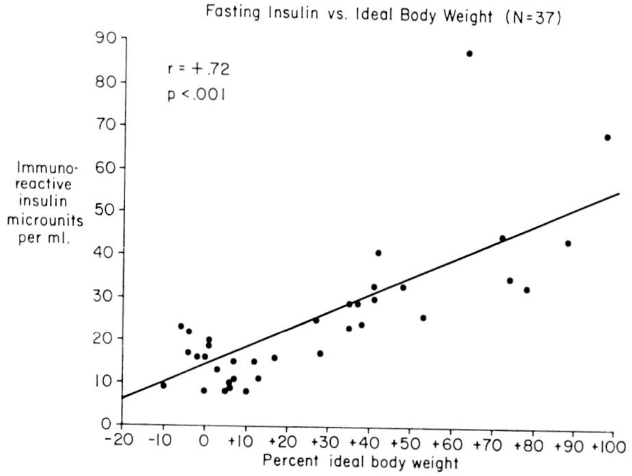

Fig. 1. Relationship between obesity expressed as percent of ideal body weight and basal serum immunoreactive insulin (IRI) levels.

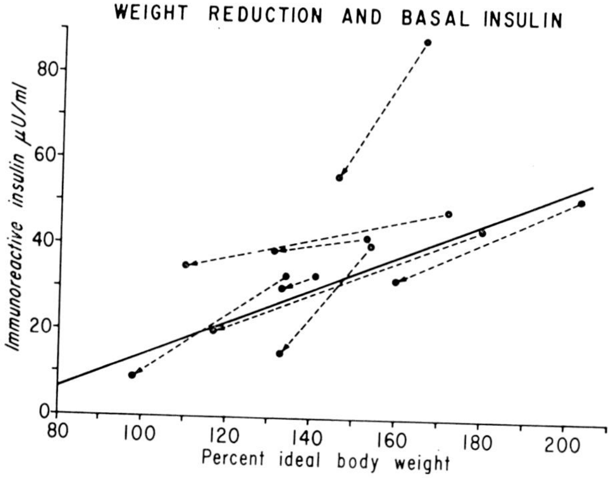

Fig. 2. Changes in basal serum immunoreactive insulin (IRI) levels following weight reduction in obese subjects compared to regression line for body weight and basal IRI.

the resting or basal state. The basal IRI level appears to influence the amount of insulin released from the pancreatic islet in both nondiabetic and diabetic subjects. The increment in IRI levels reached after glucose and glucagon (Porte and Bagdade, 1970), and tolbutamide (Bagdade *et al.*, in preparation) have been shown to be directly related to the basal or pre-stimulated IRI level. Thus obese subjects with high basal IRI and even mild to moderately severe glucose intolerance will have higher stimulated IRI levels than non-obese subjects with normal carbohydrate tolerance (Fig. 3).

Since obesity exerts such a profound effect on both basal and stimulated insulin secretion, this influence must be eliminated when insulin responses of patients of differing weights and therefore with differing basal IRI are compared. The method we employ to eliminate the effects of obesity on IRI levels is expressing the changes in IRI as a percentage of the basal level (Bagdade *et al.*, 1967). When the effects of obesity are eliminated mathematically in this way, the great disparity in IRI levels in the obese and non-obese, and apparent 'hyperinsuli-

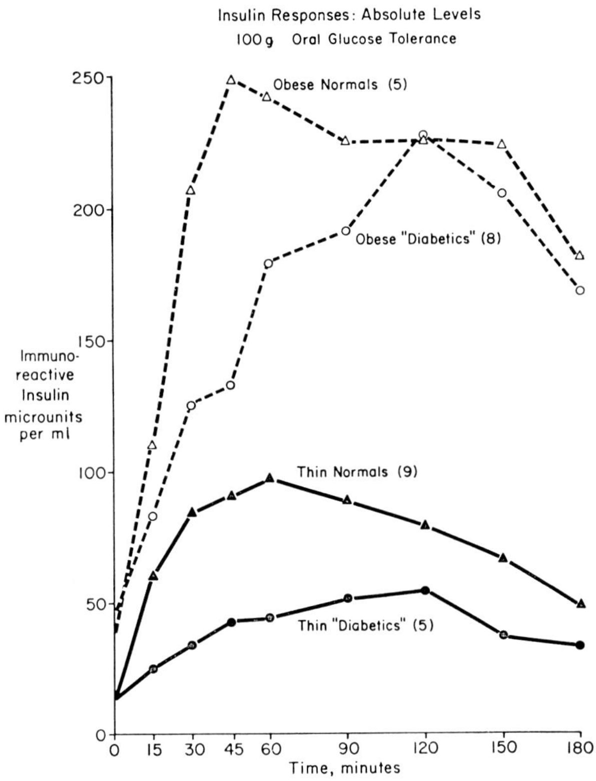

Fig. 3. A comparison of absolute serum immunoreactive insulin levels (IRI) in obese and thin non-diabetic and diabetic subjects during 3-hr oral (100 g) glucose tolerance tests.

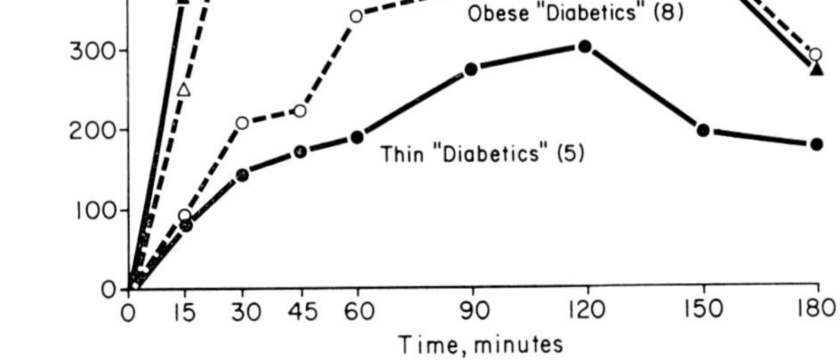

Fig. 4. A comparison of the percentage changes in serum immunoreactive insulin levels (IRI) in obese and thin nondiabetic and diabetic subjects during 3-hr oral (100 g) glucose tolerance tests.

nism' previously observed in both obese groups, is no longer present (Fig. 4). The responses of the two diabetic groups are strikingly similar: the absence of an early IRI peak and a marked delay in achieving the maximal relative increment above the basal level. These findings indicate that both thin and obese subjects with markedly different basal IRI must promptly increase circulating IRI at least 5–7 times in order to normally assimilate the ingested glucose load. Furthermore, the relative and not the absolute increment in IRI appears to be the critical determinant of glucose tolerance.

A variety of factors appear to influence the capacity of the pancreas to maintain this hypersecretory state in response to the stress of obesity (Porte and Bagdade, 1970). Most important among these is the presence of the gene for diabetes mellitus. Thus, similar to the state of peripheral insulin resistance introduced in the cortisone-glucose tolerance test, the presence of obesity also stresses the secretory reserve of the pancreatic β-cell and may unmask the latent diabetic patient and possibly explain the high frequency of glucose intolerance observed in the obese population (Ogilvie, 1935). That some degree of secretory decompensation may occur with time is also suggested by the association shown between the frequency of glucose intolerance and the duration of obesity (Fig. 5). The adult-onset diabetic patient who

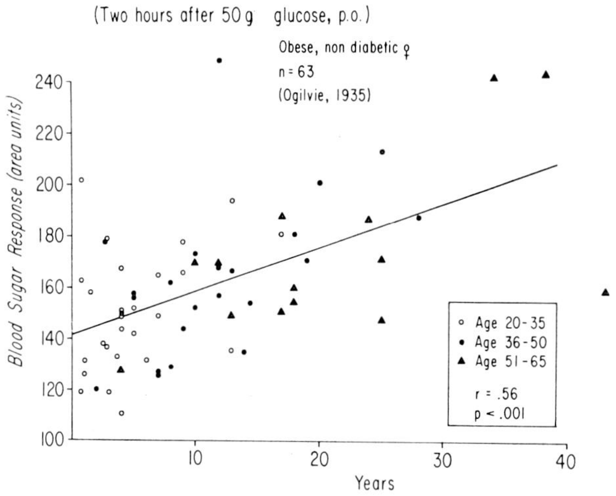

Fig. 5. Relationship between duration of obesity and frequency of glucose intolerance expressed as abnormal 2-hr postprandial glucose values.

develops symptomatic diabetes during a period of weight gain is encountered frequently. Following weight reduction and theoretically decreasing the stress of obesity on the secretory capacity of the genetically-deficient pancreatic β-cell of the diabetic patient, hyperglycemia and other clinical and chemical evidence of the diabetic syndrome may disappear.

Results of our recent studies which compare glucose tolerance, basal IRI, and insulin responses to oral glucose in massively obese diabetic and nondiabetic subjects before and after weight reduction emphasize the importance of weight control in the management of diabetic patients. Interesting differences in the IRI response to glucose were observed in the diabetic and nondiabetic subjects after weight reduction. While glucose tolerance improved significantly in the subjects shown in Figure 6, the nondiabetic achieved this improvement with a smaller IRI response than that evoked to the same glucose challenge prior to weight reduction. In contrast, the IRI response of the diabetic patient increased after weight reduction. These findings indicate that, even prior to weight loss, the nondiabetic subject fully

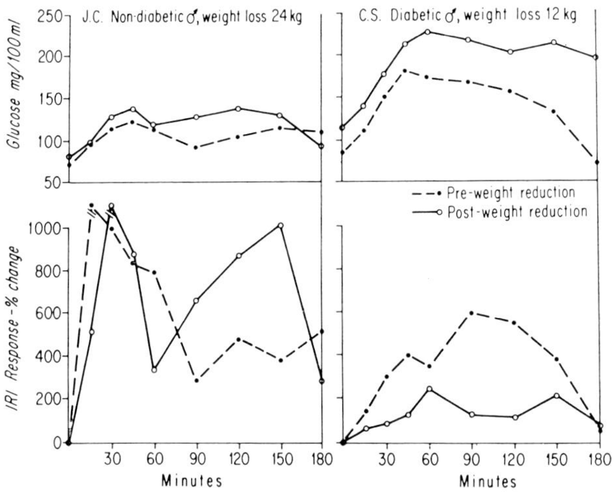

Fig. 6. Comparison of changes in glucose tolerance and the percentage changes in serum immunoreactive insulin levels (IRI) during 3-hr oral (100 g) glucose tolerance tests in obese diabetic and nondiabetic subjects before and after weight reduction.

compensates for the degree of insulin antagonism present in his adipose tissue stores by appropriately increasing both basal and stimulated IRI.

Prior to weight reduction, the diabetic patient on the other hand, while apparently able to normally elevate basal IRI, was unable to release sufficient insulin in response to the glucose stimulus to overcome the degree of peripheral insulin antagonism posed by his adipose mass. However, with the shrinkage of his adipose tissue mass and probable decrease in tissue insulin resistance that accompanied weight loss, the basal IRI level decreased, and he was able to achieve a sufficiently greater relative increase in IRI to improve glucose tolerance.

An abnormality in the regulation of lipolysis leading to increased basal FFA levels was formerly believed to characterize the diabetic (Bierman *et al.*, 1958) and obese states (Gordon, 1960; Dole, 1956). Recently reported studies from our laboratory (Bagdade *et al.*, 1969) indicate that in the nondiabetic obese subject and non-obese diabetic basal lipolysis, reflected by basal FFA and glycerol levels, is quite normal. These observations indicate that neither obesity nor mild diabetes alone is associated with an abnormality in the regulation of lipolysis. Only in the obese subjects who also demonstrated glucose intolerance were elevated basal FFA and glycerol levels observed; the degree of elevation was directly related to the severity of glucose intolerance. These observations do not support the earlier hypothesis (Randle *et al.*, 1963) that plasma FFA elevation plays an important role in the genesis of carbohydrate intolerance.

However, when a patient is both obese and diabetic, the regulation of fat mobilization becomes impaired. The fact that this abnormality becomes manifest in the obese diabetic despite the presence of increased and apparently normal basal IRI suggests that other as yet unidentified mechanisms contribute to the ineffective control of basal lipolysis.

The effects of obesity on diabetes may be summarized schematically (Fig. 7). With the adipocyte enlargement that is characteristic of the obese state, there is an associated decrease in sensitivity to insulin's metabolic actions. This acquired and apparently reversible state of insulin antagonism results in compensatory β-cell hypersecretion, and an increase in both basal and stimulated insulin levels. In the obese diabetic patient with a decrease in β-cell secretory reserve, an appropriate compensatory increase in IRI appears to be achieved in the secretion of only basal and not stimulated IRI. These alterations result in glucose intolerance.

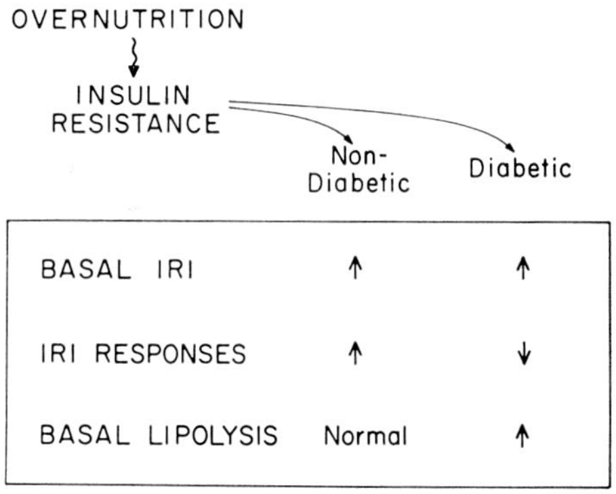

Fig. 7. Summary of a few of the metabolic effects of obesity on diabetes mellitus.

Although basal IRI levels are apparently normal in both the thin and obese diabetic subject, only in the obese diabetic is there any evidence of defective regulation of basal lipolysis, reflected by an elevation of basal FFA and glycerol levels.

REFERENCES

Bagdade, J. D., Bierman, E. L. and Porte, D., Jr. (1967): The significance of basal insulin levels in the evaluation of the insulin response to glucose in diabetic and nondiabetic subjects. *J. clin. Invest.*, *46*, 1549.

Bagdade, J. D., Bierman, E. L. and Porte, D., Jr.: Basal and stimulated insulin levels: A comparison of the insulinogenic effects of oral glucose and intravenous tolbutamide in nondiabetic and diabetic subjects (In preparation).

Bagdade, J. D., Porte, D., Jr. and Bierman, E. L. (1969): The interaction of diabetes and obesity on the regulation of fat mobilization in man. *Diabetes*, *18*, 759.

Bierman, E. L., Bagdade, J. D. and Porte, D., Jr. (1968): Obesity and diabetes: the odd couple. *Amer. J. clin. Nutr.*, *21*, 1434.

Bierman, E. L., Dole, V. P. and Roberts, T. N. (1958): An abnormality of non-esterified fatty acid metabolism in diabetes mellitus. *Diabetes*, *7*, 189.

Dole, V. P. (1956): A relation between non-esterified fatty acids in plasma and the metabolism of glucose. *J. clin. Invest.*, *35*, 150.

Gordon, E. S. (1960): Nonesterified fatty acids in blood of obese and lean subjects. *Amer. J. clin. Nutr.*, *8*, 740.

Ogilvie, R. F. (1933): The islands of Langerhans in 19 cases of obesity. *J. Path. Bact.*, *37*, 473.

Ogilvie, R. F. (1935): Sugar tolerance in obese subjects. A review of 65 cases. *Quart. J. Med.*, *4*, 435.

Porte, D., Jr. and Bagdade, J. D. (1970): Human insulin secretion: an integrated approach. *Ann. Rev. Med.*, *21*, 219.

Randle, P. J., Garland, P. B., Hales, C. N. and Newsholme, E. A. (1963): The glucose fatty-acid cycle: its role in insulin sensitivity and the metabolic disturbances of diabetes mellitus. *Lancet*, *1*, 785.

Salans, L. B., Knittle, J. L. and Hirsch, J. (1968): The role of adipose cell size and adipose tissue insulin sensitivity in the carbohydrate intolerance of human obesity. *J. clin. Invest.*, *47*, 153.

Simms, E. A. H., Holden, R. A., Horton, E. S., Gluck, C. M., Goldman, R. F., Kelleher, P. C. and Rowe, D. W. (1968): Experimental obesity in man. *Trans. Ass. Amer. Phycns.*, *81*, 153.

HYPERLIPEMIA AND DIABETES

EDWIN L. BIERMAN

Department of Medicine, University of Washington School of Medicine, and Veterans Administration Hospital, Seattle, Wash., U.S.A.

Hyperlipemia (hypertriglyceridemia) and diabetes mellitus are often associated. Recently a pathophysiological scheme was proposed to describe their possible interrelationships by the use of Venn diagrams (Bierman and Porte, 1968). All individuals who have hyperlipemia and/or glucose intolerance can be depicted as enclosed within a series of circles used to define these abnormalities (Fig. 1). The term endogenous lipemia describes a group of patients with hypertriglyceridemia after an overnight fast on normal diets, who increase their plasma triglyceride concentration (arbitrarily at least 40–50 %) on high carbohydrate, fat-free diets. On *ad libitum* diets their hypertriglyceridemia results from the accumulation of large, turbidity-producing, very low-density (α-2 or pre-β) lipoproteins, originating predominantly in the liver; dietary fat particles ('chylomicrons', 'primary particles') are not demonstrable.

Such patients with endogenous lipemia often have glucose intolerance (described by the area of overlap of the circles); however some do not (Glueck *et al.*, 1969). On the other hand, the majority of patients with clinically apparent glucose intolerance ('diabetes mellitus') do not have hypertriglyceridemia, the incidence apparently not exceeding 30 % (Albrink *et al.*, 1963; Sterky *et al.*, 1963; New *et al.*, 1963; Bierman and Porte, 1968). A quantitative relationship between the degree of glucose intolerance and the magnitude of hypertriglyceridemia has been difficult to establish since little or no significant correlation between them has been observed (Reaven *et al.*, 1963; Carlson and Wahlberg, 1966; Albrink and Davidson, 1966; Reaven *et al.*, 1967; Belknap *et al.*, 1967; Glueck *et al.*, 1969).

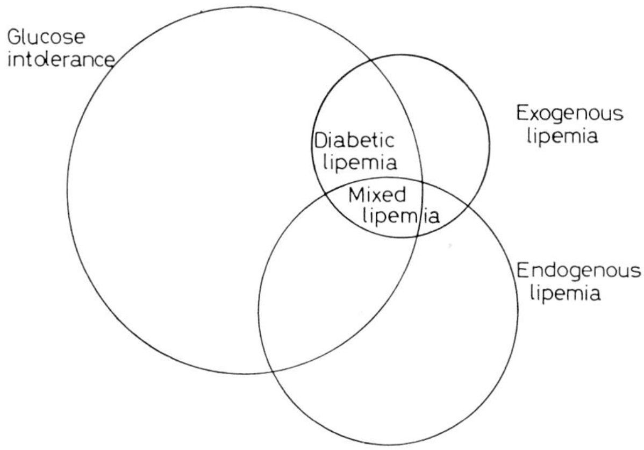

Fig. 1. Hypertriglyceridemia.

The increase of plasma triglyceride in response to substitution of a high carbohydrate diet for a normal diet is not a unique feature of patients with endogenous lipemia, since both normal and diabetic subjects, as well as those with endogenous lipemia, appear to approximately double plasma triglyceride levels as a result of this isocaloric dietary manipulation (Bierman and Hamlin, 1961; Belknap *et al.*, 1967; Porte and Bierman, 1968; Glueck *et al.*, 1969) (Fig. 2). Clearly, however, the actual triglyceride levels reached will be considerably

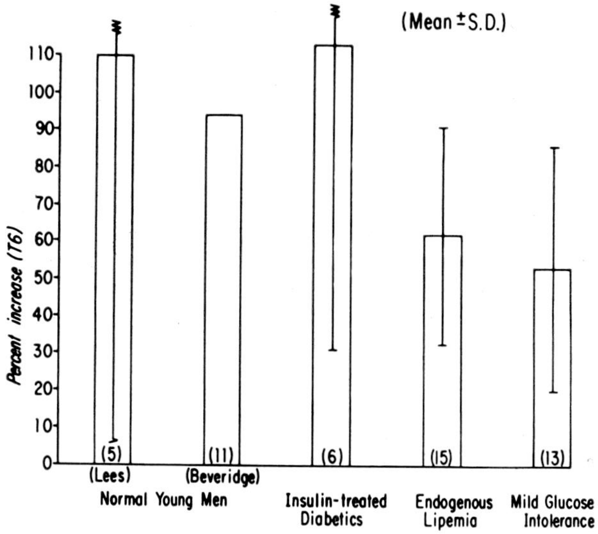

Fig. 2. Overlapping areas of lipemia and glucose intolerance.

exaggerated in patients with endogenous lipemia since the magnitude of the increment on a high-carbohydrate diet appears to be directly related to the basal plasma triglyceride level on a normal or a high-fat diet (Bierman and Porte, 1968; Bierman *et al.*, 1965; Farquhar *et al.*, 1966; Glueck *et al.*, 1969).

Thus the abnormality in this type of lipemia appears to be related to the regulation of triglyceride levels on any diet. Abnormally high triglyceride influx rates into the circulation often can be demonstrated by kinetic studies (Reaven *et al.*, 1967; Porte and Bierman, 1969; Nikkila, 1969). Although both carbohydrate and free fatty acids are the major precursors for endogenous triglyceride production, there is no evidence that fatty acid flux is accelerated in this disorder; plasma free fatty acid levels are usually within the normal range (Fredrickson and Lees, 1966; Nikkila, 1969). The precise nature of the regulatory defect, however, remains unknown.

All patients with endogenous lipemia will show an increased pre-beta lipoprotein band by paper electrophoresis (Lees and Fredrickson, 1965), with no chylomicron or lipid-staining material at the origin. This lipoprotein pattern (Type IV) (Fredrickson *et al.*, 1968) is frequently associated with endogenous lipemia; however, not all subjects with this pattern have endogenous lipemia as defined by (1) at least a 40% increase in triglyceride on a high carbohydrate, low fat diet, and (2) absence of chylomicrons in plasma obtained after an overnight fast (presumably an index of removal efficiency) by the more sensitive PVP flocculation method (Bierman *et al.*, 1962; Bierman *et al.*, 1965; O'Hara *et al.*, 1966).

The other major pathophysiologic type of lipemia is exogenous lipemia. This term describes a group of patients that are characterized by a primary difficulty in the metabolism and removal of triglyceride-rich lipoproteins from the circulation. As a result, their plasma triglyceride levels are increased by dietary fat ingestion and thus dietary fat particles (chylomicrons) predominate in the circulation after an overnight fast. Triglyceride levels are decreased (arbitrarily at least 50%) when a high carbohydrate, fat-free diet is substituted for a normal diet. Postheparin plasma lipolytic activity (PHLA) is usually low. This activity presumably reflects tissue lipoprotein lipase, a group of closely associated enzymatic activities apparently directly related to the assimilation of triglyceride-rich lipoproteins (Bierman *et al.*, 1970). Regardless of activity, impaired triglyceride clearance can be demonstrated by turnover measurements (Porte and Bierman, 1969).

The circle that represents exogenous lipemia overlaps the other two. Some of these patients have severe diabetes and the subset 'diabetic lipemia' (Fig. 1) is represented in the area of overlap between exogenous lipemia and glucose intolerance. Since the exogenous lipemia observed in these chronically insulin-deficient diabetic patients is reversed entirely by insulin therapy, severe diabetes associated with insulin deficiency appears to cause this form of lipemia (Bagdade *et al.*, 1967*a*). The diabetic lipemia syndrome also has been observed as a complication of acute pancreatitis (Bagdade, 1969) and during prolonged treatment with high doses of corticosteroids (Bagdade *et al.*, 1970). Brief withdrawal of insulin from juvenile diabetics can reproduce the reduction in PHLA and lead to reciprocal increases in triglyceride levels (Bagdade *et al.*, 1968*a*). Diabetic lipemia is usually not associated with ketoacidosis, however profound ketoacidosis may supervene as an independent event (Bierman *et al.*, 1966). Even when ketoacidosis occurs, fatty acid mobilization does not appear to make a major contribution to the lipemia, since treatment of one such patient with nicotinic acid in sufficient quantity to lower free fatty acid levels by 70% and transiently reverse ketoacidosis (Porte, 1969) did not appear to influence plasma triglyceride levels (Bagdade *et al.*, 1967*a*). Consonant with this clinical observation, no increase in hepatic triglyceride output could be demonstrated in chronically diabetic dogs (Basso and Havel, 1970) or rats (Heimberg *et al.*, 1967). In contrast, a contribution of free fatty acids to plasma triglycerides has been suggested for the acute diabetic state, produced experimentally by anti-insulin serum, in which presumably the liver remains transiently insulinized and a reduction of plasma triglycerides by nicotinic acid can be demonstrated (Gross and Carlson, 1968).

Exogenous lipemia may occur secondary to other disorders which are associated with an acquired reduction in PHLA, *e.g.* hypothyroidism (Porte *et al.*, 1966), dysgammaglobulinemia (Glueck *et al.*, 1969), or in a primary familial form associated with a congenital decrease in adipose tissue lipoprotein lipase (Harlan *et al.*, 1967). These individuals demonstrate exogenous lipemia without glucose intolerance and would be represented in the circle outside of the area of overlap.

This convenient and graphic representation of the entire spectrum of glucose intolerance and hypertriglyceridemia may be helpful to our understanding. For example, there appears to be a large group of individuals who have features of both exogenous and endogenous lipemia and are represented in the overlapping zone ('mixed lipemia'). The accumulation of both chylomicrons and pre-β lipoproteins in plasma is usually evident on paper electrophoresis as a Type V lipoprotein pattern. However, fasting chylomicronemia is extremely variable and may be inconstant (Havel, 1970). Plasma TG levels show no consistent change in response to substitution of dietary carbohydrate for fat, since dietary chylomicrons may be cleared from plasma concomitant with increased endogenous production of pre-β lipoproteins. Many patients with mixed lipemia appear to have glucose intolerance and may have clinical diabetes (Fredrickson *et al.*, 1968; Glueck *et al.*, 1969). In a few of these patients, diabetic treatment may reverse the exogenous component, unmasking endogenous lipemia. However, many patients with mixed lipemia cannot yet be defined as distinctive clinical entities (Havel, 1970).

Thus, although hyperlipemia and diabetes overlap in several clinical syndromes, only in the case of diabetic lipemia has any causal relation between the two been shown. Rather, the association between mild glucose intolerance and endogenous lipemia appears to be mediated by a common close association with environmental factors of which obesity appears to be the most important (Bierman and Porte, 1968). In addition to the well-recognized concurrence between glucose intolerance and obesity (Bierman *et al.*, 1968), correlations between plasma triglyceride levels and adiposity are manifold; they have been observed in both sexes, at all ages, in a variety of subject groups using several different indices of adiposity, such as relative weight, ponderal index, skin-fold thickness, weight gain in adult life, and actual measurements of per cent body fat (Albrink and Meigs, 1964; Feldman *et al.*, 1963; Hollister *et al.*, 1967; Evans and Ostrander, 1967; Grace and Goldrick, 1968; Ford *et al.*, 1968; Rifkind *et al.*, 1968). This relationship between adiposity and plasma triglyceride may be mediated in part by the resistance to the peripheral action of insulin imposed by adiposity with resultant compensatory hyperinsulinism (Bagdade *et al.*, 1967*b*). Hyperinsulinism appears to be the normal response to insulin antagonism due to a variety of causes such as estrogens (Hazzard *et al.*, 1969), uremia (Bagdade *et al.*, 1968*b*), liver disease (Megyesi *et al.*, 1967), and growth hormone (Beck *et al.*, 1965); (Fig. 3) (Porte and Bagdade,

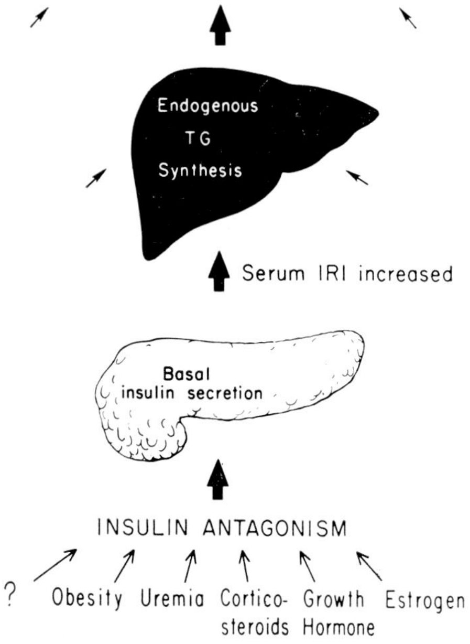

Fig. 3. Mean plasma triglyceride response to substitution of a high-carbohydrate (fat-free) diet for a normal diet.

1970). Elevated serum immunoreactive insulin levels (IRI), both in the basal state and after challenge with glucose, have been found to be closely related to triglyceride levels in normal subjects and subjects with endogenous lipemia studied under controlled dietary conditions (Table I). The reason for this relationship is not clear; however, it is possible that insulin may be one of several factors (Nikkila, 1969) promoting hepatic triglyceride synthesis and thus aggravating the accumulation of endogenous triglyceride-rich lipoproteins in plasma of subjects with endogenous lipemia. In concordance with this hypothesis, obese subjects (with or without endogenous lipemia) during caloric maintenance after a period of weight reduction have been shown to markedly decrease both triglyceride levels and insulin levels (Bierman and Porte, 1968; Levy and Glueck, 1969; Bagdade *et al.*, 1968).

The role of excessive fatty acid mobilization in the association between glucose intolerance and endogenous lipemia is unknown. Increased plasma free fatty acid levels do not appear

TABLE I

Correlation between serum insulin and triglyceride levels

Subjects	n	Correlation coefficient		Reference
		Basal IRI	IRI levels, oral glucose	
Mixed	18		.53	Sailer, Bolzano, Sandhofer, *et al.*, 1968
,,	20		.68	Ford, Bozian and Knowles, 1968
Non-lipemic	37	.44		Bagdade, 1968
,,	196		.30	Abrams, Jarrett, Keen, *et al.*, 1969
Endogenous lipemia	16	.42		Bierman, Porte and Bagdade, unpubl.
,,	15		.47	Farquhar, Frank, Gross *et al.*, 1966
,,	33		.51	Reaven, Lerner, Stern *et al.*, 1967
,,	20		.38	Glueck, Levy and Fredrickson, 1969

to be a characteristic feature of either; however, higher free fatty acid levels, which could theoretically provide additional substrate for hepatic triglyceride formation, become apparent when obesity and glucose intolerance coexist (Bagdade *et al.*, 1969). On the other hand, the accelerated fatty acid mobilization commonly associated with severe diabetes (Bierman *et al.*, 1957) when sympathetic stimulation is superimposed (Porte, 1969), does not appear to increase hepatic triglyceride release, but rather preferentially contributes to ketoacidosis (Basso and Havel, 1970).

Hopefully, this pathophysiologic differentiation of lipemic disorders will enhance our understanding of their interrelationships with glucose intolerance. It appears that there are groups of etiologically distinct disorders which may overlap with glucose intolerance for a variety of reasons; a direct causal relationship need not be inferred. For example, the association between mild glucose intolerance and endogenous lipemia may be mediated through a common association with the aggravating factor, adiposity, and its consequence, hyperinsulinism.

REFERENCES

ABRAMS, M. E., JARRETT, R. J., KEEN, H., BOYNS, D. R. and CROSSLEY, J. N. (1969): Oral glucose tolerance and related factors in a normal population sample. *Brit. med. J.*, *1*, 599.

ALBRINK, M. J. and DAVIDSON, P. C. (1966): Impaired glucose tolerance in patients with hypertriglyceridemia. *J. Lab. clin. Med.*, *67*, 573.

ALBRINK, M. J., LAVIETES, P. H. and MAN, E. B. (1963): Vascular disease and serum lipids in diabetes mellitus. *Ann. intern. Med.*, *58*, 305.

ALBRINK, M. J. and MEIGS, J. (1964): Interrelationship between skinfold thickness, serum lipids and blood sugar in normal men. *Amer. J. clin. Nutr.*, *15*, 255.

BAGDADE, J. D. (1969): Diabetic lipemia complicating acute pancreatitis. *Lancet*, *2*, 1041.

BAGDADE, J. D., BIERMAN, E. L. and PORTE, D., JR. (1967*a*): Diabetic lipemia: a form of acquired fat-induced lipemia. *New Engl. J. Med.*, *276*, 427.

BAGDADE, J. D., BIERMAN, E. L. and PORTE, D., JR. (1967*b*): Significance of basal insulin levels in the evaluation of the insulin response to glucose in diabetic and nondiabetic subjects. *J. clin. Invest.*, *46*, 1549.

BAGDADE, J. D., BIERMAN, E. L. and PORTE, D., JR. (1968): Hyperinsulinism - a metabolic consequence of obesity. *Diabetes*, *17*, *Suppl. 1*, 315.

BAGDADE, J. D., PORTE, D., JR. and BIERMAN, E. L. (1968*a*): Acute insulin withdrawal and the regulation of plasma triglyceride removal in diabetic subjects. *Diabetes, 17*, 127.

BAGDADE, J. D., PORTE, D., JR. and BIERMAN, E. L. (1968*b*): Hypertriglyceridemia: a metabolic consequence of chronic renal failure. *New Engl. J. Med., 279*, 181.

BAGDADE,J. D., PORTE, D., JR. and BIERMAN, E. L. (1969): The interaction of diabetes and obesity on the regulation of fat mobilization in man. *Diabetes, 18*, 759.

BAGDADE, J. D., PORTE, D., JR. and BIERMAN, E. L. (1970): Steroid-induced lipemia. *Arch. intern. Med., 125*, 129.

BASSO, L. V. and HAVEL, R. J. (1970): Hepatic metabolism of free fatty acids in normal and diabetic dogs. *J. clin. Invest., 49*, 537.

BECK, P., SCHALCH, D. S., PARKER, M. L., KIPNIS, D. M. and DAUGHADAY, W. H. (1965): Correlative studies of growth hormone and insulin plasma concentrations with metabolic abnormalities in acromegaly. *J. Lab. clin. Med., 66*, 366.

BELKNAP, B. H., AMARAL, J. A. P. and BIERMAN, E. L. (1967): Plasma lipids in mild glucose intolerance. I. The response of plasma triglycerides to high carbohydrate feeding and the effect of tolbutamide therapy. In: *Tolbutamide After Ten Years*. ICS No. 149 Excerpta Medica, Amsterdam.

BELKNAP, B. H., BAGDADE, J. D., AMARAL, J. A. P. and BIERMAN, E. L. (1967): Plasma lipids in mild glucose intolerance. II. A double blind study of the effect of tolbutamide and placebo in mild diabetic outpatients. In: *Tolbutamide After Ten Years* ICS No. 149. Excerpta Medica, Amsterdam.

BIERMAN, E. L., BAGDADE, J. D. and PORTE, D., JR. (1966): A concept of the pathogenesis of diabetic lipemia. *Trans. Ass. Amer. Phycns, 79*, 348.

BIERMAN, E. L., BAGDADE, J. D. and PORTE, D., JR. (1968): Obesity and diabetes: the odd couple. *Amer. J. clin. Nutr., 21*, 1434.

BIERMAN, E. L., DOLE, V. P. and ROBERTS, T. N. (1957): An abnormality of non-esterified fatty acid metabolism in diabetes mellitus. *Diabetes, 6*, 475.

BIERMAN, E. L., GORDIS, E. and HAMLIN, J. T. III (1962): Heterogeneity of fat particles in plasma during alimentary lipemia. *J. clin. Invest., 41*, 2254.

BIERMAN, E. L. and HAMLIN, J. T. III (1961): The hyperlipemic effect of a low-fat high-carbohydrate diet in diabetic subjects. *Diabetes, 10*, 432.

BIERMAN, E. L. and PORTE, D., JR. (1968): Carbohydrate intolerance and lipemia. *Ann. intern. Med., 68*, 926.

BIERMAN, E. L., PORTE, D., JR., BAGDADE, J. D. and HAZZARD, W. R. (1970): Lipoprotein lipase and plasma triglyceride. In: *Proceedings of the Second International Symposium on Atherosclerosis.* Editor: R. Jones. Springer, Heidelberg.

BIERMAN, E. L., PORTE, D., JR., O'HARA, D. D., SCHWARTZ, M. L. and WOOD, F. C., JR. (1965): Characterization of fat particles in plasma of hyperlipemic subjects maintained on fat-free high-carbohydrate diets. *J. clin. Invest., 44*, 261.

CARLSON, L. A. and WAHLBERG, F. (1966): Serum lipids, intravenous glucose tolerance and their interrelation studied in ischemic cardiovascular disease. *Acta med. scand., 180*, 307.

EVANS, J. G. and OSTRANDER, L. D. (1967): Fasting serum-triglycerides concentration and distribution of subcutaneous fat. *Lancet, 1*, 761.

FARQUHAR, J. W., FRANK, A., GROSS, R. C. and REAVEN, G. M. (1966): Glucose, insulin, and triglyceride responses to high and low carbohydrate diets in man. *J. clin. Invest., 45*, 1648.

FELDMAN, E. B., BENKEL, P. and NAYAK, R. V. (1963): Physiologic factors influencing circulating triglyceride concentration in women: age, weight gain, and ovarian function. *J. Lab. clin. Med., 62*, 437.

FORD, S., BOZIAN, R. C. and KNOWLES, H. C. (1968): Interactions of obesity, and glucose and insulin levels in hypertriglyceridemia. *Amer. J. clin. Nutr., 21*, 904.

FREDRICKSON, D. S. and LEES, R. S. (1966): Familial hyperlipoproteinemia. In: *The Metabolic Basis of Inherited Disease*. Editors: J. B. Stanbury, J. B. Wyngaarden and D. S. Fredrickson. McGraw-Hill, New York.

FREDRICKSON, D. S., LEVY, R. I. and LEES, R. S. (1967): Fat transport in lipoproteins – an integrated approach to mechanisms and disorders. *New Engl. J. Med., 276*, 34.

GLUECK, C. J., KAPLAN, A. P., LEVY, R. I., GRETEN, H., GRALNICK, H. and FREDRICKSON, D. S. (1969*a*): A new mechanism of exogenous hyperglyceridemia. *Ann. intern. Med., 71*, 1051.

GLUECK, C. J., LEVY, R. I. and FREDRICKSON, D. S. (1969*b*): Immunoreactive insulin, glucose tolerance, and carbohydrate inducibility in Types II, III, IV, and V hyperlipoproteinemia. *Diabetes, 18*, 739.

Grace, C. S. and Goldrick, R. B. (1968): Fibrinolysis and body build. *J. atheroscler. Res.*, *8*, 705.
Gross, R. C. and Carlson, L. A. (1968): Metabolic effects of nicotinic acid in acute deficiency in the rat. *Diabetes*, *17*, 353.
Harlan, W. R., Winesett, P. S. and Wasserman, A. J. (1967): Tissue lipoprotein lipase in normal individuals and in individuals with exogenous hypertriglyceridemia and the relationship of this enzyme to assimilation of fat. *J. clin. Invest.*, *46*, 239.
Havel, R. J. (1969): Pathogenesis, differentiation and management of hypertriglyceridemia. In: *Advances in Internal Medicine*, Vol. 15, p. 117. Editor: G. H. Stollerman. Yearbook Medical Publishers, Chicago.
Hazzard, W. R., Spiger, M. J., Bagdade, J. D. and Bierman, E. L. (1969): Studies on the mechanism of increased plasma triglyceride levels induced by oral contraceptives. *New Engl. J. Med.*, *280*, 471.
Heimberg, M., Van Harken, D. R. and Brown, T. O. (1967): Hepatic lipid metabolism in experimental diabetes. II. Incorporation of (1-C-14) palmitate into lipids of the liver and of the d $<$ 1.020 perfusate lipoproteins. *Biochim. biophys. Acta (Amst.)*, *137*, 435.
Hollister, L. E., Overall, J. E. and Snow, H. L. (1967): Relationship of obesity to serum triglyceride, cholesterol, and uric acid, and to plasma-glucose levels. *Amer. J. clin. Nutr.*, *20*, 777.
Lees, R. S. and Fredrickson, D. S. (1965): Differentiation of exogenous and endogenous hyperlipemia by paper electrophoresis. *J. clin. Invest.*, *44*, 1968.
Levy, R. I. and Glueck, C. J. (1969): Hypertriglyceridemia, diabetes mellitus, and coronary vessel disease. *Arch. intern. Med.*, *123*, 220.
Megyesi, C., Samols, E. and Marks, V. (1967): Glucose tolerance and diabetes in chronic liver disease. *Lancet*, *1*, 1051.
New, M. I., Roberts, T. N., Bierman, E. L. and Reader, G. G. (1963): The significance of blood lipid alterations in diabetes mellitus. *Diabetes*, *12*, 208.
Nikkila, E. A. (1969): Control of plasma and liver triglyceride kinetics by carbohydrate metabolism and insulin. In: *Advances in Lipid Research*, Vol. 7, p. 63. Academic Press, New York.
O'Hara, D. D., Porte, D. Jr. and Williams, R. H. (1966): The use of constant composition polyvinylpyrrolidone (PVP) columns to study the interaction of fat particles with plasma. *J. Lipid Res.*, *7*, 264.
Porte, D. Jr. (1969): Sympathetic regulation of insulin secretion. *Arch. intern. Med.*, *123*, 252.
Porte, D. Jr. and Bagdade, J. D. (1970): Human insulin secretion: an integrated approach. *Ann. Rev. Med.*, *21*, 105.
Porte, D. Jr. and Bierman, E. L. (1969): The effect of heparin infusion on plasma triglyceride *in vivo* and *in vitro* with a method for calculating triglyceride turnover. *J. Lab. clin. Med.*, *73*, 631.
Porte, D. Jr., O'Hara D. D. and Williams, R. H. (1966): The relation between post-heparin lipolytic activity and plasma triglyceride and myxedema. *Metabolism*, *15*, 107.
Reaven, G., Calciano, A., Cody, R., Lucas, C. and Miller, R. (1963): Carbohydrate intolerance and hyperlipemia in patients with myocardial infarction without known diabetes mellitus. *J. clin. Endocr.*, *23*, 1013.
Reaven, G. M., Lerner, R. L., Stern, M. P. and Farquhar, J. W. (1967): Role of insulin in endogenous hypertriglyceridemia. *J. clin. Invest.*, *46*, 1756.
Rifkind, B. M., Gale, M. and Lawson, D. (1968): Serum cholesterol and triglyceride levels and adiposity. *Cardiovasc. Res.*, *2*, 143.
Sailer, S., Bolzano, K., Sandhofer, F., Spath, P. and Braunsteiner, H. (1968): Triglyceridespiegel und Insulinkonzentration im Plasma nach oraler Glukosegabe bei Patienten mit primärer kohlenhydratinduzierter Hypertriglyceridämie. *Schweiz. med. Wschr.*, *98*, 1512.
Sterky, G., Larsson, Y. and Persson, B. (1963): Blood lipids in diabetic and non-diabetic schoolchildren. *Acta paediat. (Uppsala)*, *52*, 11.

ASPECTS OF LIPID METABOLISM IN RELATION TO THE PATHOGENESIS OF DIABETES MELLITUS

EDUARDO COLL-GARCÍA and VIRGILIO BOSCH

Cátedra de Patología General y Fisiopatología, Instituto de Medicina Experimental, Facultad de Medicina, Universidad Central de Venezuela, Caracas, Venezuela

When plasma lipid determinations became available about 70 years ago, it was demonstrated that the well-known grayish color of blood and the milky aspect of serum in diabetics was in fact due to hyperlipemia. It is now known that diabetes and hyperlipemia are associated very frequently, suggesting some pathogenic relationship between them. It has been clearly established that, as a consequence of absolute or relative insulin deficiency, there is a series of metabolic changes depending on the reduction of glucose oxidation by the diabetic cell, changes which can be corrected by insulin administration. Among them are the block of triglyceride synthesis, increased mobilization and oxidation of fatty acids, the development of ketosis, and an increase in cholesterol synthesis (Siperstein, 1960).

On the other hand, as a consequence of their studies on the so-called 'glucose fatty acid cycle', Randle *et al.* (1964) have considered that the crucial question in relation to human diabetes is whether or not an enhanced rate of release of fatty acids from glycerides is responsible for insulin insensitivity and, if so whether or not the latter is responsible for impaired glucose tolerance and loss of beta cell function. Although the 'glucose fatty acid cycle' has been questioned by some investigators (Pelkonen *et al.*, 1968), there is considerable evidence from *in vitro* studies (Bowman, 1962; Garland *et al.*, 1962) to support this hypothesis. Furthermore, Schalch and Kipnis (1965) have shown in humans that the circulating level of non-esterified fatty acids may be an important factor in regulating the glucose tolerance and insulin responsiveness of the intact organism.

A third possibility concerning the coexistence of diabetes and hyperlipemia, has been proposed by Bierman and Porte (1968), who consider that it is not necessary to make the assumption of a causal relation between these two conditions, since other kinds of interactions are possible. They suggest that diabetes may not cause endogenous lipoproteinemia, nor lipemia cause carbohydrate intolerance, but that they appear to be two etiologically distinct disorders that may become associated as a result of the common aggravating factor, obesity.

For all these considerations it is of interest to study glucose tolerance and insulin secretion in apparently healthy persons with normal values of fasting blood glucose but high plasma triglyceride levels. The subjects included in this report were all asymptomatic, with no clinical evidence of ischemic heart disease or other forms of atherosclerosis, and with triglyceride levels above 160 mg/100 ml plasma. For each case studied, a control was selected of the same sex and approximately the same age and weight.

All subjects were on diets containing more than 200 g of carbohydrate during the days before testing. A blood sample was taken from an antecubital vein after an overnight fast for determining triglycerides (Van Handel and Zilversmit, 1957), phospholipids (Svanborg and Svennerholm, 1961) and cholesterol (Abel *et al.*, 1952) in heparinized plasma. Blood glucose was measured by Somogyi-Nelson's method (Nelson, 1944) and plasma lipoproteins were studied by means of paper electrophoresis (Lees and Fredrickson, 1965). Plasma non-esterified fatty acids (NEFA) were determined by Dole's procedure (Dole, 1956) and plasma insulin by radioimmunoassay according to Hales and Randle (1963). After the initial blood sample was taken, glucose tolerance was studied by a standard 100 g oral test, drawing subsequent blood samples at 30, 60 and 120 minutes after the ingestion of glucose. The height and weight was recorded in each case in order to determine the presence and degree of obesity by calculating the ponderal index (Steinkamp *et al.*, 1965) and by comparison with normal weight tables from an insurance company.

Eighteen hyperglyceridemic subjects were studied following the procedure outlined above. Five were female and 13 male, aged between 18 and 56 years, average age 37.0 years. The average age for the control group was 36.8 years. The ponderal index was 12.2 ± 0.11 in the hyperglyceridemic group and 12.5 ± 0.08 in the controls; the difference is not statistically significant and there were no persons with more than 25% excess weight in either of the two groups.

The results of plasma lipid determinations are shown in Table I. It can be observed in this table that the average concentration of plasma triglycerides is greater than that of cholesterol, which is characteristic of type IV hyperlipemia in Fredrickson's classification (Fredrickson, 1967), a type defined by an increase of pre-β lipoproteins on paper electrophoresis of plasma. Analysing the individual cases by this method, it was found that 13 subjects belonged to this type, one was of type III and the others of type II.

TABLE I

Plasma lipids in control and hyperglyceridemic subjects

	Triglycerides (mg/100 ml)	Phospholipids (mg/100 ml)	Cholesterol (mg/100 ml)	NEFA (μEq/l)
Controls (18)	79 ± 8	224 ± 13	214 ± 15	334 ± 94*
Hypertriglyceridemic (18)	392 ± 65**	360 ± 28**	296 ± 29	639 ± 86**

* Mean ± S.E.M.
** Difference between means is significant, with $P < 0.01$.
In parenthesis, number of subjects in each group.

All glucose tolerance curves were normal in the control group, according to the criteria of Fajans and Conn (Fajans, 1960). On the contrary, in the hyperlipemic subjects, although the fasting values were normal in all cases, the average curve for the group shows higher values at all the other points, as can be seen in Figure 1.

Insulin secretion during the glucose tolerance test was higher in the hypertriglyceridemic subjects, as shown in Figure 2. According to Welborn *et al.* (1966), this secretion can be expressed as a '2-hour insulin area', which is the surface under the insulin curve plotted against time and indicates the mean insulin level during the two hours observed. The area obtained for the hyperlipemic group (381 ± 43 μUnit-hours) was clearly greater than that observed in the controls (230 ± 25 μUnit-hours; $P < 0.02$).

None of the cases included in the group of hyperglyceridemic subjects was markedly obese, all of them being below 25% excess weight. In order to assess the relationship in them between obesity and insulin secretion, they were divided into two groups according to their ponderal index and percentage of excess weight. The first group comprised the non-obese subjects, with a ponderal index of 12.3 or more and between 85 and 115% of ideal body weight; the second group included moderately obese people, between 15 and

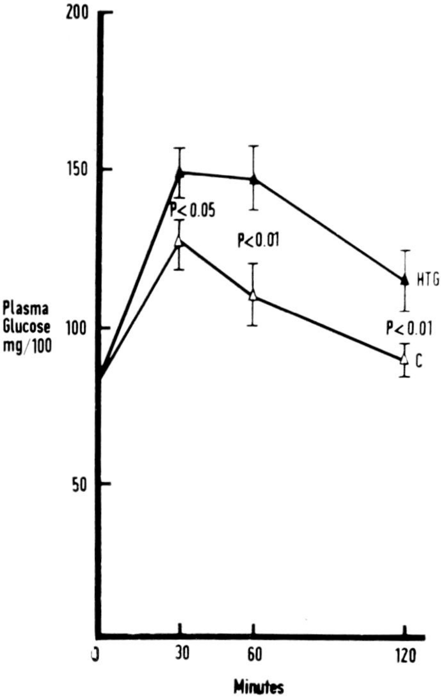

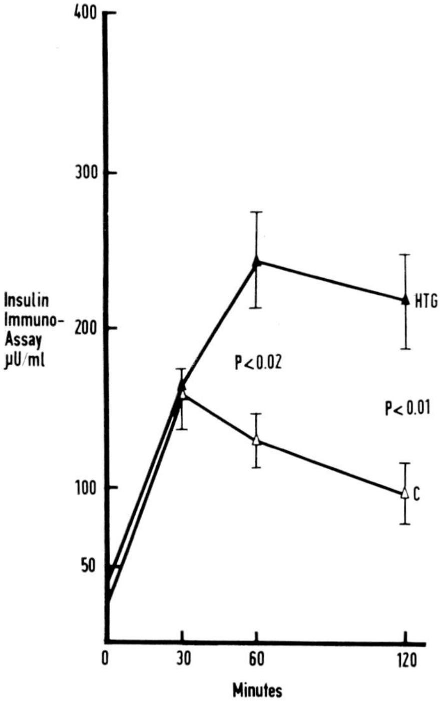

Fig. 1. Mean blood glucose values in hypertriglyceridemic subjects (HTG) and controls (C) after oral administration of glucose (100 g). Horizontal bars represent S.E.M.

Fig. 2. Mean plasma insulin curves in hypertriglyceridemic subjects (HTG) and controls (C) after oral administration of glucose (100 g). Horizontal bars represent S.E.M.

25% overweight. Although the second group shows a greater insulin secretion, the difference is not very marked, as depicted in Figure 3, and in both groups there is a clear hypersecretion of insulin when compared with the controls. The insulin area obtained for the non-obese group (350 $\pm$ 59 μUnit-hours) was not statistically different from that of the overweight cases (441 $\pm$ 66 μUnit-hours; $P < 0.4$).

Another study related to this problem has been carried out in pregnant rats. In these animals a marked hyperlipemia accompanied by an increase in the plasma non-esterified fatty acids (NEFA) towards the end of gestation has been reported by MacKay and Kaunitz (1963). This hyperlipemia was primarily due to an increase in the very low density of pre-β lipoproteins, similar to the findings in many of the patients reported above. It has been recently shown by Bosch *et al.* (1971) that the factors contributing to the hyperlipemia of the pregnant rat are diminished ability to clear administered chylomicron preparations and decreased post-heparin plasma lipoprotein lipase (LPL) activity on the one hand, and an increase in the rate of lipolysis of adipose tissue with a resultant elevation of plasma NEFA on the other. Since triglycerides are formed in the liver from fatty acids mobilized from the fat depots (Havel, 1961), an increased rate of mobilization of fatty acids should result in increased synthesis of very low-density lipoproteins, which appear in higher than normal concentrations in plasma.

Adult Sprague-Dawley rats weighing 250–300 g before the beginning of pregnancy were used. The animals were kept in individual cages and fed *ad libitum* on a locally made rat chow. They were allowed to mate for a period of 24 hours, after which the males were

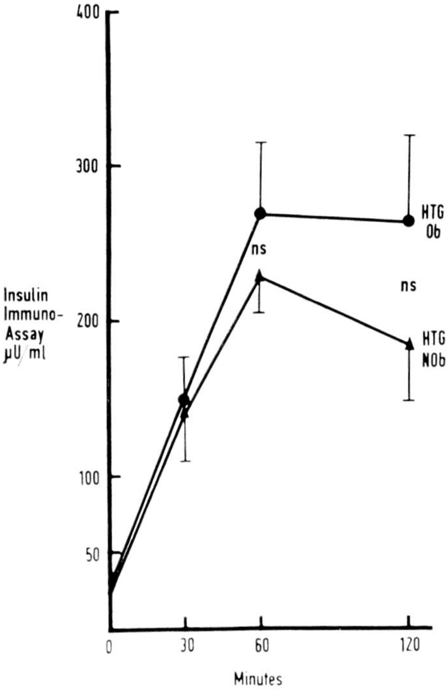

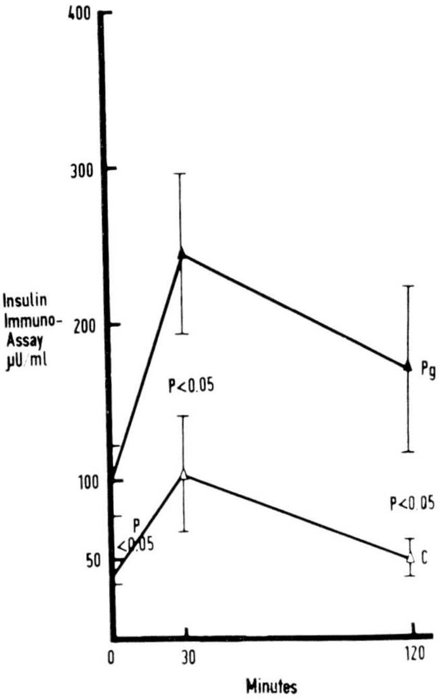

Fig. 3. Mean plasma insulin curves in moderately obese (HTG Ob) and non-obese (HTG NOb) hyperglyceridemic subjects after oral administration of glucose (100 g). Horizontal bars represent S.E.M.

Fig. 4. Mean plasma insulin curves in pregnant rats (Pg) and controls (C) after oral administration of glucose (250 mg/100 g body weight). Horizontal bars represent S.E.M.

removed from the cages. Twelve rats during the 3rd week of pregnancy and 10 controls matched by age and weight were fasted for 18–20 hours. Each rat was then given 250 mg glucose dissolved in 1 ml of water per 100 g body weight by gavage. Blood samples were obtained from the tail at 0, 30 and 120 minutes after the glucose load. Plasma was separated by centrifugation and glucose was measured by a micromethod using glucose-oxidase (Clinton Laboratories, Los Angeles, Calif.) and 0.02 ml of plasma; insulin was determined by radioimmunoassay using Milner's modification (1969) of the double antibody procedure of Hales and Randle (1963). At the end of the 2-hour tolerance test, the rats were anesthetized with ether and blood was taken by cardiac puncture in order to obtain heparinized plasma for determining triglycerides (Van Handel and Zilversmit, 1957), phospholipids (Svanborg and Svennerholm, 1961) and cholesterol (Abel *et al.*, 1952). Plasma NEFA were also determined by Dole's method and plasma lipoproteins were studied by means of paper electrophoresis (Lees and Fredrickson, 1965).

Table II summarizes the results of plasma lipid determinations in both groups studied. Paper electrophoresis showed an increase in pre-β lipoproteins.

Blood glucose values were very similar in pregnant and non-pregnant rats. Insulin measurements showed higher basal values in the pregnant animals and insulin secretion was markedly elevated during the glucose tolerance test, as can be seen in Figure 4.

The associations between the blood sugar and plasma insulin responses to oral glucose and the level of fasting plasma triglycerides can be interpreted in several ways. Bierman and Porte (1968) consider that if obesity reflects a state of relative insulin resistance only

TABLE II

Plasma lipids in control and pregnant rats

	Triglycerides (mg/100 ml)	Phospholipids (mg/100 ml)	Cholesterol (mg/100 ml)	NEFA (μEq/l)
Controls (10)	43 ± 8	109 ± 15	45 ± 6	245 ± 16*
Pregnant (12)	195 ± 32**	99 ± 9	57 ± 6	688 ± 12**

* Mean ± S.E.M.
** Difference between means is significant, with $P < 0.01$.
In parenthesis, number of animals in each group.

partially compensated by increased plasma insulin levels, and if insulin promotes hepatic triglyceride synthesis, as suggested by some studies (Salans and Reaven, 1966), then obesity could be expected to exacerbate (but not cause) both endogenous lipemia and carbohydrate intolerance. Abrams *et al.* (1969) proposed that the prevailing insulin levels of an individual, as indicated by the response to oral glucose, may determine the level of fasting triglycerides.

The coexistence of high blood glucose values and increased insulin secretion suggests the possible existence of factors which oppose the peripheral action of the hormone and it is conceivable that the plasma glycerides are capable of determining in some way the response to oral glucose. There is general agreement that primary diabetes in the human is a metabolic disorder genetically determined, although it is not possible at the present moment to define what is the defect, or defects, that are inherited. Randle *et al.* (1964) have suggested that the primary event in the development of diabetes might be an abnormality in glyceride metabolism which leads to greater release of fatty acids in adipose tissue and muscle. According to the hypothesis of the 'glucose fatty acid cycle', glucose metabolism exerts an inhibitory effect on the release and oxidation of fatty acids in adipose tissue and muscle, but this relationship is reciprocal, and the release and oxidation of fatty acids from glyceride stores inhibits the glucose uptake and metabolism in muscle, and perhaps also in adipose tissue.

If it is considered that the diabetic syndrome may be genetically heterogeneous, and that different factors could contribute to its development in different cases, it is apparent that the etiology of diabetes mellitus in man still presents an unsettled question. Many conflicting explanations can be found in the current literature, and it is not possible to find a clear-cut answer; nevertheless, the results presented in this and in other similar studies suggest that the alterations in lipid metabolism might have some pathogenic implications in human diabetes.

ACKNOWLEDGMENTS

It is a pleasure to thank the Consejo de Desarrollo Científico, Universidad Central de Venezuela, and the Fundación Vargas for financial help for this work. The authors also wish to acknowledge the valuable collaboration and efficient technical assistance of Miss Emilia Pérez Ayuso, Miss Carmen Rivas Figueroa and Mrs. María Rodríguez.

REFERENCES

ABELL, L. L., LEVY, B. B., BRODIE, B. B. and KENDALL, F. E. (1952): A simplified method for the estimation of total cholesterol in serum and demonstration of its specificity. *J. biol. Chem., 195*, 357.
ABRAMS, M. E., JARRETT, R. J., KEEN, H., BOYNS, D. R. and CROSSLEY, J. N. (1969): Oral glucose

tolerance and related factors in a normal population sample. II. Interrelationship of glycerides, cholesterol, and other factors with glucose and insulin response. *Brit. med. J.*, *1*, 599.

BIERMAN, E. L. and PORTE, D., JR. (1968): Carbohydrate intolerance and lipemia. *Ann. intern. Med.*, *68*, 926.

BOSCH, V., POSNER, I., CAMEJO, G., ARREAZA, C., MARTUCCI, A. D. and MENDEZ, H. (1971): Hyperlipaemia in research animals. *Acta cient. venez.*, *22*, *Suppl. 2*, 149.

BOWMAN, R. H. (1962): The effect of long-chain fatty acids on glucose utilization in the isolated perfused rat heart. *Biochem. J.*, *84*, 14.

DOLE, V. P. (1956): A relation between non-esterified fatty acids in plasma and the metabolism of glucose. *J. clin. Invest.*, *35*, 150.

FAJANS, S. S. (1960): Diagnostic tests for diabetes mellitus. In: *Diabetes*, p. 389. Editor: R. H. Williams. Hoeber, New York.

FREDRICKSON, D. S., LEVY, R. I. and LEES, R. S. (1967): Fat transport in lipoproteins. An integrated approach to mechanisms and disorders. *New Engl. J. Med.*, *276*, 34, 94, 148, 215 and 273.

GARLAND, P. B., NEWSHOLME, E. A. and RANDLE, P. J. (1962): Effect of fatty acids, ketone bodies, diabetes and starvation on pyruvate metabolism in rat heart and diaphragm muscle. *Nature, (Lond.)* *195*, 381.

HALES, C. N. and RANDLE, P. J. (1963): Immunoassay of insulin with insulin-antibody precipitate. *Biochem. J.*, *88*, 137.

HAVEL, R. J. (1961): Conversion of plasma free fatty acids into triglycerides of plasma lipoprotein fractions in man. *Metabolism*, *10*, 1031.

LEES, R. S. and FREDRICKSON, D. S. (1965): Differentiation of exogenous and endogenous hyperlipemia by paper electrophoresis. *J. clin. Invest.*, *44*, 1968.

MACKAY, D. G. and KAUNITZ, H. (1963): Studies of the generalized Shwartzman reaction induced by diet. VI. Effects of pregnancy on lipid composition of serum and other tissues. *Metabolism*, *12*, 990.

MILNER, R. D. (1969): Plasma and tissue insulin concentrations in foetal and postnatal rabbits. *J. Endocr.*, *43*, 119.

NELSON, N. (1944): A photometric adaptation of the Somogyi method for the determination of glucose. *J. biol. Chem.*, *153*, 375.

PELKONEN, R., MIETTINEN, T. A., TASKINEN, M. R. and NIKKILA, E. A. (1968): Effect of acute elevation of plasma glycerol, triglycerides and FFA levels on glucose utilization and plasma insulin. *Diabetes*, *17*, 76.

RANDLE, P. J., GARLAND, P. B., HALES, C. N. and NEWSHOLME, E. A. (1964): The glucose fatty acid cycle and diabetes mellitus. *Ciba Found. Coll. Endocr.*, *15*, 192.

SALANS, L. B. and REAVEN, G. M. (1966): Effect of insulin pretreatment on glucose and lipid metabolism of liver slices from normal rats. *Proc. Soc. exp. Biol. Med. (N.Y.)*, *122*, 1208.

SCHALCH, D. S. and KIPNIS, D. M. (1965): Abnormalities in carbohydrate tolerance associated with elevated plasma non-esterified fatty acids. *J. clin. Invest.*, *44*, 2010.

SIPERSTEIN, M. D. (1960): The lipid derangements in diabetes. In: *Diabetes* p. 102. Editor: R. H. Williams. Hoeber, New York.

STEINKAMP, R. C., COHEN, N. L., GAFFEY, W. R., MCKEY, T., BRON, G., SIRI, W., SARGENT, T. and ISAACS, E. (1965): Measures of body fat and related factors in normal adults. A simple clinical method to estimate body fat and lean body mass. *J. chron. Dis.*, *18*, 1291.

SVANBORG, A. and SVENNERHOLM, L. (1961): Plasma total lipids, cholesterol, triglycerides, phospholipids and free fatty acids in a healthy Scandinavian population. *Acta med. scand.*, *169*, 43.

VAN HANDEL, E. and ZILVERSMIT, D. B. (1957): Micromethod for the direct determination of serum triglycerides. *J. Lab. clin. Med.*, *50*, 152.

WELBORN, T. A., RUBENSTEIN, A. H., HASLAN, R. and FRASER, R. (1966): Normal insulin response to glucose. *Lancet*, *1*, 280.

INDEX OF AUTHORS

SUBJECT INDEX

Prepared by W. van Westering, M.D., Amsterdam